# Medical and Psychosocial Aspects of Chronic Illness and Disability

## Third Edition

### Donna Falvo, RN, PhD, CRC

Adjunct Professor

Rehabilitation Psychology and Counseling

Allied Health Sciences, School of Medicine

The University of North Carolina

at Chapel Hill

**JONES AND BARTLETT PUBLISHERS**

*Sudbury, Massachusetts*

BOSTON    TORONTO    LONDON    SINGAPORE

*World Headquarters*
Jones and Bartlett Publishers
40 Tall Pine Drive
Sudbury, MA 01776
978-443-5000
info@jbpub.com
www.jbpub.com

Jones and Bartlett Publishers
Canada
2406 Nikanna Road
Mississauga, ON L5C 2W6
CANADA

Jones and Bartlett Publishers
International
Barb House, Barb Mews
London W6 7PA
UK

**Library of Congress Cataloging-in-Publication Data**
Falvo, Donna R.
Medical and psychosocial aspects of chronic illness and disability / Donna Falvo.—3rd ed. p. ; cm.
Includes bibliographical references and index.
ISBN 0-7637-3166-8 (casebound)
1. Chronic diseases. 2. Chronically ill—Rehabilitation. 3. Chronic diseases—Social aspects.
4. Chronic diseases—Psychological aspects.
[DNLM: 1. Chronic Disease. 2. Disabled Persons—psychology.
3. Disabled Persons—rehabilitation. 4. Social Adjustment. WT 500 F197m 2005] I. Title.
RC108.F35 2005
616'.044–dc22
2004017494

**Production Credits**
Acquisitions Editor: Kevin Sullivan
Production Director: Amy Rose
Associate Production Editor: Tracey Chapman
Associate Editor: Amy Sibley
Associate Marketing Manager: Emily Ekle
Cover Design: Anne Spencer
Manufacturing Buyer: Amy Bacus
Composition: Bill Noss Graphic Design
Printing and Binding: Malloy, Inc.
Cover Printing: Malloy, Inc.

Printed in the United States of America
09 08 07 06 05    10 9 8 7 6 5 4 3 2 1

**Dedication**

This book is dedicated to the memory of

Dr. Alan Woolf,

A man of science, presence, integrity, strength, and honor

## About the Author

Donna Falvo, R.N., Ph.D., CRC is Adjunct Professor at the University of North Carolina at Chapel Hill School of Medicine, Division of Rehabilitation Psychology and Counseling. She is a Registered Nurse, Licensed Psychologist, and Certifed Rehabilitation Counselor. She has over 30 years serving as teacher, clinician, and researcher. A former Professor and Coordinator of Rehabilitation Counseling, Rehabilitation Institute, Southern Illinois University, she was named a Mary Switzer Scholar in 1986, and elected to Sigma XI National Scientific Research Society in 1995. She was elected President of the American Rehabilitation Counseling Association in 1998 and currently serves on the Editorial Board of the *Rehabilitation Counseling Bulletin*. She is the author of over 40 articles and book chapters and, in addition to authoring the two previous editions of *Medical and Psychosocial Aspects of Chronic Illness and Disability,* she is author of the book *Effective Patient Education: A Guide to Increased Compliance,* also in its third edition.

# Acknowledgments

Special thanks to the following people who generously volunteered their time to read, review, critique, and discuss various sections of the book. Their dedication and commitment to individuals with chronic illness and disability is greatly appreciated by the author as well as by the individuals they serve.

Eileen Burker, PhD, CRC
Associate Professor
Department of Allied Health
  Science
Divison of Rehabilitation
  Psychology and
  Counseling
School of Medicine
The University of North
  Carolina at Chapel Hill

Catherine T. Calvert, PhD,
  CRC
Rehabilitation Counselor
North Carolina Jaycee Burn
  Center
University of North
  Carolina Hospitals
Chapel Hill, North Carolina

Patrick P. Carone, MD
Psychiatrist
Carolina Rehabilitation and
  Surgical Associates
Cary, North Carolina

Stacy Carone, EdD, CRC
Assistant Professor
Department of Allied Health
  Science
Division of Rehabilitation
  Psychology and
  Counseling
School of Medicine
The University of North
  Carolina at Chapel Hill

Richard E. Falvo, PhD
Adjunct Professor
Cell & Molecular Physiology
School of Medicine
The University of North
  Carolina at Chapel Hill

Ernest Grant, RN, MSN
Outreach Coordinator
North Carolina Jaycee Burn
  Center
University of North
  Carolina Hospitals
Chapel Hill, North Carolina

Dawn E. Kleinman, MD
Dermatologist
Alamance Skin Center
Burlington, North Carolina

Fred Price, RN, MBA (c)
Nurse Manager
North Carolina Jaycee Burn
  Center
University of North
  Carolina Hospitals
Chapel Hill, North Carolina

Dianne Rawdanowicz
Rehabilitation Counselor
N.C. Division Vocational
  Rehabilitation Services
Department of Health and
  Human Services
Raleigh, North Carolina

Stephanie J. Sjoblad, AuD
Clinic Director
Audiologist/ Assistant
  Professor
Allied Health Sciences
Division of Speech/Hearing
School of Medicine
The University of North
  Carolina at Chapel Hill

# Preface

In its third edition, *Medical and Psychosocial Aspects of Chronic Illness and Disability* has been revised and updated. Certain sections, such as those on conditions of the nervous system have been substantially expanded. Added to the end of each chapter are brief case studies to stimulate discussion. Cases are hypothetical and not based on any specific case or individual.

This book is designed for nonmedical professionals and students who have little prior medical knowledge but who work with individuals with chronic illness and disability and need to have an understanding of medical conditions, their implications, and need to have an understanding of medical terms. It is designed as a reference book for professionals in the field as well as a textbook for students. The book continues to use a functional approach to understanding a number of medical conditions. In an attempt to reinforce this approach, an Appendix on Functional Limitations has been added (Appendix E).

Chronic illness and disability impact all areas of individual's and their family's lives. Only by understanding an individual's total experience with chronic illness and disability and how all areas of their life are affected are professionals fully able to help them reach their goals. The focus of the book is to help professionals and students understand medical and psychosocial aspects of chronic illness and disability and how they affect an individual's functioning in all areas of life, including psychological and social impact, impact on activities of daily living, and on vocational function. — *DRF*

# Table of Contents

# CHAPTER 1

# Psychosocial and Functional Aspects of Chronic Illness and Disability

## IMPACT OF CHRONIC ILLNESS AND DISABILITY

The impact of chronic illness and disability is far-reaching, extending beyond the individual to all those with whom the individual has contact. Chronic illness and disability affect all facets of life, including social and family relationships, economic well-being, activities of daily living, and recreational and vocational activities. Although several factors influence the extent of impact, every chronic illness or disability requires some alteration and adjustment in daily life. The extent of impact is dependent on:

- the nature of the condition
- individuals' pre-illness/disability personality
- the meaning of the illness or disability to individuals
- individuals' current life circumstances
- the degree of family and social support

Reactions to chronic illness and disability vary considerably. Some individuals with chronic illness or disability place less importance on the condition and associated limitations than do able-bodied members of society. Social groups establish their own standards with regard to idealized physical and emotional traits, roles, and responsibilities. Individuals with chronic illness or disability who do not fit the socially determined norm may find that, regardless of their strengths and abilities, they continue to be regarded in the context of societal views rather than their own.

People vary in their tolerance to symptoms, their functional limitations, and their general ability to cope with chronic illness and disability. Consequently, one must consider the effect of the diagnosis, symptoms, and treatment on all aspects of individuals' lives, specifically on their capacity to function within their environment.

Functional capacity goes beyond specific tasks and activities. It also includes significant events and relationships with family, friends, employers, and casual acquaintances. No relationship exists in isolation. Just as individuals' reactions to illness or disability influence the reactions of others, so the reactions of others affect individuals' self-concept and perception of their own strengths and abilities.

Participation in family, social, and work activities assumes interaction and the capacity to perform a variety of activities. As interactions or capacities change, or as they become limited or restricted, roles and relationships also change. Although some changes and adjustments may be made with relative ease, others can have repercussions in many areas of daily life. The meaning and importance that individuals and their families attribute to associated changes influence the ability to accept the condition and to make necessary adjustments. The medical condition itself is only one factor that determines individuals' ability to function effectively.

## DISEASE AND ILLNESS

Words are powerful conveyers of concepts (Smart, 2001). Using a standard definition of terms facilitates communication and understanding of what each term implies. The term **disease** is derived from the *medical model*, which refers to changes in the structure or function of body systems. The medical model focuses on the treatment and elimination of symptoms. The term **illness** refers to individuals' perception of their symptoms and how they and their families respond to these symptoms (Morof Lubkin & Larsen, 2002). It is important to understand both concepts. Professionals working with individuals with chronic illness or disability must understand the symptoms, limitations, and progression of a condition in order to facilitate individuals' adaptation to their condition and to maximize their potential for functioning. Insight into the medical nature of a condition helps guide professionals in assessments and interventions, as well as in understanding the physical consequences the individual is experiencing (Dudgeon, Gerrard, Jensen, Rhodes, & Tyler, 2002). It is also important for professionals to have insights into individuals' perception of their condition and the personal relevance and meaning it has for them so that interventions can be directed toward meeting specific needs (Shaw, Segal, Polatajko, & Harburn, 2002). There must be an understanding of individuals' strengths, resources, and abilities as well as of the symptoms and limitations associated with the condition if one is to effectively assess the impact of the condition on their daily lives and goals in relationship to the tasks they perform at home, at work, and in their social environment.

Other terms helpful to understanding the impact of chronic illness or disability on individuals are *acute* and *chronic*. **Acute** refers to the sudden onset of symptoms that are short term and that incapacitate individuals for only a short time. **Chronic** refers to symptoms that last indefinitely and that have a cause that may or may not be identifiable. Some conditions that begin acutely but are not resolved become ongoing and chronic. A chronic condition requires individuals to reorient their overall lifestyle to accommodate manifestations of the condition. It requires them to adapt to the realization that life as they previously knew it has changed. They are then faced with the task of reorienting values, beliefs, behaviors, and goals to adapt to that reality.

The course of an illness over time, including the actions taken by individuals, their families, and health professionals working with them to manage or shape the course of the condition, is called a **trajectory** (Corbin, 2001). The concept is important to professionals working with individuals with chronic illness and disability because it implies a continuum and emphasizes the social and environmental impact on the condition.

## IMPAIRMENT, DISABILITY, AND HANDICAP

Although sometimes used interchangeably, the terms *impairment*, *disability*, and *handicap* have separate meanings and describe different concepts. To promote the appropriate use of these terms, in 1980 the World Health Organization established the *International Classification of Impairment, Disability, and Handicap*, which defined these concepts.

- **Impairment** refers to the loss or abnormality of psychological, physical, or anatomical structure or function at the system or organ level that may or may not be permanent and that may or may not result in disability.
- **Disability** refers to an individual limitation or restriction of an activity as the result of an impairment.
- **Handicap** refers to the disadvantage to the individual resulting from an impairment or disability that presents a barrier to fulfilling a role or reaching a goal (World Health Organization, 1980).

Although impairments cause some degree of disability in most people (e.g., spinal cord injury), the degree to which they result in disability is also determined by individual circumstances. What may appear to be a relatively minor disruption of function may actually have major consequence for the life of the individual affected. For example, loss of a little finger may be more disabling for a concert pianist than it would be for a heavy equipment operator. Spinal cord injury resulting in paraplegia has a different impact for someone who is an accountant than it would have for someone who is a laborer. Determining the extent of disability and resulting handicaps includes considering the condition in the context of each individual's life and particular circumstances without imposing preconceived ideas about how disabling or handicapping the condition is.

## STRESS IN CHRONIC ILLNESS AND DISABILITY

Change is an unavoidable part of life. Change of job, change of home, change of family composition, or changes brought about through the normal aging process are all common experiences. Depending on individuals' perception and the circumstances involved, change may be positive or negative, but it always requires some adjustment or adaptation and thus produces a certain degree of stress.

Chronic illness and disability produce significant change and consequently stress because individuals must deal with a change of customary lifestyle, loss of control, disruption of physiological processes, pain or discomfort, and potential loss of role, status, independence, and financial stability. When individuals have confidence in their ability to maintain control over their destiny and when they believe that changes, although inevitable, are manageable, stress is less pronounced. When their perceptions of the changes associated with chronic illness or disability seem insurmountable or beyond their ability to cope, stress can be overwhelming.

The degree of stress associated with chronic illness or disability often is related to the degree of threat it represents to individuals. Potential threats of chronic illness or disability include:

- threats to life and physical well-being
- threats to body integrity and comfort as a result of the illness or disability itself, the diagnostic procedures, or treatment
- threats to independence, privacy, autonomy, and control
- threats to self-concept and fulfillment of customary roles
- threats to life goals and future plans

- threats to relationships with family, friends, and colleagues
- threats to the ability to remain in familiar surroundings
- threats to economic well-being

The response to the stresses imposed by the threat of chronic illness or disability depends on perceptions of the impact the condition has on various areas of life, as well as on individuals' capacity to cope.

Stress cannot be easily quantified, but it can be interpreted from the behaviors exhibited by those experiencing chronic illness or disability. When demands exceed psychological, social, or financial resources, stress may be manifested in a variety of ways, such as noncompliance with recommended treatment, self-destructive behaviors such as substance abuse, hostility, depression, or other harmful responses.

Individuals in the same situation do not necessarily experience the same degree of stress, and the amount of change or adjustment required is not necessarily an indicator of the amount of stress perceived. Those who are able to adapt and cope effectively and mobilize resources are more successful in managing stress and achieving more stable outcomes.

## COPING STYLE AND STRATEGIES

Coping is a constellation of many acts rather than a single act, is constantly changing, and is highly individualized. Coping mechanisms are learned and developed over time. Individuals use them to manage, tolerate, or reduce the stress associated with significant life events and to attempt to restore psychological equilibrium after a stressful or traumatic event. Everyone has developed a variety of coping mechanisms through his or her

life experiences, and each individual has a predominant coping style to reduce anxiety and restore equilibrium when confronted with a stressful situation. Coping is manifested through behavior. Coping behavior is *effective* and *adaptive* when it helps individuals reduce stress and attain their fullest potential. It is ineffective and *maladaptive* when it inhibits growth and potential or contributes to physical or mental deterioration.

Coping may be required not only for dealing with the initial diagnosis, but also for subsequent events. Conditions that are progressive with compounding limitations necessitate ongoing coping and adjustment to incorporate additional changes into daily life.

Individuals cope with illness and disability in different ways. Some actively confront their condition, learning new skills or actively engaging in treatment to control or manage the condition. Others defend themselves from stress and the realities of the diagnosis by denying its seriousness, ignoring treatment recommendations, or refusing to learn new skills or behaviors associated with the condition. Still others cope by engaging in self-destructive behavior, actively continuing behavior that has detrimental effects on their physical condition.

Effective coping must be viewed in the context of each individual's personal background and experiences, life situation, and perception of circumstances. Individuals tend to use coping strategies that have worked successfully for them in the past. When old strategies are no longer effective or are not appropriate to the new situation, new coping strategies must be implemented to neutralize events surrounding the chronic illness or disability and to adjust to any associated limitations. Effective coping enables individuals to attain emotional equilibrium, to achieve a positive mental outlook, and to avoid incapacitation from fear, anxiety, anger, or depression. However, coping does not occur in a vacuum. The social milieu in which individuals find themselves can facilitate or discourage effective coping. In general, an optimum environment is one that helps individuals gain a sense of control by actively participating in decision making and taking responsibility for their own destiny as much as possible.

Coping strategies are subconscious mechanisms that individuals use to cope with stress. All individuals have predominant coping strategies to reduce anxiety and restore equilibrium when confronted with stress. The strategies they used in the past are often those employed when they are confronted with the stress of chronic illness or disability. The use of coping strategies reduces anxiety, helping individuals assume balance and productivity in their lives. Although these strategies can be helpful, overuse can be detrimental.

## Denial

The diagnosis of chronic illness or disability and the associated implications can be devastating and anxiety provoking. *Denial* is a coping strategy some individuals use to negate the reality of a situation. In the case of chronic illness or disability, individuals may deny that they have the condition by avoiding recommended treatment or by denying implications of the condition. In the early stages of adjustment, denial may be beneficial in that it enables individuals to adjust to the painful reality of their situation at their own pace, preventing excessive anxiety. When denial continues, however, it can prevent individuals from following medical recommendations or from learning new skills that would help them reach their maximum potential.

Denial of the chronic illness or disability can have far-reaching effects on others if, by denying the condition, individuals place others at risk. For example, proper precautions can greatly reduce the spread of some contagious diseases, such as tuberculosis or HIV infection. Individuals in active denial of their tuberculosis or its ramifications may neglect to take tuberculosis medications regularly, and those with HIV infection may have unprotected sex, putting others in jeopardy. Some individuals may put others at risk by denying their limitations, such as individuals who are legally blind but continue to drive even though driving has been prohibited.

## Regression

In regression, individuals revert to an earlier stage of development and become more dependent, behave more passively, or exhibit more emotionality than would normally be expected at their developmental level. In the early stages of chronic illness or disability, returning to the state of dependency experienced in an earlier stage of development can be therapeutic, especially if treatment of the condition requires rest and inactivity. When individuals continue in a regressive mode, however, it can interfere with adjustment and the attainment of a level of independence that would allow them to reach maximum functional capacity.

## Compensation

Individuals using compensation as a coping strategy learn to counteract functional limitations in one area by becoming stronger or more proficient in another. Compensatory behavior is generally highly constructive when new behaviors are directed toward positive goals and outcomes. For example, someone who is unable to maintain his or her level of physical activity because of limitations associated with his or her condition may turn to creative writing or other means of self-expression. Compensation as a coping strategy can be detrimental, however, when the new behaviors are self-destructive or socially unacceptable. For example, someone who experiences disfigurement as a result of his or her disability may become promiscuous as a way of compensating for the perception of physical unattractiveness.

### Rationalization

As a coping strategy, rationalization enables individuals to find socially acceptable reasons for their behavior or to excuse themselves for not reaching goals or not accomplishing tasks. Although rationalization can soften the disappointment of dreams unrealized or goals unreached, it can also produce negative effects if it becomes a barrier to adjustment, prevents individuals from reaching their full potential, or interferes with effective management of the medical condition itself.

### Diversion of Feelings

One of the most positive and constructive of all coping strategies can be the diversion of unacceptable feelings or ideas into socially acceptable behaviors. Those with chronic illness or disability may have particularly strong feelings of anger or hostility about their diagnosis or the circumstances surrounding their condition. If their emotional energy can be redefined and diverted into positive activity, the results can be beneficial, making virtue out of necessity and transforming deficit into gain. As with all coping strategies, diversion of feelings can have negative effects if feelings of anger or hostility are chan-

neled into negative behaviors or socially unacceptable activities.

## EMOTIONAL REACTIONS TO CHRONIC ILLNESS OR DISABILITY

Sudden, unexpected, or life-threatening chronic illness or disability engenders a variety of reactions. How individuals view their condition, its causes, and its consequences greatly affects what they do in the face of it. They may view their condition as a challenge, an enemy to be fought, a punishment, a sign of weakness, a relief, a strategy for gaining attention, an irreparable loss, or an uplifting spiritual experience. Although emotional reactions vary, the following are common.

### Grief

Grief is a normal reaction to loss. Individuals with chronic illness and disability may experience loss of a body part, loss of function, role, or social status, or other perceived losses that lead to a reaction of grief. Although the grieving and the progression through stages of grief vary from person to person, a common initial reaction is shock, disbelief, or numbness during which the diagnosis or its seriousness may be denied or disputed. As individuals acknowledge the reality of the situation, the grief reaction may become more pronounced.

After repeated confrontations with elements of loss, normal adaptation results in a gradual change in emphasis and focus that enables individuals to accept the loss emotionally and to make the adjustments and adaptations that are necessary to reestablish their place within the everyday world. When the grief reaction is prolonged, individuals may develop a pathological grief reaction, which may become more disabling than the chronic illness or disability itself.

## Fear and Anxiety

Individuals normally become anxious when confronted with threat. A chronic illness or disability can pose a threat because of the potential loss of function, love, independence, or financial security. Threat causes anxiety. Some individuals fear the unknown or unpredictability of a condition, which provokes anxiety. For others, hospitalizations that immerse them in a strange and unfamiliar environment away from home, family, and the security of routine produce anxiety. When conditions are life-threatening, fear and anxiety may be associated not only with loss of function, but also with loss of life. Fear and anxiety associated with chronic illness or disability can place individuals in a state of panic, rendering them psychologically immobile and unable to act. Helping them regain a sense of control over their situation through information and shared decision making can be an important step in reducing anxiety and facilitating rehabilitation.

## Anger

Individuals with chronic illness or disability may experience anger at themselves or others for perceived injustices or the losses associated with their condition. They may believe that their chronic illness or disability was caused by negligence or that their condition was avoidable. If they perceive themselves as victims, anger may be directed toward the persons or circumstances they blame for the condition or situation. If they believe that their own actions were partly to blame for the chronic illness or disability, anger may be directed inward.

Anger can also be the result of frustration. Individuals may vent frustration and anger by showing hostility toward those who have no relationship to the development of the chronic illness or disability and no influence over its outcome. Anger may also be an expression of the realization of the seriousness of the situation and its associated feelings of helplessness. At times, anger may not be openly expressed but rather expressed through quarreling, arguing, complaining, or being excessively demanding in an attempt to gain some control. Helping individuals express anger in appropriate ways and enabling them to experience a sense of control over their situation can help to resolve anger, which could otherwise be detrimental to successful rehabilitation.

## Depression

With the realization of the reality, seriousness, and implications of the chronic illness or disability, individuals may experience feelings of depression, helplessness and hopelessness, apathy, and/or dejection and discouragement. Signs of depression include sleep disturbances, changes in appetite, difficulty concentrating, and withdrawal from activity. Not all individuals with chronic illness or disability experience significant depression, and, in those who do, depression may not be prolonged. The extent to which depression is experienced varies from person to person. Prolonged or unresolved depression can result in self-destructive behaviors, such as substance abuse or attempted suicide. Individuals with prolonged depression should be referred for mental health evaluation and treatment.

## Guilt

Guilt can be described as self-criticism or blame. Individuals or family members may feel guilt if they believe they contributed to, or in some way caused, the chronic illness or disability. Those who develop lung cancer or emphysema after years of tobacco use, or those who receive a spinal cord injury from an accident that occurred because they were driving while intoxicated, may experience guilt because of the role they played. In other instances, they may experience guilt because they feel their chronic illness or disability places a burden on their family or because they are unable to fulfill former roles.

Family members may experience guilt because of anger or resentment they have toward the individual with a disability. Guilt may also be associated with blame. Family members may actively demonstrate scorn or contempt toward the individual with chronic illness or disability, causing him or her to feel more guilty.

Guilt may be expressed or unexpressed and can occur in varying dimensions. It can be an obstacle to the successful adjustment to the condition and its limitations. Self-blame or blame ascribed by others is detrimental not only to the individual's self-concept, but also to rehabilitative efforts as a whole. Guilt that affects rehabilitation potential or well-being is an indication that referral to appropriate professionals for evaluation and treatment may be appropriate.

## CHRONIC ILLNESS AND DISABILITY THROUGH THE LIFE CYCLE

Development is not static or finite. It is a continual process from infancy to old age and death. Each developmental stage is associated with certain age-appropriate behaviors, skills, and developmental tasks that allow psychological and cognitive transition from one stage to another. Individuals' age and developmental stage influence their reactions to chronic illness

or disability and the problems and consequences they experience.

Each developmental stage of life has its own particular stresses or demands, apart from those experienced as a result of illness or disability. Chronic illness and disability at various stages of development can affect the independence, self-control, and life skills associated with these different developmental stages. Since the needs, responsibilities, and resources of adults differ from those of children, the impact of chronic illness or disability in later years differs from its impact in young adulthood.

Family members and others generally adjust their behavior to accommodate and to interact appropriately with individuals as they pass from one developmental stage to the next. When individuals experience chronic illness or disability, however, others may modify expectations of age-appropriate behavior, and these modified expectations may interfere with the individual's mastery of the normal skills required to meet the challenges of future developmental stages.

All aspects of development are related. Each developmental stage must be understood within the context of the individual's past and current experience. Those with chronic illness or disability must be considered in the context of their developmental stage and the way in which the changes and limitations associated with their condition influence the attitudes, perceptions, actions, and behaviors characteristic of that stage. Stages of development serve as a guideline not only in assessing individuals' functional capacity, but also in determining potential stressors and reactions.

Problems and stresses at different developmental stages are similar whether individuals have a chronic illness or disability or not. Although there are no clear lines of demarcation between life stages and all individuals develop at different rates, there are some commonalities associated with different life stages.

Ideally, those with chronic illness or disability should be encouraged to progress through each stage of development as normally as possible, despite their condition. Those whose emotional, social, educational, or occupational development has been thwarted may be more handicapped by their inability to cope with the subsequent challenges of life than by any limitations experienced because of the illness or disability per se.

## Chronic Illness or Disability in Childhood

Although the majority of children with chronic illness or disability and their families adapt successfully, these children are at increased risk of emotional and behavioral disorders (Gledhill, Rangel, & Garralda, 2000). In early life, children develop a sense of trust in others, a sense of autonomy, and an awareness and mastery of their environment. During these years, they begin to learn communication and social skills that enable them to interact effectively with others. They also learn that limits are set on their explorations, expressions of autonomy, and behaviors. Important to their development is a balance between encouraging initiative and setting limits consistently.

Chronic illness or disability can impede the attainment of normal developmental goals. Repeated or prolonged hospitalizations may deprive children of nurturing by a consistent and loving caregiver. The physical limitations of the condition or treatment may prevent normal activities, socialization, and exploration of the environment. In some cases, overly protective family members may restrict activities or prohibit the child from expressing emotions normally. In other instances, overly

sympathetic parents may condone inappropriate behaviors rather than correct them.

Conditions affecting the development of communication skills may also affect children's interaction with the environment, as well as their future development. *Congenital conditions* (conditions present at birth) or conditions that occur in early childhood require adjustments throughout the life cycle. These limitations must be confronted and compensated for with every new aspect of normal development. Awareness of normal developmental needs enables professionals working with these children to facilitate experiences that foster normal development and to enhance children's ability to reach their full potential.

For most children, entering school expands their world beyond the scope of their family. Before children attend school, the values, rules, and expectations they experience are, for the most part, largely those expressed within the family. As they enter school, however, they are exposed to a larger social environment. Not only do they learn social relationships and cooperative interactions, but they also begin to develop a sense of initiative and industry. Children gradually become aware of their special strengths. As new skills begin to develop, school-age children gain the capacity for sustained effort that eventually results in the ability to follow through with tasks to completion. Approval and encouragement by others and acceptance by peers help them build self-confidence, further enhancing development.

When children with chronic illness or disability enter school, they may not need specific special education placement, but they may require coordinated school interventions to maximize attendance and facilitate educational and social growth. School-related problems may be reflected in these children's psychological well-being, their interaction with other children, or their academic performance. When physical or cognitive limitations affect their ability to perform the skills normally valued at their developmental stage, acceptance by peers may be affected. School attendance may be disrupted by the need for repeated absences, resulting in the inability to interact on a consistent basis within the peer group, which may diminish social interactions.

In an attempt to shield the child from hurt and emotional pain, family members may further isolate the child from social interactions, creating the potential for reduced self-confidence. The reluctance of sympathetic family members to allow the child to participate in activities in which there may be failure can interfere with the child's ability to accurately evaluate his or her potential. Encouragement of social interactions and activities to the degree possible enables the child to develop the skills and abilities that are needed for later integration into the larger world.

## Chronic Illness or Disability in Adolescence

Perceptions of and interactions with peers become increasingly important as adolescents further define their identity apart from membership in their family. With the need to establish independence, adolescents begin to emancipate themselves from their parents and may rebel against authority in general. Physical maturation brings about a strong preoccupation with the body and appearance. Adolescents' need to be attractive to others often becomes paramount. Awareness of and experimentation with sexual feelings present a new dimension with which the adolescent must learn to cope. Dating and expression of sexuality are important aspects of maturation. Thus any alteration

in physical appearance caused by a chronic illness or disability can influence adolescents' perception of body image and self-concept, thwarting the expression of sexual feelings.

Adolescents with physical disabilities may also be at risk for secondary disabilities associated with psychosocial factors (Anderson & Klarke, 1982; Stevens, Steele, Jutai, Kalnins, Bortolussi, & Biggar, 1996). An illness or disability during adolescence can disrupt relationships with peers, resulting in delayed social and emotional development. Limitations imposed by the condition, its treatment, or the sympathetic and protective reactions by family members may become barriers to the attainment of independence and individual identity. Parents may be overprotective to the point of infantilizing the adolescent, thus decreasing self-esteem and self-confidence.

In some instances, certain characteristics of normal adolescent development, such as rebellion against authority or the need to be accepted by a peer group, can interfere with the treatment necessitated by a chronic illness or disability. If adolescents deny the limitations associated with their disability or ignore treatment recommendations, there can be further detrimental effects on physical and functional capacity.

## Chronic Illness or Disability in Young Adulthood

In young adulthood, individuals establish themselves as productive members of society, integrating vocational goals, developing the capacity for intimate relationships, and accepting social responsibility. When a chronic illness or disability develops, its associated limitations, rather than the individual's interests or abilities, may define his or her social, vocational, and occupational goals.

Physical limitations may also inhibit individuals' efforts to build intimate relationships or to maintain the relationships they have already established. At this developmental stage, established relationships are likely to be recent, and the level of commitment and willingness to make necessary sacrifices may vary. Depending on the nature of the condition, procreation may be difficult or impossible, or, if the individual already has young children, child-care issues may be the source of additional concerns in light of the functional limitations inherent in a specific chronic illness or disability. Young adults who have not fully gained independence or left their family of origin by the time of the onset of their chronic illness or disability may find gaining independence more difficult. In some cases the family's overprotectiveness may prevent them from having experiences appropriate to their own age group.

## Chronic Illness or Disability in Middle Age

Individuals in middle age are generally established in their career, have a committed relationship, and are often providing guidance to their own children as they leave the family to establish their own careers and families. At the same time, middle-aged individuals may be assuming greater responsibility for their own elderly parents, who may be becoming increasingly fragile and dependent. During middle age, individuals may begin to reassess their goals and relationships as they begin to recognize their own mortality and limited remaining time.

Illness or disability during middle age can interfere with further occupational development and may even result in early retirement. Such changes can have a significant impact on the economic well-being of individuals and their families, as well as on their identity, self-concept, and self-esteem. It may be necessary to alter established roles and associated responsibilities within the family. At the same time, individuals' partners, even when the relationship is long term, may be reevaluating their own life goals. They may perceive chronic illness or disability as a violation of their own well-being, and they may choose to leave the relationship. Responsibilities for children and aging parents provide additional financial and emotional stress to that experienced as a result of illness or disability.

## Chronic Illness or Disability in Older Adulthood

Ideally, older adults have adapted to the triumphs and disappointments of life and have accepted their own life and imminent death. Although physical limitations associated with normal aging are variable, older adults often experience diminished physical strength and stamina, as well as losses of visual and hearing acuity. Illness or disability during older adulthood can pose physical or cognitive limitations in addition to those due to aging. The spouse or significant others of the same age group may also have decreased physical stamina, making physical care of individuals with chronic illness or disability more difficult. When older adults with chronic illness or disability are unable to attend to their own needs or when care in the home is unmanageable, they may find it necessary to surrender their own lifestyle and move to another environment for care and supervision. Many individuals in the older age group live on a fixed retirement income, and the additional expenses associated with chronic illness or disability place significant strain on an already tight budget. Not all older individuals, of course, have retirement benefits, savings, or other re-sources to draw on in time of financial need.

## OTHER ISSUES IN CHRONIC ILLNESS AND DISABILITY

### Self-Concept and Self-Esteem

*Self-concept* is tied to self-esteem and per-sonal identity. It can be defined as individ-uals' perceptions and beliefs about their own strengths and weaknesses, as well as others' perceptions of them. *Self-esteem* can be defined as "the evaluative compo-nent of an individual's self concept" (Corwyn, 2000, p. 357). It is often thought of as the assessment of one's own self-worth with regard to attained qualities and performance (Gledhill et al., 2000).

Self-concept influences the perceptions of others about an individual. A negative self-concept can produce negative re-sponses in others, just as a positive self-concept can increase the likelihood that others will react in a positive manner. Individuals' self-esteem is related to their self-concept and how others respond to them. Consequently, self-concept has a significant impact on interactions with others and on the psychological well-being of the individual.

### Body Image

Body image, an important part of self-concept, involves individuals' mental view of their body with regard to appearance and ability to perform various physical tasks. It is influenced by bodily sensations, social and cultural expectations, and reac-tions of and experiences with others (White, 2000). Body image also changes over time as one's appearance, capabilities, and functional status change over the life cycle. It is influenced by each individual's personal conception of attractiveness,

which is also determined by social and cultural influences. Body image is related to both self-concept and self-esteem.

Chronic illness or disability forces an individual to alter his or her self-image to accommodate associated changes. Factors influencing the degree of alteration include:

- the visibility of change
- the functional significance of the change
- the speed with which change occurred
- the importance of physical change or associated functional limitations to the individual reactions of others (Moore et al., 2000).

The degree to which an altered self-image is perceived by the individual in a negative way influences social and intra-personal interactions, functional capacity, and success or failure in the workplace (Cusack, 2000).

The extent to which individuals incor-porate change into their body image is also dependent on the meaning and sig-nificance of the change to the individual. The degree of physical change or disfigure-ment is not always proportional to the reaction it provokes. Change considered minimal by one individual may be con-sidered catastrophic by another.

Changes do not have to be visible in or-der to alter body image. Burn scars on parts of the body normally covered by clothing or the introduction of an artifi-cial opening or stoma such as with colo-stomy may cause significant alteration in body image even though physical changes are not readily apparent to others.

The concept of body image is complex and individually determined. Body image is not only the way individuals perceive themselves, but also the way they perceive others as seeing them. Negative views of one's body can be a barrier to psycholog-ical well-being, social interactions, functional capacity, and workplace adjustment. Consequently, the ultimate goal is to help individuals adapt to changes brought about by chronic illness or disability, integrating those changes into a restructured body image that can be assimilated and incorporated into daily life.

## Stigma

*Stigma* is a significant factor in many chronic illnesses and disabilities. Despite efforts to create a heightened awareness of the negative impact of prejudice and stereotypes, and despite changes in social and public policy that have helped to reduce the stigma associated with chronic illness or disability, it still exists for many individuals with chronic or disabling conditions.

Acceptable standards of appearance, activities, and roles are socially determined. Individuals who deviate from societal expectations of what is acceptable are often labeled as different from the majority and, thus, often stigmatized. The degree of stigma varies from setting to setting, from disability to disability, and from person to person. Conditions that are particularly anxiety provoking or threatening are likely to have more stigma attached. Stigma results in discrimination, social isolation, disregard, depreciation, devaluation, and, in some instances, threats to safety and well-being. Gender and/or race or ethnic background can be additional sources of prejudice and subsequent stigma, causing additional stress and creating additional barriers to effective functioning (Nosek & Hughes, 2003).

Stigma can have a profound impact on the ability to regain and maintain functional capacity and on acceptance of one's illness or disability. Stigma not only affects self-concept and self-esteem, but it also produces barriers that prohibit individuals from reaching their full potential. In an effort to avoid stigma, individuals may deny, minimize, or ignore their condition and/or treatment recommendations, even though it is detrimental to their welfare. Although efforts to reduce or obliterate stigma in society should continue, stigma is most likely to be overcome through individual effort. It is possible to reduce the negative impact of societal stigma by helping individuals establish a sense of their own intrinsic worth, despite the characteristics of their medical condition.

## THE IMPACT OF UNCERTAINTY

Uncertainty in the lives of individuals with chronic illness and disability can exist for a variety of reasons, but it is often related to concerns about an unknown future, erratic symptoms, the unpredictability of the progression of the disease, or ambiguous symptoms. Some chronic illnesses and disabilities have an immediate and permanent impact on functional capacity, whereas in others the course of the illness or disability is more variable. Deterioration may occur slowly over the span of several years or rapidly within months. Some conditions have periods of remission, when symptoms become less noticeable or almost nonexistent, only to be followed by periods of unpredictable exacerbation, when symptoms become worse. In some cases, the same condition progresses at different rates for different individuals, rapidly for some and slowly for others. In some conditions, it is difficult to determine when or if the condition will reach the point of severe disability or whether a dramatic change of functional capacity will take place.

Uncertainty of prognosis or progression of the condition can make planning and prediction of the future difficult. This unpredictability can be frustrating for affected individuals as well as for those around them. There may be reluctance to plan for the future at all, so that inability to predict the future becomes more disabling than the actual physical consequences of the condition itself. In other instances, given the unpredictability of their condition, individuals may elect to follow a different life course than they would have otherwise chosen. Decisions not to have children, to cut down on the number of hours spent in the work environment, or to suddenly relocate to a different part of the country may be misinterpreted by those unaware of the individual's condition or its associated unpredictability. For those conditions in which symptoms or residual effects are unapparent to others, such decisions may be met with misunderstanding or criticism. Criticisms of such decisions may be particularly distressing to individuals who do not wish to disclose or share intimate details of their condition with the casual observer.

Insecurity about the course of the condition may also cause those closest to the individual to withdraw emotional interactions or support in an attempt to protect themselves from potential future loss. Thus uncertainty poses particular challenges for individuals and their families and can be a source of stress. Living in the present, rather than dwelling on events that may or may not occur, can help to reduce stress and anxiety and enhance the quality of life.

## INVISIBLE DISABILITIES

Some chronic illnesses or disabilities have associated physical changes that can be objectively assessed by others or have functional limitations that necessitate the use of adaptive devices. The *visibility* of a condition has often been associated with

stigmatization and marginality (Livneh & Wilson, 2003). Other conditions, such as diabetes or cardiac conditions, have no outward signs that alert casual observers to an individual's condition. The term *invisible disability* refers to these latter conditions. Because there are no outward physical signs or other cues to indicate limitations associated with chronic illness or disability, others have no basis on which to alter their expectations of the individual's functional capacity. Although this lack of reaction can be positive (in the sense that it prevents others from acting out of prejudice or stereotypes), it can also be negative in the sense that it can enable individuals to deny or avoid acceptance of their condition and its associated implications.

The degree to which a condition remains invisible may be a function of the closeness of the observer's association with the individual. Although casual acquaintances may not notice limitations, those more closely involved with the individual in day-to-day activities may more readily observe them. However, some conditions under normal circumstances may offer no visible signs or cues, no matter how close another person is with the affected individual.

The unapparent aspect of the limitation in invisible disability may be a unique element related to individuals' adjustment and acceptance of their limitation. Without environmental feedback to create a tangible reality of the condition, individuals with invisible disability may postpone adaptation or ignore the medical treatment or recommendations necessary to control the condition and prevent further disability.

## SEXUALITY

Human sexuality is more than genital acts or sexual function. It is intrinsic to a person's sense of self (Hordern & Currow, 2003). It is an ever changing, lived experience, affecting the way individuals view themselves and their body (Hordern, 2000). Sexuality encompasses the whole person and is reflected in all that individuals say and do. It is an important part of identity, self-image, and self-concept. Each person is a sexual being with a need for intimacy, physical contact, and love. Chronic illness or disability can have many effects on sexuality and can influence all phases of sexual response (McInnes, 2003).

The expression of sexual urges is one form of sexuality. Chronic illness or disability can affect sexual expression because of physical limitations, depression, lack of energy, pain, alterations in self-image, or the reactions of others. In some conditions, the main barrier to sexual expression may be problems with self-concept and body-image; in other conditions, physical changes may present physical barriers that affect sexual function directly.

Regardless of the type of limitations associated with chronic illness or disability, sexual expression continues to be an important function that should be addressed (McBride & Rines, 2000). In some instances, it may be necessary to help individuals overcome their own misperceptions and fears in order to establish a means for sexual expression. In other instances, individuals may need assistance to overcome barriers or to learn methods of sexual expression different from those used previously. In any case, sexual adjustment is a significant element in the restoration of an individual's maximal functional capacity.

## FAMILY ADAPTATION TO CHRONIC ILLNESS AND DISABILITY

The family is the social network from which individuals derive identity and with whom they feel strong psychological bonds. "Family" has different meanings for different people and is not always based on blood or law. Family provides protection, socialization, physical care, support, and love. Each individual within the family structure plays some role that is incorporated into everyday family life.

Chronic illness or disability has an emotional and economic impact on families as well as on individuals. Family reactions to chronic illness and disability may be similar to those experienced by the individual and may include shock, denial, anger, guilt, anxiety, and depression. Families must make adaptations, adjustments, and role changes both as a unit and as individual family members. The way in which families react and adapt to chronic illness and disability affects an individual's subsequent adjustment. Whether families foster independence or dependence, show acceptance or rejection, or encourage or sabotage compliance with restrictions and recommended treatments has a profound effect on individuals' ultimate functional capacity.

When a family member is no longer able to perform certain functions, families may react in various ways. There may be a strong desire to be a "normal" family again. Family members with prior expectations for the individual's future or "what he or she might have been" may experience anger, resentment, or disappointment if they see chronic illness or disability interfering with the achievement of their expectations.

Family members can also act as advocates for the individual. They may need to become more involved with health professionals and service agencies or may need to be increasingly assertive to obtain necessary services. If individuals with chronic illness or disability require significant care or therapies to be administered at home, family members may become fatigued because of the extra responsibility and work required, especially if respite services are limited.

Families, like individuals, have differing resources, depending on their life circumstances, previous experiences, and the personalities involved. Individual family members may be called upon to provide not only emotional support but also physical care, supervision, transportation, or a variety of other services necessitated by the individual's condition. In addition, changes in roles or financial circumstances due to chronic illness or disability may alter the goals and plans of other family members, such as a sibling's plans for college or a parent's retirement plans. The amount of care and attention required by individuals with chronic illness or disability may create emotional strain among family members, resulting in feelings of resentment, antagonism, and frustration. Role change and ambiguity may make it necessary to redefine family relationships as new and unaccustomed duties and responsibilities arise.

## QUALITY OF LIFE

Successful rehabilitation means more than helping individuals reach their maximum functional capacity. It also means helping them achieve and enhance their quality of life. *Quality of life* is subjective in nature and has no universal meaning. No two people define the term in quite the same way. Although some see it as optimal functioning at the highest level of independence, others may place greater emphasis on life itself, regardless of level of function. Only the individual can determine the personal meaning of this term. Individual value systems, cultural backgrounds, spiritual perspectives, and the

attitudes and reactions of those within the environment all influence the interpretation of quality of life.

As already stated, perceptions of the same condition and its impact vary from individual to individual (Burker, Carels, Thompson, Rodgers, & Egan, 2000; Crews, Jefferson, Broshek, Barth, & Robbins, 2000). People with similar conditions, symptoms, and limitations may perceive their condition in totally different manners. Determining factors are the characteristics of the condition and its treatment, the age and developmental stage of the individual, the degree of limitation and the extent of disability experienced, and how characteristics of the condition affect the individual's definition of quality of life. Symptoms or limitations that one individual accepts and adapts to may be overwhelming and intolerable to another.

Because of the ambiguous nature of the concept, it is difficult to assess quality of life (Bishop & Feist-Price, 2001). Attempts to discover and accurately measure quality of life have caused considerable confusion and resulted in the creation of multiple indicators, ranging from physiologic parameters to the ability to return to work to the ability to participate in social activities and the number of psychological problems experienced by the individual. In addition, studies of quality of life have often identified discrepancies between the judgment of service providers and that of the consumer regarding quality-of-life outcomes (Leplege & Hunt, 1997).

Individuals' perception of quality of life is among the main determinants of demand for services, compliance with treatment, and satisfaction with treatment and services provided. How some individuals assess the impact of their condition on their quality of life is determined by the degree to which they feel control over their life circumstances or destiny. Accurate knowledge about their condition and treatment, together with active participation in decision making about the management of the condition, can enable individuals with chronic illness and disability to make judgments that will enable them to enhance their quality of life in terms of their own needs, goals, and circumstances.

## ADHERENCE TO PRESCRIBED TREATMENT AND RECOMMENDATIONS

Most chronic illnesses or disabling conditions require ongoing treatment, medical supervision, or restrictions on activity to control the condition or to prevent complications. However, many individuals with chronic illness or disability fail to follow the recommendations prescribed, imperiling their own well-being (Dunbar-Jacob et al., 2000; Graham, 2003). Neglecting to take medications as prescribed, resisting restriction of activities, or engaging in behaviors that are likely to cause complications can significantly influence individuals' medical prognosis and functional capacity (Dolder, Lacro, Leckband, & Jeste, 2003; Schmaling, Afari, & Blume, 2000; Vergouwen, Bakker, Katon, Verheij, & Koerselman, 2003; Zygmunt, Olfson, Boyer, & Mechanic, 2002). The best rehabilitation plan is of little value if individuals do not follow the treatments designed to control their symptoms or disease or to prevent complications or progression of the disease (Kovac, Patel, Peterson, & Kimmel, 2002; Loghman-Adham, 2003).

Although individuals who purposely behave in a way that makes their condition worse seem irrational, there are a number of explanations for nonadherent behavior. Illness or disability elicits many responses from individuals and their families. Different reactions, experiences, and motives direct behavior and can help or hinder adherence with treatment recommendations.

Individuals' lives are guided by a set of norms and values—expressed or unexpressed. Each individual has a personal, unique perspective on health, illness, and medical care itself. Thus each individual understands the meaning of illness, the consequences ascribed to adherence to recommendations, and treatment recommendations and their implications differently. Whereas some individuals react mildly to a condition that may devastate another, others display considerable emotional and physical discomfort with conditions that most people consider minor. Obviously, various psychosocial factors determine individuals' reactions to illness and, consequently, their reactions to the recommendations and advice given.

Chronic illness or disability disrupts the way individuals view themselves and the world, and it can produce distortions in thinking. Most individuals initially experience a feeling of vulnerability and a shattering of the magical belief that they are immune from illness, injury, or even death. With this realization, they may lose their sense of security and cohesiveness. Life may seem a maze of inconveniences, hazards, and restrictions. Nonadherence to recommendations may be an attempt to exert self-determination, to regain a sense of autonomy and control, and to claim some mastery over their individual destiny. In other instances, resistance to treatment recommendations may be a denial of the condition itself.

Nonadherence can also be a reflection of an individual's feelings about his or her life circumstances. For some individuals, having a chronic illness or disability is not a positive role; for others, it may be far preferable to the social role they held previously. Some may vacillate between the wish to be independent and the wish to remain dependent. Chronic illness or disability can be a means of legitimizing dependency, as well as a means of increasing the amount of attention received. Subsequently, individuals may be reluctant to return to former roles and obligations. Motivation to retain the sick role is at times greater than the motivation to gain optimal function. As a result, ultimate rehabilitation is hampered.

Failure to adhere to recommendations can also be a response to guilt that has been incorporated into the reaction to or beliefs about illness or disability. If health and well-being are perceived as rewards for a life well lived, illness or disability may be viewed as punishment for real or imagined actions of the past. Adherence to medical advice may be perceived as interference with a punishment believed to be deserved. In other instances, individuals may feel guilty because they believe that the illness or disability is a direct result of their own negligence or overt actions. Guilt or shame at being different may also hinder adherence to treatment recommendations. Some individuals may attempt to hide their condition from others and, thus, fail to follow recommendations that they fear may call attention to their condition.

The impact of chronic illness or disability on individuals' general economic well-being can also affect their ability and willingness to follow treatment recommendations. Many occupations offer fringe benefits, such as paid sick days or even time off with pay in which to seek medical care, but other occupations provide no such benefits. In the latter instances, days taken off from work because of illness or medical appointments can

decrease income. The economic consequences of chronic illness or disability may also cause a reverse reaction. If an individual is receiving disability benefits and has little opportunity for satisfactory employment, he or she may not follow recommendations that would increase his or her capacity to return to work and thereby decrease or eliminate benefits.

Finally, as already discussed, quality of life is a relative concept, uniquely defined by each individual. If treatment recommendations result in pain, discomfort, or inconvenience greater than the benefit perceived by the individual in terms of his or her own subjective definition of the quality of life, compliance with prescribed recommendations may not be perceived as worth the psychological, social, or physical cost. Treatment can sometimes, but not always, be adjusted to make adhering to recommendations more palatable. Individuals' right to self-determination must be carefully balanced with the assurance that the choice of nonadherence is based on information and full understanding of the consequences.

Some individuals readily adjust to the challenges, limitations, and associated behavioral changes necessitated by chronic illness or disability. Many individuals, however, actively sabotage treatment and recommendations, to their own detriment. In such instances, professionals' goals should be to attempt to understand these individuals' underlying problems and motivations and to help them make necessary adjustments and adaptations. Rather than criticize them for disinterest, lack of motivation, or failure to follow recommendations, it is important to identify the barriers that prohibit adherence and to recognize that such reactions may indicate difficulty in accepting the condition or adapting recommendations to their own unique way of life.

## PATIENT (CLIENT AND FAMILY) EDUCATION

Although medical care, support, and auxiliary services are important aspects of helping individuals reach their maximum potential, successful management of chronic disease or disability requires considerable individual and family effort. Regardless of the complexity of the condition, many individuals are now expected to carry out treatments in their home rather than depend on medical personnel in health care settings. Individuals' understanding of their condition and treatment is one of the basic components of self-determination and responsible care. Not only must they understand how to integrate regimens into daily routines and how to carry out daily care activities, but they must also understand preventive health care measures to retain function and prevent further disability or health problems (Falvo, 2004). Because of increasing public awareness of the need for individuals to accept this greater responsibility and self-determination, a number of programs and counseling services have been established to help clients and their families reach this goal.

## STAGES OF ADAPTATION AND ADJUSTMENT

A host of personal, social, and environmental experiences, demands, supports and resources, and coping strategies interact to influence adaptation outcomes (Livneh, 2001). The process of adjustment includes a search for meaning in the experience and an attempt to regain control and self-determination over events that affect one's life. Most individuals with chronic illness and disability experience some loss, either a direct physical loss or a more indirect loss of the ability to participate in some previously performed activity. Regardless of the nature of the loss, a variety of reactions may take place while individuals attempt to make necessary adaptations and changes.

Stages of adjustment are individual and varied. The shock of diagnosis and its consequent implications may have a numbing effect, so initially individuals may demonstrate little emotional reaction. As the reality of the situation becomes clear, they may experience a sense of hopelessness and despair, mourning for a self, a role, or a function that is lost. They may experience feelings of anger, which alternate with depression. Many individuals go through a period of mourning and bereavement similar to that experienced when a loved one is lost. Mourning is a natural reaction to loss and allows time for reflection and reestablishment of emotional equilibrium. As individuals begin to appraise their condition realistically, examine the limitations that it imposes, and adjust to the associated losses, they may gradually seek alternatives and adaptations to become integrated into a broader world.

The ultimate goal of adjustment is acceptance of the condition and its associated limitations, along with a realistic appraisal and implementation of strengths. As individuals accept their condition, they attain their maximal functional capacity. The amount of time that individuals need to reach acceptance is dependent on personality, the reaction of family and significant others, life circumstances, available resources, and the types of challenges that confront them. Some individuals never reach acceptance. Maladjustment and nonacceptance are characterized by immobility, marked dependency, continued anger and hostility, prolonged mourning, or participation in detrimental or self-destructive activities.

Just as coping mechanisms are vital parts of human nature, serving to protect against stress, reduce anxiety, and facilitate adjustment, overuse or maladaptive use of coping mechanisms can postpone or inhibit adjustment.

## FUNCTIONAL ASPECTS OF CHRONIC ILLNESS AND DISABILITY

The functional effects of chronic illness or disability are many and varied. Each individual has different needs, abilities, and circumstances that determine how chronic illness or disability affects his or her functional capacity. The extent to which the condition is handicapping depends to a great extent on individuals' perception of the condition, the environment, and the reactions of family, friends, and society in general. The severity of the condition as measured by diagnostic tests does not always indicate the severity of functional impairment. Also, individuals' ability to function is not always directly correlated with the severity of the condition itself.

Professionals working with individuals with chronic illness or disability need to understand the potential limitations or restrictions associated with a specific condition or treatment in order to help individuals and their families make appropriate changes. The effects of chronic illness and disability are far-reaching; they include psychological, social, and vocational effects, and changes and adjustments in both general lifestyle and activities of daily living. The medical diagnosis per se is not as important as the degree to which function in each area of an individual's life is affected. The interactive nature of function between each of the areas determines the extent to which individuals reach their maximal potential. A focus on any one area without full consideration of the impact of the illness or disability on all other areas can dilute the effectiveness of rehabilitative efforts. Thus understanding and working effectively with individuals who have a chronic illness or disability requires a broad outlook that goes beyond medical diagnosis. The most important factor is the individual's ability to function with the condition within his or her environment and all areas of his or her life.

### Psychological Issues in Chronic Illness and Disability

Individuals react both cognitively and emotionally to events that involve them. These reactions, in turn, affect the further course of those events. Psychological factors are ever present in all aspects of chronic illness and disability and influence individuals' response to their condition; sometimes these factors are part of the symptoms of the condition. They affect not only individuals' adjustment and subsequent functional capacity, but also the outcome and prognosis.

### Lifestyle Issues in Chronic Illness and Disability

Lifestyle comprises daily tasks and activities of daily living within an individual's environment. It includes the ability to perform tasks related to grooming, housekeeping, and preparing meals. It also includes activities related to transportation, daily schedules, rest or activity, recreation, sexuality, and privacy. At times, limitations in performing the activities of daily living result from environmental considerations that serve as barriers to effective functioning. Modifications such as widening doorways to permit the passage of a wheelchair, placing handrails in a bathroom, or installing more effective lighting may be required to increase functional capacity. Other lifestyle modifications may be necessary because of the additional tasks and time commitments related to medical treatment of a specific condition. In some instances, restrictions of diet or activity may require a considerable lifestyle change. Continued treatments, medical appointments, and related activities may require significant alteration of the daily schedule.

## Social Issues in Chronic Illness and Disability

The social environment can be defined as individuals' perceived involvement in personal, family, group, and community relationships and activities. Social well-being is based on emotionally satisfying experiences in social activities with those within the individual's social group. Chronic illness and disability often lead to changes in social status. Individuals may find themselves in a socially devalued role. As a result, they may experience changes in social relationships or interactions, or they may have to limit the number of social activities, all of which can result in social isolation. Even when individuals with chronic illness or disability attempt to remain socially active, they may have difficulty entering community facilities because of environmental barriers or because of prejudice or stereotyping.

Many factors contribute to an individual's adaptation or adjustment to the social limitations associated with a particular medical condition. Individuals' perception or misperception of the reactions of others in social groups may determine the level of acceptance that they receive. The degree to which they are able to adapt, accept, and adjust to their functional limitations is determined in part by their interactions with others in their environment, as well as by their interpretation of the reactions of others.

## Vocational Issues in Chronic Illness and Disability

The significance of work in the rehabilitation of people with chronic illness and disability has been well documented (Cunningham, Wolbert, & Brockmeier, 2000). Work involves more than remuneration for services rendered and does not necessarily include only activity related to financial incentives. Work provides a sense of contribution, accomplishment, and meaning to life (Ben-Shlomo, Canfield, & Warner, 2002; Bond et al., 2001; Corrigan, Bogner, Mysiw, Clinchot, & Fugate, 2001). Consequently, loss of the ability to work extends beyond financial consequences to social and psychological well-being. It also means the loss of a socially valued role. For many individuals, work is not only a major part of their identity, but also a source of social interaction, structure, and purpose in life.

The degree to which chronic illness and disability affect individuals' ability and willingness to work depends on a variety of factors in addition to the limitations imposed by the illness or disability itself (Young & Murphy, 2002). Other factors include the nature of the work, the physical environment of the work setting, and the attitudes of employers and coworkers. Psychosocial variables may also complicate functional capacity and, thus, the rehabilitation process. At times, individuals with chronic illness or disability may continue to perform the same work they performed before the onset of the condition. At other times, certain work tasks, environmental conditions, or work schedules must be modified to accommodate the limitations imposed by the chronic illness or disability. If modifications cannot be made in these cases, individuals must change employment. Some individuals must assume disability status because appropriate modifications cannot be made or because their limitations are severe. Job stress or the attitudes of employers or coworkers can significantly interfere with individuals' ability to return to the work force. Problems with transportation to and from work because of limitations caused by the condition may also make a return to work more difficult. In other instances, the time required to carry out treatment recommendations related to the condition may make completing a full day at work virtually impossible.

Individuals' capacity to function at a job can depend on cognitive, psychomotor, and attitudinal factors, as well as on the physical aspects of the illness or disability. Accurately assessing individuals' capacity to return to work consists of more than evaluating physical factors. Individuals' fear of reinjury, vocational dissatisfaction, or legal issues can also hamper return to work. Their ability to relate to and interact with others within the work environment must also be considered. Interests, aptitudes, and abilities are always pivotal factors in determining vocational success, regardless of limitations. Effective rehabilitation that enables individuals to function effectively in their job often involves the interdisciplinary efforts of many types of medical and nonmedical professionals to conduct assessment, evaluation, therapy, and vocational guidance.

## REFERENCES

Anderson, E. M., & Klarke, L. (1982). *Disability in adolescence*. London: Methuen.

Ben-Shlomo, Y., Canfield, L., & Warner, T. (2002). What are the determinants of quality of life in people with cervical dystonia? *Journal of Neurology and Neurosurgical Psychiatry, 72*, 608–614.

Bishop, M., & Feist-Price, S. (2001). Quality of life in rehabilitation counseling: Making the philosophical practical. *Rehabilitation Education, 15*(3), 201–212.

Bond, G. R., Resnick, S. G., Bebout, R. R., Drake, R. E., Xie, H., & McHugo, G. J. (2001). Does competitive employment improve nonvocational outcomes for people with severe mental illness? *Journal of Consulting Clinical Psychology, 69*, 489–501.

Burker, E. J., Carels, R. A., Thompson, L. F., Rodgers, L., & Egan, T. (2000). Quality of life in patients awaiting lung transplant: Cystic fibrosis versus other end-stage lung diseases. *Pediatric Pulmonology, 30*, 453–460.

Corbin, J. (2001). Introduction and overview of chronic illness and nursing. In R. Hyman and J. Corbin (Eds.), *Chronic illness: Research and theory for nursing practice* (pp. 1–15). New York: Springer.

Corrigan, J. D., Bogner, J. A., Mysiw, J. W., Clinchot, D., & Fugate, L. (2001). Life satisfaction after traumatic brain injury. *Journal of Head Trauma Rehabilitation, 16*, 543–555.

Corwyn, R. F. (2000). The factor structure of global self esteem among adolescents and adults. *Journal of Research and Personality, 34*, 357–379.

Crews, W., Jefferson, A., Broshek, D., Barth, J., & Robbins, M. (2000). Neuropsychological sequelae in a series of patients with end-stage cystic fibrosis: Lung transplant evaluation. *Archives of Clinical Neuropsychology, 15*, 59–70.

Cunningham, K., Wolbert, R., & Brockmeier, M. B. (2000). Moving beyond the illness: Factors contributing to gaining and maintaining employment. *American Journal of Community Psychology, 28*(4), 481–493.

Cusack, L. (2000). Perceptions of body image: Implications for the workplace. *Employee Assistance Quarterly, 15*(3), 23–29.

Dolder, C. R., Lacro, J. P., Leckband, S., & Jeste, D. V. (2003). Interventions to improve antipsychotic medication adherence: Review of recent literature. *Journal of Clinical Psychopharmacology, 23*(4), 389–399.

Dudgeon, B. J., Gerrard, B. C., Jensen, M. P., Rhodes, L. A., & Tyler, E. J. (2002). Physical disability and the experience of chronic pain. *Archives of Physical Medicine and Rehabilitation, 83*(2), 229–235.

Dunbar-Jacob, J., Erlen, J. A., Schlenk, E. A., Ryan, C. M., Sereika, S. M., & Doswell, W. M. (2000). Adherence in chronic disease. *Annual Review of Nursing Research, 18*, 48–90.

Falvo, D. R. (2004). *Effective patient education: A guide to increased compliance*. Boston: Jones and Bartlett.

Gledhill, J., Rangel, L., & Garralda, E. (2000). Surviving chronic physical illness: Psychosocial outcomes in adult life. *Archives of Disease in Childhood, 83*(2), 104–110.

Graham, H. (2003). A conceptual map for studying long-term exercise adherence in a cardiac population. *Rehabilitation Nursing, 28*(3), 80–86.

Hordern, A. (2000). Intimacy and sexuality for women with breast cancer. *Cancer Nursing, 23*(3), 230–236.

Hordern, A. J., & Currow, D. C. (2003). A patient-centered approach to sexuality in the face of life-limiting illness. *Medical Journal of Australia, 179*(Suppl. 6): S8–S11.

Kovac, J. A., Patel, S. S., Peterson, R. A., & Kimmel, P. L. (2002). Patient satisfaction with care and behavioral compliance in end-stage renal disease patients treated with hemodialysis. *American Journal of Kidney Disease, 39*(6), 1236–1244.

Leplege, A., & Hunt, S. (1997). The problem of quality of life in medicine. *Journal of the American Medical Association, 278*(1), 47–50.

Livneh, H. (2001). Psychosocial adaptation to chronic illness and disability: A conceptual framework. *Rehabilitation Counseling Bulletin, 44*(3), 150–160.

Livneh, H., & Wilson, L. M. (2003). Coping strategies as predictors and mediators of disability-related variables and psychosocial adaptation: An exploratory investigation. *Rehabilitation Counseling Bulletin, 46*(4), 194–208.

Loghman-Adham, M. (2003). Medication noncompliance in patients with chronic disease: Issues in dialysis and renal transplantation. *American Journal of Managed Care, 9*(2), 155–171.

McBride, K. E., & Rines, B. (2000). Sexuality and spinal cord injury: A road map for nurses. *SCI Nursing, 17*(1), 8–13.

McInnes, R. A. (2003). Chronic illness and sexuality. *Medical Journal of Australia, 179*(5), 263–266.

Moore, G. M., Franzcp, N., Hennessey, P., Kunz, N. M., Ferrando, S., & Rabkin, J. G. (2000). Kaposi's sarcoma: The scarlet letter of AIDS. The psychological effects of a skin disease. *Psychosomatics, 41*(4), 360–363.

Morof Lubkin, I., & Larsen, P. A. (2002). *Chronic illness: Impact and interventions.* Boston: Jones and Bartlett.

Nosek, M. A., & Hughes, R. B. (2003). Psychosocial issues of women with physical disabilities: The continuing gender debate. *Rehabilitation Counseling Bulletin, 46*(4), 224–233.

Schmaling, K. B., Afari, N., & Blume, A. W. (2000). Assessment of psychological factors associated with adherence to medication regimens among adult patients with asthma. *Journal of Asthma, 37*(4), 335–343.

Shaw, L., Segal, R., Polatajko, H., & Harburn, K. (2002). Understanding return to work behaviours: Promoting the importance of individual percep- tions in the study of return to work. *Disability Rehabilitation, 24*(4), 185–195.

Smart, J. (2001). *Disability, society, and the individual.* Gaithersburg, MD: Aspen.

Stevens, S. E., Steele, C. A., Jutai, J. W., Kalnins, I. V., Bortolussi, J. A., & Biggar, W. D. (1996). Adolescents with physical disabilities: Some psychosocial aspects of health. *Journal of Adolescent Health, 19*, 157–164.

Vergouwen, A. C., Bakker, A., Katon, W. J., Verheij, T. J., & Koerselman, F. (2003). Improving adherence to antidepressants: A systematic review of interventions. *Journal of Clinical Psychiatry, 64*(12), 1415–1420.

White, C. A. (2000). Body image dimensions and cancer: A heuristic cognitive behavioural model. *Psych-Oncology, 9*, 183–192.

World Health Organization. (1980). *International classification of impairments, disabilities, and handicaps: A manual of classification relating to the consequences of disease.* Geneva, Switzerland: Author.

Young, A., & Murphy, G. A. (2002). A social psychology approach to measuring vocational rehabilitation intervention effectiveness. *Journal of Occupational Rehabilitation, 12*, 175–189.

Zygmunt, A., Olfson, M., Boyer, C. A., & Mechanic, D. (2002). Interventions to improve medication adherence in schizophrenia. *American Journal of Psychiatry, 159*(10), 1653–1664.

# CHAPTER 2

# Conditions of the Nervous System: Part I
## *Conditions of the Brain*

## NORMAL STRUCTURE AND FUNCTION OF THE NERVOUS SYSTEM

The nervous system consists of the central nervous system and the peripheral nervous system (Table 2–1). The nervous system is a complex network that serves as the communication center for the body. It controls and coordinates activities and functions throughout the body by sending, receiving, and sorting electrical impulses. Disruption of any part of the nervous system affects body function in some way, either internally or externally. Specifically, functions of the nervous system include the following:

1. Organizing and directing motor responses of the voluntary muscle system, enabling the body to move more effectively as a whole and to achieve purposeful movement. This coordination of voluntary muscle makes possible complex activities such as walking or playing a piano, as well as activities as simple as maintaining muscle tone and posture while at rest.
2. Monitoring and recognizing stimuli within the environment and interpreting changes as information to be observed or acted upon. This function makes possible reflex action such as pulling away one's hand from a hot surface as well as perceiving music being played in the next room.
3. Monitoring and coordinating internal body states so that internal organs function as a unit, internal body constancy is maintained, and protective action is taken. For example: in response to lack of oxygen, breathing becomes more rapid; in response to cold, the body shivers; when threat or danger is encountered, the heart beats more rapidly.

---

**Table 2–1** The Nervous System

---

I. Central nervous system
  A. Brain
  B. Spinal cord
II. Peripheral nervous system
  A. Afferent (sensory)
  B. Efferent (motor)
    1. Somatic nervous system
    2. Autonomic nervous system
      a. Sympathetic nervous system
      b. Parasympathetic nervous system

---

The nervous system also controls cognitive functions, such as learning and remembering, feeling emotion, reasoning,

25

generating and relaying thoughts, and displaying the general personality traits that are characteristic of how each individual responds to stimuli.

## Nerve Cells

Specialized cells called *neurons* are the functional units of the nervous system. Neurons transmit messages to and from the brain. They consist of a cell body and processes or *nerve fibers* that extend beyond the cell body. In most cases a single long nerve fiber, called an *axon,* conducts nerve impulses (and information) away from the cell body to other neurons. Smaller, shorter nerve fibers, called *dendrites*, conduct nerve impulses toward the cell body after receiving information from other neurons. Fibers that carry information from parts of the body to the brain are called *afferent neurons* (sensory neurons). Fibers that carry information from the brain to other parts of the body are called *efferent neurons* (motor neurons).

Surrounding neurons is a fatty sheath called *myelin*, which, much like the covering of electrical cords, provides insulation, thus helping electrical impulses flow smoothly and reliably. Information is passed from neuron to neuron by both electrical and chemical impulses. The electrical impulse, which has been picked up by the dendrites, is passed through the cell body to the axon. The electrical impulse moves down the full length of the axon till it reaches its tip. At the tip of the axon are tiny processes that release chemicals known as *neurotransmitters*, which, through chemical means, transfer the impulse from one neuron to another across the space between the two neurons. This space is called the *synapse*. The electrical impulse, through the vehicle of neurotransmitters, then moves to the next neuron's dendrites, and the process begins again

(Figure 2–1). After neurotransmitters are released, they are either taken up again by the neuron or destroyed.

Longer axons are generally grouped in bundles. When transmitting impulses within the central nervous system, these bundles are referred to as *tracts*. Those bundles located outside of the central nervous system are referred to as *nerves*.

## The Central Nervous System

The *central nervous system* is made up of the brain and spinal cord, which are both protected by bony coverings. On the interior of the bony coverings are three membranes (*meninges*) that provide additional protection:

- The *dura mater* is the outer membrane, lying most closely to the bony covering of the brain and spinal cord.
- The *arachnoid membrane* is the middle membrane, a cobweb-like membrane.
- The *pia mater* is the inner membrane that lies next to the brain and spinal cord.

Between each of the membrane layers are spaces. The space between the dura mater and the inner surface of the bony covering is the *epidural space*. The space between the dura mater and arachnoid membrane is the *subdural space*, and the space between the arachnoid membrane and the pia mater is the *subarachnoid space*.

The central nervous system is also protected and cushioned by *cerebrospinal fluid* (CSF), which is formed by specialized capillaries called the *choroid plexus* in inner chambers within the brain called *ventricles*. The CSF bathes the brain and spinal cord. It circulates from the ventricles into the subarachnoid space; then it flows to the back of the brain, down around the spinal cord, and then flows back to the brain, where it is reabsorbed into the blood

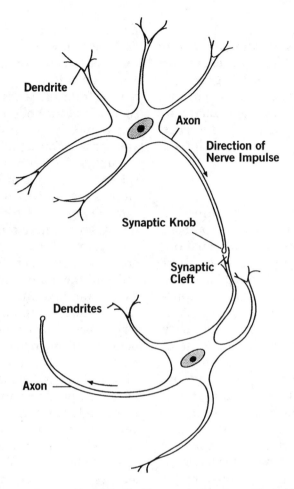

**Figure 2–1** The Neuron. *Source:* Reprinted with permission from M. J. Miller, *Pathophysiology: Principles of Disease*, p. 369. © 1983, W. B. Saunders Company.

through the arachnoid membrane. The amount of CSF produced and absorbed is equally balanced, so that under normal conditions it remains constant within the central nervous system.

Another protective device is the *blood-brain barrier*, a structural arrangement of capillaries that selectively determine which substances can move from the blood into the brain. Whereas substances such as oxygen and glucose are necessary to brain survival and, consequently, move freely across the blood-brain barrier, most potentially harmful substances, such as

toxins, are prevented from crossing into the brain.

The central nervous system is composed of white matter and gray matter. The *white matter* makes up the inner part of the brain and the outer portion of the spinal cord and consists of myelin (covered) axons that conduct nerve impulses. It is called white matter because of its whitish appearance due to the myelin covering. *Gray matter* makes up the thin outer layer of the brain and the inner portion of the spinal cord. Small segments of gray matter are also embedded deep within certain parts of the white matter of the brain. Gray matter consists of groups of neuron cell bodies. It is called gray matter because of its grayish appearance. The gray matter of the brain receives, sorts, and processes nerve messages, and the gray matter of the spinal cord serves as a center for reflex action (automatic response to stimuli).

### The Brain

The brain, which is directly connected to the spinal cord, serves as the primary center for the integration, coordination, initiation, and interpretation of most nerve messages. The brain regulates and monitors many unconscious body functions, such as heart rate and respiration, and also coordinates most voluntary movements. In addition, it is the site of consciousness and intellectual function.

The brain is protected by the bony covering of the skull (*cranium* or *cranial bones*). The largest part of the brain, the *cerebrum*, is covered with a thin outer layer of gray matter called the *cortex*, which contains billions of nerve cells. The cortex has three specialized areas that serve three major functions:

1. The *motor cortex* coordinates voluntary movements of the body.
2. The *sensory cortex* is responsible for the recognition or perception of sensory stimuli, such as touch, pain, smell, taste, vision, and hearing.
3. The *associational cortex* is involved in cognitive functions, such as memory, reasoning, abstract thinking, and consciousness.

The cerebrum is divided into two halves, called hemispheres: the *right hemisphere* and the *left hemisphere*. The two hemispheres communicate with each other. Dividing the hemispheres and connecting specific areas within them are bundles of nerve fibers called the *corpus callosum*. Each hemisphere has centers for receiving information and for initiating responses. The left hemisphere mostly receives information from and sends information to the right side of the body, and the right hemisphere mostly receives information from and sends information to the left side of the body. Deep within the cerebral hemispheres are groups of gray matter called *basal ganglia*, which are part of the *extrapyramidal system*. (*Extrapyramidal* denotes nerve fiber tracts that lie outside the pyramidal tract, a relatively compact group of nerve fibers that originate from cells in the outer layer of the brain.) Extrapyramidal function is concerned with postural adjustment and gross voluntary and automatic muscular movements. Basal ganglia help to maintain contractile tone in muscles in the trunk and extremities, enabling individuals to maintain balance and posture and engage in movement such as walking. The basal ganglia also play a role in enabling individuals to react swiftly, appropriately, and automatically to stimuli that demand an immediate response, such as, after tripping, enabling the individual to adjust movement in order to avoid a fall.

Each hemisphere of the cerebrum is divided into lobes that contain areas related to specific functions. The *frontal lobe* is located in the front of each hemisphere and contains motor areas that initiate voluntary movement and skilled movements, such as those involved in writing. Other areas in the frontal lobe control higher intellectual functions such as foresight, analytical thinking, and judgment. The *parietal lobe* is located in the middle of each hemisphere and is primarily the sensory area, integrating and interpreting sensation such as touch, pressure, pain, and temperature. Some memory functions are also located in the parietal lobe, espe-

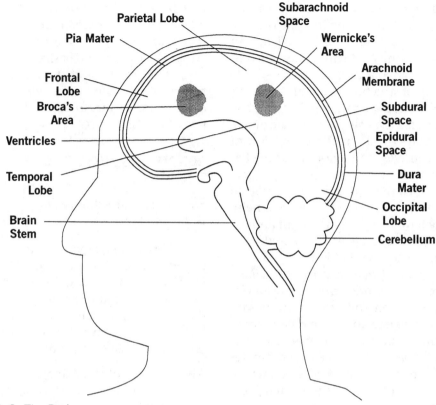

**Figure 2–2**  The Brain.

cially those responsible for storage of sensory memory. The *temporal lobe* is located under the frontal and parietal lobes and is primarily responsible for the interpretation of and distinction between auditory stimuli. The *occipital lobe* is located at the back or posterior portion of each hemisphere. It is the primary area for reception and interpretation of visual stimuli.

Several parts of the cerebrum are involved in language function, which involves receiving, interpreting, and integrating visual and auditory stimuli as well as expressing thoughts in a coordinated way so that others may comprehend it. Language function is located in the left hemisphere of the cerebrum in most individuals, whether they are right- or left-handed. An area located over the temporal

and parietal lobes, called *Wernicke's area*, is the major area responsible for *receptive function*, or the ability to integrate visual and auditory information in order to understand a communication received. An area located in front of the temporal lobe and in the frontal cortex is called *Broca's area*, which contributes to expressive function, or the ability to integrate and coordinate words so that the meaning can be comprehended (Figure 2–2).

A structure known as the *thalamus* lies within the center of the brain. The thalamus acts as a relay station that sorts, interprets, and directs sensory information. Below the thalamus is the *hypothalamus*, which coordinates neural and endocrine activities. It helps regulate the body's internal environment and behaviors that are important to survival, such as eating, drinking, and reproduction. Below the hypothalamus is the *pituitary gland*, an endocrine gland that will be discussed in more detail in a later chapter.

A group of structures consisting of both gray and white matter surrounding the thalamus is called the *limbic system*. The limbic system plays a role in the expression of instincts, drives, and emotions as well as the formation of memories. A band of gray matter called the *hippocampus* is involved in learning and long-term memory, helping to determine where important and relevant aspects of facts will be stored.

Beneath the occipital lobe of the cerebrum is a structure called the *cerebellum*. The cerebellum is primarily responsible for the coordination and integration of voluntary movement and for maintenance of equilibrium, posture, and balance. The cerebellum also regulates and coordinates fine movements of the extremities, which have been initiated by the frontal lobe.

The *brain stem*, located beneath the cerebellum at the base of the brain just above the spinal cord, acts as a relay station, transmitting nerve impulses between the spinal cord and the brain. The brain stem is the primary center of involuntary functions. Control of vital organ functions such as regulation of heartbeat or respiration occurs in the brain stem. Areas in the brain stem also regulate the diameter of blood vessels, consequently helping to control blood pressure. Reflex actions, such as coughing and swallowing, are controlled in the brain stem. The brain stem also contains scattered groups of cells, called the *reticular formation*, that are involved in the initiation and maintenance of wakefulness and alertness.

The brain requires both oxygen and nourishment in the form of *glucose* to function and survive. Oxygen and glucose are transported to the brain by blood car-ried by four major arteries, two *carotid arteries* and two *vertebral arteries*. The vertebral arteries join to form the *basilar artery*. The carotid and basilar arteries then connect at the base of the brain to form the *circle of Willis*, from which *cerebral arteries* branch out to carry blood to the rest of the brain.

## CONDITIONS AFFECTING THE BRAIN

### Traumatic and Atraumatic Brain Damage

The brain, like any other tissue, needs oxygen in order to function. Anything that interferes with the brain's ability to get oxygen or causes damage to the brain directly will impact its ability to function effectively. The manifestations of brain damage are dependent on:

- the cause of the damage
- the area of the brain damaged
- the extent of the damage

Generally, brain damage is classified as one of two types:

1. *Atraumatic* (nontraumatic) brain damage caused by interference with oxygen reaching the brain (such as with choking, carbon monoxide poisoning, or infection) or problems within the brain itself (such as stroke, or structural problems within the brain or blood vessels in the brain)
2. *Traumatic* brain injury (TBI), caused by an outside force that impacts the head hard enough to cause damage to the brain

Both *atraumatic* (nontraumatic) and *traumatic brain damage* are considered *acquired brain injuries* because they occur after birth and are not the result of genetic disorder, birth trauma, or degenerative disease.

### Atraumatic Brain Damage

*Atraumatic brain damage, as just explained*, refers to conditions in which the brain has sustained damage due to conditions other than traumatic injury. Specifically, *atraumatic brain damage* is caused by conditions that cause restriction or interference with blood and oxygen reaching parts of the brain. When a part of the brain receives no oxygen (**anoxia**) or too little oxygen (**hypoxia**), the tissue can die. Examples of conditions that can cause atraumatic brain damage are stroke, congenital malformations (such as *arteriovenous malformations*, in which blood vessels are abnormal at birth), **aneurysms** (a weakened area in an artery located in the brain that then balloons out and can rupture), infections or inflammation of the brain or surrounding membranes (such as *meningitis* or *encephalitis*), or other conditions that deprive the brain of oxygen, such as strangulation, near drowning, or inhalation of noxious gases.

### Stroke (Cerebral Vascular Accident)

Stroke, also known as **cerebral vascular accident**, is a sudden alteration in brain function resulting in weakness or paralysis in a body part as well as other neurological deficits due to decreased blood flow to a part of the brain. Stroke is usually the culmination of progressive disease that has occurred over the course of many years. Heart disease or *ischemic vascular disease* (arteriosclerosis), **hypertension** (high blood pressure), and diabetes are often associated with stroke. There are three main causes of stroke:

1. The most common cause is blocking of a cerebral artery by a clot (**thrombus**) that has formed inside the artery, a condition referred to as *cerebral thrombosis*. Formation of the thrombus blocks blood flow to an area of the brain. Because brain tissue needs the oxygen contained in blood to survive, tissue that cannot obtain needed nourishment because of the blockage dies within a short period of time. This tissue death is called an **infarct**. The amount of damage depends on how large an area of the brain has been deprived of blood supply from the clot.

2. Another cause of stroke is **embolism**. In this case a clot forms in another part of the body and then breaks off, traveling through the blood to the brain and lodging in one of the cerebral arteries. Again, when the clot occludes blood flow to a part of the brain, surrounding brain tissue dies.

3. A third cause of stroke is *hemorrhage*, which occurs because of rupture of a blood vessel. A common cause of cerebral hemorrhage is **hypertension** (high blood pressure). When blood vessels are weakened because of disease, such as with arteriosclerosis, or because of congenital weakness as with an aneurysm, increased pressure may cause the blood vessel to burst. Death of brain tissue occurs in this instance not only because a certain area of the brain has been deprived of oxygen, but also because the escaped blood compresses brain tissue against the skull, causing further damage.

The amount and degree of function lost as the result of stroke depends on:

- the side of the brain affected
- the specific area of the brain that has been damaged
- the amount of damage that has occurred

Often after stroke, in addition to the initial damage to an area of the brain, surrounding brain tissue becomes **edematous** (swells), causing additional deficits. Although death of brain tissue causes permanent damage, areas of the brain that have only experienced swelling may recover, and function in these areas may be restored. Consequently, individuals experiencing stroke may not know the extent of permanent functional limitations until months after the stroke as occurred.

At times, temporary blocking of the cerebral arteries causes slight, temporary neurological deficits. These "ministrokes" are referred to as **transient ischemic attacks (TIAs)**. Although neurological deficits experienced from TIAs are usually temporary, their occurrence forewarns of the possibility of a larger stroke unless treatment controls the underlying condition.

### Infections of the Central Nervous System

Any infection of the brain or the membranes that surround the brain and spinal cord can cause serious neurological effects, some of which may be permanent.

Meningitis. **Meningitis** refers to an inflammation of the **meninges** (membranes surrounding the brain and spinal cord). It can be caused by bacteria, viruses, or other organisms. There are many types of meningitis. The specific name given to the meningitis infection is frequently related to its cause or location. For instance, *cerebral meningitis* refers to meningitis of the brain, whereas *cerebrospinal meningitis* refers to meningitis of both the brain and spinal cord. *Meningococcal meningitis* (commonly known as *spinal meningitis*) is caused by a bacterium that settles in the lining of the throat and is spread easily through respiratory secre-

tions. The organism is relatively common. Normally the lining of the throat is sufficient to act as a barrier to the bacteria; however, when the barrier is insufficient, the infecting organism invades the bloodstream and reaches the meninges, causing them to become inflamed. The organism also gains access to the cerebrospinal fluid and begins to multiply.

The hallmark of meningitis is its rapid onset. Individuals with meningitis are usually acutely ill, initially with fever and flu-like symptoms. Within a short period of time they develop severe headache, neck rigidity, and discomfort when exposed to bright lights. If the cause is bacterial in origin, prompt treatment with antibiotics reduces the chance of disease progression. The use of medication and prompt treatment has greatly reduced the number of fatalities from meningitis; however, if it occurs in individuals whose physical state is weakened or if diagnosis and treatment are delayed, it can still be fatal. Although most individuals with meningitis recover completely, some may have residual neurological deficits such as deafness, paralysis, or cognitive difficulties.

Encephalitis. **Encephalitis** is an inflammation of the brain due to direct invasion of an organism. It may be caused by an endemic virus, such as the West Nile virus, a mosquito-borne virus (Huhn, Sejvar, Montgomer, & Dworkin, 2003; Marfin & Gubler, 2001), or it may be secondary to another infection, such as measles or chickenpox. Some individuals with encephalitis may experience severe headache, stiff neck, and coma. There is no adequate treatment for encephalitis, except for maintaining comfort and preventing complications. The symptoms can subside in a few weeks, leaving no permanent damage; however, the condition can also be life-threatening. Some individuals develop irreversible neurological changes as a result of encephalitis.

Although meningitis or encephalitis and resulting deficits can occur in any age group, children and older adults, or those with compromised immune systems, are often the most susceptible to more severe manifestations of these diseases.

### Traumatic Brain Injury

*Traumatic brain injury* is broadly defined as an injury to the brain from external forces, such as vehicular accidents, falls, violence, or sports or recreational events (NIH Consensus Development Panel on Rehabilitation of Persons with Traumatic Brain Injury, 1999). It is not degenerative, is not the result of a disease, and is not congenital in origin. Damage to the brain occurs from a blow to the head that is hard enough to cause the brain to move within the skull, or from an impact that fractures the skull, injuring the brain directly.

Almost two million people, of all ages, sustain brain injury each year in the United States. TBI can cause myriad effects, including physical, cognitive, emotional, and behavioral deficits that impact every aspect of an individual's life. This wide range of deficits presents unique challenges to rehabilitation of individuals with TBI.

### Types of Traumatic Brain Injury

There are two types of traumatic brain injuries:

- *Open or penetrating head injury*
- *Closed head injury*

*Open (penetrating) injuries* refer to injuries in which the skull is fractured (such as with a blow to the head in which the skull is broken) or penetrated (such as with a gunshot wound). Functional impairments experienced with open or penetrating injury may be more localized and are usually related to the specific area of the brain affected. At times, functional impairments in open head injury may be more extensive if additional damage is sustained. For example, in addition to the trauma to the brain itself, bone fragments from the injury may also lacerate and injure the brain, blood vessels, or **meninges** (lining surrounding the brain).

In *closed head injury* (such as a blow to the head or violent shaking of the head, as in shaken baby syndrome), the skull is not fractured; rather, the brain is damaged because the head has been hit with sufficient force that the brain slams against the other side of the skull or twists within the skull, causing shearing of blood vessels or nerve fibers throughout the brain. This is called *diffuse axonal injury*. Injury is caused to the brain both from the external force as well as from movement of the brain within the skull. The initial impact to the brain is called the *coup*, and the impact of the brain on the opposite side of the skull is called the *contre coup*. Functional limitations associated with closed head injury depend on where and how much shearing occurred in the brain and may be more diffuse because of the more extensive damage to the brain itself.

Additional injury may occur as an indirect result of **edema** (swelling) of the brain, hemorrhage, or the formation of a **hematoma** (sac filled with blood) within the skull as a direct result of the injury itself. Bleeding within the cranial vault is referred to as *intracranial hemorrhage*. Because the brain is confined within the skull, there is no space available for expansion if swelling or bleeding should occur. As a result, swelling or bleeding compresses the brain, increasing intracranial pressure and interfering with brain function.

Unless recognized and treated promptly, these events can cause additional permanent brain damage or death.

Bleeding and blood clots compress the brain, increasing intracranial pressure. An *epidural hematoma* is bleeding that occurs in the space between the outer membrane of the brain (the dura mater) and the skull. Although bleeding generally occurs rapidly, it may not be recognized immediately. Individuals who have been injured may carry on a lucid conversation, only to slip into drowsiness and unconsciousness hours later. Epidural hematomas carry a high mortality rate because they may not be immediately recognized and consequently not immediately treated.

A *subdural hematoma* is a hemorrhage that occurs in the space beneath the dura mater. Although symptoms may be apparent immediately, they may also appear more gradually, becoming evident days or even weeks after the injury. In both instances, immediate action is essential to stop the bleeding and to relieve the intracranial pressure before permanent damage to the brain occurs.

### Measuring the Severity of Traumatic Brain Injury

A variety of instruments are available to measure the severity of TBI. These instruments are used to predict the condition of the individual after discharge and can be useful measures for rehabilitation services after hospitalization (Wagner, Hammond, Grigsby, & Norton, 2000).

Brain injuries are classified as:

- mild
- moderate
- severe

One basis of classification is the length of time the individual is unconscious after injury and the depth of unconsciousness or coma. The length of unconsciousness is also used as a predictor of prognostic outcome. Generally, the longer the period of unconsciousness, the more severe the injury to the brain and the greater subsequent residual effects. An instrument called the *Glasgow Coma Scale* (Jennet, Snoek, Bond, & Brooks, 1981) has become widely accepted as a classification system for rating the seriousness of brain injury. The scale is used to assess the level of consciousness on a continuum ranging from alert to coma state. Scores are assigned according to the level of response in each of three areas: eye opening, motor response, and verbal response (Table 2–2). Scores ranging from 3 to 15 may be obtained. The lower the score, the deeper the level of unconsciousness. The Glasgow Coma Scale provides a means whereby individuals' level of consciousness can be assessed systematically. An initial assessment provides a baseline from which changes in neurological status can be measured. The scale is usually used in the early postinjury period in the emergency and critical care units.

Another scale used to measure level of brain injury is the *Rancho Los Amigos Cognitive Scale*. The scale basically describes levels of arousal and cognitive functioning. It measures increasing levels of consciousness, so it often is used to give a gross indication of stages of recovery after brain injury. The range of the scale is from 1 to 8, with higher scores indicating higher functional level. In the treatment and rehabilitation phase after injury, individuals may remain at one level of unconsciousness or coma for an extended period of time or may move from one level of consciousness to the next. The Ranchos Los Amigos Scale of Cognitive Function, as a measure of cognitive function, is usually used to assess changes in the level of consciousness during the postinjury period and as a broad indicator of the extent to which independent functioning is possible. In this way a specific treatment can be instituted to promote appropriate behavior as the individual moves through different levels (Table 2–3).

**Table 2–2** The Glasgow Coma Scale

| Category | Score |
| --- | --- |
| Eyes open | |
| Never | 1 |
| To pain | 2 |
| To verbal stimuli | 3 |
| Spontaneously | 4 |
| Best verbal response | |
| None | 1 |
| Incomprehensible sounds | 2 |
| Inappropriate words | 3 |
| Disoriented and converses | 4 |
| Oriented and converses | 5 |
| Best motor response | |
| None | 1 |
| Extension (decerebrate rigidity) | 2 |
| Flexion abnormal (decorticate rigidity) | 3 |
| Flexion withdrawal | 4 |
| Individual localizes pain | 5 |
| Individual obeys | 6 |

*Source:* White & Likavec (1992).

The *Disability Rating Scale* (Rappaport, Hall, Hopkins, Belleza, & Cope, 1982) is also used to estimate functional capacity after brain injury. The scale evaluates individuals on eight categories of disability and their ability to function. The highest possible score is 30. The lower the individual scores on the Disability Rating Scale the better. Functional ability is scored on the following areas:

- Level of arousal, awareness, and responsiveness
- Cognitive skills needed for self-care

**Table 2–3** Rancho Los Amigos Scale of Cognitive Functioning

| | |
| --- | --- |
| Level I | No response to sounds, light, or touch. |
| Level II | Generalized response to stimuli, such as responding to a loud noise but not turning toward the noise. Movement is not consistent and does not appear to have a purpose. When eyes are open, they do not appear to be focusing on anything in particular. |
| Level III | Localized response. The individual begins to open eyes and look at specific objects. The head turns in the direction of sound. Simple commands are followed, such as "squeeze my hand." |
| Level IV | Confusion and agitation. The individual becomes very restless and agitated regardless of the circumstances. Conversation may at times appear to be coherent. The individual may become verbally abusive. |
| Level V | Confused, with conversation often not making sense. The individual appears confused although may be able to follow simple instructions. The individual seems less agitated but may become frustrated. |
| Level VI | Confused, but verbal responses are appropriate. Some memory problems regarding recent events may be present. Capable of most self-care activities. Some judgment and problem-solving difficulties, but the individual is often aware of this deficit. |
| Level VII | Automatic, appropriate response. Oriented with little or no confusion. Lacks insight and problem-solving skills. |
| Level VIII | Purposeful and appropriate. Independent. Can process new information and problem-solve. |

- Dependence on others
- Psychosocial adaptability, including flexibility and ability to adapt to different people and situations

*Levels of Traumatic Brain Injury*

*Mild brain injuries* constitute about 70 percent of all TBIs (Busch & Alpern, 1998) and are characterized by a traumatically induced disruption of brain function in which there is at least one of the symptoms as listed in Table 2–4. Individuals with mild brain injuries have a Glasgow Rating of 10 or above and may have few if any outer signs of brain injury or no detectable anatomic damage to the brain. As a result, the brain injury itself may be undiagnosed and consequently untreated (Clements, 1997). Individuals with mild brain injury may experience subtle but disruptive symptoms that persist months or even years after the initial injury. This group of symptoms has come to be known as *postconcussion syndrome* and can consist of symptoms such as headache, **vertigo** (dizziness), **tinnitus** (ringing in the ears), sleep disturbance, depression, irritability, reduced attention span, or memory impairment. Because with mild brain injury there often are few, if any, objective signs of brain damage, individuals experiencing these symptoms may have their credibility questioned, and they may be labeled as malingerers (Koch, Merz, & Torkelson Lynch, 1995). Cognitive deficits associated with mild brain injury may cause individuals considerable distress and adversely affect both social and occupational functioning.

*Moderate brain injury* is defined by a Glasgow Coma Scale score of 9 to 12. Individuals with moderate brain injury may have loss of consciousness for a few minutes or several hours. There may be confusion or disorientation that lasts for a few days or several weeks. Physical, cognitive, or psychosocial deficits may last for weeks to months or may be permanent.

---

**Table 2–4** Manifestations of Mild Brain Injury

---

Individual experiences at least one of the following:

1. Brief loss of consciousness (30 minutes or less)
2. Brief period of time after the injury during which the individual feels stunned and disoriented
3. Loss of memory for events occurring immediately before or after the injury, lasting no longer than 24 hours
4. Temporary neurological deficit
5. Initial Glasgow Coma Scale score of 13–15.

---

*Source*: Berrol (1992).

*Severe brain injury* is defined as a Glasgow Coma Scale score of 8 or less. Individuals with severe brain injury remain in a coma for an extended period of time, ranging from days to months. **Coma** is defined as prolonged unconsciousness in which there is little, if any, meaningful response from the individual and he or she is unable to be awakened. Individuals are said to be in a *vegetative state* when they react to painful stimuli and may open their eyes in response to stimulation but have no meaningful response with the environment (Giacino & Zasler, 1995). The more severe the injury, the more severe the permanent consequences or deficits experienced. Thus the potential consequences of brain injury vary tremendously, depending on the type of injury and the area of brain damaged as well as factors that existed before the event.

*Conditions Associated with Traumatic Brain Injury*

*Posttraumatic epilepsy* is experienced by some individuals after TBI. In the early postinjury period, seizures may be related to increased intracranial pressure or other direct results of injury. Seizures occurring later may be due to the formation of scar tissue in the brain and may occur over a year after the initial injury.

Individuals with TBI may also develop *posttraumatic hydrocephalus*, in which there is interference with reabsorption of CSF. Posttraumatic hydrocephalus can cause increasing neurological or functional deterioration. It may be treated by surgically implanting a shunt in the brain to divert and drain the CSF. The prognosis for individuals who develop posttraumatic hydrocephalus is variable.

## Right-Sided Versus Left-Sided Brain Damage

Although the manifestations of brain damage vary, the outward signs and symptoms of closed head injury or of stroke are frequently related to which side of the brain has been damaged.

### Left-Sided Damage

The most visible sign of left-sided brain damage, regardless of the underlying cause, is right-sided motor and sensory paralysis. For individuals who are right-handed, implications for everyday tasks such as feeding themselves, dressing, writing, or a number of other activities are significantly affected. For most people, regardless of whether they are right- or left-handed, the language center, which processes verbal symbols, is located in the left side of the brain. Consequently, individuals with left-sided damage will most probably have problems with verbal and/or written communication. (See aphasia, described below.) Although they may be able to understand more than they can speak or write, often they also have difficulty understanding verbal and/or written communication. However, even though individuals may have difficulty with speech and language, their ability to learn and communicate should not be underestimated. By the same token, individuals' ability to understand speech should not be overestimated. In general, short, concise statements are more successfully communicated than long, complicated ones.

In general, besides having problems with language, individuals with left-sided brain damage tend to be slow, hesitant, anxious, and disorganized when presented with a new or unfamiliar situation. Reassurance and frequent reinforcement for tasks performed correctly help reduce anxiety and enhance the individuals' ability to perform.

### Right-Sided Damage

The most visible sign of right-sided brain damage is left-sided motor and sensory paralysis. Invariably, right-sided brain damage is also accompanied by some degree of damage to visual perception or visual-motor integration. Spatial-perceptual deficits can include loss of depth perception or lack of awareness of stimuli on the left side of the body, causing difficulty with navigation within the environment. For instance, individuals may miss the table with a glass when putting it down, or bump into a doorway when attempting to go through it. Since those with right-sided brain damage have difficulty processing visual cues, an uncluttered and structured environment prevents distraction and enhances their ability to perform. Ability to read may also be compromised because of the inability to move down the page without skipping lines.

Memory impairment may also be present so that individuals are unable to recognize familiar people or places. In other instances memory impairment is manifest as disorientation in familiar environments, so that individuals may require specific instructions about how to get from place to place. In other instances, memory impairment results in individuals misplacing personal items and then concluding that someone else must have taken them.

Because language function is often not affected, the abilities of individuals with right-sided brain damage may be overestimated. Individuals themselves may be disinhibited and unaware of deficits and may overestimate their own abilities to perform tasks, acting quickly and impulsively. As a result of diminished self-awareness, they may tend to set unrealistic goals and appear insensitive to the needs of others. In other instances, individuals may have difficulty decoding nonverbal cues from others and as a result may be oblivious to others' reactions or feelings.

## Functional Consequences of Brain Damage

Because the brain is responsible for so many functions, damage to the brain, whether *traumatic* or *atraumatic*, can have a profound impact on all areas of an individual's life. Regardless of whether brain damage is caused from an accident, a blow to the head, stroke, infection of the brain, exposure to toxins, or lack of oxygen, manifestations of brain damage may affect many functions. The effects experienced from brain damage depend on which part of the brain was damaged and the extent of the damage incurred. In gen-

eral, potential consequences of brain damage can be broken down into four categories (Groswasser & Stern, 1998):

1. Motor control and perception
2. Communication effects
3. Cognitive changes
4. Personality change and affective response

### Motor and Perceptual Consequences of Brain Damage

The motor and perceptual consequences of brain damage depend on whether the damage was diffuse or local. Functional impact can affect any of the following areas:

1. Movement, coordination, or balance
2. Visual-spatial relations
3. Perception
4. Vision and hearing
5. Touch, taste, and smell
6. Eating and swallowing
7. Endurance
8. Bowel and bladder function

In addition, individuals with brain damage may also experience seizure disorders and, in some instances, persistent pain.

#### Movement, Coordination, or Balance

Whether brain damage is atraumatic (such as stroke) or traumatic (such as from a gunshot), damage confined to one hemisphere of the brain will result in symptoms related to the extent of damage and which hemisphere was affected. Because one side of the brain controls the opposite side of the body, damage to one hemisphere of the brain affects function of the body on the opposite side. Consequently, right cerebral damage can cause paralysis or weakness of the left side of the body (*left hemiplegia*) that affects the left arm and leg, whereas left cerebral damage can result in paralysis or weakness of the right side of the body (*right hemiplegia*) that affects the right arm and leg. The resulting paralysis or weakness interferes with the individual's ability to walk so that he or she may need assistive devices such as a cane, walker, brace, or in some instances a wheelchair.

When individuals experience diffuse *axonal injury*, such as in closed head injury, changes of movement affecting both sides of the body may be present. Individuals may experience problems with muscle coordination (**ataxia**) that affect balance, causing them to walk with an unsteady gait or to lurch from side to side as they walk. They may experience other motor changes, including **dyskinesia** (abnormal movements) or **dystonia** (abnormal muscle tone). Dystonia can consist of too little tone (**flaccidity** or **hypotonicity**), which decreases the ability to move, or too much muscle tone (**spasticity** or **hypertonicity**), which heightens reflexes or abnormal movements.

Even when the motor function of muscles remains intact and muscle strength, coordination, and sensation are normal, there may be reduced ability to organize and sequence specific muscle movements to perform a task (**apraxia**).

Individuals with apraxia are aware of what they want to do and how to do it, but they are unable to organize muscle movements to perform the task. Consequently, a number of tasks, from dressing and eating to performing higher-level activities, may be affected.

### Visual-Spatial Relations

Visual-spatial deficits cause problems with depth perception and judgment of distance, size, position, rate of movement, form, and the relation of parts to wholes. Visual-spatial changes as a result of brain damage interfere with the ability to interpret visual information accurately. Consequently, there may be difficulty orienting position and navigating movement within the environment, or individuals may demonstrate inappropriate judgment of space or distance or the relationship of the distance between two objects. As a result, they may appear careless or clumsy, frequently bumping into furniture, having difficulty navigating doorways, knocking items off tables or counters, or missing the table when attempting to put a glass down. Visual-spatial deficits can affect other activities of daily living as well. For example, individuals may find it difficult to read because they continue to lose their place on the page, or they may have difficulty dressing because they confuse the inside and outside of clothes as well as left and right. Because of difficulty judging distances, individuals with even minor visual-spatial deficits may have difficulty driving a car.

### Perception

Perceptual problems affect the ability to understand or interpret stimuli or objects within the environment. Depending on what part of the brain is damaged, many different perceptual problems may occur. Although some perceptual problems may improve over time, others will be permanent.

There may be loss of comprehension of sensations (**agnosia**) in which individuals lose the ability to recognize familiar things such as words, faces, or objects. Some individuals, especially those with brain damage localized to the right side, may experience a condition called **anosognosia** (one-sided or unilateral neglect) in which body parts or objects on one side of the body are ignored. For instance, an individual with anosognosia may shave only one side of his face, or only put on one shoe. In some instances, anosognosia is visual, so that there is an inability to perceive objects on either the right or left of the central field of vision. In these instances, individuals may bump into things on the ignored or neglected side of their body. Sometimes, signals from all senses on one side of the body are involved so that individuals may not recognize their own arm or leg or are unresponsive to verbal stimuli that originate from one side of the body. Nonresponsiveness to verbal stimuli on the impaired side is different from merely losing hearing in one ear. All stimuli on the affected side are ignored, while stimuli on the individual's unaffected side evoke a response.

### Vision and Hearing

Visual problems may be present even though the eye itself is not injured. When the part of the brain that receives, perceives, or interprets nerve impulses from the eye has been damaged, visual deficits may still be present. These can include total blindness, **diplopia** (double vision), blurred vision, visual field loss such as cuts in the peripheral field of vision (*blind spots*), **hemianopia** (loss of vision in half the visual field), or color blindness.

As with vision, even though the ear has not been damaged directly, hearing deficits may be present if the area of the brain responsible for receiving, perceiving, or interpreting sound has been damaged (**sensorineural hearing loss**). Individuals may experience ringing in the ears (**tinnitus**) as well as partial or total loss of hearing.

### Touch, Taste, and Smell

Brain damage that involves the parts of the brain responsible for sensation can lead to a variety of abnormalities, such as decreased feeling or absence of feeling in various body parts. These changes may result in numbness (**anesthesia**), the inability to feel pain (**analgesia**), or the inability to sense movement of body parts. Individuals may also experience abnormal sensations (**paresthesia**) such as pain, tingling, or burning in various locations in their body.

If the olfactory nerve or corresponding area of the brain has been damaged, there may be no sense of smell (**anosmia**). Although loss of sense of smell may not appear to be a deficit that significantly affects the ability to function, it can affect the ability to detect hazards such as smoke, gas leaks, or other important warning signs. Lack of sense of smell also affects the ability to taste. Inability to taste may affect the individual's will to eat and consequently affect his or her nutritional status as well as the ability to detect food that is spoiled.

### Eating and Swallowing

Swallowing reflexes may be affected so that individuals have difficulty swallowing (**dysphagia**) and in some instances difficulty with chewing. The gag reflex may also be impaired so that there is increased susceptibility to choking. Because of difficulty with swallowing or performing chewing movements, food may be pocketed in one side of the mouth, increasing the risk of gagging or choking. This can be dangerous because of the risk of **aspiration** (food or liquid entering the lungs rather than the stomach). When individuals are unable to swallow food because of swallowing difficulty, a special diet consisting of pureed food may be needed or tube feedings may be necessary to prevent aspiration into the lungs. In addition, because of difficulty or inability to swallow, saliva may build up in the mouth, causing the individual to drool.

## Endurance

After brain damage individuals may experience extreme mental and physical fatigue when completing both physical and mental tasks, especially when tasks are unfamiliar or require significant concentration. Physical and mental activities that, prior to injury, were easy for the individual to complete may also be exhausting to complete after the injury. Sleep patterns may be altered so that quality of sleep is affected, compounding the problem. Tasks may be performed better earlier in the day, since performance levels can deteriorate later in the day due to fatigue.

## Bowel and Bladder Function

In some instances control of bladder or bowel function may be lost (**incontinence**) after brain damage. At times problems are caused by the individual's inability to recognize the need to urinate or defecate. In other instances, individuals are unable to urinate at will or to completely empty the bladder when urinating. There may be need for bladder and/or bowel retraining, or the need for individuals to wear or utilize a *catheter* (tube inserted into the bladder to drain urine).

## Posttraumatic Seizures

Seizures may be experienced in the period immediately after the brain damage. They can be mild or severe, temporary or permanent. In some instances, seizures occurring in the immediate postdamage phase resolve after swelling of the brain recedes. In many other cases, however, individuals continue to have seizures, a condition called *posttraumatic epilepsy*.

## Communication Consequences

Brain damage can affect all forms of communication, including the ability to speak, comprehend, or convey language through either written or verbal means. **Speech** refers to the physical ability to produce sounds and/or movement of the lips, tongue, or other structures that are used to produce language. **Language** refers to how words, as symbols, are put together to convey and understand concepts. The ability to use and understand words (language) is controlled in the brain. In addition, the ability to use certain muscles that enable individuals to form words and project speech is controlled within the brain. When the area of the brain that controls either speech or language is damaged, limitations may occur.

Motor difficulty in structures related to speech may affect the individual's ability to speak. Coordination and accuracy of movement of the muscles, lips, tongue, or other parts of the speech mechanism may be impaired secondary to weakness or paralysis of the muscles needed to speak. This condition is called **dysarthria**. Impairment may range from speech that is slightly slurred to speech that is unintelligible. Paralysis or weakness of muscles may also cause vocal cord dysfunction, which in turn can affect voice quality.

Other motor problems can cause *articulation disorders* in which there is no significant weakness or lack of coordination for reflexive action but rather the inability to position and sequence muscle movements. For example, individuals may be able to scrape a food particle off their teeth with their tongue, but they may be unable to coordinate the muscles that move the tongue to produce a phonetic sound. This condition is known as *apraxia of speech*.

Another communication consequence of brain damage may be the inability to comprehend or use language (**aphasia**). Aphasia can affect either verbal or written communication. It results from dysfunction of the language centers in the brain, rather than impairment in the musculature involved in producing speech. Although there are a number of types of aphasia, two common categories are:

- **nonfluent** (**expressive** or **motor**) aphasia
- **fluent** (**receptive** or **sensory**) aphasia

**Broca's aphasia** is a type of *nonfluent aphasia* characterized by misarticulation, laborious speech, hesitancy, and reduced vocabulary and grammar. Individuals may be able to understand and read simple material; however, as the complexity or length of the message increases, difficulty becomes more apparent. Although they are able to comprehend, they may have difficulty expressing thoughts in speech and writing because of difficulty putting words and sentences together logically. Word-finding difficulties (**dysnomia**) are also common. Reading ability may be better than writing ability. Speech may be labored, slow, and/or difficult to understand, and small connecting words, such as prepositions, may be omitted.

**Wernicke's aphasia** is a type of *fluent aphasia* in which there is effortless speech, relatively normal grammatical structure, and increased verbal output, but with reduced information content, so that what the individual says makes little sense. Auditory and reading comprehension is usually poor. Individuals with Wernicke's aphasia are typically unaware of their communication difficulties.

In some instances individuals may experience **global aphasia**, in which there is severe difficulty communicating because of both the inability to use language (to use words and organize them into coherent sentences) and severe difficulty understanding language, either written or spoken.

Language impairment may differ depending on the area of the brain damaged. Because the center of language function is located in the left cerebral hemisphere for most individuals, communication deficits can occur when damage involves the left side of the brain. Individuals with right cerebral damage often have language function left intact.

### Cognitive Consequences

Brain damage can alter a variety of cognitive skills:

- Memory
- Attention and concentration
- Self-awareness
- Problem solving and decision making
- Information processing and concept formation
- Judgment

### Memory

Memory encompasses the ability to store and retrieve information. Memory problems affect the individual's ability to recognize and recall people, places, facts, and concepts as well as to problem-solve, form goals, organize, and plan. Memory for both new and old information may be affected.

Several types of memory exist:

1. Immediate memory lasts only seconds or minutes unless converted into short-term memory. An example of immediate memory is remembering a phone number long enough to dial the number, but then not committing it to memory for later use.

2. Short-term memory lasts from minutes to hours, but it is then lost if not converted to long-term memory. An example of short-term memory may be learning facts for a test but not committing the facts to long-term memory for continued use.

3. Long-term memory is memories that are stored and are able to be retrieved in the future, whether after weeks or years.

A variety of memory problems may be experienced after brain damage. Some individuals may be able to remember facts but are unable to remember how to do specific tasks. For instance, an individual may be able to remember the names and birthdates of family members but be unable to remember how to operate a washing machine. Some individuals experience *retrograde amnesia* in which they are unable to remember things that occurred prior to the time of brain damage. Individuals with *remote memory impairments* may have forgotten their own personal history so they do not recognize family members, or they may not be able to remember what type of work they had been engaged in prior to brain damage.

After brain damage individuals can have difficulty remembering or learning new information so that they are unable to acquire new memories or recall recent conversations and events. In some instances individuals make up answers to questions, or make up situations or events (**confabulation**). This results not from faulty memory but from the tendency to juxtapose unrelated memories together. At other times, in conversation, individuals may get stuck on one theme, repeating a question, phrase, or concept again and again (**perseveration**). Perseveration can also pertain to tasks that the individual repeats over and over, such as continuing to wipe the same spot on a counter until someone intervenes.

Individuals with brain damage may be unable to remember skills that were once very familiar. For instance, they may be unable to complete simple daily tasks, such as dressing, because they are unable to remember the steps involved or because, after completing the first steps of the task, they forget their original goal.

Memory problems can be the most limiting of all of the potential cognitive consequences of brain damage because they affect the individual's ability to learn, store, and retrieve information. The ability to profit from experience is often limited as well. Consequently, individuals may continue to make the same mistakes over and over, since the ability to apply what was learned from past experience is usually diminished. The ability to generalize from one situation to another may also be impaired. Therefore, what is learned in one setting may not be able to be transferred to another. For example, an individual who has learned a skill in a rehabilitation setting may be unable to perform that skill in his or her own home.

### Attention and Concentration

After brain damage individuals may find it difficult to focus attention and to concentrate on a specific activity. Consequently, they may be unable to follow a train of thought or perform multiple step instructions. They may have difficulty focusing on one task, may be easily distracted, or may be unable to "shift gears" from one task to another. Individuals with brain damage may find it difficult to perform multiple tasks at one time, such as writing down messages or notes while talking on the phone, or carrying on a conversation while polishing furniture.

*Self-Awareness*

Individuals with brain damage may have limited ability to recognize or understand the limitations they are experiencing. They may lack insight into the appropriateness of their behavior and may be unaware of the impact certain aspects of their behavior have on people, remaining oblivious to subtle reactions or emotional cues from others. Because they may be unaware of their deficits, they may be unable to assess the extent of their disability and may therefore set unrealistic goals. There may also be an inability to monitor and adjust their own actions according to feedback from others. When they do receive feedback, they may discount it because they disagree with others' observations regarding their behavior or performance.

*Problem Solving and Decision Making*

Planning and organizing and therefore problem solving may be difficult after brain damage. Sequencing tasks may be problematic. For example, when preparing a meal, individuals may not recognize that food items that take more time to cook should be prepared first. Consequently, they may fully prepare the mashed potatoes before even starting to make the meatloaf. In other instances individuals may have difficulty following steps in order. For instance, when dressing they may put on their slacks before they put on underwear or put their socks on over their shoes.

There may be the inability to recognize problems as they occur, and if a problem is identified, the inability to generate alternative solutions or to select a solution when one is presented. Individuals may consider only immediate information rather than looking at the situation as a whole. For example, if they want to visit a friend in another city, they may recognize that they can take a train to get there, but they may not be able to consider how they would obtain money for the train fare, how they would obtain a ticket, or how they would get to the train station. Because individuals with brain damage sometimes have difficulty thinking or planning for the future, reasoning and decision making may be more difficult. For instance, they may see no need to go to the grocery store for supplies if they are not currently hungry.

There may also be lack of ability to initiate and sustain activity. Performance can become inconsistent, so that tasks performed well on one day may not be performed well on subsequent days. Individuals with damage to the left side of the brain may find problem solving especially difficult. When presented with a new problem, they may respond slowly and in a cautious, disorganized fashion. In most instances, it is helpful to divide tasks into smaller steps to avoid confusion. Individuals may need frequent feedback throughout even simple tasks such as dressing to be assured that the task is being performed correctly.

*Information Processing*

Even when hearing and vision are unimpaired, more time may be needed to synthesize verbal or visual input. There may be delayed response to visual and/or verbal stimuli, so that individuals may find it difficult to maintain pace in a social setting. In some instances comprehension of input itself may be severely disrupted. Information-processing information may be disrupted not only in terms of speed, but also in the ability to sequence and categorize information, so that there is difficulty understanding concepts. As a result, abstraction may be difficult, and individuals may tend to think only in concrete terms and cues and stimuli may be taken literally. For instance, in money exchange, the phrase "Do you have anything smaller?" may be taken quite literally by individuals with brain damage because they are unable to distinguish between "smaller" as referring to denomination and "smaller" as referring to size.

### Judgment

Judgment may be impaired because of loss of ability to learn from experience, problem-solve, self-monitor, or interpret cues from other individuals or the environment. Individuals may demonstrate a rigidity of response that precludes alternative responses. For instance, because of the inability to recognize the need to adjust plans or to plan alternative activities, an individual who had planned to go swimming may proceed with his or her plans, even though the weather has become cold and rainy. Lack of judgment can also cause individuals to endanger themselves or others when they attempt to perform tasks or engage in situations for which they have limited skills. They may behave impulsively and act quickly without thinking or without anticipating the consequences of their behavior.

### Personality Change and Affective Response

The psychosocial effects of brain damage pose not only serious limitations for individuals but can also be the most difficult challenge for family and friends to face. Potential psychosocial effects can consist of the following:

- Personality changes
- Anger or irritability
- Nonconformance to social norms
- Apathy and depression
- Loss of self-esteem

### Personality Changes

Personality changes associated with brain damage may be slight or extreme, but they can be severely disabling. Individuals who were very meticulous and precise prior to brain damage may become careless and sloppy post damage. Individuals who were once jovial and outgoing may, after brain damage, become quiet and withdrawn. Such behavior may at first be misinterpreted by others as laziness, disinterest, or uncooperativeness rather than as a symptom of the condition itself. In other instances individuals who, prior to damage, had been calm and tolerant may, post damage, be emotionally explosive, demonstrating outbursts of anger or episodes of severe anxiety. Social interactions are often affected by these personality changes, so that individuals are unable to maintain relationships. Once personality changes are recognized as symptoms associated with brain damage, compensatory behaviors can be learned to overcome them.

### Anger or Irritability

Aggressive behavior displayed after brain damage may be the result of frustration, but it can also be a direct physiologic consequence of damage to the brain itself. Aggression can be expressed actively or passively, verbally or physically. There may be decreased patience or overreaction to stresses in the environment, or individuals may be more sensitive to environmental stimuli and may become distracted or react to stimuli with irritation. Because individuals with brain damage may have low frustration tolerance, aggressive behaviors and emotional outbursts can be common. Individuals may have sudden mood swings, turning from happy to sad or complacent to volatile with little or no provocation.

### Nonconformance to Social Norms

Disinhibition can also be a consequence of brain damage, so that there are inadequate social skills to function effectively within the environment. As a result, individuals may make rude or embarrassing remarks to others, exhibit inappropriate sexual behavior in public, or make inappropriate sexual remarks. They may misinterpret gestures of others, such as a hug, as an indication that the individual desires a more passionate encounter. In some instances individuals with brain damage may have heightened sexual drive and become overdemanding sexually.

Substance abuse is frequently a contributor to accidents that result in TBI. If substance abuse or dependence was a problem prior to injury, it may also contribute to problems post injury. Because of the stress of adjusting to changes associated with brain damage, lack of self-awareness and insight, and inability to recognize cues from the environment, substance abuse may become problematic post injury. Since individuals with brain damage are more sensitive to the effects of alcohol or drugs, use often further impairs cognitive, psychomotor, and psychosocial skills, making it more difficult for them to integrate into the community or into the workplace. In addition, drugs and alcohol may interact with other prescribed medications, causing serious effects. Individuals with brain damage are also more prone to seizures. Alcohol and drugs can lower the seizure threshold, increasing the risk of seizures for these individuals. As individuals with brain damage achieve greater levels of independence, the likelihood of substance abuse increases. Assessment of alcohol and/or drug use should be ongoing throughout the rehabilitation process.

### Apathy and Depression

Depression is a natural reaction to the loss experienced with many disabilities, whether loss is related to cognitive, motor, sensory, social, or vocational functions. At times it may be difficult to discern the extent to which depression is the direct consequence of physiologic damage to the brain or a personal reaction to losses associated with the disability. As individuals become increasingly aware of losses, restrictions, and alterations in lifestyle, they may go through a grieving process that leads to depression. As a consequence, they may become increasingly withdrawn and have difficulty taking initiative to interact socially with others.

### Loss of Self-Esteem

After brain damage some individuals have no memory of what they were like prior to injury. Others may develop an increasing awareness of their disability or an awareness that they are unable to perform the tasks they performed previously. They may recognize the role changes they are experiencing and may sense that their status has changed within the family, social, and work setting. This loss of status may diminish their self-image, so that they become preoccupied with feelings of worthlessness and grief.

### Treatment and Management of Brain Damage

Comprehensive, individualized interdisciplinary treatment and rehabilitation provided by a diverse team of professionals are necessary to achieve both short-term goals and global outcomes. Interventions are directed at preventative, restorative, and compensatory strategies. The course of recovery and rehabilitation of individuals with brain damage is variable, but it is almost always lengthy, lasting from months to years. The rate of recovery may vary over time. Physicians involved in the care of individuals with brain damage usually include a primary physician such as an *internist* or *family physician*, as well as specialists such as a *neurologist, neurosurgeon,* and *physiatrist.* Other health professionals involved in the individual's care, treatment, and/or rehabilitation may include *nurses, respiratory therapists, physical therapists, dietitians or nutrition specialists, speech/language pathologists, audiologists, pharmacists, occupational therapists, recreational therapists, clinical or counseling psychologists, neuropsychologists, cognitive retrainers, social workers,* and *rehabilitation counselors.*

### Initial Treatment

The initial treatment for individuals experiencing brain damage, whether from traumatic or atraumatic causes, is intended to stabilize the condition and enhance the recovery process by preventing complications from occurring. Damage to the brain can cause increased muscle tone, paralysis, or weakness. If these changes are left untreated, permanent deformities such as **contractures** (deformity and immobility of a joint due to permanent contraction of a muscle) can occur, which could interfere with the individual's future function. Because individuals are kept immobile in the initial stages after brain damage, they are also susceptible to other complications, such as pneumonia, pressure sores, urinary tract infection, and blood clots. Should these complications

arise, potential for recovery could be compromised. Consequently, in the initial stages of treatment special attention is given to maintaining nutritional status and preventing complications from occurring.

Along with traumatic brain damage, there is often damage to at least one other major organ system. These injuries may include spinal cord injury, musculoskeletal injury, or injury to internal organs. Treatment of any complicating associated injury is necessary to prevent deterioration, which could jeopardize recovery, rehabilitation, and in some instances survival. In the case of atraumatic damage, direct treatment of any underlying conditions (such as hypertension, infection in the case of meningitis, or diabetes in the case of stroke) is also important to stabilize the condition and prevent further damage from occurring.

*Neurosurgical procedures* are sometimes indicated in the immediate treatment phase of brain damage. Careful observation is essential to detect early signs of increased intracranial pressure due to swelling of the brain or intracranial bleeding, which, unless relieved, could cause additional damage or death. Treatment of increased intracranial pressure can be surgical or nonsurgical. Surgical intervention may involve placing a shunt that allows excess CSF to drain into the general body circulation. If individuals with traumatic brain damage have an open skull fracture, surgery may be necessary to remove fragments of bone or other foreign materials and to repair the skull. If increased intracranial pressure is caused by a blood clot (e.g., a subdural or epidural hematoma) or hemorrhage, two small holes may be placed into the skull (*burr holes*) and the blood clot removed or the bleeding controlled. In some instances individuals may undergo a **craniotomy**, a surgical procedure in which the skull is surgically opened and the clot or foreign object removed or bleeding controlled through the surgical incision. Nonsurgical interventions for increased intracranial pressure consist of giving medications to remove fluid and to decrease swelling of the brain or prevent further clot formation. If individuals have an aneurysm or malformed arteries or veins, surgery to remove the aneurysm or correct the malformation may be performed.

### Postacute Treatment and Rehabilitation

After the condition has stabilized, appropriate postacute treatment requires early and active intervention by the interdisciplinary team. In the early treatment phases after brain damage, *physical therapy* may focus on activities to prevent joint and muscular complications. *Physical therapists* work with individuals early after the initial phase of brain damage to provide range-of-motion exercise to extremities, thus preventing deformity, as well as later in the recovery period to assist with ambulation. Later, physical therapy may be directed toward helping individuals improve balance, muscle control, and ambulation as well as other physical movements. Individuals who experience **hemiplegia** (paralysis on one side of the body) may need special instruction in ambulation techniques (*gait training*). Depending on the extent of permanent damage to the brain, individuals may use assistive devices to perform a variety of functions and activities. Braces or splints may be necessary to help them increase functional capacity and become independent. Individuals with paralysis of an arm may be taught to use special tools such as a plate guard to keep food from sliding off the plate, or special eating utensils or other tools designed to help in daily living activities. If there is paralysis of

an upper extremity, the weight of the paralyzed arm can cause separation of the arm from the shoulder joint (**subluxation**). To prevent this from occurring, individuals with this condition may wear a sling to support the arm.

Individuals with brain damage may need assistance to increase their awareness or orientation to time, place, and persons. *Occupational therapy* can help individuals with brain damage integrate available sensory information so that they can use it as a basis for motor activity and increase their ability to perform the activities of daily living. For example, helping them learn skills and use assistive devices for such daily activities as maintaining personal hygiene, dressing, and eating may be a focus of therapy.

*Speech and language therapies* may focus on the mechanical difficulties of speech, the formation and execution of language, or the development of alternative communication systems. *Speech and language therapists* may help individuals with both verbal and nonverbal communication. They may focus on speech or language acquisition or on conversational skills training. The *speech therapist* can also help individuals with brain damage develop social skills that relate to communication, such as techniques to structure the environment so that communication effectiveness is maximized. In some instances, alternative methods of communication, such as writing or using a picture board, may be used. If individuals have impaired swallowing capabilities, *speech pathologists* may also be involved in helping them learn how to swallow again. In some instances, speech pathologists may also be involved in cognitive remediation.

*Clinical or counseling psychologists* may conduct psychotherapy or counseling with the individual with brain damage and/or family members in order to facilitate the adjustment process. *Neuropsychologists* may be involved in neurological assessment. Some neuropsychologists may also be involved in cognitive retraining or remediation, helping individuals with brain damage learn ways to compensate for areas of lost cognitive function.

Often cognitive changes, rather than physical changes, hamper effective daily functioning. In these instances, *cognitive remediation* strategies designed to ameliorate sensory/perceptual, language-related, and problem-solving deficits may be a major focus of the rehabilitation effort. The goal of therapy is to return individuals with brain injury to as much independent functioning as possible in as many areas as possible. Cognitive strengths and weaknesses are identified through observation and *neuropsychological assessment*. How cognitive abilities and limitations in areas such as memory, organizational ability, reasoning, or judgment affect individuals' ability to function in the environment is evaluated, and cognitive strategies are devised to help them compensate for their condition or improve it. Individuals are then helped to transfer these strategies from the clinical setting to their own environment. In some instances, depending on the individuals' life circumstances and the extent of the brain damage, long-term supportive care may be needed.

Most individuals who have experienced brain damage should abstain from alcohol or drugs that have not been medically prescribed. The use of alcohol and other substances can increase the potential for seizures after brain damage. In addition, the combination of alcohol or drugs when taken with prescribed medications can have dangerous effects. Furthermore, alcohol and other substances may accentuate any existing residual from brain damage, increasing the chances of additional accident or injury as well as preventing individuals from functioning to their maximal capacity.

Several approaches are utilized for individuals with brain damage after they are medically stable, including *home-based programs*, *outpatient rehabilitation programs*, *community reentry programs*, *day treatment*, *residential community reentry or transitional living programs*, or *neurobehavioral programs*. These programs offer individuals therapies designed to improve functioning or to help them develop social skills, or they may provide care and supervision for individuals who require some assistance in meeting basic needs, as in a *supported living program* or *independent living center*.

## Functional Implications of Brain Damage

### Psychological Issues in Brain Damage

The emotional reactions experienced by individuals after brain damage can range from depression to mood swings or psychosis (Busch & Alpern, 1998). Although the extent of personality change or other psychological symptoms varies from individual to individual, it is safe to assume that whether damage is mild or severe, some psychological symptoms will be experienced. Symptoms may differ at different phases of recovery. Those in the early stages of recovery may deny the extent of their limitations. Later they may experience feelings of frustration because of difficulty with memory or because they are unable to perform tasks they were once able to perform. Later feelings of anger, grief, anxiety, or helplessness may occur, or there may be feelings of worthlessness or guilt.

Because of the damage sustained, some individuals are no longer able to comprehend the world around them or respond to it in the same way they did before. They may show loss of emotional control in the form of emotional lability, suddenly switching from laughing to crying or crying to laughing when there is no apparent cause. At times emotional lability is expressed as prolonged crying that, rather than being caused by depression or sadness, is instead a direct result of damage to the brain. If emotional lability exists, the family may need support and guidance in dealing with the individual's outbursts. The emotional reaction can often be diverted if the individual's attention can be directed to another activity.

Individuals may demonstrate impulsivity with regard to money, sex, drugs, or interactions with others. In some instances there may be outbursts of verbal or physical aggression. They may lose sensitivity to the impact of their behavior on others. In instances in which individuals are aware of their behavior, they may become self-conscious and anxious, avoiding contact with others, or they may become overcautious and hypervigilant.

Personality traits that were present prior to brain damage may become exaggerated after the damage has occurred, or there may be dramatic personality change, so that an individual who was quiet and passive prior to brain damage may become boisterous and aggressive after his or her injury. A person who was once self-directed and took initiative may become apathetic and unable to complete tasks independently.

Counseling and/or psychotherapy is an important part of total rehabilitation in most disabling conditions, and it can be used to treat depression, reduce denial, increase self-esteem, or help individuals form realistic goals. However, the work may be challenging if the individual has lost the capacity for insight or is unable to participate in abstract reasoning. Counseling may be directed toward providing emotional support for both individuals and their family and toward helping all involved adjust and relate to each other in the context of the changes brought about by brain damage.

In the case of TBI, substance abuse is often a contributor to the original accident that caused the injury. After the injury has occurred, individuals may continue in the same pattern of substance abuse behavior they were involved with prior to the injury. Consequently, substance abuse evaluation should be conducted routinely and treatment instituted as needed. Substance abuse may also be a maladaptive means of coping with the stress and depression individuals experience following brain damage. In either case, the effects of alcohol or other drugs further impair individuals' functioning ability and also have the potential to interact with other medications an individual may be taking. In addition, substance abuse may precipitate a seizure, which the individual is already more prone to experience. Abstinence is, therefore, the best policy for individuals with TBI. Some individuals may believe that substance use has been a significant part of their social relationships. In these instances, they may need to learn other circumstances under which to engage in social activity and should be encouraged to participate in social and recreational activities that do not involve alcohol or other drugs.

Role changes as a result of injury impact not only the individual but also on his or her family. Often because of changes in temperament, behavior, and personality, there is a disruption in family cohesion and feelings of entrapment by family members. Depending on the extent of role change, individuals may feel diminished social status, social isolation, and consequently loss of self-esteem. Often the physical ramifications and residuals of the injury are less troublesome for family and friends than the associated behavioral and personality changes caused by the brain damage. Personality changes may put a strain on family relationships.

### Social Issues in Brain Damage

After brain injury, social relationships are often drastically altered. No relationship is more significantly altered than that of the family. Brain damage dramatically and permanently impacts not only the individual experiencing it but also the whole family system. Severe brain damage produces prolonged stress in the family. Not only must the family cope with profound physical, cognitive, and emotional changes in the individual, but the stress of caregiving and the financial burden can be extreme. Because brain damage, whether traumatic or atraumatic, occurs suddenly, neither the family nor the individual has the opportunity to prepare for the emotional and economic impact. Normal family development is disrupted and any prior family stress exacerbated.

The family also has significant influence on how the individual reacts to the damage and its residual effects. Depending on the circumstances of the injury, family members may place blame on the individual or others, may be angry, or may express other negative emotions that can have a negative impact on the individual and his or her rehabilitation potential. Family members may misinterpret personality change or specific behaviors as deliberate or spiteful and coming from deepseated anger toward the family, or they may assume the individual could control behavior if he or she wanted to. Individual family members may feel trapped and may be resentful of the caregiving role they now assume, reminding the individual with brain damage of their dependence, or they may belittle the individual.

In other instances, glad to have the individual home again, the family may encourage or enforce dependence.

Family structure may be altered because the individual's condition may alter the roles and functions of other family members. In many cases, individuals who were once self-sufficient and living independently may, post injury, need support and care from a spouse or other family member. Depending on the severity of the brain damage, the personality and coping ability of the caregiver, and the previous relationship between the individual and the family, the situation can breed resentment and stress, which in turn can have a negative impact on rehabilitation potential. Even when the spouse or other family members willingly assume responsibility and do not consider their responsibility a burden, most still undergo tremendous emotional turmoil as they adjust to changes in the individual with brain damage. The primary caregiver may neglect his or her own physical and emotional needs, as well as the needs of other family members. In some instances the behavior of the individual with brain damage may make even simple social interactions embarrassing, so that the family eventually feel it is easier to stay within their home environment and they become increasingly socially isolated. Marital relationships can begin to deteriorate. Determining premorbid family function can be helpful in identifying problems and working toward solutions. If there was significant marital strain prior to brain damage, the stress after damage will only be increased.

Support, counseling, education about the nature of the disability and how to cope with the individual's behavior, and identification of support resources can be of considerable help in restoring family functioning. Members should be given the opportunity to work through their feelings and be assured that their feelings are natural. Emphasis should be placed on maintaining the well-being of self and others in the family unit as well as attending to the needs of the individual with brain damage. Overall, the individual and family should be assisted in attaining realistic expectations and directed to pursuing reasonable goals.

### Lifestyle Issues in Brain Damage

The complexity of brain damage is extensive and impacts general activities of daily living. The degree to which home modifications or assistance in independent living is needed will depend on the affected individual's physical, cognitive, and perceptual limitations. Although the goal of rehabilitation is to assist individuals to achieve as much independence in as many areas as possible, because of issues of problem solving, judgment, and impulse control with brain damage, safety can also be an issue.

The nature of the accommodations, modifications, and assistive devices used in the home depends on the physical limitations caused by brain damage. For example, if the individual experiences paralysis of an upper extremity, items kept in cabinets and cupboards should be moved for ease of reach, or special adaptive devices may be needed for eating or to assist in dressing. In the case of limitation in lower extremities, bathroom modifications such as a raised toilet seat, grab bars, and a bench in the shower or tub may be needed, or doorways may need to be modified to accommodate a wheelchair. In other instances, adaptive devices such as a leg brace may be needed.

The capability of individuals after brain damage to operate a motor vehicle is dependent not only on their physical ability but also on their cognitive and emotional limitations, which could harm not only the individual but also the general public. Driving is a complex task, requiring organizational ability, problem solving, decision-making ability, reflex actions, visual-motor skills, coordination, and physical manipulation. Limitation in any of these areas could affect individuals' ability to drive. If a seizure disorder is present, the problem is compounded. Thus a comprehensive assessment may be needed to evaluate the individual's capability to drive. Since the facilities and professionals qualified to provide this type of assessment may be limited except in urban areas, such an evaluation may not be available to all who need it (Handler & Boland Patterson, 1995).

Because in some instances eating behavior is also affected, eating habits, weight gain or loss, and nutrition may need to be monitored. In some cases, individuals may refuse to eat; in other instances there may be a constant urge to eat without feeling full. Specific strategies to ensure adequate nutrition and weight stabilization may need to be implemented. For instance, there may be a need to institute a regular schedule for individuals so that they take meals at the same time each day. If there are problems with eating or swallowing or if tube feedings are necessary, privacy should be provided.

Memory problems can interfere with individuals' ability to perform even small tasks of daily living. Encouraging individuals to keep a note pad of scheduled events, appointments, and important information can help them remember specific events. Strategically placing notes in the home or at work can help individuals remember specific tasks that may otherwise be overlooked, such as turning off the lights or closing the door.

Almost inevitably, brain damage will cause cognitive, psychological, and sometimes physical changes that in some way affect sexuality (Dombrowski, Petrick, & Strauss, 2000). Sensory-motor changes can cause erectile dysfunction in males, and motor changes can cause spasticity or ataxia that can affect sexual behavior. Cognitive changes that inhibit or regulate emotional responses can result in disinhibition, impaired judgment, or impaired impulse control, which also can affect sexual activity. Psychological factors such as depression or decreased self-esteem can decrease sex drive. The anxiety or emotional reactions of the individual's sexual partner may also adversely affect sexual function and drive.

A primary issue impacting sexual activity may be social isolation and limited social contacts. Individuals with brain damage may have lost friends and contacts, or they may not have had a sexual partner at the time of the injury. When opportunities to increase social interaction do occur, they may, in their desire to be accepted, be anxious to be accepted and thus become vulnerable and are taken advantage of. Individuals with brain damage who do not have a sexual partner may need to learn acceptable outlets through which they can express sexual needs.

Some individuals with brain damage may experience disinhibition, impairment in judgment, or inability to control sexual impulses. In these instances, they may engage in socially inappropriate behaviors, such as inappropriate sexual advances or responses, or masturbation in public. Individuals may need help in learning to interpret social and environmental cues and in learning more socially appropriate ways of expressing sexual need.

Individuals or family members may be reluctant to bring up sexual problems; in some instances the individual with brain damage may be unaware that a problem exists. Talking openly about sexuality and

assessing specific sexuality issues in the context of their specific values enables individuals to discuss specific concerns and to identify ways to adapt to changes in sexuality. In addition, identifying specific sexuality issues can lessen the effects of problem areas (Hibbard Buffington, 1996).

### Vocational Issues in Brain Damage

Return to work for individuals with brain damage involves many factors. Because of the wide variations in disability related to brain damage, no one model can be applied to all individuals. The changes that may occur present unique challenges. The degree to which individuals with brain damage are able to maintain employment depends on the extent of the damage and associated functional limitations as well as on their prior background, age at the time brain damage occurred, preinjury education, occupation, and work history (Keyser-Marcus et al., 2002; Kreutzer et al., 2003; Wagner, Hammond, Sasser, & Wiercisiewski, 2002). Personal motivation and support from family are also important factors in determining the individual's rehabilitation potential.

Factors that seem most related to the ability to return to work and to maintain employment after brain damage are the severity of the damage, age, and work history prior to brain damage (Felmingham, Baguley, & Crooks, 2001; Wagner, Hammond, Sasser, Wiercisiewski, & Norton, 2000). As the severity of brain damage increases, the rate of return to work decreases. Persons with greater disability have been shown to require more extended time and more extensive rehabilitation services before placement (Malec, Buffington, Moessner, & Degiorgio, 2000). Although the majority of individuals with mild brain damage may be able to return to work, individuals with moderate and severe brain damage have poorer outcomes (Fabiano & Daugherty, 1998). Even when job placement is accomplished, for individuals with moderate to severe disability, job retention may be difficult. The type of occupation they were in before the injury also appears to influence return to work outcome, with the highest rate of return to work being among persons with higher decision-making jobs (Orr, Walker, Marwitz, & Kreutzer, 2003). Age also appears to be a significant determinant of return to work. Generally, the older the individual is at the time of injury, the less likely he or she is to return to work (Rothweiler, Temkin, & Dikmen, 1998). Lastly, work history prior to brain damage appears to be related to ability to return to work post damage. Those individuals with poor work history prior to experiencing brain damage are more likely to have more problems returning to work after brain damage has occurred (Rubin & Roessler, 2001).

Cognitive deficits and psychosocial difficulties may have greater impact on return to work than physical limitations. Individuals who retain average to above-average intellectual abilities and interpersonal skills after brain damage occurs are often better able to compensate for other limitations and maintain or gain employment. For others, however, the levels of interpersonal functioning and cognitive self-awareness are often limited. Brain damage may result in drastic changes in personality and personal ability as well as in impaired self-awareness, which is also a frequent contributor to employment problems. Individuals who experience emotional lability may have more difficulty in the workplace and with coworkers.

Memory impairment may be a debilitating effect of brain damage. Individuals with memory problems may forget what they have learned and thus may not be able to benefit from experience. Helping them find alternative ways to perform tasks and to develop strategies to reduce, organize, and retrieve information can reduce the disabling effects of memory impairment. Since individuals may have difficulty organizing their day, implementing structured routines, using written notes or lists, or using audiotaped reminders may help improve performance. Usually notes or lists will be most effective if information is kept simple with no extraneous details. Too much information may cause the individual to become overwhelmed and confused.

Individuals with brain damage may not be aware of their deficits and may overestimate their abilities. Judgment may also be affected. Poor self-awareness or inaccurate self-perception can be a contributor to employment problems. Individuals may be unable to recognize job errors and may consistently rate their performance more highly than it is rated by their employer. Consequently, there may be limited benefit from feedback.

The ability to communicate verbally or in writing or to comprehend words and concepts influences all aspects of job selection, training, and performance. Special considerations need to be given to limitations in the ability to communicate. Visual-perceptual skills are integral to many jobs, both skilled and unskilled. The ability to perceive detail and to scan, match, or accurately perceive patterns may affect a number of daily life activities, including reading, driving, and navigating the environment.

Motor skills limitations affecting finger dexterity or eye-hand or eye-foot coordination may also be present. When these limitations exist, work involving precision or operation of various tools or equipment may be difficult. Individuals who have experienced paralysis of one of the upper extremities may be limited in their ability to lift, carry, or pull or push. If one of the lower extremities has been affected, they may require assistive devices, such as a cane, walker, braces, or in some instances a wheelchair. Consequently, ambulation may be restricted to short distances. Ambulation on uneven surfaces should be avoided; if a wheelchair is used, environmental modifications may be required. One should also consider that they perform tasks less quickly and have less physical stamina and endurance. Often individuals may be able to perform a task well if they are allowed to take their time, rather than feeling pressured to rush. Thus competitive environments in which speed is a priority may not be the best environments for individuals with brain damage and may actually decrease their quality of work.

Brain damage is not a progressive condition, and unless there is accompanying chronic illness that produces additional symptoms or that increases the chance of another stroke occurring, the individual's overall life expectancy is not affected. Brain damage is, however, a lifelong disability. Just as the rehabilitation needs of individuals vary, depending on the age at which the damage occurred, so will rehabilitation needs change over the individual's lifetime. Consequently, ongoing monitoring and contact with individuals may be necessary to help them maintain maximum potential in the workplace.

In some instances, supported employment or job coaching may be appropriate. In other instances, performance-based feedback or prompts may be sufficient to help the individual maintain employment. Returning to gainful employment represents a series of complex challenges because of the number, complexity, and interaction of problems, all of which may contribute to difficulty in maintaining long-term employment. Mon-

itoring performance as well as maintaining communication with the employer can contribute to job retention. Helping individuals learn compensatory strategies, providing appropriate workplace accommodations, and educating employers about the nature of brain damage and its consequences can greatly increase the chances of successful job placement.

## Cerebral Palsy

Damage to the brain before, during, or shortly following birth results in a condition known as **cerebral palsy**. Cerebral palsy is not a disease, but rather a complex of symptoms covering a wide number of functional impairments. It is characterized by chronic disorders of movement or posture. It may be accompanied by seizure disorders, sensory impairment, and cognitive limitation (Nelson, 2003). No two people with cerebral palsy are alike. Cerebral palsy is not progressive, communicable, or inherited. The condition is also not curable, since once damage to the brain is sustained, damage is permanent. However, different therapies and training programs can help individuals manage symptoms and increase their functional capacity. Consequently, therapies are designed to enhance individuals' abilities rather than to reverse the condition.

### Causes of Cerebral Palsy

The cause of cerebral palsy varies. It can be caused by:

- a birth injury in which the infant experiences direct damage to the brain, such as from ruptured blood vessels or compression of the brain
- exposure of the mother to toxic chemicals while pregnant or infectious disease experienced by her during pregnancy

- other causes, such as Rh or A-B-O blood type incompatibility between parents of the infant
- lack of oxygen to the brain of the fetus before birth or shortly after birth due to conditions such as umbilical cord strangulation, prolonged labor (which stresses the fetus), or premature separation of the placenta from the uterus

### Characteristics of Cerebral Palsy

The word *cerebral* refers to the brain. The word *palsy* refers to movement or posture. One characteristic of cerebral palsy is the inability to totally control and coordinate movement. The type of cerebral palsy and symptoms experienced depends on the location and extent of the damage to the brain. Some individuals have minor, barely detectable symptoms, while others have severe functional disability. Depending on the type of cerebral palsy, individuals may experience a number of symptoms affecting movement. One symptom may be **spasticity**, in which there is abnormality of muscle tone resulting in muscle stiffness and exaggerated muscle contraction. Spasticity interferes with dexterity and the ability to perform various muscle movements. Some individuals with cerebral palsy experience **ataxia** (disorder in the accuracy of muscle movement), which affects balance and coordination of gait. Still others have **dyskinesia** (unwanted, involuntary muscle movements), which interferes with the ability to conduct purposeful movements or causes movement when none is desired. Some individuals have a combination of spasticity, ataxia, and dyskinesia.

Abnormal movements may include purposeless, jerky, or abrupt movements (**athetosis**), especially of the upper extremities; or slow, continuous writhing movements (**choreoathetosis**). In rare instances, **atonia**, in which there is lack of muscle tone, and muscle flaccidity may be present.

Although cerebral palsy primarily affects muscle control, the brain is responsible for many other activities as well. Consequently, additional manifestations resulting from cerebral palsy may include visual or hearing impairments, perceptual disorders, seizures, communication difficulties, mental retardation, learning difficulties, or behavioral disorders, depending on the parts of the brain affected.

### Classification of Cerebral Palsy

Clinically, cerebral palsy is classified according to the type, location, and degree of movement manifestations and to the tone of muscles at rest. Clinical types of cerebral palsy based on classification of movement are as follows:

1. *Spastic cerebral palsy*, in which individuals experience high muscle tone (**hypertonia**) so that muscles and joints are tight and stiff, limiting movements in areas of the body that are affected. Individuals often experience an increase in hypertonia with activity and interference with residual motor function.
2. *Ataxic cerebral palsy*, in which individuals have difficulty with balance and coordination.
3. *Athetoid cerebral palsy*, in which individuals exhibit uncoordinated, jerky, or twisting movements in affected body parts, particularly in fingers and wrists.
4. *Mixed-type cerebral palsy*, in which individuals experience manifestations of more than one clinical type of cerebral palsy.

Cerebral palsy can also be classified according to the location of manifestations:

1. **Hemiplegia** indicates that manifestations are found on only one side of the body, such as an arm and a leg on the right side.
2. **Quadriplegia** indicates that manifestations affect all four extremities.
3. **Paraplegia** indicates that manifestations only affect the legs.
4. Other classifications, such as **monoplegia,** in which only one limb is involved, and **triplegia,** in which three limbs are involved, are rare.

Another way of classifying cerebral palsy is by degree:

1. *Mild cerebral palsy* describes manifestations that affect only fine motor movement.
2. *Moderate cerebral palsy* describes manifestations that affect general muscle movement, fine motor movement, and clarity of speech so that activities of daily living and communication may be affected but the individual is still able to function.
3. *Severe cerebral palsy* describes manifestations that significantly affect the ability to walk, use the hands, or to communicate so that ability to function in activities of daily living and/or communicate is extensively compromised.

Lastly, cerebral palsy may be classified according to muscle tone at rest:

1. **Isotonic**, in which muscle tone is normal
2. **Hypertonic**, in which there is increased muscle tone
3. **Hypotonic**, in which there is decreased muscle tone

### Management of Cerebral Palsy

Management of cerebral palsy is directed toward providing functional supports to individuals based on the specific symptoms exhibited so that functional capacity can be enhanced and additional disability prevented. Although cerebral palsy itself is not progressive, altered tone and/or activity of muscles may cause conditions that result in additional limitations and disability, such as **contractures** (loss of range of motion or fixation of a joint) or **scoliosis** (lateral curvature of the spine). Consequently, in addition to helping individuals reach their maximum functional capacity, management of cerebral palsy is also directed toward preventing conditions that could impede function.

All aspects of symptom management should be directed toward giving individuals the opportunity to control and manage their own situation as much as possible. Major goals of management often include maintaining joint range of motion to prevent contractures and other deformities, and increasing muscle control and coordination to help individuals counteract abnormal postures.

Interventions begin at an early age and include a number of services, depending on the specific needs and symptoms of the individual. *Physical therapy* may be instituted to increase and enhance motor skill and balance. *Occupational therapy* may be utilized to help individuals learn how to manage activities of daily living as well as other daily functions. *Orthotics* in the form of prescribed braces or splints may be used to help prevent or correct deformity. Braces can help individuals improve functional mobility as well as appearance. The type of brace depends on the type of disability experienced.

Medical interventions may also be involved in the management of cerebral palsy. In some instances medications may be prescribed to promote muscle relaxation when excessive muscle spasticity or excessive muscle tone is present. Anticonvulsant medications may be prescribed if individuals also have a seizure disorder associated with cerebral palsy. *Orthopedic surgery* may be needed to correct joint deformities or to lengthen muscles or tendons in order to decrease muscle spasm.

The best management of complications is through prevention. Contractures can be prevented through regular passive exercise or surgical intervention to lengthen the muscles that are contracted. Bowel and bladder incontinence can be managed through training programs that help individuals establish dietary control and a regular evacuation schedule, as well as programs to increase awareness of the sensory stimuli that indicate a need for evacuation. Individuals may decrease their dental problems through training in oral hygiene and regular dental care. A specific program of weight bearing and muscle activity as well as a diet adequate in calcium can help to prevent osteoporosis. Training that helps individuals increase posture control and the use of braces and splints can retard the development of degenerative joint disease and scoliosis. Training to help individuals develop improved breathing patterns, coughing, and lung expansion can decrease the chances of aspiration and consequently respiratory infection.

Adequate rest at night as well as establishment of rest periods throughout the day can decrease fatigue. Evaluating individuals' total energy output and adjusting their tasks and schedules to fit their needs can help preserve energy and prevent excessive fatigue.

### Complications of Cerebral Palsy

Because of the manifestations of cerebral palsy, a variety of complications that are secondary to the condition itself can alter the individual's functioning ability or well-being. Contractures can limit both passive and active joint movement and can interfere with self-care, walking, and sitting. Some individuals with cerebral palsy also experience bowel and bladder incontinence because of their inability to attend or respond to sensory stimulus indicating the need to urinate or defecate. Other individuals may experience dental problems that are exacerbated by their inability to brush their teeth adequately. Because of insufficient muscle activity, some individuals may be more prone to osteoporosis, which in turn can cause pain and increase susceptibility to fractures. Poorly aligned joints may predispose them to degenerative joint disease, resulting in pain and increased immobility. In some instances, if individuals have poorly supported sitting posture, **scoliosis** (lateral curvature of the spine) may occur, compromising breathing as well as the function of internal organs. If coughing and swallowing ability is insufficient, aspiration of food or fluids may place individuals at risk of respiratory infections or pneumonia.

Although not necessarily a complication, fatigue secondary to manifestations of cerebral palsy can also interfere with individuals' ability to function efficiently. Because they may experience difficulty with motor control and coordination, more energy may be expended to carry out even routine motor activities. Involuntary movement or spasticity may also increase the amount of energy expended. As a result, individuals with cerebral palsy may become fatigued more easily.

### Psychosocial Issues in Cerebral Palsy

Although data regarding the psychosocial adjustment of adults with cerebral palsy are limited, cerebral palsy as a developmental disability poses many of the same problems as other developmental disabilities. Misunderstanding of the condition by parents, teachers, or others with whom individuals with cerebral palsy come in contact can perpetuate a sick and dependency status rather than one of empowerment. How individuals with cerebral palsy were treated in childhood can influence their self-perception and functioning in adulthood. With any type of developmental disability there is the risk of overprotectiveness by parents and others, which can impede the individual's emotional development by restricting access to experiences that are vital to the development of adequate coping strategies. As a result, children may learn, at an early age, to use maladaptive behavior to achieve goals. If this behavior is continued into adulthood, it may impede the individual's ability to integrate effectively into the larger social milieu. When children have been kept overly dependent on parents, have been given little responsibility for home chores, have not been confronted with the typical consequences of behavior, or have not learned acceptable means of expressing emotions, lack of experience and mature social development can serve as a handicapping factor in adulthood.

In other instances, children who have often been the focus of a wide variety of services and activities from an early age may continue these expectations into adulthood, demonstrating a sense of egocentricity that may limit positive social interactions and lead to further social isolation. If these behaviors persist into adulthood, they may become more of an impediment to social integration than the manifestations of the condition itself. At times brain damage associated with cerebral palsy may also create behavior deficits that can interfere with the development and maintenance of social relationships.

For adolescents with cerebral palsy, opportunities to participate in social activities, information related to sexuality, and opportunities to participate in sexual exploration and relationships may have been limited. In addition, adolescents with cerebral palsy may have a distorted body image and a low self-concept, which can affect their social competence, dating, and sexual behavior. Although individuals with cerebral palsy, as adolescents as well as adults, experience normal desires, they may lack the skills necessary to fulfill those needs. In addition to barriers of inadequate information, skill, or opportunity for appropriate sexual expression, they may also experience physical barriers because of their disability that make sexual expression more difficult.

Communication issues for individuals with cerebral palsy can include hearing or auditory comprehension problems, visual disorders, or speech deficits. Individuals with communication problems as the result of cerebral palsy may have grown up in an environment in which family, friends, and others became accustomed to their adaptive communication methods. In adulthood, however, when relationships change and higher standards of performance are expected, communication may become increasingly difficult. For instance, those unfamiliar with the individual or with cerebral palsy itself may misinterpret problems with hearing or unintelligible speech as lack of cognitive ability. In other instances, because the individual may be difficult to understand, acquaintances may begin to avoid interactions with the individual who then becomes socially isolated. Depending on the severity and type of cerebral palsy, decreased mobility, problems with eating, or problems with personal hygiene may further restrict the individual's social interactions.

### Vocational Issues in Cerebral Palsy

Cerebral palsy is not a progressive condition, and there is no progressive deterioration as a direct result of the cerebral palsy itself. However, it is a lifelong condition. Consequently, follow-up throughout the individual's life may be necessary. As individuals age with their disability, additional limitations may develop. For instance, fatigue is a consideration for individuals with cerebral palsy, regardless of age. However, as individuals become older, endurance for the same activities once performed may be decreased.

Long-term goals are appropriate and desirable. The degree to which individuals are able to achieve their goals in a specified occupation will be dependent on their physical, psychosocial, and language abilities, as well as on their motivation and social support. Specific skills and abilities may be enhanced with compensatory measures and/or with practice. Since the functional limitations associated with cerebral palsy are individual, specific vocational limitations will be dependent on the symptoms each individual experiences. In some instances, verbal communication is severely impaired, and in other cases it may be totally unaffected. Some individuals may have limited mobility or ambulation problems; others may have significant difficulty with mobility or ambulation. Whereas some individuals will be ambulatory, others may require a wheelchair. In some instances individuals may have difficulty concentrating or remembering, and in other instances individuals' cognitive abilities are unaffected.

Since most jobs require some degree of social skill, when individuals have difficulty in this area, social skills training may be beneficial (Salkever, 2000). Matching the work setting to the individual's specific needs, interests, and abilities is important for anyone with a disability; however, in the case of cerebral palsy, attention to these factors may be even more important to increase the potential for vocational success.

## Epilepsy

Epilepsy is a chronic disorder of the nervous system. It is not a disease, but rather a symptom of an underlying neurological condition in which neurons in the brain create abnormal electrical discharges that cause **seizures** (temporary loss of control over certain body functions). There is no single cause of epilepsy, and it can affect anyone at any age. It can be caused by a number of conditions in which function of the brain has been affected, such as head injury or stroke. Sometimes, however, no clear-cut cause can be identified. In this case, epilepsy is considered as *idiopathic*.

Although the essential feature of epilepsy is recurrent seizures, not all seizures are due to epilepsy. Seizures can occur as a result of a temporary dysfunction of the brain brought on by certain conditions, even though there are no permanent changes in brain function. Acute conditions such as **meningitis** (infection of the covering of the central nervous system), diabetic coma, **hypoxia** (too little oxygen to the brain), and drug intoxication or withdrawal can all cause temporary disturbed brain function resulting in a seizure. If the underlying cause of brain dysfunction is reversible so that no permanent alteration of brain function exists and seizures do not recur, individuals are not considered to have epilepsy. The term *epilepsy* is reserved for individuals with recurring seizures and with a chronic abnormality of the brain that results in seizures.

### Classification of Seizures

Individuals with epilepsy can exhibit a variety of seizures with varying symptoms, ranging from muscle spasms or confusion to total loss of consciousness. Seizures can be mild or severe, can occur frequently or rarely, and can change their pattern of occurrence over time. Depending on the type, seizures usually last only seconds to minutes. Between seizures most individuals are able to function normally.

Seizures are classified according to the part of the brain that demonstrates abnormal electrical activity and the type of seizure experienced. Classification of seizures is important so that appropriate management and treatment can be determined.

Seizures are classified as *generalized*, in which nerve cells discharge abnormally throughout the brain, or *partial*, in which the abnormal nerve cell discharge is limited to one specific part of the brain (Browne & Holmes, 2001). Although there are many classifications of seizures related to epilepsy, common types of seizures are listed in Table 2–5. What follows is a brief description of common types of seizures.

### Generalized Tonic-Clonic Seizure (Grand Mal)

An abnormal discharge of nerve cells throughout the brain results in a *generalized tonic-clonic* seizure, sometimes called a grand mal seizure. Some individuals experience an **aura** (warning sign) immediately before the seizure begins. They may see a flash of light, have an unusual taste in the mouth, or have other unusual sensations. As the seizure develops, individuals lose consciousness and fall down, entering a *tonic* state in which there is generalized body rigidity. Muscles then enter a *clonic* state so that the whole body un-

dergoes rapid, jerky movements. The teeth are clenched tightly together and control of the bladder or the bowel may be lost. The seizure generally lasts less than a few minutes. When the seizure ends, consciousness is gradually regained, but individuals may experience confusion, difficulty in speaking, and headache. Although postseizure symptoms usually disappear within several hours, the fatigue experienced may be overwhelming, often necessitating an extended period of rest or sleep.

---

**Table 2–5** Common Types of Seizures Associated with Epilepsy

---

Generalized seizures
   1. Tonic-clonic (grand mal)
   2. Absence (petit mal)

Partial seizures
   1. Simple-partial (focal)
   2. Complex-partial (psychomotor)

---

Although a tonic-clonic seizure may be frightening to those who witness it, individuals experiencing the seizure are usually in no imminent danger unless there are hard, sharp, or hot hazards within the immediate environment. No attempt should be made to move individuals experiencing a seizure except when necessary to protect them from such hazards. To avoid injury, there should be no attempt to restrain individuals during a tonic-clonic seizure, to pry open clenched teeth, or to place hard objects in the individual's mouth. Individuals should be placed on their side during a seizure so that secretions can drain from the mouth and do not compromise the airway.

### Absence Seizure (Petit Mal)

Like tonic-clonic seizures, *absence seizures* are classified as generalized, because nerve cells discharge throughout the brain. Children most commonly experience this type of seizure. Absence seizures are characterized by brief blank spells or staring spells and a loss of awareness of the surroundings. The seizure generally lasts for only seconds. The individual does not fall, and there are usually no outward motor manifestations of absence seizures, although abnormal blinking or slight twitching may occur occasionally. Because of the limited visible symptoms of the seizure, those around the individual may misinterpret absence seizure as daydreaming or inattentiveness.

When children experience frequent absence seizures, school performance may be disrupted. Because there may be no significant signs that are easily observed during the seizure, the seizure disorder may not be diagnosed, and poor school performance may be attributed to other causes. Recognition of symptoms and appropriate diagnosis are crucial to enable children to achieve maximum school potential. Absence seizures may disappear spontaneously with age, although some individuals who have had absence seizures later go on to develop tonic-clonic seizures.

### Partial Seizures

When nerve cells discharge in an isolated part of the brain, partial seizures occur. One type of partial seizure is a *focal seizure*, in which there is no loss of consciousness and symptoms are very localized, depending on the part of the brain affected. One type of focal seizure, a *Jacksonian (simple-partial) seizure*, begins with convulsive symptoms in one part of the body, such as a hand or foot. The convulsive muscle movement then progresses in an orderly manner up the extremity. Jacksonian seizures can remain limited to one part of the body or can go on to develop into full-blown tonic-clonic seizures.

Other types of partial seizures may have more complex symptoms. *Complex-partial (psychomotor)* seizures are characterized by a loss of awareness of the surroundings. Individuals may pace, wander aimlessly, make purposeless movements, and utter unintelligible sounds. The seizure can last up to 20 minutes, with mental confusion lasting for a few minutes after the seizure is over. Observers may misinterpret symptoms of complex-partial seizures, often attributing the symptoms to alcohol, drug abuse, or mental illness.

### Status Epilepticus

*Status epilepticus* is a term used to describe seizures that are prolonged or that come in rapid succession without full recovery of consciousness between seizures. It is a medical emergency that can be life–threatening and consequently requires immediate medical attention and treatment (Lowenstein & Alldredge, 1998).

### Diagnosis of Epilepsy

Individuals who are having a seizure for the first time usually undergo medical evaluation by a *neurologist* to determine whether the seizure is a symptom of an acute medical or neurological illness that can be treated and resolved or a symptom of a chronic neurological problem that will require ongoing treatment for control. Extensive physical examination and blood tests are usually part of initial screening, as well as a detailed history of the precipitating factors that appeared to trigger the seizure.

When individuals have more than one seizure, or when other symptoms or history indicate that epilepsy may be the cause of seizure activity, a more extensive medical evaluation is conducted. A primary diagnostic tool for evaluating individuals after seizures is *electroencephalography* (EEG), a noninvasive procedure in which the electrical activity of the brain is recorded on a graph. *Magnetic resonance imaging* (MRI), a noninvasive procedure in which rapid detailed pictures of body structures are produced, may also be used to identify structural anomalies in the brain that may be related to seizures.

### Treatment and Management of Epilepsy

Treatment of epilepsy is dependent on the cause of the seizure activity and the types of seizures experienced. Generally individuals who have had only a single seizure are not considered to have epilepsy. Although they may be thoroughly evaluated in an attempt to determine the cause of the seizure, they usually are only monitored and not given medication (Willmore, 1998). If the seizures are caused by a tumor, scar tissue, or another abnormality that can be corrected, surgical intervention to remove or repair the abnormality may be indicated. In most instances, however, when epilepsy is diagnosed, the standard treatment of most types of seizures is the regular use of one or more *anticonvulsant* or *antiepileptic* medications.

Although medications do not cure epilepsy, they can effectively control seizures and enable many individuals to carry on full and productive lives. Successful control of seizures, however, requires the individual's strict, long-term compliance with medication instructions. The anticonvulsant medications used to treat epilepsy are also not without side effects, and toxic effects are common during long-term treatment. Depending on the medication, side effects can include gum overgrowth,

nausea, dizziness, clumsiness, visual difficulty, or fatigue.

Once medication for treatment of seizures has begun, it is generally maintained for at least two years, regardless of whether the individual has remained seizure free (Browne & Holmes, 2001). If there have been no recurrent seizures after this time, the physician may consider withdrawing the medication. Individuals who have had no additional seizures after beginning the medication, or who have experienced side effects, may be tempted to alter or discontinue their medication. The consequences could be dangerous and at times life-threatening. Consequently, individuals should never attempt to alter or discontinue their medication without consulting their physician.

The medication prescribed is based on the type of seizure and on whether more than one type of seizure is experienced. The general goal of treatment with medication is to maximize control of seizures without causing toxic side effects, such as liver damage or bone marrow suppression. The physician periodically monitors levels of the medication in the blood. Based on medication blood level and its effectiveness in controlling seizure activity, the physician may alter medication dosages accordingly. Measuring the blood levels of the anticonvulsant also helps the physician monitor individuals' compliance with the medication regime as well as identify any toxic effects.

In some cases, even when individuals are compliant with taking anticonvulsant medications, seizures remain uncontrolled. Many of these individuals experience several seizures a month or, at times, several seizures a day, despite following a strict treatment regimen of medication. When seizures are severely disabling and cannot be controlled by medication, surgery may be recommended to treat epilepsy. Under these circumstances, surgery may involve removing a portion of the brain structure, resecting a portion of the brain, or disconnecting the affected portion from the rest of the brain. Surgery itself may leave residual effects. The amount of disability experienced, if any, after this type of surgery depends on individual circumstances. Anticonvulsant medications may still be needed even after surgery.

Alcohol can lower the seizure threshold and therefore precipitate seizures. Alcohol and antiepileptic medications may also interact and cause untoward effects. Consequently, individuals with epilepsy should consult their physician about alcohol use.

Individuals with epilepsy should be helped to identify factors that may trigger a seizure. They should also avoid activity that would be hazardous if a seizure should occur, such as swimming alone or operating heavy equipment. A medical identification bracelet should be worn by individuals with epilepsy at all times.

The general prognosis for individuals with epilepsy depends on the type of seizure, the underlying cause, the administration of appropriate treatment, and the individual's willingness and ability to follow the prescribed treatment regimen. If their condition is accurately diagnosed and appropriately treated, most individuals with epilepsy can live active, productive lives. Prompt detection and early medical intervention can greatly improve the ability to control seizures and enhance the general quality of life for the individual with epilepsy.

### Psychosocial Issues in Epilepsy

Individuals with epilepsy may face many psychological and psychosocial challenges. They must learn to deal with the uncertainty of whether and when another seizure will occur. No matter how well controlled seizures are, individuals live with the possibility, even if remote, that another seizure will occur. The time, place, and social circumstances under which a seizure may occur are unknown. If individuals experience a seizure in public, they risk feelings of embarrassment and onlookers' potential misperception of the seizure. Individuals may feel they have no control over their lives and behavior. At times, even when seizures are adequately controlled, anxiety over the possibility of having a seizure or other psychosocial dysfunction may be the most disabling factor associated with the condition. As a result, individuals may have difficulty establishing interpersonal relationships, building self-esteem, and obtaining or maintaining employment.

The family is crucial in the adjustment of individuals with any disability. Adjustment and emotional development depend on when the diagnosis of epilepsy is made and the reaction of the individual's family to it. When epilepsy is diagnosed in childhood, parental feelings of fear, anxiety, guilt, overprotectiveness, or mourning can affect not only the child's ability to accept his or her disability but also his or her self-concept and social adjustment. Overly protective parents may foster dependency in their child. Children may learn to use their condition as an excuse for inactivity or avoidance of responsibility. When they are teenagers, concerns related to whether they will drive a car, participate in sports, or engage in dating may cause additional stress and lessening of self-esteem.

Diagnosis of epilepsy in adulthood can also disrupt interpersonal and family relationships. The impact on individuals' social identity may be threatened, so that they go to great lengths to conceal their disability in order to avoid potential rejection. Partners of individuals with epilepsy may be fearful of observing a seizure or may be concerned that the disorder is hereditary. Because of anxiety and misinformation, they may be unwilling to learn more about the condition or to provide the support that the individual with epilepsy needs.

Sexual activity, in most cases, need not be affected by epilepsy (Frazer & Gumnit, 1990). Although some medications used to treat seizures may have some effect on libido, most do not. Psychological issues of low self-esteem or poorly developed social skills may produce greater limitations. Individuals may be reluctant to form intimate relationships because of the fear of having a seizure. Counseling may be necessary to help them overcome this fear so that appropriate intimate relationships can be established.

Between seizures, epilepsy is an invisible disability. Unless individuals are having a seizure, there are no outward signs of disability. Although considerable effort has been devoted to educate the public about the condition, misinformation and lack of acceptance still exist, and epilepsy continues to carry a stigma for many individuals. In some cultures, historical misconceptions about epilepsy have linked it to demonic possession and insanity. In other instances people with epilepsy were not permitted to participate in various events because of their diagnosis. Attitudes have changed in recent years as the result of public education programs, improved placement of individuals with epilepsy into the world of work, and increased ability to control seizures. In many instances, however, individuals with epilepsy may still experience unjust restrictions that deny them access to participation in routine activities. The stigma and shame associated with epilepsy may cause individuals and/or their family to deny or minimize the condition. Individuals may try to pass as someone without a disability because of anticipated rejection due to real or perceived public attitudes.

Operating a motor vehicle has a direct impact on independence and social well-being. Inability to drive can limit social interaction, educational experiences, and employment opportunities. In most instances, individuals with epilepsy can drive without significant risk of accident if their seizures are controlled with medication.

In the past, individuals with epilepsy were restricted from driving motor vehicles because of concerns for public safety as well as personal safety. Although today most states permit individuals with epilepsy to obtain driver's licenses, the length of time they must be seizure free in order to obtain the license varies from state to state. State laws do not always take into account individual differences; some make blanket rules that apply to all individuals with epilepsy regardless of their personal circumstances.

Alcohol consumption is frequently an activity at social occasions. Individuals with epilepsy should always consult their physician about alcohol consumption, especially in regard to taking alcohol when they are also taking anticonvulsant medication; however, each individual situation must be considered.

Sports activities are also an important means of socializing as well as helping individuals build self-confidence and self-esteem. In some situations, restrictions on participation in various activities are placed on individuals with epilepsy even though no basis for limiting the activities exists. Although some individuals' seizures may be precipitated by fatigue or other sports-related circumstances, others may have a reduced incidence of seizures with exercise. Consequently, authorities should consider the individual's specific circumstances rather than issuing blanket restrictions; each case should be considered individually. Restrictions may be necessary for specific activities that present a hazard should a seizure that involves loss of consciousness take place. For instance, individuals with epilepsy should not swim alone. Activities such as flying an airplane, rock climbing, or other activities in which a seizure could cause severe and possibly fatal consequences should also be avoided. In most instances applying common sense enables individuals to participate in activities while also avoiding potential hazards.

Even when seizures are relatively well controlled, individuals may still fear having the "occasional" seizure and the physical and social consequences it may bring. In addition to the embarrassment of having a seizure in public, individuals may also fear injury. Injury during a seizure while performing routine tasks, such as setting clothes on fire from gas stoves or falling in the bathtub, can occur. Consequently, individuals may need help in establishing commonsense safety precautions for activities of daily living. Family, friends, and coworkers should also be informed about appropriate procedures if a seizure occurs.

Despite control of seizures, individuals may still feel the weight of their restrictions on the freedoms, activities, and events that others take for granted. For instance, in most states individuals are required to report that they have epilepsy when applying for a driver's license. They may be required to obtain a written statement from the physician to verify that they can return to regular activities after a seizure occurs. If flickering lights precipitate seizures, they may need to avoid certain theaters, bars, or other places that use strobe lights for decoration or effect. Taking medication regularly as prescribed, obtaining proper rest, and

reducing stress are other self-management issues individuals with epilepsy must consider. The stress, uncertainty, restrictions, isolation, and difficulty with employment all require adjustment and coping skills if individuals are to achieve their full potential.

### Vocational Issues in Epilepsy

Most individuals with epilepsy have the same range of IQ as the general population, unless other conditions that affect intellectual function are involved. However, individuals with epilepsy experience both unemployment and underemployment (Bishop, 2004; Fisher, 2000). Many problems in the workplace for individuals with epilepsy continue to be related to misperceptions and stigma rather than physical limitations. Although some individuals with epilepsy, especially epilepsy associated with head trauma, may have neuropsychological limitations that can affect employment, many do not. Consequently, special consideration must be given to each individual situation.

Epilepsy is a chronic condition that requires a continuous relationship with the medical community. Medication is, of course, a major part of treatment and requires close medical supervision. Multiple medications may be needed to control seizures, and the medications themselves may have associated side effects. Individuals must be diligent in taking medication because missed doses may precipitate a seizure. When individuals are in denial of their condition, their denial may be manifest as poor compliance with medication, which in turn causes poor seizure control and may consequently affect employment potential.

Because of the chance of an unpredictable loss of consciousness that may place individuals with epilepsy or others at risk of injury, some occupations, such as airplane pilot or interstate truck driver, may be unrealistic for the individual to pursue. Understanding how seizures affect job function is critical. It is important to assess the type and number of seizures individuals have, the degree to which seizures are controlled with medication, and how compliant individuals are in following the treatment regimen. Determining the situational patterns to seizures (such as a regular time when seizures occur) or the factors that precipitate seizures (such as fatigue, stress, or flickering lights) is important to help individuals avoid or alter situations in which seizures may occur. If fatigue tends to precipitate a seizure, care should be taken so the individual does not become overly fatigued. Likewise, if seizures are related to the individual's sleep pattern, he or she may be unable to work on a rotating shift. It is also helpful to know if individuals experience an aura and if they consequently would be able to remove themselves from dangerous situations before the seizure begins. Finally, individuals who experience seizures should probably not work alone in an isolated environment, especially if the environment imposes some threat of danger if a seizure should occur.

Employers who fear risk of lawsuits arising from workplace injuries may be overly conservative with restrictions for employees with epilepsy. However, many jobs once thought to be inappropriate for individuals with epilepsy may not be contraindicated if proper safety equipment is used. In addition, many states have specific regulations protecting employers from excessive liability if injury occurs even though adequate safety precautions were maintained. Work potential can be maximized with continued education of employers, adequate safety precautions, and consideration of individual needs.

## DIAGNOSTIC PROCEDURES USED FOR CONDITIONS OF THE NERVOUS SYSTEM

### Skull Roentgenography (X-ray)

*Roentgenograms (radiographic studies* or *X-rays)* of the skull provide visualization of the bones making up the skull as well as structures such as the sinuses. They are helpful in identifying fractures or other abnormalities of surrounding structures. X-ray films are usually taken by a *radiology technician.* The films are then read and interpreted by a **radiologist** (physician who specializes in radiology).

### Computed Tomography (CT Scan, CAT Scan)

A noninvasive radiographic technique called *computed tomography* is a test that applies computer technology and digital imaging techniques to X-ray studies to produce images of cross-sections of the body. Unlike conventional roentgenography, CT shows one "slice" of the structure being studied at a time, in sequence. On regular X-ray films, bone (e.g., the skull) can block the view of parts lying behind it (e.g., the brain). CT scans show both the bone and the underlying tissue and are able to detect abnormalities that could not be visualized on plain X-rays.

A scan of the head by CT can detect tumors and blood clots inside the brain. It can also reveal an enlargement of the ventricles of the brain due to inadequate drainage of CSF (**hydrocephalus**), as well as other types of abnormalities in the brain and skull. It can also be used to identify tumors or other sources of pressure on the spinal cord.

Individuals who are undergoing a scan by CT are placed within a large cylinder that contains an X-ray tube and a receptor. Usually a special substance (*contrast medium*) is administered to the individual intravenously to highlight certain structures and make the results more readable. The tube is rotated around the individual. X-rays are sent from the tube to the receptor, which measures the amount of radiation that each body tissue or organ absorbs during each rotation. A computer converts this information to a visual image on a screen. Images are monitored on a video screen and later photographed for more careful study by the *radiologist*, a physician who has been specially trained in the field of radiology and who reads and interprets results from radiological testing.

## Magnetic Resonance Imaging (MRI)

*Magnetic resonance imaging* (MRI) is a noninvasive procedure that may be used to obtain detailed information about body organs, especially soft tissue. It is used in disorders of the brain to diagnose or evaluate conditions such as brain tumors, aneurysms or malformations of blood vessels, strokes, multiple sclerosis, hydrocephalus, or abscesses. It may also be useful in determining the extent of TBI. In spinal cord injury, MRI may be used in conjunction with regular X-ray films, *myelograms*, and scans obtained by CT to identify spinal cord compression, swelling, or bleeding. In addition, MRI is very sensitive in detecting conditions such as herniated disk or other destructive conditions of the spine.

During the test individuals are placed in a narrow cylinder. When in the cylinder, a strong magnetic field of radio waves causes biological substances in the body (*protons*) to change their alignment and become aligned in a certain direction. When the radio waves are discontinued, the protons return to their normal position. The change is recorded electronical-

ly, and a computer translates the degree of change into highly detailed images that help physicians distinguish between normal and abnormal body tissues.

Although the procedure is relatively safe, it may be contraindicated for some individuals. Because of the confining nature of the cylinder used for the test, individuals with claustrophobia, those who are confused or agitated, or those with severe mental retardation may be unable to be tested. Likewise, individuals who are extremely obese may not be able to be placed within the cylinder. Open MRI machines that do not require individuals to be placed into a confining cylinder are available at some medical facilities. Because of the use of magnetic force in conducting an MRI, the test may be contraindicated for individuals with cardiac pacemakers, metal implants, or other metal fragments such as shrapnel because of potential injury.

## Brain Scan (Brain Nuclear Scan)

Brain scan, also sometimes called brain nuclear scan, uses *radionuclides* (*radioisotopes*) to identify changes in brain tissue, including tumors, **infarction** (death of tissue), infection, or blockage of blood vessels in the brain. A small amount of the radioactive material (radionuclide) is injected intravenously. The radioactive material localizes in areas of the brain that are abnormal. A small camera records the concentration of radioactive material that has accumulated in various parts of the brain. These data are then transcribed by a computer to form images on film. The scan is usually performed by a *radiologist* or *nuclear medicine technician*.

A refinement of nuclear scanning is the *single photon emission computed tomography* (SPECT). This test uses computer methods similar to that of a CT scan (described above), and a scanning camera rotates around the body recording images of collections of radionuclides in areas of abnormality. SPECT scans are used to examine blood flow to the brain.

The radiation hazard in nuclear scanning is very slight because the dosage of the radionuclide is very small and the duration of the exposure brief. In many instances nuclear scanning can provide useful information so that more dangerous, invasive tests can be avoided.

## Positron Emission Transaxial Tomography (PET Scan)

In order to study the biochemical or metabolic activities in cells of body tissue, *positron emission transaxial tomography* may be used. Individuals are injected with or inhale a biochemical substance tagged with a *radionuclide*. When the particles from the radionuclide combine with particles normally found in the cells of certain tissues, they emit special rays (*gamma rays*) that a scanner can detect. The scanner then translates these emissions into color-coded images. PET scans are able to assess chemical activities in body tissue, especially those related to blood flow and metabolism. Consequently, information from the PET scan not only shows the structure of an area of the body, but it also provides information about how body tissues function. In the brain, this type of scan can be used to evaluate tumors or disorders that may alter cerebral metabolism, such as Parkinson's disease, multiple sclerosis, or epilepsy.

## Cerebral Angiography

Abnormalities of circulation in the brain can be visualized radiographically through *cerebral angiography*. Because blood vessels cannot be readily observed on regular X-rays, a contrast dye must be injected in order to view vessels on X-ray films. Cerebral angiography is considered an invasive procedure because a catheter is inserted into an artery and radiopaque dye is injected. A series of X-ray films are then taken. The test enables physicians to identify blockages that may be interfering with blood flow to certain parts of the brain.

## Lumbar Puncture (Cerebrospinal Fluid Analysis, Spinal Tap)

When a laboratory analysis of an individual's CSF is needed, a *lumbar puncture* is done. To remove the fluid, a physician inserts a needle into the subarachnoid space of the spinal column at the lumbar area. The test may be done to determine whether there is blockage of the flow of spinal fluid, to detect any bleeding, to detect infection, such as *encephalitis* or *meningitis*, or to identify other central nervous system disorders. Although a lumbar puncture is often performed for diagnostic purposes, it can also be done for therapeutic reasons, such as to reduce increased pressure or to instill medications. It is often performed in an outpatient setting under local anesthesia.

## Electroencephalography (EEG)

A graphic recording of electrical activity of the brain (*brain waves*) can be obtained through *electroencephalography* (EEG). The procedure is helpful in identifying tumors, seizure disorders, and other types of brain dysfunction, such as drug intoxication, or determining brain function after brain injury. It may also be used to evaluate sleep disorders.

EEG is a noninvasive procedure in which electrodes are placed in various areas of the scalp and connected to a machine that records brain waves graphically. It may be performed by a physician or by a specially trained technician. The test is usually evaluated by a *neurologist* (physician who is trained to diagnose and treat conditions of the nervous system).

### Neuropsychological Tests

Neuropsychological tests are procedures that are used to assess major functional areas of the brain and to describe the impact of brain dysfunction on many areas of an individual's life, including emotional, social, educational, and vocational areas, to name a few. The tests are performed by a *clinical neuropsychologist*, an individual with advanced graduate training in the field of neuropsychology. Information gained from these tests may be used for diagnosis, monitoring of changes, or treatment planning. In addition to assessing cognitive processes, most neuropsychological tests also assess perceptual and motor skills. Neuropsychological tests can be used to assess memory, abstract reasoning, problem solving, spatial abilities, and emotional and personality consequences of brain damage or dysfunction.

Examples of commonly used neuropsychological tests are the Wechsler Intelligence Scales, the Wechsler Memory Scales, the Halstead-Reitan Neuropsychological Test Battery, and the Luria Nebraska Neuropsychological Battery.

## PSYCHOSOCIAL ISSUES IN NERVOUS SYSTEM CONDITIONS INVOLVING THE BRAIN

Individuals with conditions involving the brain experience many of the same issues as individuals with other types of disability. Conditions involving the brain are often compounded, however, by emotional and cognitive changes that can interfere with individuals' capabilities. Unlike other chronic illnesses or disabilities, conditions involving the brain often affect individuals' social and behavioral responses, and their impact can be great for both the individual and the family. Fuller discussion of psychosocial issues in conditions affecting the nervous system can be found in Chapter 3.

## CASE STUDIES

### Case I

Mr. T. is a 35-year-old auto parts salesman who was injured in an automobile accident when his car was hit head-on by a driver who was intoxicated. The driver of the other car was only slightly injured; however, Mr. T. sustained a closed head injury. When admitted to the trauma unit, his Glasgow Coma Scale was recorded as 9. He remained in a coma for eight days.

Mr. T. stayed at the trauma center for four weeks before being transferred to a rehabilitation center. While at the rehabilitation center, he worked on learning how to walk, talk, and regain physical strength and endurance. Residuals from his head injury include mild dysarthria. In addition, he has developed a seizure disorder, having experienced several grand mal seizures for which he is currently receiving medication, which appears to control the seizures.

### Questions

1. What other potential residual effects might you expect resulting from Mr. T.'s brain injury, in addition to those mentioned?
2. How might Mr. T.'s seizure activity affect his rehabilitation potential?
3. Given Mr. T.'s residuals from his head injury, what aspects of his former oc-

cupation as an auto parts salesman would you expect to be affected by his injuries?

4. What specific accommodations would you expect Mr. T. to need because of his injury?

## Case II

When Mr. G., a night watchman at a gas plant, had his annual physical, he was found to have severe hypertension (high blood pressure). After ongoing monitoring and evaluation, he received a diagnosis of hypertension and was placed on antihypertensive medication. Because Mr. G. experienced no symptoms, however, he often failed to take his medication as prescribed, and he finally stopped taking it altogether. Several weeks later he collapsed at work, was taken to the emergency department by ambulance, and was diagnosed with left cerebral damage from a stroke. After several weeks of hospitalization and rehabilitation, he returned home, but it was unclear whether or not he would be able to return to work.

### Questions

1. What residual effects of left-sided cerebral damage might you expect Mr. G. to have?
2. Although obviously you would need more detailed information about Mr. G.'s functional capacity to determine whether or not he might be able to return to work, how might manifestations from left-sided brain damage affect Mr. G.'s ability to be a night watchman at a gas plant?
3. What psychosocial issues might you consider in Mr. G.'s case?

## REFERENCES

Berrol, S. (1992). Terminology of post-concussion syndrome. *Physical Medicine and Rehabilitation; State of the Art Reviews, 6,* 1–19.

Bishop, M. (2004). Determinants of employment status among a community-based sample of people with epilepsy: Implications for rehabilitation interventions. *Rehabilitation Counseling Bulletin, 47*(2), 112–120, 122.

Browne, T. R., & Holmes, G. L. (2001). Epilepsy. *New England Journal of Medicine, 344*(15), 1145–1151.

Busch, C. R., & Alpern, H. P. (1998). Depression after mild traumatic brain injury: A review of current research. *Neuropsychology Review, 8*(2), 95–108.

Clements, A. D. (1997). Mild traumatic brain injury in persons with multiple trauma: The problem of delayed diagnosis. *Journal of Rehabilitation, 63,* 3–5.

Dombrowski, L. K., Petrick, J. D., & Strauss, D. (2000). Rehabilitation treatment of sexuality issues due to acquired brain injury. *Rehabilitation Psychology, 45*(3), 299–309.

Fabiano, R. J., & Daugherty, J. (1998). Rehabilitation considerations following mild traumatic brain injury. *Journal of Rehabilitation, 64*(14), 9–11.

Felmingham, K. L., Baguley, I. J., & Crooks, J. (2001). A comparison of acute and postdischarge predictors of employment 2 years after traumatic brain injury. *Archives of Physical Medicine Rehabilitation, 82*(4), 435–439.

Fisher, R. S. (2000). Epilepsy from the patient's perspective: Review of results of a community-based survey. *Epilepsy and Behavior, 1*(Suppl.1), S9–S14.

Frazer, C., & Gumnit, R. J. (1990). Sexuality and the person with epilepsy. In Gumnit, R. J. (Ed.), *Living well with epilepsy* (pp. 105–108). New York: Demos Publications.

Giacino, J., & Zasler, N. (1995). Outcome after severe traumatic brain injury: Coma, the vegetative state, and the minimally responsive state. *Journal of Head Trauma Rehabilitation, 10,* 40–56.

Groswasser, Z. & Stern, M. J. (1998). A psychodynamic model of behavior after acute central nervous system damage. *Journal of Head Trauma Rehabilitation, 13*(1), 69–79.

Handler, B. S., & Boland Patterson, J. (1995). Driving after brain injury. *Journal of Rehabilitation, 61,* 43–49.

Hibbard Buffington, A. L. (1996). Sexuality issues among survivors of traumatic brain injuries. *Journal of Applied Rehabilitation Counseling, 27*(1), 45–48.

Huhn, G. D., Sejvar, J. J., Montgomer, S. P., & Dworkin, M. S. (2003). West Nile virus in the United States: An update on an emerging infectious disease. *American Family Physician, 68*(4), 653–660.

Jennet, B., Snoek, J., Bond, M. R., & Brooks, N. (1981). Disability after severe head injury: Observations on the use of the Glasgow outcome scale. *Journal of Neurology and Neurosurgical Psychiatry, 44*, 285–293.

Keyser-Marcus, L. A., Bricout, J. C., Wehman, P., Campbell, L. R., Cifu, D. X., Englander, J., High, W., & Zanfonte, R. D. (2002). Acute predictors of return to employment after traumatic brain injury: A longitudinal follow-up. *Archives of Physical Medicine Rehabilitation, 83*(5), 635–641.

Koch, L., Merz, M. A., & Torkelson Lynch, R. (1995). Screening for mild traumatic brain injury: A guide for rehabilitation counselors. *Journal of Rehabilitation, 61*, 50–56.

Kreutzer, J. S., Marwitz, J. H., Walker, W., Sander, A., Sherer, M., Bogner, J., Fraser, R., & Bushnik, I. (2003). Moderating factors in return to work and job stability after traumatic brain injury. *Journal of Head Trauma Rehabilitation, 18*(2), 128–138.

Lowenstein, D. H., & Alldredge, B. K. (1998). Status epilepticus. *New England Journal of Medicine, 338*, 970–976.

Malec, J. F., Buffington, A. L., Moessner, A. M., & Degiorgio, L. (2000). A medical/vocational case coordination system for persons with brain injury: An evaluation of employment outcomes. *Archives of Physical Medicine Rehabilitation, 81*(8), 1007–1015.

Marfin, A. A., & Gubler, D. J. (2001). West Nile encephalitis: An emerging disease in the United States. *Clinical Infectious Disease, 33*(10), 1713–1719.

Nelson, K. B. (2003). Can we prevent cerebral palsy? *New England Journal of Medicine, 349*(18), 1765–1769.

NIH Consensus Development Panel on Rehabilitation of Persons with Traumatic Brain Injury. (1999). Rehabilitation of persons with traumatic brain injury. *Journal of the American Medical Association, 282*(10), 974–983.

Orr, M. R., Walker, W. C., Marwitz, J. H., & Kreutzer, J. (2003). Occupational categories and return to work after traumatic brain injury. *Archives of Physical Medicine Rehabilitation, 84*(9), E5.

Rappaport, M., Hall, K. M., Hopkins, K., Belleza, T., & Cope, D. N. (1982). Disability rating scale for severe head trauma: Coma to community. *Archives of Physical Medicine and Rehabilitation, 63*, 118–123.

Rothweiler, B., Temkin, N. R., & Dikmen, S. S. (1998). Aging effect on psychosocial outcome in traumatic brain injury. *Archives of Physical Medicine and Rehabilitation, 79*(8), 881–887.

Rubin, S. E., & Roessler, R. T. (2001). *Foundations of the vocational rehabilitation process* (5th ed.). Austin, TX: Pro-Ed.

Salkever, D. S. (2000). Activity status, life satisfaction, and perceived productivity for young adults with developmental disabilities. *Journal of Rehabilitation, 66*(3), 4–13.

Wagner, A. K., Hammond, F. M., Grigsby, J. H., & Norton, H. J. (2000). The value of trauma scores: Predicting discharge after traumatic brain injury. *American Journal of Physical Medicine Rehabilitation, 79*(3), 235–242.

Wagner, A. K., Hammond, F. M., Sasser, H. C., & Wiercisiewski, D. (2002). Return to productive activity after traumatic brain injury: Relationship with measures of disability, handicap, and community integration. *Archives of Physical Medicine Rehabilitation, 83*(1), 107–114.

Wagner, A. K., Hammond, F. M., Sasser, H. C., Wiercisiewski, D., & Norton, H. J. (2000). Use of injury severity variables in determining disability and community integration after traumatic brain injury. *Journal of Trauma, 49*(3), 411–419.

White, R. J., & Likavec, M. J. (1992). The diagnosis and initial management of head injury. *New England Journal of Medicine, 327*(21), 1507–1510.

Willmore, L. J. (1998). Epilepsy emergencies: The first seizure and status epilepticus. *Neurology, 51*(Suppl. 4), S34–S38.

# CHAPTER 3

# Conditions of the Nervous System: Part II
## *Conditions of the Spinal Cord and Peripheral Nervous System and Neuromuscular Conditions*

## NORMAL STRUCTURE AND FUNCTION OF THE SPINAL CORD AND PERIPHERAL NERVOUS SYSTEM

### The Spinal Cord

The spinal cord is part of the central nervous system (see Chapter 1) and extends from the brain stem to the lower part of the back. Bony coverings called *vertebrae* surround the spinal cord and protect it. This bony covering as a whole forms the *vertebral column*. The vertebral column consists of 7 *cervical vertebrae* located in the neck area; 12 *thoracic vertebrae* located in the upper and middle back; and 5 *lumbar vertebrae* located in the lower back. The *sacrum* located below the lumbar vertebrae consists of *fused* (joined) bone. At the tip of the sacrum is the *coccyx*, or tailbone.

The spinal cord conducts impulses to and from the brain. The outer white matter of the spinal cord, which consists of bundles or tracts of myelinated fibers of sensory (*afferent*) and motor (*efferent*) neurons, conveys electrical impulses up and down the spinal cord between the peripheral nervous system (those nerves lying outside the central nervous system) and the brain. In most instances, sensory information traveling up the right side of the spinal cord crosses over to the left side of the brain, so, for example, the left hemisphere of the brain would interpret pain in the right hand. Conversely, motor impulses originating in the left brain cross to the right side of the spinal cord and initiate a response to the right side of the body. Because of this crossover effect, damage on one side of the brain typically causes symptoms on the opposite side of the body.

The inner gray matter of the spinal cord, which is composed of cell bodies and unmyelinated neurons, acts as a coordinating center for reflex and other activities, such as voluntary movements and control of internal functions. A reflex center in the gray matter of the spinal cord is where sensory and motor neurons connect. This part of the spinal cord serves as a center for spinal reflexes. A *reflex* can be defined as an automatic response to a given stimulus. Spinal reflexes control not only muscle reflexes but also the reflexes of internal organs.

The gray matter within the spinal cord resembles an H. The projections of the H are named according to the direction to which they project. The *posterior horns* extend toward the back, and the *anterior horns* project toward the front. Cerebrospinal fluid, which nourishes and protects the spinal cord, fills both the *central canal*, located within the center of the gray matter, and the subarachnoid space surrounding the outer portion of the spinal cord.

Motor (*efferent*) impulses originate in the motor cortex of the brain, extend down the spinal cord through *descending tracts*, and exit through motor spinal nerve roots that extend through openings between the vertebrae that surround the spinal cord. Sensory (*afferent*) impulses from the body enter the spinal cord through spinal nerve roots that also extend through openings between vertebrae and then travel up *ascending tracts* in the spinal cord to the brain.

Spinal nerve roots are named for the vertebral level from which they exit. For example, the nerve roots that leave the spinal cord at the cervical level are labeled C-1 through C-8, and the nerve roots that leave at the thoracic level are labeled T-1 through T-12. The sensory (*afferent*) nerves carry body sensations into the sensory nerve roots (*posterior roots*) at the back of the spinal cord, where they are then carried up the spinal cord to the brain. Motor (*efferent*) impulses travel from the brain down the spinal cord and exit from motor nerve roots (*anterior roots*) at the front of the spinal cord. Motor nerve fibers then carry impulses to the voluntary muscles in the body.

Many types of neurons work together to transmit impulses through the spinal cord. Sensory impulses entering the spinal cord at the lumbar region are relayed vertically to the brain through a number of connecting sensory neurons. Motor impulses from the brain to the peripheral nerves, however, are conducted through two separate categories of motor neurons. *Upper motor neurons* originate in the brain and are contained entirely within the central nervous system. *Lower motor neurons*, although originating in the central nervous system, have fibers extending to the *peripheral nerves* in voluntary muscles. Dysfunction of either upper or lower motor neurons can generally affect the voluntary muscles. The location of the dysfunction determines the nature of the disorder.

## The Peripheral Nervous System

A nerve is a bundle of fibers outside the central nervous system that transmits information between the central nervous system and various parts of the body. The *peripheral nervous system* consists of all nerves that extend from the brain and spinal cord. In order to function effectively, the peripheral nerves must be connected to the central nervous system. Some peripheral nerves connect directly to the brain (*cranial nerves*), and others connect directly to the spinal cord (*spinal nerves*). Cranial and spinal nerves are essential links between the rest of the body and the central nervous system.

The 12 pairs of peripheral nerves that connect and transmit messages directly to the brain are called *cranial nerves*. Some cranial nerves contain only sensory fibers, whereas others contain both sensory and motor fibers. Cranial nerves mediate many aspects of sensation and muscular activity in and around the head and neck. Cranial nerves and their related functions are illustrated in Table 3–1.

Peripheral nerves that connect and transmit messages directly to the spinal cord are called *spinal nerves*. There are 31 pairs of spinal nerves. Each nerve divides and then subdivides into a number of branches. Nerves at each level travel to specific parts of the body, conveying information between those areas and the

**Table 3–1** Cranial Nerves and Related Functions

| Cranial Nerve | Area of Function |
|---|---|
| I. Olfactory | Smell |
| II. Optic | Vision |
| III. Oculomotor | Movement of eye muscles |
| IV Trochlear | Eyelids |
| V. Trigeminal | Sensation in head, face, and teeth, motor activity of chewing |
| VI. Abducens | Pupil dilation, focusing of lens |
| VII. Facial | Taste, sensation of external ear, control of salivary glands, tears, muscles in facial expression |
| VIII. Vestibulocochlear | Sensation of sound, balance, orientation of head |
| IX. Glossopharyngeal | Swallowing, sensation of pain, taste, touch from tongue and throat |
| X. Vagus | Heartbeat, digestion, speech, swallowing, respiratory function, gland functions |
| XI. Accessory | Movement of head and shoulders, muscles of pharynx and larynx in throat, production of voice sounds |
| XII. Hypoglossal | Tongue movement, speech, swallowing |

central nervous system. Spinal nerves and their related functions are illustrated in Table 3–2.

Nerves control both voluntary and involuntary functions in the body. Nerves that control *voluntary* functions (such as movement of the muscles in the extremities) are called *somatic* nerves. Nerves that are concerned with the control of involuntary functions are part of a subcategory of the peripheral nervous system called the *autonomic nervous system.*

The autonomic nervous system integrates the work of vital organs, such as the heart and lungs. Its primary function is to coordinate the activity of internal organs so that they can make adaptive responses to changing external situations in order to maintain internal equilibrium. Nerve fibers monitor the activities of internal organs as well as changes in the external environment. When changes are necessary to maintain internal **homeostasis** (equilibrium), or to protect the body, the autonomic nervous system stimulates immediate, involuntary responses. For example, in response to a speck of dust in the eye, tears are produced. In response to a fearful situation, the heart beats faster.

**Table 3–2** Spinal Nerves and Related Functions

| Spinal Nerve | Area of Function |
|---|---|
| Cervical (C1-C8) | Back of head, neck, shoulders, arms, hands, diaphragm |
| Thoracic (T1-T12) | Chest, back, regions of abdomen |
| Lumbar (L1-L5) | Lower back, parts of thighs and legs |
| Sacral (S1-S5) | Regions of thighs, buttocks, legs, bowel, bladder, genital function |

The autonomic nervous system is divided into two subsystems:

1. The sympathetic nervous system
2. The parasympathetic nervous system

These two systems work together and in opposition to control internal organs and regulate their function. Hormones and emotions can affect both systems.

The sympathetic nervous system becomes active during stress and emergencies. It prepares the body for action, deepening respirations, making the heart beat faster, dilating the pupils, stimulating production of stress hormones, and increasing blood supply to the large muscles of the body. The parasympathetic nervous system dominates when the body is at rest. It activates mechanisms that focus on body conservation, such as decreasing the heart rate and constricting the pupils of the eye. The parasympathetic nervous system is also an important component of sexual arousal in both males and females.

## CONDITIONS AFFECTING THE SPINAL CORD

### Spinal Cord Injuries

Spinal cord dysfunction can result from a number of causes. Most often, it is due to injuries from motor vehicle accidents, sports injuries, falls, or violence such as gunshot wounds. Other causes of spinal cord dysfunction are compression of the cord from conditions such as herniated disc, spinal tumors, infectious disorders such as polio or tetanus, degenerative disorders such as multiple sclerosis, or congenital disorders such as spina bifida.

Ultimately spinal cord dysfunction results in some combination of sensory, motor, or reflex deficit. When the spinal cord is injured, transmission of impulses between the brain and other parts of the body below the level of injury are inter-

rupted. Consequently, some damage to motor, sensory, or reflex function below the injury occurs. There may be numbness, complete paralysis, or exaggerated, absent, or diminished reflexes below the level of the injury. The extent of functional impairment or loss depends on the part of the spinal cord injured and whether the cord is bruised, compressed, or severed. For instance, in some cases, swelling, bleeding, or a tumor may compress the cord without severing it. In these instances, removal of the source of compression can, at times, restore function. When the spinal cord is severed, however, transmission of nerve impulses may be permanently lost or impaired.

When the spinal cord is completely severed (*complete spinal cord injury*), there is no nerve function below the level of the injury and hence no voluntary motor or sensory function below that level. If severance is not complete (*incomplete spinal cord injury*), some motor or sensory function below the level of the injury may be intact. In these instances, one portion of the spinal cord may be nonfunctional while another portion maintains some function; or certain nerve tracts may still be functioning, but in an abnormal way. The term ***paraparesis*** refers to partial paralysis and indicates that some function remains below the level of the injury. Sometimes even when the spinal cord is not completely severed, all motor and sensory function below the level of the injury may be lost if the remaining nerves are destroyed from lack of blood supply, degeneration, or compression. In general, the higher the level of spinal cord injury, the greater the functional impairment.

### *Manifestations of Spinal Cord Injury*

Symptoms of spinal cord injury specifically reflect the level of the injury and

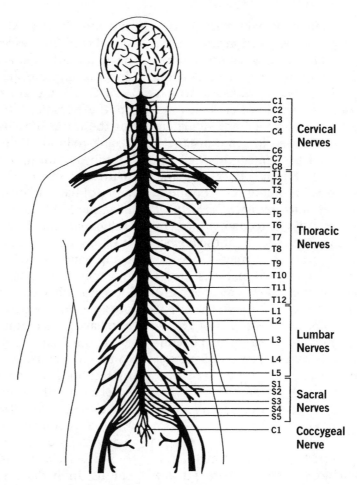

**Figure 3–1** Spinal Nerves. *Source:* Reprinted with permission from M. J. Miller, *Pathophysiology: Principles of Disease*, p. 380. © 1983, W. B. Saunders Company.

the function of the neurons involved (Figure 3–1). If spinal nerves are unable to transmit messages between the central nervous system and the peripheral nervous system, function below the level of injury will be disrupted. The degree of functional loss is dependent on the degree to which the spinal cord is injured. For example, if the *afferent nerve roots* in the *ascending tracts* (*sensory tracts*) are injured, some sensory loss below the level of injury will exist. If *efferent nerve roots* in the *descending* (*motor tracts*) are injured, some motor loss below the level of injury is expected. When both sensory and motor tracts are injured, as with complete severance of the spinal cord, both motor loss and sensory loss occur below that level.

Ambulation is affected to some degree regardless of the level of injury, with the exception of injury at the *sacral level* (S-2 through S-4), in which ambulation may return to normal. Individuals with spinal cord injuries above T-12 usually require a wheelchair for ambulation. At lower levels of injury, ambulation for short distances may be possible with braces or crutches.

Most individuals lose voluntary control of bladder and bowel function after spinal cord injury. Bladder evacuation may be accomplished through external collection devices such as *condom catheters*, which may be used for men; however, there is no equivalent device for women. *Indwelling catheters* are still used in some instances for both men and women, although because of the risk of urinary tract infection, this practice is becoming less common. When feasible, *intermittent catheterization* several times a day is recommended. In lower-level injuries, such as at the *lumbar level*, bladder evacuation may be accomplished by applying external pressure to the lower abdomen. Bowel management may be accomplished through the use of suppositories or rectal stimulation; however, the individual may still be concerned about involuntary bowel movements in public.

### Spinal Cord Injuries at the Cervical Level (C-1 through C-8)

Diving accidents, motor vehicle accidents, or a blow to the head with a heavy object may cause fractures of the cervical vertebrae. An injury to the spinal cord at the *cervical level* (C-1 through C-8) results in **quadriplegia** (paralysis of both upper and lower extremities). Injuries at C-1 or C-2 are often fatal because the functioning of all muscles, including the muscles of respiration, is lost. Individuals who survive these injuries require ventilatory support in order to breathe and are totally dependent on others for self-care. Individuals with injuries at C-3 or C-4 also have compromised ventilatory capacity and will also require special respiratory equipment, as well as be dependent on others for self-care; however, at this level of injury individuals may be able to manipulate a wheelchair through the use of a mouth stick. Most individuals with spinal cord injuries at C-4 or above must have an attendant for personal care, dressing, and transfers.

At C-5, some gross movement of the upper extremities is possible, such as bending the arm at the elbow. Individuals may be able to hold a light object between the thumb and finger, or they may be able to maneuver small objects with the assistance of hand splints. Assistance will still be required for most activities; however, individuals may be capable of transfer on their own with the assistance of special equipment. Total independent living is probably not feasible, but independent electrical wheelchair ambulation may be possible. Individuals with injury at C-6 also have gross motor movement of upper extremities and may be able to retain some independence in self-care, such as by feeding and dressing with the aid of special orthotic equipment. Propelling a wheelchair manually may be possible with a modified hand rim, although many individuals continue to operate a motorized chair. With the use of hand splints, individuals may also be able to write. Independent transfer from bed to chair or to a car may also be possible, as well as driving with the use of special adaptive devices.

Individuals with C-7 injuries are capable of straightening their arm and are able to sit up in bed, dress themselves, and transfer, so almost total independence with some adaptations in the environment may be achieved. Fine motor movements of the hands are impaired, but writing may be possible with the use of a special device that can be strapped to the hand. Driving is possible with hand controls. With C-8 injuries individuals have some sensation in their hands and may become totally independent with modified environment and some adaptive devices.

### Spinal Cord Injuries at the Thoracic Level (T-1 through T-12)

Spinal cord injuries occurring at T-1 or below result in **paraplegia** (paralysis of the lower extremities). Upper extremities, for the most part, are unimpaired, with the exception of T-1 injuries, in which there may be slight weakness and some loss of flexibility in the hands. Individuals with injury between T-1 and T-3 may need a brace or other support to maintain posture in an upright position because even though the upper extremities are functional, the muscles of the trunk are paralyzed. In most cases, individuals with injuries at T-1 through T-12 are able to attain total independence in self-care, wheelchair ambulation, and transfer. Individuals with injury at T-7 to T-12 may be able to walk with the use of long leg braces; however, because of the strenuous nature of the activity, ambulation may only be possible for short distances.

### Spinal Cord Injuries at the Lumbar Level (L-1 through L-5)

Many of the muscles of mobility are intact with L-1 through L-5 injuries. All upper body muscles and many of the leg muscles are functional. Ambulation with braces and/or use of cane or crutches may be possible, especially for short distances. Individuals are able to gain total independence in care, although hand controls still may be necessary for operating a motor vehicle. Although bowel and bladder function are still impaired, reflex emptying of bowel and bladder may be possible.

### Spinal Cord Injuries at the Sacral Level (S1 through S-4)

Ambulation is usually possible with little or no equipment. Bowel and bladder function may still be impaired to some degree.

## Treatment and Management of Spinal Cord Injury

### Initial Treatment of Spinal Cord Injury

The initial treatment of spinal cord injuries focuses on preventing further injury, stabilizing individuals' physical condition, and in some instances performing surgery to realign the spinal column or achieve decompression of the spinal cord. Many individuals with spinal cord injuries, especially those who received the injury as the result of an accident, will have other injuries, such as fractures, injury to internal organs, or brain injuries, that further complicate their care.

Individuals with injuries to the *cervical spine* are usually placed in skeletal traction to immobilize the spine. In some instances, individuals may have cervical orthoses, such as a *halo brace* (Figure 3–2), in which metal pins are inserted into the skull and attached to a metal "halo" that surrounds the head. The "halo" is attached with two metal rods to a "vest" worn on the torso of the individual. The halo brace is used to allow mobility while keeping the head and neck in proper position. Traction is usually not used to stabilize and immobilize thoracic or lumbar fractures because there is no effective way to provide it.

### Postacute Treatment and Rehabilitation

After the condition has been stabilized and acute medical needs met, individuals are usually transferred to a rehabilitation unit, where they learn skills or learn to use adaptive devices that will help them to achieve the maximum level of inde-

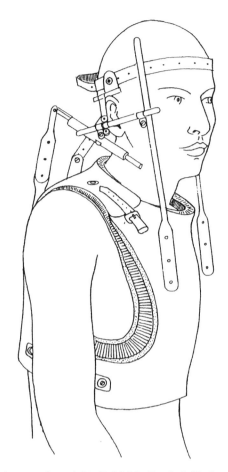

**Figure 3–2**  Halo Brace. *Source:* Copyright © 1999. Rachel Clarke.

pendence. A wide variety of health professionals are usually involved in this phase of rehabilitation, including *physiatrists, physical therapists, rehabilitation nurses, occupational therapists, orthotists, psychologists, social workers,* and *rehabilitation counselors*.

Physical therapy begins as soon as possible to prevent deformities such as **contractures** (permanent contractions of a muscle so that a joint becomes fixed or immobile) or footdrop, as well as to build strength. An immediate treatment goal is to have individuals with either **paraplegia** (involvement of lower extremities) or **quadriplegia** (involvement of all four extremities) placed into an upright position as soon as possible to prevent complications such as respiratory problems from occurring. A *tilt board* or *circular bed* is used to accomplish this goal. Individuals are strapped securely to the tilt board or circular bed while in a prone position. The board is then gradually raised or the circular bed rotated until the individual is upright.

As the individual's condition stabilizes, treatment is directed toward teaching self-care. Most individuals with spinal cord injury become mobile with a wheelchair. Many types of wheelchairs are available with a variety of options, including detachable armrests and footrests, removable back panel, a lapboard, and a carryall bag. Power-operated wheelchairs are available for individuals who have little or no use of their upper extremities. These chairs are battery operated and can be controlled with a switch adapted to the particular individual's ability. Because of the size of the battery-operated wheelchairs, they are heavy and therefore difficult to transport.

Individuals are taught a variety of self-care skills, including dressing, hygiene, and grooming. It may be necessary to install specific adaptive devices, such as grab bars and a raised toilet seat, in the home. Because most spinal cord injuries affect bladder and bowel function, instructions in catheter care and bowel retraining are usually necessary.

### Potential Complications Associated with Spinal Cord Injury

Individuals with spinal cord injury are at risk of developing additional health problems that could result in a secondary disability and consequently additional functional limitations. The extent of the risk is related to the level of injury. In general, the higher the level of injury, the greater the risk of developing secondary disabling conditions. It is therefore imperative that individuals with spinal cord injuries, family members, and professionals working with them are aware of the risk and use prevention strategies to lessen the risk.

### Altered Symptoms of Illness

Because of the lack of sensation that accompanies most spinal cord injuries, as well as the interruption to nerve pathways, symptoms of various conditions unrelated to the spinal cord injury itself may be not be recognized, and consequently may not receive prompt treatment. For example, because pain is not felt, appendicitis may not be discovered until the appendix ruptures. In some instances symptoms may be expressed differently in individuals with spinal cord injury than in individuals without spinal cord injury. For example, those without spinal cord injury may experience severe flank pain in response to a kidney infection; however, individuals with spinal cord injury may, instead, experience an abrupt increase in spasticity. As a result, the symptom may not be recognized as being related to kidney infection and the kidney infection may not be immediately diagnosed and treated. Individuals with spinal cord injuries, caregivers, and professionals should be made aware of this alteration of symptom presentation and should be alerted to report or investigate new symptoms or accentuated old symptoms as soon as they are noted.

### Pressure Sores (Decubitus Ulcers)

One of the most common complications associated with spinal cord injury is pressure sores (**decubitus ulcers**), which result from lack of blood supply to a body pressure point, such as the buttocks, sacrum, heel, or back. Pressure sores develop when continuous pressure is exerted to a body part over time (Pires & Adkins, 1996; Woolsey & McGarry, 1991). Pressure on a body part interferes with blood supply, eventually resulting in breakdown and ulceration of the skin. Because individuals with spinal cord injury are often immobile, areas of pressure on certain bony prominences are more likely to develop. Since these individuals usually have no sensation below the level of injury, they are unable to feel pressure, and because of the paralysis they are unable to easily shift their weight to relieve the pressure. Inadequate skin care, irritation, and nutritional deficiency can further contribute to the development of the problem. Pressure sores may appear to be small on the surface, but the depth of the ulcer may be more extensive. Untreated pressure sores can progress from redness to breakdown of the skin, infection, and eventually death (**necrosis**) of skin tissue, which could extend through the tissue all the way to the bone. Thus pressure sores are not only debilitating but can be potentially life-threatening.

Individuals with spinal cord injury must be aware of the risk of pressure sores and the importance of monitoring their skin. Education about the importance of decreasing the amount of pressure on bony prominences by regularly changing position, maintaining good nutrition, and following good skin care is an important part of the rehabilitation process. A number of prescribed wheelchair cushions are available that can help distribute pressure to prevent skin breakdown and endurance in a wheelchair. In addition to having the correct cushion prescribed, individuals with spinal cord injury should also be helped to learn how to position them properly.

### Urinary Tract and Bowel Complications

Urinary tract infections are the second highest reported complication of spinal cord injury. Because the bladder is emptied in abnormal ways, it may not empty often enough or may not empty completely. When this happens, the urine left in the bladder acts as a reservoir for infection. Because individuals with spinal cord injury are generally unable to control their bladder, they may need to have a *catheter* inserted into the bladder to drain

urine and prevent incontinence. The bladder and its contents normally contain no pathologic organisms, but there is always the potential for the introduction of infectious organisms when a catheter is inserted. For individuals with spinal cord injury, urinary tract infections can be a serious, debilitating, and, at times, life-threatening problem. Untreated urinary tract infection can lead to **pyelonephritis** (infection of the kidney) and, in severe cases, **septicemia** (infection in the blood).

Because of the inactivity after paralysis, the amount of calcium in the blood increases. As a consequence, the risk of developing kidney stones (**renal calculi**) is increased. The stone may form in the kidney itself or may lodge in the **ureters** (tubes leading from the kidney to the bladder) so that they obstruct urine flow, causing urine to back up into the kidneys (**urinary reflux**), and eventually causing damage to the kidney itself.

Education of individuals with spinal cord injury about the urinary tract and the risk of infection or stone formation and how to decrease this risk is crucial to preventing secondary urinary tract complications. In addition, individuals with spinal cord injury should be made aware of the importance of self-monitoring and promptly reporting symptoms they may be experiencing so that prompt diagnosis and treatment may be instituted.

Secondary conditions related to bowel elimination may also be problematic. Incontinence of fecal material may not only contribute to skin breakdown and urinary tract infection, but may result in social isolation if individuals become concerned about the probability that incontinence will occur. Other problems may relate to **impaction** (fecal matter that becomes hardened and is unable to be evacuated) or in some instances to a condition called

**paralytic ileus**, in which the intestine ceases to function.

Individuals can decrease the risk of these conditions by establishing a pattern of regular elimination, monitoring diet and fluid intake, and learning specific techniques for enhancing optimal bowel function.

### Contractures

**Contractures** (loss of range of motion, or fixed deformity of a joint) may occur in paralyzed limbs if the joints are not moved through their regular range of motion. Contractures of the upper extremities in individuals with quadriplegia can interfere with the use of assistive devices. If individuals with paraplegia or quadriplegia develop contractures of the hip or knee, it may be difficult to assume adequate positioning in a wheelchair. Regularly moving the joints through the full range of motion through passive exercises conducted by another person, or by using special equipment, can prevent contractures from occurring. In addition, proper wheelchair seating as well as positioning of joints can help reduce risk of contractures.

### Spasticity

**Spasticity** refers to the exaggerated involuntary movement of paralyzed muscles. Although spasticity may be absent immediately after injury, it can occur long after individuals leave the rehabilitation facility. Because communication between the *peripheral nervous system* and the brain is interrupted by spinal cord injury, signals received by the *peripheral nerves* are "short–circuited." Rather than traveling to the brain to be interpreted and appropriately adapted, they instead return from the spinal cord directly to the muscle. The resulting muscle contraction can some-

times be violent and can occur with even slight stimulation. Spasticity can be debilitating, not only because it is disruptive and can potentially cause embarrassment to the individual, but also because in some instances it can be so strong that it causes individuals to fall from their wheelchairs. Spasticity can also contribute to the formation of contractures. Although in some instances spasticity can be useful to help individuals perform certain functions such as shifting position or standing, more often it is a source of discomfort. When spasticity is a cause of concern, individuals may be helped to learn a program of stretching that may help diminish occurrences. In other instances medications may be used to reduce spasticity; however, generalized weakness, the side effects of sedation, or other side effects may make this treatment less desirable. In severe cases when other treatments are ineffective in controlling spasticity, individuals may resort to surgery, such as **rhizotomy** (surgical resection of a nerve root) to relieve spasticity.

### Osteoporosis

Bone is a dynamic substance that is continually depositing and reabsorbing calcium. The combined stress of weight bearing and muscle pull that occurs with normal activity helps bones maintain their calcium content. Inactivity can contribute to softening and weakening of bones (**osteoporosis**). Individuals with spinal cord injury have an increased rate of calcium removal from the bone and are consequently more susceptible to fractures, which could be caused from falls but also from a simple activity such as a wheelchair transfer. Calcium that is excreted through the urinary system can also contribute to urinary tract stones, as noted above. In some instances calcium is deposited in soft tissues so that function of the joint or muscle is disrupted.

Adequate diet, passive exercise and strength-building exercises, and electrical stimulation to the muscles can be used to help reduce risk. In addition, proper training in safety procedures when operating a wheelchair and transferring can help prevent falls and potentially broken bones if osteoporosis is present.

### Cardiac and Respiratory Problems

In the initial stages after injury, individuals are susceptible to **thrombophlebitis** (formation of blood clots in the legs) or **pulmonary embolism** (a blood clot that travels to the lungs), a serious and potentially life-threatening disorder. As the individual's condition stabilizes, this condition becomes less of a treat. In the initial period after injury, individuals may also experience a condition called **orthostatic hypotension**, in which blood pressure becomes significantly lower when the individual is moved from a flat to upright position.

Although these conditions become less prominent after the first month, individuals with spinal cord injury continue to be more prone to respiratory disorders, especially conditions such as pneumonia that can be debilitating as well as life-threatening. Individuals with high cervical or high thoracic injuries, because of weakened chest muscles, have more difficulty expanding the lungs and clearing respiratory secretions. Consequently, they are more susceptible to infection of the lungs.

Individuals with spinal cord injury also have a more sedentary lifestyle, which can affect the cardiovascular system. Because of the increased susceptibility to cardiovascular conditions, they should refrain from smoking or using tobacco products or drinking alcohol excessively.

Good nutrition, an exercise program, and weight control are also important in preventing cardiovascular disease. Because of the increased risk of cardiovascular conditions, individuals should have regular medical examinations and comprehensive health care programs that accommodate their needs.

### Autonomic Dysreflexia

**Autonomic dysreflexia** is an abnormal reflex condition characterized by a sudden rise in blood pressure, profuse sweating, and headache as the result of excessive neural discharge from the autonomic nervous system. It may be triggered by events as simple as overdistension of the bowel or bladder. Unless the individual receives immediate treatment to decrease the blood pressure, there is risk of stroke. Autonomic dysreflexia commonly occurs in individuals who have experienced an injury to the upper spinal cord. Identifying and preventing the situations or conditions that trigger autonomic dysreflexia are important to prevention.

### Other Neurological Complications

**Diaphoresis** (profuse sweating) and **paresthesia** (abnormal painful sensations below the level of injury) are other potential sequelae of spinal cord injury.

### Sexual Dysfunction

Nerves to the genital region are almost always affected to some degree by spinal cord injury. This does not mean, however, that other aspects of sexuality, such as sexual attraction to others, sexual desire, and the need to express oneself as a sexual being, are changed. Many men and women remain sexually active after spinal cord injury; however, in most instances, modifications of sexual behavior and function may need to be made.

Genital function is controlled by the parasympathetic and sympathetic nervous systems as well as by motor nerves and will be dependent on the level of injury and on whether the injury is complete or incomplete. Consequently, the higher the level of injury, the more significantly will genital function be affected. Most individuals with spinal cord injury, both males and females, will have little sensation directly in the genital area. Because mobility is affected, they will also need to alter their technique in sexual performance.

Many males, regardless of level of injury, continue to have reflex erections, and in many instances erection can be produced through manual stimulation. The ability to produce an erection through psychological arousal is absent in most men with spinal cord injuries; however, they may have a weakened sexual response due to psychological stimuli. Some individuals have used techniques such as penile implants to achieve intercourse. Ejaculation is absent for most men with spinal cord injury, or, if it does occur, individuals experience retrograde ejaculation, so that semen is deposited into the bladder rather than externally. As a result, fertility in males is significantly affected, especially males with complete severance of the spinal cord. Some techniques, such as *electro ejaculation*, in which ejaculation is stimulated through electrical means, have been used so that sperm can be obtained for artificial insemination.

Females with spinal cord injury are still able to engage in sexual intercourse, but lubrication in response to psychological arousal is usually absent. Menses typically are absent the first months after injury; however, with the return of menstruation, in most instances female fertility is unal-

tered. Consequently, women who do not wish to become pregnant need to use some form of contraception. When women with spinal cord injury become pregnant, they are able to carry the pregnancy to term, although because of altered sensation, it may be more difficult for them to determine when labor begins.

### Psychosocial Issues in Spinal Cord Injury

Spinal cord injury interrupts and alters not only physical functioning, but psychosocial functioning as well. Individuals with spinal cord injury, in addition to experiencing changes in movement and sensation, decreased mobility and independence, and changes in bowel and bladder functioning and sexual functioning, also experience altered self-concept and in many instances loss of self-esteem. Frustrated goals, loss of self-regard, or loss of the illusion of omnipotence and control can result in internalized anger, anxiety, and guilt. To a great degree, how individuals adjust will be related to how they conceptualize the losses they experience, to their individual coping style and to the amount and type of social support available.

Although depression is common after spinal cord injury, it is not universal and is not necessary for adjustment to occur (Cushman & Dijkers, 1991). Some individuals are more likely to exhibit depressive symptoms after spinal cord injury than others. Those who had difficulty coping with stress prior to the injury or who had a history of substance abuse or relationship problems demonstrate increased difficulty adjusting after injury, whereas those who have greater personal resources and demonstrated optimal adjustment prior to injury are more likely to display adequate adjustment after injury (Elliot & Frank, 1996).

Lack of social support is strongly associated with depressive symptoms after spinal cord injury (Rinala, Young, Hart, Clearman, & Fuhrer, 1992). Outward displays of depressive symptoms may result in avoidance by others. Thus the individual becomes isolated, which in turn causes more depression. In general, individuals who demonstrate a greater internal locus of control also demonstrate less psychosocial distress and better adaptation (Livneh, 2000).

Not only must individuals with spinal cord injury incorporate new behaviors and mobility techniques in order to function, but they must also continually adapt to their changing environment. Although spinal cord injury causes radical changes in mobility and independence, most individuals are able to return to their community, and many to their own home with environmental modifications. The degree of successful reentry into the community is largely dependent on the individual's social support, access to adequate housing and transportation, and the availability of quality attendant care if needed.

In some instances, establishing new relationships and/or reestablishing or maintaining old ones may be difficult. Relationships may need to be reexamined and redefined. Significant others may experience many of the same or parallel reactions and losses as the individual with spinal cord injury. The sudden incapacity of a family member or significant other due to spinal cord injury may result in shock, denial, anger, or depression in other family members. If they think the cause was avoidable or blame the individual or others for the injury, they may exhibit hostility, pessimism, anxiety, and higher levels of social distress. Family relationships may be strained if family caregivers experience stress related to finances or to

helping individuals with activities of daily living and self-care. Family members and significant others may need the same degree of help and support as those individuals with spinal cord injury so that they can cope with the condition and in turn offer support to the individual. Role obligations may need to be shifted, negotiated, and shared.

The focus of many rehabilitation programs for spinal cord injury is on helping individuals attain maximum functionality related to self-care activities or employment, with less attention being given to recreational activities that could enable individuals to become active in a larger social sphere. The lack of structured peer recreation activities and peer support can lead to social isolation and prevent individuals from living effectively with their disability (McAweeney, Forchheimer, & Tate, 1996). After spinal cord injury, the level of participation in social and recreational activities will be dependent on the attitude and interests of the individual, the number of recreational opportunities and resources available, and the degree of access to appropriate adaptative devices and adequate sources for equipment repair. Adaptive devices that enable individuals with spinal cord injury to participate in many sports and other recreational activities are available; however, adequate transportation, quality attendant care if needed, and other environmental restrictions must also be considered.

Increased access to public buildings, businesses, and services enables individuals with spinal cord injury to participate more fully in a broader range of community activities and to explore and pursue a number of social roles; however, architectural and attitudinal barriers still exist. Consequently, in order to live most effectively with their disability, individuals with spinal cord injury must also learn to assert the importance of their own needs and advocate for themselves.

Because of the physical needs resulting from spinal cord injury, individuals must modify their daily routines to function effectively in personal, social, or occupational spheres. For example, extra time may be needed for daily activities related to personal hygiene. Individuals may need to conform daily routines to a structured bowel and bladder program. Transportation, or moving from one place to another, may require extra time and planning. Awareness of the demands involved in routine self-care will help individuals establish and adjust daily routines so that they can participate in social and occupational activities.

Individuals with spinal cord injury continue to be sexual beings. Sexual adjustment is an integral and necessary part of total psychological adjustment. Changes in sexual functioning as a result of spinal cord injury may be a source of extreme frustration for adults. Those who experience spinal cord injury in adolescence or preteen years may have added challenges with acceptance, self-worth, and self- esteem. Discussion and accommodation of sexual needs as well as reassurance that sexual expression is still possible in their life are an important part of rehabilitation.

Individuals should be provided with opportunities to obtain accurate and complete information about sexual activity in spinal cord injury, and information should be provided in the context of their personal values.

### Vocational Issues in Spinal Cord Injury

Unless individuals with spinal cord injury have an associated brain injury, they should experience no cognitive deficits. The level of injury determines, to a great extent, the amount and kind of activity in which they are able to engage and what assistive devices or special accommodations may be needed. Individuals with very low spinal cord injuries (sacral or lumbar level) may be able to walk short distances with the assistance of braces and crutches, whereas those with higher levels, such as at the thoracic level, will probably require a wheelchair for mobility; individuals with cervical injuries will require a powered chair. When the injury is in the cervical area, they will have limited ability to use the upper extremities, and at the highest levels of injury they will be unable to use the upper extremity at all. Consequently, special adaptive equipment will be required to use a telephone, computer, or other equipment that requires hand use.

Environmental barriers such as steps, table heights, and width of doorways will need to be considered in the work environment. Since many individuals with spinal cord injury also have difficulty with temperature regulation, the work environment should be climate controlled.

The individual's preinjury education and vocational interests and skills, as well as his or her functional capacity after injury, are important considerations in vocational placement. Age or the presence of financial disincentives are also factors that influence the individual's employment status.

Spinal cord injury is a lifetime disability. Consequently, periodic checkups should be instituted to identify those who are experiencing difficulty or encountering new barriers to access in the workplace, so that appropriate accommodations can be instituted (Roessler, 2001).

### Spina Bifida

**Spina bifida** is one of several different congenital conditions known as *neural tube* *defects.* These defects involve incomplete development of the brain, spinal cord, and/or coverings of these structures. Other neural tube defects besides spina bifida are **anencephaly**, in which infants are born with underdeveloped brains and incomplete skulls, and **encephalocele**, in which infants are born with a hole in the skull through which brain tissue protrudes. In most cases infants with either of these conditions do not survive, or if they do, they experience severe mental retardation.

Spina bifida, however, does not involve the brain but rather the spinal column and is a condition in which one or more vertebrae are left open so that the spinal cord is exposed.

### Types of Spina Bifida

There are three types of spina bifida:

- **Spina bifida occulta** refers to an opening in one or more vertebrae of the spinal column. This is the mildest form of spina bifida, which does not involve any damage to the spinal cord. Many individuals with this form of spina bifida may be unaware that their condition even exists.
- Spinal **meningocele** refers to a more serious type of spina bifida. In this form of the condition the **meninges** (protective coverings around the spinal cord) protrude through the opening in the spinal column. The protruding part is called a meningocele and contains only the meninges, not portions of the spinal cord. In some cases surgery can correct this problem so that there is little or no damage to the nerves of the spinal cord. In other instances, however, individuals with a spinal meningocele may have residual effects resulting from spinal cord damage.

- **Myelomeningocele**, the most common and most severe form of spina bifida, is a condition in which nerves of the spinal cord as well as the meninges protrude through the opening of the vertebrae to the outer part of the body. Because there is no protective covering for the cord and meninges, spinal fluid may leak from the protrusion, and the risk of infection is great. When this defect occurs, it usually results in **paraplegia** (paralysis of the lower extremities) as well as poor bladder and bowel control. Although surgery is usually performed immediately to correct the defect, symptoms of paralysis in the lower extremities usually persist.

### Manifestations of Spina Bifida

Manifestations of spina bifida depend on the type, the part of the spinal cord affected, and the severity of the condition. They can range from mild, in which there are few if any symptoms, to severe, in which there is muscle paralysis, loss of sensation, and loss of bowel and bladder control. Many children with the severe type of spina bifida also experience **hydrocephalus**, a condition in which fluid builds up in the brain. In cases of hydrocephalus, surgical implantation of a shunt is necessary so that the fluid can be drained to prevent excessive pressure on the brain. If hydrocephalus is not corrected, mental retardation can result.

Because spina bifida is congenital, more severe forms of the condition impinge on normal motor development. Depending on the social, economic, and psychological circumstances of the individual and his or her available resources, cognitive development could also be affected. Although the condition itself is not progressive, problems associated with the condition may increase over time. For example, in more severe cases when paralysis is present, uneven posture compounded by vertebral abnormalities may lead to **scoliosis** (lateral S-shaped curvature of the spine). Scoliosis can lead to respiratory problems, impede effective functioning of other internal organs, and decrease endurance. Paralysis and associated bowel and bladder problems can also predispose individuals to develop **decubitus ulcers** (pressure sores). In addition, bowel and bladder problems increase the potential for chronic urinary tract infections.

Adult males with more severe forms of spina bifida may have difficulty maintaining erection and may have difficulties with fertility. Conversely, females may be capable of engaging in sexual relations and have normal fertility, but sensation to the genital area may be absent.

### Treatment and Management of Spina Bifida

Since the condition is obvious at birth, treatment is usually instigated within 24 hours of birth. Treatment depends on the extent of the neurologic problems, the level of the lesions, and any complications, such as hydrocephalus or infection, that may be present. The early surgical interventions that are available today have significantly increased the survival rate of people with spina bifida, as well as their quality of life. In addition, greater awareness of the potential for complications has enabled health care personnel to treat the symptoms of complications as soon as they occur and also to take active measures to prevent complications from occurring.

### Psychosocial Issues in Spina Bifida

Spina bifida, as a congenital condition, produces important variances in life ex-periences that have a potential impact on the psychological and social development of the child. The degree to which the child achieves maturity and independence in later life is largely shaped by the biological, psychological, and social experiences of childhood.

When a child is born with a congenital disability, common parental reactions include denial, guilt, anxiety, rejection, anger, or overprotectiveness. If, during this vulnerable time, parents are not provided with necessary support, parent-infant attachment and bonding may be altered, leading to disorders of parenting. Child-rearing style has a profound effect on the child's personality development. Parents who do not establish norms and expectations for a child's behavior may create a psychosocial disability that has a greater impact than the physical disability associated with the congenital condition. In addition, a secondary disability of social isolation may result from the amount of time needed for medical care and hospitalization. Early intervention, active steps to promote socialization, and family counseling may help to overcome many of these problems.

A normal part of development is gradual separation of parent and child emotionally. When this does not occur because of parental overprotectiveness or overinvolvement, the child may experience prolonged dependence and the inability to take control, which, in turn, adversely affects normal development and delays or impedes his or her ability to form an independent identity. As a result, the individual may develop emotional dependence and remain in the parents' home past maturity rather than establishing his or her own living environment.

Children with spina bifida and the resulting physical limitations may not be provided the same opportunities to test their physical and intellectual capabilities as are provided to able-bodied individuals of the same age group. Doubting the child's capabilities or setting expectations that are too high or too low can also contribute to low self-esteem and increased dependence. At times, in an attempt to boost the child's self-concept, parents, teachers, and others may shower a child with attention, emphasizing or humoring unrealistic expectations. In so doing, they may foster an egocentric personality that may be more of a handicap than any physical limitation the child experiences.

During adolescence, when a normal part of development is body image and the quest for identity, the child with spina bifida may experience anxiety over appearance, acceptance by peers, and sexuality. Difficulties with interpersonal relationships may rise from limited experience in learning and practicing social skills. Helping the individual develop appropriate social skills throughout his or her development can help him or her form relationships during adolescence and adulthood.

Sexual education is important regardless of the disability or the age of its occurrence. In the case of congenital dis-ability, issues of sexuality may be ignored as the individual reaches adolescence. As a result, individuals may have limited opportunity to explore or express sexual desires.

Anticipatory guidance provided to parents from the time they are first told about their child's diagnosis can be extremely helpful in preventing many of the problems that can affect the child's psychosocial development and can help the child gain full affective and personality growth and maturity. As the child goes through each stage of development, new needs and new demands arise. Social encounters outside the home should be encouraged as well as participation in sports, camping, and other adaptive recreational events designed to promote physical independence and social maturity.

### Vocational Issues in Spina Bifida

Unless the individual has associated mental retardation because of other complications associated with spina bifida, intellectual ability should not be altered. Limitations associated with spina bifida are dependent on the severity of the condition. Those individuals with paraplegia have the same functional limitations as individuals with paraplegia from other causes. Vocational success and ability to function in society are determined primarily by the emotional and personality development achieved throughout childhood.

## Poliomyelitis and Post-Polio Syndrome

Poliomyelitis, also known as *infantile paralysis*, or *polio*, is an acute infectious viral disease that was prevalent in the United States in the first half of the twentieth century. The virus enters the body when contaminated water or food is ingested or when hands that have been contaminated with the virus touch the mouth.

Poliomyelitis affects the nerve cells that control muscles. The brain stem, spinal cord, and neuromuscular system may be affected (Salcido, 2000). The nerve cells or *motor neurons* affected by the poliovirus are located in the *anterior horn* of the spinal cord and extend to the muscles. As neurons are affected, muscle cells lose the ability to contract, resulting in paralysis. If motor cells are able to overcome the virus, paralysis may be temporary. Motor cells unable to overcome the virus, however, die, resulting in permanent paralysis or in some instances weakness of affected muscles. The extent of paralysis is unpredictable. Although the disease primarily affects children, the devastating epidemics of polio that spread across North America and Europe from the 1930s to the mid-1950s severely disabled adults as well.

In 1955 Dr. Jonas Salk developed the inactivated poliovirus vaccine which was followed in 1960 with the development of a live, attenuated oral poliovirus vaccine by Dr. Albert Sabin. As a result of the vaccines, widespread immunization against polio was begun, and polio is now nearly abolished in the United States and other countries in which an immunization program is widely available. But although poliomyelitis has been nearly eradicated in the industrialized world, the residuals of the condition experienced by those who contacted the disease prior to immunization are still present. In addition, small outbreaks continue to occur in developing countries, and a few cases continue to appear in the industrialized world as well.

### Manifestations of Poliomyelitis

Individuals in the initial stages of polio are acutely ill. Initial symptoms are usually nonspecific, such as gastrointestinal or upper respiratory symptoms accompanied by fever. Symptoms later progress to headache, stiff neck, and muscle pains. Affected muscles become paralyzed or weakened. In some individuals only a small group of muscles are affected; in others, paralysis is widespread and may include the whole body. Extremity involvement is often asymmetrical, so that one extremity may have major paralysis while the opposite limb has only slight weakness or may not be affected at all. Although muscles are paralyzed, functions of sensation, bowel and bladder control, and sexual response are left intact.

When an extremity is involved in childhood during a time of continued growth, the rate of growth of the affected extremity is delayed, resulting in a smaller extremity when full growth is reached. The legs are most frequently affected; however, sometimes all four extremities are affected, sometimes only one extremity is affected, or sometimes paralysis extends to only the lateral half of the body (**hemiplegia**), with one arm and one leg being affected. This type of polio is called *paralytic polio*. When the poliovirus affects the brain stem, the muscles that control breathing and swallowing are also affected. This is called *bulbar polio*. When respiration is affected, individuals require mechanical respiratory support such as the "iron lung."

Functional limitations resulting from polio depend on the nerves affected and the degree of damage. Individuals with affected lower extremities have difficulty with ambulation and may require a wheelchair, cane, or braces. When upper extremities are involved, self-care skills may also be affected. If the trunk muscles are affected, a muscle imbalance may result, lead to **scoliosis** (lateral curvature of the spine), which can interfere with breathing as well as the functioning of internal organs.

After the initial acute episode of poliomyelitis, some degree of function may return, but some of the residuals are permanent. The degree of residual disability is dependent on the extent of the permanent damage to nerves that has occurred.

### Manifestations of Post-Polio Syndrome

Poliomyelitis itself is not a progressive condition. Consequently, many individuals who contracted the disease 30 or more years ago adapted to residual paralysis, muscle weakness, or other symptoms and went on to live productive lives with little medical intervention needed. In the 1980s, however, individuals who had previously been diagnosed as having poliomyelitis began to seek medical advice because of new symptoms that ranged from mildly to severely debilitating. At first they were not taken seriously. Many were classified as having "emotional disturbances," or symptoms were merely attributed to "aging." As more and more individuals who had had polio sought help for new symptoms, however, their symptoms were taken more seriously and the term *post-polio syndrome* was coined to describe this phenomenon.

Post-polio syndrome is a noncontagious neurological disorder that produces a variety of symptoms in individuals who had recovered from poliomyelitis many years earlier. Common symptoms of post-polio syndrome appearing 30 to 40 years after the acute bout of poliomyelitis include:

- abnormal muscle fatigue as well as generalized fatigue
- new muscle weakness in muscles not previously affected
- muscle pain (**myalgia**) and/or joint pain
- respiratory difficulty

The cause of post-polio syndrome is unknown (Burk & Agre, 2000). It appears that most of the motor neurons originally damaged in the initial bout of polio are involved in post-polio syndrome and that most individuals who had polio are at risk to develop the syndrome. Individuals who initially had experienced severe polio seem to be at greatest risk for developing post-polio syndrome; however, individuals less severely affected initially also can experience a decline in function. Those who had been able to walk without assistive devices may require them because of post-polio symptoms. Those who had used assistive devices for ambulation may find it necessary to begin using a wheelchair.

Post-polio syndrome is progressive, so deterioration will continue. Despite increasing decline, however, individuals will not return to the level of disability they experienced when polio was in its acute state. With appropriate exercise, strength and function can be improved and deterioration slowed, if not halted.

### Diagnosis of Polio and Post-Polio Syndrome

The diagnosis of poliomyelitis in its acute state is based primarily on the medical history of the individual and on the symptoms. Spinal tap or fecal sample can be used to confirm the diagnosis. The diagnosis of post-polio syndrome is, at times, more difficult.

One step in diagnosing post-polio syndrome is to identify or eliminate other conditions that may be responsible for the symptoms. Symptoms of post-polio syndrome may be difficult to distinguish from other degenerative disorders of muscles and joints, such as osteoarthritis or osteoporosis. General medical evaluation, routine laboratory tests, *electromyographic studies* (graphic record of the contraction of a muscle as the result of electrical stimulation), and *nerve conduction studies* may help to identify and exclude other diseases. *Magnetic resonance imaging* may be used to exclude other conditions of the spine that could cause similar symptoms (Burk & Agre, 2000).

### Treatment and Management of Post-Polio Syndrome

No specific treatment is available to alter the course of post-polio syndrome. Individuals with symptoms of increasing muscle weakness, fatigue, and pain should first have a thorough physical examination by a physician to rule out other potential causes of symptoms. Treatment is largely directed toward managing symptoms and helping individuals maintain functional status and independence as long as possible. Good health practices, including proper nutrition and adequate rest, are important.

Generalized fatigue is treated with lifestyle changes consisting of energy conservation measures. Physical activities should be paced to prevent excessive fatigue. Individuals may require frequent rest periods throughout the day. Using additional assistive devices, such as a wheelchair rather than crutches, may help to conserve energy.

Mild to moderate weakness may be treated by increasing muscle strength through nonfatiguing exercise. Exercises that are tolerable and that do not contribute to more weakness and fatigue may be prescribed. Physical therapists generally instruct individuals about proper exercise protocols so that overuse and excessive fatigue can be avoided. Individuals are instructed to exercise for short intervals, to rest between bouts of exercise, and to exercise only every other day to prevent excessive muscle fatigue.

Individuals with respiratory difficulty may require noninvasive positive-pressure ventilation at night. Because individuals with post-polio syndrome are more susceptible to infectious diseases, pneumonia and influenza vaccines are usually recommended. Tobacco use should be avoided.

The use of braces to decrease mechanical stress on joints may be necessary to help muscle and joint pain. Changes in orthotics or in the mode of ambulation may be required. Moving from braces or crutches to a wheelchair can also reduce stress on joints. If the individual with post-polio syndrome is overweight, weight

reduction may be recommended to reduce fatigue and stress on muscles and joints. For those whose respiratory muscles were also affected by the initial infection, weight control can also help to prevent respiratory difficulty.

### Psychosocial Issues in Post-Polio Syndrome

Since poliomyelitis is not a progressive disease, many individuals believed their recovery to be permanent and adapted and adjusted to the functional limitations and residual effects associated with the condition, going on to lead full and productive lives. Individuals with residual disability from polio have worked for years to minimize their disability and maximize their assets. Now, however, the unexpected symptoms associated with post-polio syndrome threaten their function and independence and can be psychologically devastating.

The symptoms of this new "secondary disability" can be frightening as well as frustrating for the individual, who again must adjust and adapt to continuing functional limitations, the potential use of new assistive devices, and an alteration in lifestyle. After regaining function previously through much physical and emotional effort, being forced to deal again with disability symptoms that are much like the initial symptoms can be discouraging. Individuals may reject new assistive devices because they symbolize the loss of a physical ability that they feel they earned through great effort.

### Vocational Issues in Post-Polio Syndrome

Many individuals with poliomyelitis have achieved gainful employment and lived productive lives with residuals of polio. The onset of symptoms related to post-polio syndrome, however, may make a number of alterations necessary in the work setting. In some instances, depending on performance requirements, the individual may be unable to perform all of the job duties. Thus altering job duties or retraining for other job duties may be necessary.

Even when remaining in the current job is possible, individuals may experience increased fatigue, so that frequent rest periods may be needed, or they may need a more sedentary job structure. The ability to lift, reach, walk, or climb may be altered.

The symptoms of post-polio syndrome, whether pain, weakness, or fatigue, may necessitate additional assistive devices. Individuals who once ambulated without assistive devices may require a cane, crutches, or braces. Individuals who once used crutches or braces may require a wheelchair for ambulation. Adapting the workplace to accommodate these devices may be necessary. If, because of increased symptoms and disability, the individuals' current mode of transportation is no longer accessible, transportation to and from work may be a barrier. In addition, because of increased disability, individuals may require additional time to get ready for work.

In some instances the onset of new symptoms and increasing limitations may result in depression, which can interfere with the individual's ability to work effectively. Supportive counseling may be necessary to enable the individual to cope with increasing disability.

## NEUROMUSCULAR CONDITIONS

### Parkinson's Disease

Parkinson's disease is a slowly progressive disorder of the central nervous system, leading to progressive impairment of motor function. Although its cause remains unknown, evidence suggests that both genetic and environmental factors may play a role (Janson, Leone, & Freese, 2002; Nussbaum & Ellis, 2003). Parkinson's disease involves extensive degenerative changes in the *basal ganglia* (the gray matter imbedded in the white matter of the brain, which has a role in complex movements) and the loss of or decrease in levels of *dopamine* (a neurotransmitter) in the basal ganglia. Most of the disabling symptoms associated with Parkinson's disease are due predominantly to drastic reductions of dopamine levels in the brain. Although Parkinson's disease occurs most commonly after the age of 50 (Litvan, 1998), greater awareness and improved methods of detection have increased the number of diagnosed cases of Parkinson's disease among younger individuals.

*Secondary parkinsonism* is a term used to describe a parkinsonian syndrome in which individuals experience Parkinson-like symptoms that are due to other causes. Secondary parkinsonism can be associated with the ingestion of certain drugs (prescription or illicit) or exposure to toxic substances, such as carbon monoxide or other chemicals. Secondary parkinsonism gained attention in the early 1980s when the "designer drug" MPTP, which mimicked the action of heroin, entered the street market. A number of young adults, after taking the drug, suddenly developed permanent signs and symptoms of severe Parkinson's disease. Some medications used to treat mental illness may also produce Parkinsonlike side effects if not closely monitored.

A variety of other conditions mimic Parkinson's disease, causing similar symptoms. These symptoms are collectively called parkinsonism and should be distinguished from Parkinson's disease.

### Manifestations of Parkinson's Disease

The four most common symptoms of Parkinson's disease include:

- tremor
- muscle rigidity
- **akinesia** (complete or partial absence of movement, or difficulty with voluntary movement, especially of the extremities)
- postural instability
  (Janson et al., 2002)

In early stages of the condition, individuals may exhibit extreme slowness in initiating or maintaining movements (**bradykinesia**). Individuals who have Parkinson's disease may walk with small, shuffling steps and may have difficulty rising from a chair or bed. They may find it difficult to initiate or to stop voluntary movements. While walking, for example, they may experience *gait hesitation* and suddenly "freeze," taking seconds to regain motion; in other instances, they may continue five or six more steps beyond where they want to stop. The impairment experienced with bradykinesia can interfere with activities such as shaving, buttoning clothes, or cutting food, all of which take longer and become more difficult to perform as the disease progresses. Because Parkinson's disease affects both the central and autonomic nervous systems, some individuals may also experience urinary or bowel problems.

Individuals with Parkinson's disease are sometimes said to have a poverty of spontaneous movement. They may blink less frequently and may develop a masklike, expressionless face. They may develop difficulty swallowing (**dysphagia**), which results in saliva accumulation and drooling. Because the individual is unable to swallow quickly, the rate of swallowing decreases and eating becomes slower and more deliberate as the condition progresses. As food collects in the mouth and the back of the throat, individuals may be prone to coughing and choking episodes.

Motor changes related to Parkinson's disease may cause speech changes related to incoordination and reduced movement of the muscles that control breathing, voice, pronunciation, and rate of speaking. Volume of speech may be decreased (**hypophonia**), and there may be no verbal inflections. Individuals' ability to write may also be affected. Reduction in amplitude of movement may affect individuals' ability to write so that their handwriting gradually becomes smaller and smaller (**micrographia**) until it is no longer legible.

Tremor of a limb, usually most noticeable in one hand, is the most frequent early symptom of Parkinson's disease. The tremor intensifies when the hand rests in the lap (*resting tremor*) and diminishes with voluntary movement. The tremor is not present during sleep, however.

The posture of individuals with Parkinson's disease becomes stooped, and their arms fail to swing with their stride when they are walking. The loss of postural reflexes makes it difficult for these individuals to maintain an upright position if they are suddenly bumped, increasing the risk of falls. To keep from falling, they may inadvertently quicken their steps as if to "catch up" with their own center of gravity. Muscle tone is increased, creating muscle rigidity, which also interferes with movement and causes severe im-mobility. Because greater effort is necessary to engage in voluntary movement, fatigue is also increased.

Mental and behavioral changes do not always occur as a result of Parkinson's disease, but cognitive changes, as well as changes in emotions and behavior, can be part of the symptoms. Dementia can also occur in some individuals later in the course of the condition. Apathy, passivity, depression, and loss of initiative may be noted. Some studies indicate that depression is present in a large number of individuals with Parkinson's disease and can have more impact on quality of life than the symptoms of the condition or the side effects of treatment (Phillips, 1999a). As the individual becomes aware of his or her decreasing cognitive abilities, depression related to losses may result. The degree to which depression reflects physiologic changes rather than a reaction to the disease itself is not known.

There is no cure for Parkinson's disease. The disease is characterized by progressive debilitation, although the progression occurs slowly over years. Treatment, usually in the form of medication, physical therapy, and exercise, along with maintenance of general health, can reduce the effects of the symptoms so that the individual with this condition may remain active longer.

### Diagnosis of Parkinson's Disease

There is no single test that can be used to diagnose Parkinson's disease. Individuals with initial symptoms are usually referred to a *neurologist* (physician who specializes in the evaluation and treatment of nervous system disorders) for evaluation. Physicians usually base their diagnosis on the presence of tremor, stiffness, and slow movement. Because many other conditions may have similar symptoms in early stages of development, and because initially symptoms may be attributed to aging, misdiagnosis can frequently occur (Aminoff, Burns, & Silverstein, 1997).

### Treatment and Management of Parkinson's Disease

Currently, there is no cure for Parkinson's disease; however, the administration of a medication called *levodopa* (L-dopa) frequently decreases its symptoms. Levodopa works by helping to increase the level of the *neurotransmitter dopamine* in the brain. At first, small amounts are usually prescribed, and the dosage is then gradually increased.

Although helpful, levodopa also can have serious side effects and limited long-term efficacy (Jankovic, 1999; Janson, Leone, & Freese, 2003). Some individuals may experience side effects such as nausea or abnormal involuntary movements called **dyskinesia**. These effects are generally related to the dosage of the medication, occurring more frequently with higher dosages. In some individuals, levodopa causes mental confusion or decreases alertness.

Exercise and activity are especially important for individuals with Parkinson's disease because of the tendency of the muscles to be stiff and rigid. Muscles can **atrophy** (become smaller, or shrink) without the stimulation that exercise provides, decreasing the individual's ability for self-care. Individuals are usually encouraged to engage in a daily exercise routine, such as walking a prescribed distance, doing simple calisthenics, or doing active range-of-motion exercises. Other aspects of treatment are directed toward preventing complications. Individualized physical therapy directed toward joint mobility, correction and prevention of postural abnormalities of trunk and limbs, and maintenance of normal gait are important to help individuals maintain function as long as possible. Passive stretching of extremities, muscle massage, resistive exercises, and training are techniques used by *physical therapists* to achieve this goal.

Neurosurgical intervention as a treatment for Parkinson's continues to be explored. One technique, *deep brain stimulation*, has been used with some success at specialized clinics in Europe and North America. The procedure involves implanting an electrode into a target area of the brain. The electrode is then tunneled under the skin to an external stimulator that can be switched on or off by the person with Parkinson's disease (Phillips, 1999b). Another surgical procedure, *pallidotomy*, consists of identifying and destroying the part of the basal ganglia that secretes the substances that are believed to destroy portions of the basal ganglia. Surgical procedures appear to be most helpful for those individuals who are unable to control symptoms satisfactorily with medication.

Parkinson's disease is a chronic, lifelong condition with progressive deterioration. Because of the gradual onset and slow progression of the condition, however, with appropriate assistive devices and other therapies most individuals have many years to remain productive and functional.

### Psychosocial Issues in Parkinson's Disease

Parkinson's disease has a profound impact on the individual's life, as well as on the family. Parkinson's disease is a visible neurological disorder. Not only is it difficult for the individual to move, but there is also stooped posture, flexed arms with lack of swinging when walking, and often tremor of an extremity. One aspect of the movement disorder is lack of facial expression and spontaneous movements when talking. Because they are unable to use these sources of body language, individuals have reduced capability for nonverbal communication. They may also experience speech disturbances as a result of motor difficulties; thus both verbal and nonverbal communication may be difficult. Acquaintances or strangers as well as family members may attribute lack of expression to disinterest, dementia, or low

intellectual ability. Individuals may become stressed or frustrated by the attitudes of others and consequently begin to withdraw from social interactions or be reluctant to participate in them.

Anxiety and depression may occur from the time of initial diagnosis and may continue as symptoms progress. For individuals who had prided themselves in efficiency, communication, or manual skills, deterioration of these skills can be particularly stressful. Stress can make symptoms of Parkinson's disease worse, further contributing to the individual's social isolation. Because the disease is progressively debilitating, the individual and his or her family must continually readjust to increasing loss of functional capacity, which can also contribute to anxiety and depression. If mental deterioration, confusion, or personality changes occur, family members may have increased difficulty coping. In some instances individuals with Parkinson's disease may also demonstrate decreased initiative and impaired judgment, which can be the source of additional stress for the family. As the individual becomes more dependent on others for self-care, the social support system may become further eroded.

Information regarding sexual function in Parkinson's disease is scarce; however, sexual problems are frequently present in neurological disorders. Depression is considered a contributor to sexual problems in the general population. Consequently, since individuals with Parkinson's disease frequently experience depression, it stands to reason that some sexual problems may exist. The medications taken to treat symptoms of Parkinson's disease may also contribute to sexual dysfunction. Factors associated with many types of chronic illness can cause lack of interest in sexual activities. As the time needed for treatment and for activities of daily living, such as dressing, eating, and cleaning oneself, increases, the interest in sexual activity and the energy for it may be decreased.

Activities of daily living such as dressing or bathing can be very tiring and time consuming. Individuals should allow enough time so they don't feel rushed. Since balance is sometimes a problem, special safety precautions, such as grab bars or a tub bench or shower chair, should be used when bathing. Clearing the environment of potential hazards that could cause the individual to fall can prevent the complications that could result from the fall. Walking aids such as crutches or walkers may be useful in helping individuals avoid falls.

### Vocational Issues in Parkinson's Disease

Whether persons with Parkinson's disease can continue working is an individual decision and based on the specific circumstances. In most instances, work that is more sedentary and that does not require significant verbal communication may be continued longer than work that requires more strenuous activity. Since individuals have difficulty with balance and gait, jobs that require considerable walking, stooping, or bending should be avoided. Transportation to and from work may be the largest obstacle to maintaining employment.

Highly stressful occupations should be avoided because stress tends to increase the severity of symptoms. For some individuals, work becomes increasingly difficult and the effort to continue working may produce a tremendous strain. For these individuals, not working may bring a sense of relief from the physical and mental stress of attempting to carry out various tasks and responsibilities. For others, the inability to work may have a detrimental

effect. In most cases, individuals will be able to continue working if the work is not extremely demanding physically or does not require manual dexterity. Scheduling frequent rest periods and restructuring the workload may help to increase the total amount of work that can be done during the workday. Because stiffness and muscle rigidity are common symptoms of the condition, working in a cold environment should be avoided because of the possible increase in muscle stiffness.

## Huntington's Disease (Huntington's Chorea)

**Huntington's disease** is a progressive, genetic condition of the central nervous system in which neurons in the basil ganglia of the brain degenerate. Most individuals develop symptoms between the ages of 30 and 50 years. The condition advances slowly and progressively. Although the rate of deterioration varies from person to person, as does the rate at which symptoms appear, Huntington's disease leads to total disability and death after 15 to 20 years (Cattaneo, Rigamonti, & Zuccato, 2002).

### Manifestations of Huntington's Disease

Huntington's disease is characterized by:

- cognitive deficits
- motor impairments
- behavioral changes

Cognitive changes usually occur in the early stages, with the individual at first becoming increasingly absent-minded and having difficulty with concentration. As the condition progresses, mental deterioration (**dementia**) occurs.

Early signs of motor impairments involve movements of the fingers, which give the impression that the individual is fidgeting. As the condition progresses, movement and coordination continue to deteriorate, with **bradykinesia** (slowness of movement) and rigidity interfering with the individual's ability to walk. Jerky, involuntary movements (**chorea**) are also present. Motor difficulty also affects the individual's ability to speak and to swallow.

The individual also experiences personality change. Behavioral changes associated with the condition range from delusions to impulse-control problems.

### Diagnosis of Huntington's Disease

Diagnosis is usually based on the individual's symptoms and family history. In most instances extensive neurological testing is not necessary. Evaluation is usually done by a *neurologist* (physician who evaluates and treats neurological disorders).

### Treatment and Management of Huntington's Disease

There is no known treatment to slow progression or to cure Huntington's disease. Treatment is usually directed toward preventing complications and treating symptoms. *Physical therapy*, a major component of the treatment program, can help the individual improve or stabilize motor ability, prevent contractures, or adapt the environment to promote safety and maximum independence. *Occupational therapists* may help individuals improve coordination abilities and activities of daily living skills. *Speech therapists* may help individuals maximize their speech capability as well as their ability to swallow. In some instances cognitive retraining and memory training may be useful. Avoiding exposure to upper respiratory infections as well as other communicable diseases is also advised.

It is sometimes difficult to distinguish which behavioral symptoms are related to the condition itself and which are related to the individual's anxiety about having the condition. Psychotropic medications may be used to help alleviate or control behavioral symptoms, regardless of their cause. Medication may be prescribed for anxiety or depression, irritability, or mood swings. In some instances psychotropic medication may also be used to control some of the involuntary, jerky movements individuals may be experiencing.

A major portion of treatment is directed to assisting individuals and their families manage self-care as the condition progresses. Individual counseling, family counseling, and genetic counseling of family members may be important interventions.

### Psychosocial Issues in Huntington's Disease

Individuals and their families must cope with continuing losses, both physical and mental, as the condition progresses as well as with the knowledge that Huntington's disease is a progressive condition in which continued deterioration can be expected. The cognitive and behavioral changes for affected individuals may make it more difficult for them to cope. Individuals as well as family members may feel helpless and hopeless. As a result, they may be reluctant to participate in activities designed to maintain or improve their current level of function.

Faulty judgment and impulsivity related to behavioral changes may result in unsafe situations for the individual. Those who are in denial about their condition and their limitations may also be exposed to situations that could result in unsafe practices or injury.

As the condition progresses, individuals become less able to care for themselves and thus become more dependent on others. As communication becomes more difficult, social interactions also become more difficult, resulting in increasing social isolation. Personality changes that may produce violent or hostile behaviors further stress support systems.

Because Huntington's disease has a genetic component, family members may be under the additional stress of knowing that they may themselves be at risk for developing Huntington's disease. Counseling, education, and support can help to reduce the stress that family members may be experiencing.

### Vocational Issues in Huntington's Disease

Huntington's disease is a progressive, degenerative disease; however, in the early stages before mental deterioration and physical incapacitation are present, short-term training may be appropriate. As the condition progresses and individuals have increasing difficulty with memory, communication skills, and physical ability, sheltered employment may be the most feasible alternative.

## Amyotrophic Lateral Sclerosis (ALS; Lou Gehrig's Disease)

Amyotrophic lateral sclerosis (ALS), also sometimes referred to as Lou Gehrig's disease in memory of the baseball player who died of ALS in 1941, is a progressive, degenerative condition in which there is destruction of the motor neurons (nerve cells that convey impulses to initiate muscular contraction). Damaged portions of the nerve tracts are replaced by scar tissue or plaques.

The cause of ALS is unknown, although current medical theory suggests a multifactorial etiology that may include genetic, viral, autoimmune, and neurotoxic fac-

tors (Rowland & Shneider, 2001; Walling, 1999). Individuals are usually affected in middle or later life, with males affected more frequently than women.

### Manifestations of ALS

Symptoms of ALS depend on the area of the nervous system affected; both upper and lower extremities are affected. There are two primary forms of ALS:

- Spinal form
- Bulbar form

The spinal form of ALS is characterized by muscular weakness, muscle **atrophy** (decrease in size), spasticity, and hyperactive reflexes. Individuals may first complain of tripping, stumbling, or awkwardness when walking or running. Others may complain of difficulty with simple activities such as buttoning a shirt or picking up small objects. In the bulbar form individuals may first notice difficulty in breathing, slurring of speech or lowered volume when speaking, or difficulty with swallowing.

As the condition progresses, symptoms become worse, spreading to other parts of the body so that eventually, whether the individual first experienced the bulbar or spinal form of ALS, he or she eventually experiences all the symptoms. Individuals become increasingly weak and immobile. Progressive paralysis leads to increasing loss of function so that finally individuals are completely dependent on others for help with all activities of daily living. Excessive production of saliva and difficulty in swallowing can cause drooling. Some individuals may also experience muscle pain as a result of muscle spasticity. They may experience respiratory muscle weakness leading to breathing problems, and in later stages of the condition they may require ventilatory assistance in order to breathe. Cognitive function, sensation, vision, hearing, and bowel and bladder function are usually not affected.

### Diagnosis of ALS

There is no reliable laboratory test to detect the presence of ALS. Diagnosis is usually based on the symptoms the individual exhibits and their progression and the individual's medical history, and by ruling out other causes for the symptoms.

### Treatment and Management of ALS

There is no cure for ALS, and no effective treatment is currently available. Treatment goals are generally directed toward helping individuals and their family cope with the disability and to help the individual with ALS to remain independent as long as possible, be comfortable, and avoid complications. Treatment of symptoms is used to maintain muscle function, relieve discomfort, and forestall complications such as respiratory infections and decubitus ulcers. Medications to reduce spasticity may be used; however, these can also increase muscle weakness and cause sedation. *Physical therapy* may be helpful to maintain function and to reduce the painful symptoms brought on by muscle spasm.

*Occupational therapists* can provide support and help individuals to adapt their environment in order to maximize functioning. Individuals with speech difficulties may utilize *speech therapists* to help them learn communication techniques. *Speech pathologists* may be utilized to help individuals who have difficulty with swallowing. If individuals have breathing difficulty, *respiratory therapists* may be used to help them learn techniques in respiratory management.

### Psychosocial Issues in ALS

The social, economic, and psychological impact of the condition is substantial. It is common for individuals with ALS to experience fear, anxiety, and depression, especially as the condition progresses and the individual recognizes rapid progressive deterioration of physical function. Because of loss of mobility and increased dependency, feelings of helplessness and powerlessness are also common. Some individuals may experience discouragement and become angry as their physical limitations increase. They may experience grief with each subsequent loss of function. There may be loss in social relationships leading to social isolation.

Changes in physical appearance and physical ability may cause individuals to question their self-worth. They may feel guilty because of their increased dependence on others and may express concern and frustration over the burden they feel is being placed on family members.

Family members are also affected. Family members' roles are often modified. Since individuals with ALS need substantial help with most activities of daily living, family members most often find themselves in a caregiving role even in the early stages of the individual's condition. Expenditures for medical care and equipment can be sizeable. If the individual with ALS is also the major breadwinner, financial issues may become a major concern. Family members may quit work to assume the caregiving role, which further contributes to financial distress. Family members may also have feelings of powerlessness, anger, or anxiety about the future. They may vacillate between resentment and guilt.

Despite the significant disability individuals with ALS experience, they retain their cognitive and intellectual ability and still have needs for recreation, entertainment, and companionship. Using special techniques and equipment that enhance their functional capacity and independence in self-care can help them exert personal control over their life and thus maintain self-esteem. Since communication is usually significantly affected, equipment such as voice amplifiers, or techniques such as eye blinking if individuals' condition has progressed so that they can communicate no other way, are means to help them maintain meaningful relationships.

### Vocational Issues in ALS

As ALS progresses, activity becomes more and more difficult. The condition generally progresses fairly rapidly over a course of 3 to 5 years, although some individuals survive for up to 10 years. Many individuals live productive lives after their diagnosis is made, continuing to work despite advanced symptoms. The degree to which they are able to continue working depends on the requirements of the job and how symptoms affect their ability to perform. Older age, female gender, short time from symptom onset to diagnosis, and disease severity are key prognostic factors (del Aguila, Longstreth, McGuire, Koepsell, & van Belle, 2003).

The physical demands of work should be light and sedentary. Even if the individual is still ambulatory, a wheelchair-accessible work environment should be considered, since individuals will require a wheelchair for ambulation as the condition progresses. Transfer may become more difficult in later stages of the condition. Since communication can also be a problem, occupations in which the ability to speak makes up an important part of the job should be avoided.

## Guillain-Barré Syndrome

**Guillain-Barré syndrome** is an inflammatory condition of the *peripheral nerves* (nerves lying outside the central nervous system). The exact cause of Guillain-Barré syndrome is unknown, but symptoms are almost always preceded by an infectious illness that has occurred about 10 days before. A particular bacterium appears to be commonly involved. Because of immunological differences, not everyone who is infected with the bacterium develops Guillain-Barré syndrome. However, some individuals develop antibodies in response to the virus that attack not only the bacteria but also peripheral nerves. As a result, these individuals develop Guillain-Barré syndrome.

### Manifestations of Guillain-Barré Syndrome

The severity of Guillain-Barré syndrome varies greatly. Some individuals may have only mild muscle weakness, whereas others may become totally paralyzed and develop complications such as inability to breathe, abnormal blood pressure or heartbeat, or other conditions that can be life-threatening. An acute and progressive condition, Guillain-Barré syndrome is characterized by muscular weakness that usually begins in the lower extremities and spreads upward (*ascending paralysis*). Paralysis of both upper and lower extremities can occur, and chest and facial muscles can be affected. Breathing can be affected so that ventilatory support is needed. The amount of paralysis varies: some individuals experience only mild footdrop, whereas others develop complete paralysis. Abnormal sensations, such as numbness, tingling, or the sense of something crawling under the skin in the feet, hands, or face, may also be present. Individuals may also experience muscle aches or back pain as early symptoms.

Symptoms develop rapidly, over hours to days, or sometimes over a few weeks.

Generally, they reach their maximum intensity within 3 to 8 weeks. For the most part, the symptoms are reversible, and recovery occurs after progression of the symptoms cease. Although most individuals recover completely, the rate of recovery is variable and can take up to 2 years. In some individuals, permanent disability or even death can result. Some individuals, even though they appear to have recovered, may develop fatigue with sustained activity. Poor endurance with regard to walking or other activities of daily living can be an ongoing problem.

### Diagnosis of Guillain-Barré Syndrome

Diagnosis is usually based on symptoms and physical examination. *Electromyography* may be used to differentiate symptoms from other causes of generalized weakness.

### Treatment and Management of Guillain-Barré Syndrome

Early treatment usually requires hospitalization. Treatment is primarily symptomatic and used to treat complications that may accompany Guillain-Barré syndrome. General physical rehabilitation is started early, usually under the guidance of a *physiatrist* (physician who specializes in rehabilitation and physical medicine). *Physical therapists* are usually involved in the early stages of the condition to help individuals prevent muscle **atrophy** (shrinkage), contractures, or pressure sores. *Occupational therapists* help individuals learn how to strengthen muscles, learn energy conservation techniques, and perform activities of daily living. If speech or swallowing is affected, a *speech therapist* may be needed to help individuals improve speech patterns or facilitate swallowing.

### Psychosocial Issues in Guillain-Barré Syndrome

The initial stages of the condition can be extremely frightening. Individuals who were healthy suddenly find themselves paralyzed and unable to care for themselves. If respiration is affected and individuals are placed on mechanical ventilation, the inability to breathe in itself is frightening. In addition, individuals on a respirator are unable to communicate, further adding to apprehension and feelings of helplessness.

Even though most individuals regain function, the unpredictability of the condition and progression of symptoms lead to fear, frustration, and concern for the future. Depending on the individuals' situation and the extent of time needed to recover, financial concerns, fear of permanent disability, and fear of dependence can be extremely stressful and can have long-standing psychological effects even after the individual has recovered.

### Vocational Issues in Guillain-Barré Syndrome

Because individuals with Guillain-Barré syndrome have, in many instances, been incapacitated for a lengthy period of time, most will require an extensive period of rehabilitation that may include driver retraining, learning to pace activities, and in some instances reemployment training. Individuals may, after a certain amount of activity, continue to experience muscle aches or other sensations that interfere with normal activity. Initially they may consider returning to work on a part-time basis and anticipate the need for periodic rest periods during the day. In the case of those who require a wheelchair for a period of time after hospital discharge, architectural barriers at their employment site should be considered.

## Myasthenia Gravis

*Myasthenia gravis* is a *neuromuscular* condition characterized by muscle weakness and fatigue. It is an *autoimmune* disease in which symptoms are caused by a decrease in the *neurotransmitter acetylcholine* at the point at which nerves initiate contraction of a muscle. The eyelids, muscles of the throat, and often muscles of the extremities are affected. A common symptom is **ptosis** (drooping) of the eyelid. Speech, chewing, and swallowing may also be affected.

Diagnosis is usually based on symptoms and physical examination. Treatment with medications in most instances enables individuals to live productive lives with no significant disability.

## Muscular Dystrophy

*Muscular dystrophy* refers to a group of hereditary conditions that are characterized by progressive muscle weakness, muscle wasting, contractures of the joints, and deformity. Some forms of the condition are rapidly progressive.

Symptoms lead to impairment in ambulation and mobility and often arm function. If facial muscles or muscles of the gastrointestinal tract are affected, feeding and speech difficulties may also be present. In some forms of the condition, mental retardation may occur.

There is no specific treatment for muscular dystrophy; however, *physical therapy* is essential to help individuals prevent contractures of the joints and maintain muscle strength and maximum functional capacity.

## OTHER CONDITIONS OF THE NERVOUS SYSTEM

### Multiple Sclerosis

Multiple sclerosis is a multifaceted, progressive condition of the central nervous system with myriad physical and psychological consequences. It is one of the most common disabling neurological diseases in young adults (Confavreux, Vukusic, Moreau, & Adeleine, 2000; McDonald, 2000; Noseworthy, Lucchinetti, Rodriguez, & Weinshenker, 2000). Most experts now believe that multiple sclerosis is an *autoimmune condition* in which the body's immune system attacks segments of *myelin*, the protective sheath that surrounds and insulates message-carrying nerve fibers (*axons*) in the brain and spinal cord (Dyment & Ebers, 2002; McDonald, 2000; Wekerle & Hohlfeld, 2003). The term *multiple sclerosis* comes from the multiple areas of scarring or **sclerosis** that occur when myelin surrounding nerve fibers in the brain and spinal cord is destroyed. The scar tissue that replaces the areas of myelin that have been destroyed interferes with the transmission of nerve impulses, causing neurological deficits.

What triggers the autoimmune response, causing the body to attack myelin, is unknown. Genetic predisposition and geographic factors appear to have some role in determining susceptibility to multiple sclerosis. Individuals with northern European heritage and those living in more temperate climates appear to be more susceptible (Lutton, Winston, & Rodman, 2004). There is speculation that genetic factors alone do not increase susceptibility, but rather that the interaction of genetic predisposition with environmental factors or exposure to a virus predisposes individuals to develop the condition (Dyment et al., 2002). Multiple sclerosis most often affects young adults between the ages of 20 and 40, with about 70 percent of cases being women (Johnson & Baringer, 2001).

### Manifestations of Multiple Sclerosis

The symptoms and the extent of disability experienced with multiple sclerosis vary from individual to individual, depending on the location and extent of myelin destruction. Symptoms are diverse and unpredictable, appearing in varying combinations and patterns. Consequently, not all persons with a diagnosis of multiple sclerosis experience the same symptoms or progression of the condition.

The most common initial symptoms of multiple sclerosis are dizziness; sensory disturbances, including numbness, weakness, and spasticity, especially of the lower extremities; unsteadiness; visual problems; or poor bowel and bladder control. Weakness and fatigue frequently accompany other symptoms. Symptoms fluctuate, becoming worse at times (**exacerbation**) and better at other times (**remission**) (Antel & Bar-Or, 2003).

Loss of motor, sensory, intellectual, or emotional function may be associated with multiple sclerosis, depending on the part of the central nervous system affected. Symptoms vary greatly not only from person to person, but also from time to time in the same person. Because of the variability and fluctuation of symptoms, diagnosis of the condition is often a challenge. Before being diagnosed with multiple sclerosis, many individuals have gone from one health provider to another with a host of vague complaints and clinical symptoms that health professionals may attribute to fatigue, stress, or even laziness and withdrawal. Often, the condition is not recognized or diagnosed immediately because the symptoms have resolved by the time the individual sees a physician. Before the condition is diagnosed, individuals may experience considerable anxiety, self-doubt, and depression because of the continuing vague symptoms that cannot be explained.

As symptoms become more pronounced, permanent dysfunction in a variety of areas becomes more apparent. Symptoms may include **paresthesia** (a sensation of numbness or tingling in some part of the body); weakness of an extremity; visual disturbances, such as **diplopia** (double vision) and dimness of vision; and **vertigo** (dizziness or false sensation of circular movement). Individuals with multiple sclerosis may develop difficulty with coordination and balance (**ataxia**), a symptom that may be misinterpreted by the casual observer as indicating intoxication. There may be partial or complete paralysis of any part of the body or spasticity of muscles, especially in the lower extremities. A particular tremor of the hands, called *intention tremor*, may be present. The tremor is called *intention tremor* because it occurs only when the individual tries to engage in a purposeful activity, such as reaching for a glass.

Speech may be slurred, or there may be scanning speech, in which the individual enunciates slowly with frequent hesitations at the beginning of a word or syllable. Individuals with multiple sclerosis may also have difficulty in swallowing (**dysphagia**), which can contribute to choking.

Multiple sclerosis may also affect the genitourinary tract, causing **incontinence** (loss of control of the bladder or bowel). Some individuals may experience *urinary retention* (the inability to empty the bladder of urine). Sexual function can also be affected. Men may experience erectile dysfunction and women may experience decrease in sexual desire, lubrication problems, or inorgasmia (McCabe, McDonald, Deeks, Vowels, & Cobain, 1996). However, women with multiple sclerosis are able to become pregnant and carry pregnancy to term. There is no evidence that pregnancy causes an increase in symptoms or exacerbations of the condition (Hansell, 1995).

Some individuals experience cognitive changes as a result of multiple sclerosis, but intellectual function remains intact for many. Some individuals, however, may experience impairment in performing tasks that require conceptualization, memory, or new learning, as well as difficulty with tasks that require either rapid or precise motor responses. Some may have difficulty with abstract reasoning and problem solving. Depression is common, although the degree to which it is a reaction to the disease or a manifestation of neurological dysfunction is not known. Other individuals, rather than experiencing depression, experience an inappropriate euphoria.

### Treatment and Management of Multiple Sclerosis

The diagnosis of multiple sclerosis is based on the results of a full neurological examination and tests such as *magnetic resonance imaging*. There is no specific treatment for multiple sclerosis, nor is there a cure. Treatment is usually directed toward controlling individual symptoms and preventing exacerbations and complications. Treatment may improve symptoms somewhat or help to prevent or delay future exacerbations of symptoms, but it can have risks that must be carefully weighed by each individual. Consequently, the potential side effects of each treatment must be weighed against the potential benefit for functional capacity or delay of decline.

A variety of medications may be used to treat specific symptoms. Some medications may exacerbate symptoms or adversely affect remaining function, and some have the potential to impair memory and learning. Consequently, the type of medication prescribed varies with the individual. Medications are commonly used for bladder management, control of spasticity, or emotional symptoms.

Although some individuals with multiple sclerosis never experience urinary problems, for those who do, *anticholinergic medications*, which inhibit the actions of the parasympathetic nervous system, are sometimes helpful in relieving bladder symptoms such as frequency and urgency. Conversely, *cholinergic medications*, which stimulate the actions of the parasympathetic nervous system, may be helpful in relieving urinary retention. When urinary problems are present, individuals may be referred to a *urologist* (physician who specializes in evaluation and treatment of the genitourinary tract). Bladder training may be helpful in reducing bladder problems and in helping the individual to manage bladder control. Use of a catheter or sanitary pads may also decrease the embarrassment of possible leakage of urine. Other ways of managing bladder control are monitoring the time of day that fluids are ingested and ensuring a ready availability of restrooms to minimize the chance of accidents. If individuals have problems with urinary retention, they may be taught to insert a catheter into their bladder to drain accumulated urine.

Most patients to some degree experience spasticity. *Relaxants* or *antispasmodics* may be prescribed for muscle spasm or spasticity; however, at doses high enough to control spasticity, weakness may be exacerbated.

*Steroids* are at times prescribed, especially in acute phases of exacerbations to suppress the symptoms, but they do not affect the progression of the disease. Because of the potential harmful effects of steroids taken over extended periods of time, they are usually prescribed only on a temporary basis to decrease exacerbations, and not as ongoing therapy.

Individuals who experience depression or anxiety may have *antianxiety agents* or *antidepressants* prescribed. Since suicide rates are relatively high among individuals with multiple sclerosis (Livneh & Antonak, 1997), psychiatric consultation may also be indicated.

In general, individuals with multiple sclerosis should remain as active as they can without developing excessive fatigue. *Physical therapy* may be prescribed to help with problems of mobility or with the use of assistive devices, such as walkers, if needed. Specific exercises that help to decrease calcium loss from bones, strengthen weak muscles, and maintain muscle strength and joint mobility may also be prescribed. Physical therapy that includes massage and passive range-of-motion exercises may also be beneficial. Individuals with multiple sclerosis who experience speech problems may be referred to a *speech therapist* or may use *assistive devices*, such as a communication board and voice amplifier.

For many individuals with multiple sclerosis, exposure to heat can have a temporary adverse effect on symptoms. Environments in which body temperature is increased, such as during hot or humid weather, illness with fever, or even a hot bath, can make the individuals feel worse, although heat does not necessarily cause a worsening of the condition itself. Individuals should therefore avoid hot and humid environments.

Since there is no cure for multiple sclerosis, it is a lifetime condition. Multiple sclerosis is usually not fatal, and most individuals with the condition can expect to live a normal life span, although with varying degrees of disability. There is no formula for estimating the general outcome for all individuals. Symptoms often fluctuate with periods of **remission** (when symptoms get better) and periods of **exacerbation** (when symptoms get worse). Although the symptoms may partly resolve when the disease is in remission, exacerbations can leave permanent residual defects.

The condition and deterioration of function show no predictable pattern. The general prognosis for individuals with multiple sclerosis is unpredictable, with varying rates of progression and varying rates of disability. For some individuals (about 20 percent) the condition remains relatively stable with only mild symptoms, such as slight weakness, unsteadiness, or vision problems, and no long-term disability. The majority of individuals (about 65 percent) develop a *relapsing-remitting pattern* in which there are continuing exacerbations when symptoms become worse with periods of complete or partial remission in which there is no significant overall disability or restriction of general activity. Many of these individuals retain their mobility 20 or more years after diagnosis, with limited disability (Schapiro, Scheinberg, Weiner, & Wolinsky, 1997). For some individuals the disease progresses slowly with no remissions and gradually increasing disability. Still others experience rapid progression with total disability.

### Psychosocial Issues in Multiple Sclerosis

Most individuals with multiple sclerosis are young adults who have lived through formative years of childhood and adolescence as relatively healthy individuals and are at a stage of their life in which they are beginning to assume many social and economic responsibilities, such as choosing a career, establishing intimate personal relationships, and perhaps starting a family. When the diagnosis of multiple sclerosis has been established, the limitations and unpredictability of the condition can severely affect the individual's self-concept. Restrictions on abilities, activities, and social relationships call for significant initial psychosocial adjustment and alteration of self-concept as well as continual readjustment as exacerbations, remissions, and new disabling features of the condition occur. Consequently, the long-term experience of living with multiple sclerosis through young adulthood, middle age, and older adulthood requires not only initial acceptance of the condition but also continued flexibility and adjustment as the condition changes.

The ambiguity of the condition and the erratic nature of the symptoms produce significant stress. When the diagnosis of multiple sclerosis is finally established, individuals may react in a number of ways. Those who have been newly diagnosed may be unwilling to accept the diagnosis and continue to search for someone who will provide an alternative diagnosis. In other cases, individuals who have searched for years for an explanation for their vague and elusive neurological symptoms may feel a sense of relief at finally being given a diagnosis to explain what they have been experiencing. Others may react with shock and disbelief; still others may react with fear and anxiety. As with other chronic conditions, the individual's reaction to the diagnosis of multiple sclerosis is dependent on a number of individual factors.

As the diagnosis and implications of the condition are accepted, individuals may attempt to gain some control over the condition and its symptoms. Although they may adapt to the realization that multiple sclerosis is a lifelong condition, the unpredictability of the condition is still a source of stress. Despite planning, unforeseen exacerbations may occur, interfering with plans and activities without warning. Exacerbations can renew a sense of vulnerability, undermining optimism or enthusiasm for long-range planning and causing anxiety about the future.

Even when individuals have mild cases of multiple sclerosis, manifestations of the condition can be stressful. In mild cases, individuals may have few visible symptoms or may experience only vague symptoms of weakness or fatigue. Family, friends, or colleagues, unable to observe visible signs of disability, may be unable to understand why they cannot keep pace with others or continue to perform all the tasks in the same time frame as they were once able to do. They may be accused of being lazy or attempting to get out of activity when actually their level of energy is reduced because of the condition. As a result, they may attempt to push themselves beyond their capability or beyond what is in their own best interest with regard to management of their condition.

Bladder problems resulting from multiple sclerosis may cause embarrassment, causing the individual to withdraw from social and work activities. A variety of steps can be taken to minimize the social limitations that such problems may present, as described previously.

Although alcohol is not contraindicated for most people with multiple sclerosis, if balance problems are experienced as a result of the condition, alcohol will compound the problem. Likewise, alcohol can be dangerous when taken in combination with some medications. Consequently, individuals with multiple sclerosis should always consult their physician before deciding whether alcohol may be consumed on social occasions. Because of the wide variation of disease progression and its associated functional limitations, comprehensive evaluation of the individual's environment must be established so that adequate modifications and compensations can be made. Increasing the functional capabilities of each person has the potential to reduce the social and psychological impact of multiple sclerosis.

### Vocational Issues in Multiple Sclerosis

Many individuals with multiple sclerosis experience problems with unemployment and underemployment (Bishop, Tschopp, & Mulvihill, 2000). Educational attainment, symptom severity, and the presence of cognitive limitations appear to be significant predictors for employment status for a number of individuals (Roessler, Rumrill, & Fitzgerald, 2004). Since multiple sclerosis varies greatly among different persons, each individual's vocational potential must be considered separately. Those with mild symptoms, slowly progressive multiple sclerosis, or those who have extended periods of remission are capable of being gainfully employed for many years. Others, with more serious manifestations of the condition, can, with appropriate accommodations and assistive devices, often remain employed despite exacerbations or progression of the condition.

Mobility, communication, vision, and cognitive function are common areas that need to be addressed. The specific accommodations and needs of each individual must be evaluated. For example, those who experience symptoms requiring the use of a wheelchair will need wheelchair accommodations. Those with communication difficulties, such as slurred speech, may need other types of accommodations or considerations regarding job placement. Individuals with balance problems may need to avoid situations in which falling could be hazardous or may need a walking aid, such as a cane or crutch, that could be helpful in preventing a catastrophic fall. If vision is affected, specific accommodations related to visual needs may be warranted. If cognitive function is affected, individuals may benefit from cognitive retraining or memory enhancement programs (Roessler, Fitzgerald, Rumrill, & Koch, 2001).

Emotional stress as well as physical stress can cause a temporary worsening of symptoms. The degree of emotional stress the individual experiences on the job, as well as the level of physical activity required, should be considered. Excessive fatigue, particularly to the point of overexhaustion, should be avoided. Although individuals do not need to curtail physical activity, they should attempt to avoid pushing themselves to exhaustion. They may minimize the effects of fatigue on job productivity by learning to pace themselves so that activities are planned when energy levels are higher, such as at the beginning of the day. Individuals should also learn to moderate their pace of activities and find levels conducive to optimize energy. Frequent rest periods may be needed throughout the day. It may be important to break tasks into smaller steps, resting at intervals in between. Adapting work hours to individual needs, involving individuals in more sedentary work, or using energy-saving technology may be advisable to increase work capacity.

Because heat also affects symptoms, individuals should avoid hot and humid environments. They should avoid prolonged exposure to the sun and during hot days stay in an air-conditioned environment as much as possible.

Individuals with multiple sclerosis have increased susceptibility to complications from infectious disease. Therefore, environments in which there is significant exposure to people with colds, flu, or other infectious diseases should be avoided. Although there are limitations associated with the condition, many people with multiple sclerosis are able to continue to work with only minor adjustments. Loss of time at work during exacerbations should be expected; however, generally these episodes are not excessive. Assistive devices, new equipment, ready access to restrooms, and job restructuring can enhance the individual's ability to continue work. Specifically, environmental factors, accommodations that allow for more sedentary work, flexible schedules, and use of technology can all be instrumental in helping individuals with multiple sclerosis maintain employment.

## Central Sleep Apnea

Sleep apnea is one of the most chronic disorders of adults and the second most common breathing disorder during sleep (Drazen, 2002). Sleep apnea is characterized by frequent episodes of **apnea** (cessation of breathing) during sleep (Gottlieb, 2002). The result is daytime sleepiness, which is a significant problem because it can increase the incidence of traffic accidents (Yamamoto, Akashiba, Kosaka, Ito, & Horie, 2000). Lack of sleep also causes stress, so that affected people become irritable, undergo changes in personality, or have difficulty with memory, causing social and family disruption (Findley, Smith, Hooper, Dineen, & Suratt, 2000). It can also lead to disability because of the increased risk of **hypertension** (high blood pressure) and heart disease (Nieto, Young, Lind et al., 2000; Roux, D'Ambrosio, & Mohsenin, 2000;

Shahar, Whitney, Redline et al., 2001) and in some instances death (Drazen, 2002; Veale, Chaileux, Hoorelbeke-Ramon et al., 2000).

There are two types of sleep apnea. The most common type, *obstructive sleep apnea*, is discussed in Chapter 12. The second type of sleep apnea, *central sleep apnea*, occurs when the brain fails to send appropriate messages to the muscles needed to initiate breathing. It can be caused from stroke, infections affecting the brain stem, or neuromuscular diseases that involve respiratory muscles.

## Narcolepsy

**Narcolepsy** is a complex neurological sleep disorder involving the central nervous system that is linked to a disruption of the sleep control mechanism (Siegel, 2000). It is characterized by episodes of excessive sleepiness and uncontrollable sleep during the day (Stansberry, 2001). It can occur at any time and during any activity, such as while engaging in conversation, while driving, eating, or even when reading (Siegel, 2000).

Diagnosis is usually based on a persistent history of excessive daytime sleepiness not due to other causes and is confirmed through tests conducted at a sleep-disorders clinic. Treatment usually consists of planned short nap periods during the day, and in some instances prescription of central nervous system stimulants.

The physical, psychosocial, and vocational implications of narcolepsy can be devastating. Individuals who are not adequately diagnosed and treated have a high risk of motor vehicle accidents and may have difficulty reaching their full potential either in school or in employment (Siegel, 2000). Even with treatment, symptoms of narcolepsy may not be adequately managed. The fear of the embarrassment that may result from an attack can cause individuals to limit their social interactions. Safety concerns regarding operation of potentially dangerous equipment may be an issue if the individual's symptoms are not adequately controlled. Employers, teachers, and others coming in contact with the individual should be helped to understand the individual's condition so that if an attack does occur, symptoms will not be misinterpreted.

## Lyme Disease

**Lyme disease** is a multisystem inflammatory disease that affects the nervous system as well as the joints and muscles. It is the result of an infection caused by a type of organism called a *spirochete* and is transmitted by an infected tick. In the early stages it is characterized by a reddened area around the site of the tick bite.

Lyme disease is rarely, if ever, fatal and is not contagious. Although most people, if treated early, have no permanent disability, some individuals can go on to develop other abnormalities of the central nervous system, including gait spasticity, facial palsy, memory loss, mild confusion, joint pain, or meningitis (Hayes & Piesman, 2003).

Diagnosis is usually based on symptoms and blood tests. Early treatment with antibiotics can significantly improve outcome and prevent chronic affects.

## Bell's Palsy

Sudden partial or complete paralysis of one side of the face is characteristic of Bell's palsy (Salinas, 2002). Individuals may experience a sagging eyebrow, inability to close their eye, and drooping of one side of the mouth. Bell's palsy occurs when a nerve running from the brain to the face becomes inflamed. As the inflam-

mation progresses, the nerve swells, becomes compressed, and is no longer able to transmit signals; consequently, paralysis results. A growing body of evidence links reactivation of herpes viruses with the development of a large number of cases of Bell's palsy (Gilbert, 2002).

Although most individuals recover from Bell's palsy within a month, during the acute phase, if they are unable to close their eye, the eye may need to be protected with an eye patch, or artificial tears may need to be used. Individuals may also have anti-inflammatory steroids prescribed soon after the symptoms appear.

## DIAGNOSTIC PROCEDURES IN CONDITIONS OF THE SPINAL CORD OR NEUROMUSCULAR OR PERIPHERAL NERVOUS SYSTEM

In addition to the diagnostic procedures discussed in Chapter 2, X-ray and electromyography may be used to diagnose neuromuscular conditions or conditions involving the peripheral nerves.

### Spine Roentgenography (X-ray)

X-ray films of the spine are called *spinal X-rays* and are used to identify fractures or other abnormalities of the vertebrae and to evaluate the spaces between vertebral discs of the spinal column. X-ray films are usually taken by a *radiology technician*. The films are then read and interpreted by a **radiologist** (physician who specializes in radiology).

### Electromyography (EMG) and Nerve Conduction Velocity Studies

*Electromyography* is a procedure used to evaluate the electrical activity of certain muscles and is helpful in the diagnosis of certain muscle diseases. It may be performed by a physician, physical therapist, or specially trained technician. A small needle that is attached to an electrode is inserted into the muscle being examined, and the electrical activity of the selected muscle is recorded both at rest and during exercise. *Nerve conduction studies* are often performed in conjunction with EMG and are helpful in diagnosing conditions affecting *peripheral nerves*. For the nerve conduction portion of the procedure, a stimulating electrode that delivers a mild electrical charge is placed on the skin over a nerve. An electrode placed over a muscle records the activity of the nerve distally at the nerve-muscle junction. EMG makes it possible to identify defects in the transmission of impulses from nerves to muscles. It may be used in the diagnosis of a number of neuromuscular disorders and peripheral nerve injuries.

## GENERAL ISSUES IN NERVOUS SYSTEM CONDITIONS

Conditions of the nervous system have widespread effects. Physical deficits can prevent individuals with such disorders from performing even routine self-care. Problems with speech can alter the way individuals communicate. Emotional ability may cause difficulty in social relationships. Cognitive deficits may interfere with work as well as everyday activities such as managing finances, performing household tasks, or carrying out self-care activities.

Symptoms of some conditions of the nervous system, such as epilepsy, can be controlled with medication. Other conditions, such as multiple sclerosis and Parkinson's disease, involve progressive deterioration, and treatment focuses on controlling symptoms, preventing complications, and promoting function and independence as long as possible. When there has been permanent damage to the nervous system, such as that caused by head injury or spinal cord injury, treatment is directed toward rehabilitation and prevention of complications.

In many instances, treatment of nervous system disorders involves helping individuals to compensate for neurological deficits or to learn alternative methods of performing routine tasks. Assistive devices such as canes, braces, and wheelchairs may be indicated for individuals with special motor needs. Other means of assistance for individuals with neurological disorders that interfere with motor function are "help animals," such as dogs or monkeys that have been especially trained to retrieve various items or to perform other tasks that are difficult or impossible for an individual with a neurological disorder.

## Psychosocial Issues in Conditions of the Nervous System

### *Psychological Issues*

Adjustment to any chronic condition or disability can be difficult. Individuals with neurological disorders may face particular challenges because their disorders affect many different functional areas. As with all disabling conditions, psychological reactions are individually determined, based in part on the way the individual has dealt with life problems in the past. Individuals with traumatic brain injury, stroke, or multiple sclerosis may have cognitive and emotional impairments as well as impairment of motor function as a direct consequence of their injury or condition. Because they need to learn compensatory strategies for a number of activities and social interactions, psychological adaptation to the disorder becomes multifaceted. It is often difficult to determine the degree to which behavioral and affective changes are physiologic and the degree to which they are situationally induced.

For many neurological conditions, available treatment is limited and directed mainly toward controlling symptoms or preventing complications. As a result, individuals with these conditions may feel they have little control over the condition or their future. When conditions are progressively debilitating, as in multiple sclerosis or Parkinson's disease, individuals must continually readjust as additional functional capacity is lost. Under these circumstances, they may experience a helpless rage or bitterness because of a condition over which they have no control.

The rate of progression and degree of loss of functional capacity in many neurological conditions are often unpredictable. The uncertainty about whether disability will be minimal or will progress to severe disability can produce stress and hardship. Although wheelchair use can provide mobility and an added sense of freedom and independence, some individuals may have a negative emotional reaction to using a wheelchair, viewing it instead as a symbol of the inability to walk. In other instances, even though the disability experienced is minimal, they may grieve over the lost ability to function.

Often conditions of the nervous system not only impose permanent loss of function, but also involve complex self-concept and body image changes. Traumatic brain injury, stroke, and spinal cord injury provide no time for gradual adjustment. Individuals who had been previously active are suddenly faced with adjusting to loss of functional capacity and alteration in physical appearance.

Reactions may include hostility, anger, or withdrawal.

Individuals injured because of accidents may feel remorse or self-recrimination for failure to prevent the accident from occurring. If the accident was the fault of a third party, they may feel chronic anger toward the offender or may turn anger inward and become depressed. In some instances, the quest for retribution becomes a negative force, eroding the individual's life as he or she continually seeks some sort of justice.

By their very nature, symptoms of many neurological conditions necessitate assistance in care and function. Individuals may harbor resentment over the dependency imposed by the condition. Those who experience paralysis may feel an increased sense of vulnerability, fearing that escape from a dangerous situation or defending themselves against threat would be difficult or impossible. Their reaction may vary from overdependence to overcompensation, in which they take unnecessary risks to test or prove their independence and strength.

When there is loss of the capacity to care for basic physical needs, this loss is difficult to accept. Learning to accept necessary assistance from others for basic needs, such as feeding, personal hygiene, and bowel and bladder care, requires reconstituting views of privacy and self-reliance. Impairment of bladder and bowel control may be an especially difficult area of adjustment. Not only are such activities private and mishaps a potential source of embarrassment, but both may also be associated with the shame and humiliation experienced in early childhood when control of these most basic bodily functions was a central issue of development.

Most individuals with neurological disorders adjust and learn to be self-reliant, despite the fact that their ability to care for their basic physical needs is decreased. Those who have experienced disability as a result of an accident may turn their experience into a positive force directed toward broader social issues, such as seat belts in automobiles, helmets for motorcyclists, or laws against drunk driving. Other individuals use their experience to create public awareness of the needs of individuals with a disability and to educate others about disability issues. Just as neurological conditions have a spectrum of functional consequences, so also the adjustment of individuals with neurological conditions is highly individualized, and no two individuals with the same disability will have a reaction that is quite the same.

### Lifestyle Issues

The effects of neurological disorders on an individual's lifestyle are varied and complex. Activities of daily living are often altered so that help from family members or others is necessary. Subsequent loss of privacy for most intimate details of daily life, such as bathing or other aspects of self-care, may be part of the general condition. Even when individuals are able to manage their own personal care, the additional time required to carry out most activities may be considered a liability.

Special adaptations may have to be made within the environment, such as widening doorways for wheelchairs, lowering countertops in kitchens, raising toilet seats, and adding ramps and railings. Although not all neurological conditions require the use of a wheelchair, most require some consideration of environmental factors. For example, individuals with epilepsy may need to avoid environmental conditions such as flashing lights, which may precipitate seizures. Because

those with multiple sclerosis may be especially sensitive to hot, humid conditions, they may need to remain in a cool environment with decreased humidity. Individuals with balance or coordination problems caused by brain injury may need to avoid uneven terrain or other situations in which they may fall or be thrown off balance.

Alterations in daily schedules and routines may be necessary to allow additional time for dressing, bathing, and other self-care needs. If wheelchairs are used, the environment must be made navigable. Wheelchairs can provide more freedom of movement for those with paralysis, for those who have difficulty walking because of problems with coordination, or for those who fatigue easily and use a wheelchair to conserve energy. Freedom of movement is limited, however, if there are stairs but no elevator, if bathrooms are too small to accommodate a wheelchair, or public transportation is unequipped with lifts or mechanisms for transporting individuals in wheelchairs.

Individuals with neurological disorders can usually drive, even with paralysis, if the vehicle is equipped with special controls. If the disability includes cognitive or perceptual deficits, however, driving may not be possible. Although regulations vary from state to state, individuals with epilepsy may have to demonstrate that they have been seizure free or that medication has adequately controlled their seizures over a number of months or years before they are permitted to drive a motor vehicle.

When fatigue exacerbates the symptoms of a neurological disorder, as in multiple sclerosis, or when fatigue is part of the symptomatology, as in post-polio syndrome, it may be necessary to space out activities or to arrange for frequent rest periods during the day. It is sometimes helpful to divide activities that were once completed in a short amount of time into a series of smaller tasks, allowing rest periods in between.

A number of nervous system conditions can lead to sexual difficulties. Generally, physiologic responses require an intact nervous system. Sexual function may be most disrupted by conditions involving the spinal cord. Although women with a spinal cord injury are still capable of intercourse, sensory loss in the genitals is common in both men and women. Men may still experience reflex erections but are usually incapable of psychologically stimulated erections. Reproductive function may also be a concern after spinal cord injury. Women with such an injury generally remain fertile and are capable of conceiving and delivering a child. However, men with spinal cord injury may be infertile because of the inability to ejaculate, retrograde ejaculation, or decreased sperm formation.

Sexual intercourse may be more difficult in conditions involving spasticity, such as cerebral palsy or multiple sclerosis. In some instances, the stimulation and arousal experienced as part of sexual excitement may make the spasms worse. In other instances, special arrangements for positioning or other technical assistance may be necessary for sexual intercourse to occur.

Sexuality is more than genital acts of sex. Some form of sexual expression is possible for almost all individuals with a disability. Individuals may need to learn new forms of sexual expression to meet their needs, or in other instances they may need to learn to control sexual expression. For instance, individuals with quadriplegia may be helped to learn alternate means of sexual expression, or individuals with brain damage who exhibit sexual disinhibition may be helped to learn how to use appropriate social behaviors.

Although loss or alteration of sexual function is initially a severe blow to self-esteem and sense of attractiveness, individuals can express sexual feelings and needs through a variety of alternate means. Those with neurological disorders can develop long-term intimate relationships that include love, respect, and mutually satisfying expression of sexual feelings.

The financial impact of many neurological conditions can be devastating. The cost of medical care, rehabilitation, assistive devices, and environmental restructuring can be significant. The financial adjustments that must be made have a significant impact on the individual's general lifestyle. Assistance by various social agencies can help reduce the financial burden and reduce the stress caused by these concerns.

### Social Issues

Many factors associated with disorders of the nervous system can affect social function. A supportive environment, including the family, plays an instrumental role in individuals' response to disability. Misinterpretation or misperception of the individuals' disability and associated functional limitations, however, can act as a barrier to effective social interaction and personal adjustment.

Although some functional limitations associated with neurological conditions are visible, such as the mobility restrictions indicated by use of a wheelchair, others are not so readily recognizable. For example, the fatigue experienced in multiple sclerosis, the visual or perceptual problems experienced because of brain damage, or the difficulty with bladder control in spinal bifida may create a conflict of expectations when others do not understand the reason behind certain behaviors. Those who do not understand the consequences of multiple sclerosis may interpret fatigue as laziness or attempts to avoid work. Visual and perceptual problems associated with brain injury may be interpreted as clumsiness. Individuals with spina bifida who need ready access to a restroom may be viewed as having a neurotic preoccupation with the location of restroom facilities. The consequences of stroke, which may involve emotional lability or memory, attention, or judgment problems, may be perceived by others as rudeness, insensitivity, or irresponsibility rather than manifestations of the condition itself. The gait disturbance or slurred speech associated with multiple sclerosis may be viewed by others as a sign of intoxication.

In addition to the stigma often attached to disability, some conditions have associated myths or misinformation attached. Individuals with epilepsy, for example, may encounter social stigma because of outdated and erroneous beliefs about the cause or meaning of the seizures they experience. Seizures can be frightening for those who observe them. Lack of understanding may cause people to avoid social contact with individuals with epilepsy so as to avoid the possibility of witnessing a seizure. Misunderstanding may also cause people to avoid individuals with cerebral palsy with communication difficulties because they want to avoid the discomfort of attempting to understand what the individual is saying.

All chronic illness and disability affect family members and social interactions. Family members may become overly protective, shielding individuals from responsibility. Individuals may be excluded from family problems or decision making. In other instances family members may find it difficult to express anger toward their family member with a disability, instead coddling the individual or hiding their own displeasure over the individual's actions.

Some of the symptoms or behaviors manifested in the neurological condition may be more troublesome to the individual exhibiting the symptom than to those around them. Individuals may fear becoming a burden on family members and consequently withdraw from close personal interactions, while family members, willing and anxious to provide help and support, are hurt at what they view as the individual's rejection of their attempts to help. In other instances, individuals may assume that others would not want to interact with them because of their disability, when actually they are greatly admired by others because of their ability to cope.

Wheelchair use may also affect social function. Because not all social events or situations are accessible to individuals using a wheelchair, they may either avoid an activity or make special arrangements to attend it. Although most public places have made provisions for accessibility, some are more desirable than others. For example, a multilevel historic site may only be accessible to individuals in wheelchairs through a back entrance or freight elevator. In order to reach a stage for presentation, individuals may need to be "pushed" up a ramp rather than negotiate the ramp themselves. In addition, different angles of eye contact can create multiple emotional impacts for individuals in wheelchairs, who must continually look upward at their peers. This can produce an impression of differing social stature, both in the individuals and in those with whom they engage in conversation.

Social interaction difficulties associated with neurological disorders may be manifest in poor social performance, social anxiety, and low self-esteem. Individuals with such a disorder may experience considerable frustration, as well as lowered self-esteem and self-assurance, in the struggle to cope with social demands. Some neurological conditions result in impaired capacity for social perceptiveness, distractibility, an absence of social initiation, or behavioral problems (e.g., disinhibition or impulsivity). These symptoms can significantly affect individuals' ability to interact effectively in social settings. In these instances, social skills training or continuing supervision or prompting in the social setting can help individuals to integrate more fully into social situations.

## Vocational Issues in Conditions of the Nervous System

The capabilities of individuals with nervous system conditions vary widely, depending on the nature of the condition. For progressive conditions or conditions characterized by remissions and exacerbations, such as multiple sclerosis, ongoing evaluation of limitations and remaining function is necessary. For other conditions, such as spinal cord injury or traumatic brain injury, in which the damage is permanent but not progressive, initial evaluation of capabilities and remaining function may suffice.

Brain damage affects a number of functions, all of which should be assessed. Not only should cognitive functions, such as memory, problem-solving ability, and spatial and temporal orientation, be assessed, but also motor abilities, such as coordination, balance, speed of performance, and muscle dexterity.

The degree of job stress is a factor to be considered for those with a number of neurological conditions. In some instances, stress in the workplace may add to fatigue that is already a consequence of the condition itself. In other instances, stress may precipitate symptoms, as it does in epilepsy or multiple sclerosis. Moreover, when individuals who experience poor motor speed or decreased processing ability as a result of disability are rushed or feel stressed, the quality of their work may suffer.

When communication skills are affected by a neurological condition, alternate means of communicating in the workplace or job modifications may be needed. In many instances, even though individuals' communication may be difficult to understand, patience and practice allow coworkers to establish basic patterns of communication that make interchange in the workplace possible.

Some conditions have specific characteristics that must be considered in an assessment of the workplace. For example, for individuals with epilepsy it is important to assess the degree to which seizures are controlled and to identify whether any stimuli in the work environment could precipitate seizures. Hot, humid environments should be avoided by individuals with multiple sclerosis. Individuals with high thoracic spinal cord injuries or cervical injuries often experience difficulty with heat regulation and consequently should avoid extremes of temperature. In addition, because of the loss of sensation in the extremities, situations in which there is a possibility of burns or frostbite should be avoided. Individuals with spinal cord injuries, multiple sclerosis, or Parkinson's disease may be especially susceptible to upper respiratory problems. Consequently, the extent to which there is exposure to pollutants or upper respiratory infections, which could threaten respiratory function, should be considered.

Accessibility of the workplace should be evaluated if individuals use a wheelchair or other assistive devices and environmental factors could interfere with mobility. Availability of elevators as opposed to stairs, desk or workbench height, width of doorways, and size of bathrooms are all important environmental considerations.

In addition to the disability itself, a variety of other factors that could interfere with reaching full vocational potential should be considered. The availability of transportation, the additional time required for various activities, and the attitudes of coworkers can determine individuals' success or failure in the workplace. In all instances, a realistic appreciation of the individual disability is crucial. Because of the complexity and multifactorial aspects of nervous system conditions, each person and his or her specific needs and abilities should be considered. Expectations for performance may be too high or too low and may not match the individual's abilities. Consequently, viewing the individual as an individual with specific needs and abilities rather than putting him or her in a category is crucial for vocational success.

## CASE STUDIES

### Case I

Mr. G., a 27-year-old male, experienced a spinal cord injury (T-10) when he fell off a roof while working as a self-employed carpenter. He had been interested in being a carpenter since he could remember, and he wanted to follow in the footsteps of both his father and grandfather. He had attended high school, where he enrolled in building trades courses and mechanical drawing classes. He married his high school sweetheart several years after high school, and they now have two children. Mrs. G., who has been working as a legal secretary since their marriage, was devastated by the accident; however,

with the help of family who live nearby she has begun to adjust to the permanence of her husband's injury. Mr. and Mrs. G. live in a rural community of 2,000, and it is 170 miles from the nearest city. After the acute phase of the injury, Mr. G. was transferred to a rehabilitation center in the city where his vocational potential will be established.

### Questions

1. What types of limitations would you expect Mr. G. to experience given his level of injury?
2. What types of adaptive devices will Mr. G. most likely need to achieve his greatest level of independence?
3. What types of alternative vocational choices might Mr. G. have, given his occupation and training?
4. What lifestyle issues may need to be considered?
5. How does Mr. G.'s family status influence his rehabilitation goals?
6. What specific issues would you address when working with Mr. G. to establish his rehabilitation plan?

### Case II

Ms. L. is a 32-year-old female who has recently been diagnosed with multiple sclerosis. Ms. L. had sought medical attention for several years before the diagnosis was made because she experienced double vision, weakness in her extremities, and dizziness. Because she was also going through a separation and divorce at the same time, her symptoms were attributed to "stress and depression," and antidepressant medications were prescribed. When her symptoms became worse and additional testing was conducted, the diagnosis was made. The weakness in Ms. L.'s legs has continued, so that she has some difficulty walking and has collapsed several times. She has significant blurring of vision, and she has had some numbness and weakness in her right hand, which is her dominant hand. Ms. L. lives alone. She has a master of science degree in education and has continued to work as a sixth-grade teacher, although she wonders how much longer she will be able to continue. She is currently in remission; however, she has had exacerbations about every 3 months. She currently lives in a suburb of a large metropolitan city but questions whether she should consider moving to her hometown, a small midwestern city, where she can be closer to her parents.

## Questions

1. What issues specifically related to Ms. L.'s age and life situation should be considered in working with her to develop a rehabilitation plan?
2. What specific issues in the diagnosis of multiple sclerosis should be considered?
3. Are there accommodations that Ms. L. would need either at home or in her job to enable her to maintain her maximum level of independence?
4. Will symptoms of her multiple sclerosis prevent her from continuing employment? What issues would you discuss?

## REFERENCES

Aminoff, M. J., Burns, R. S., & Silverstein, P. M. (1997). Update on Parkinson's disease. *Patient Care, 31*(10), 12–14, 16, 19–20, 23–25.

Antel, J. P., & Bar-Or, Amit. (2003). Do myelin-directed antibodies predict multiple sclerosis? *New England Journal of Medicine, 349*(2), 107–109.

Bishop, M., Tschopp, M. K., & Mulvihill, M. (2000). Multiple sclerosis and epilepsy: Vocational aspects and the best rehabilitation practices. *Journal of Rehabilitation, 66*(2), 50–55.

Burk, J., & Agre, J. C. (2000). Characteristics and management of postpolio syndrome. *Journal of the American Medical Association, 284*(4), 412–413.

Cattaneo, E., Rigamonti, D., & Zuccato, C. (2002). The enigma of Huntington's disease. *Scientific American, 287*, 93–97.

Confavreux, C., Vukusic, S., Moreau, T., & Adeleine, P. (2000). Relapses and progression of disability in multiple sclerosis. *New England Journal of Medicine, 343*(20), 1430–1437.

Cushman, L. A., & Dijkers, M. (1991). Depressed mood during rehabilitation of persons with spinal injury. *Journal of Rehabilitation, 57*, 35–38.

del Aguila, M. A., Longstreth, W. T. Jr., McGuire, V., Koepsell, T. D., & van Belle, G. (2003). Prognosis in amyotrophic lateral sclerosis: A population-based study. *Neurology, 60*(5), 813–819.

Drazen, J. M. (2002). Sleep apnea syndrome. *New England Journal of Medicine, 346*(6), 390.

Dyment, D. A., Cader, M. Z., Willer, C. J., Risch, N., Sadovnick, A. D., & Ebers, G. C.(2002). A multigenerational family with multiple sclerosis. *Brain, 125*(7), 1474–1482.

Dyment, D. A., & Ebers, G. C. (2002). An array of sunshine in multiple sclerosis. *New England Journal of Medicine, 347*(8), 1445–1447.

Elliot, T. R., & Frank, R. G. (1996). Depression following spinal cord injury. *Archives of Physical Medicine and Rehabilitation, 77*, 816–823.

Findley, L., Smith, C., Hooper, J., Dineen, M., & Suratt, P. M. (2000). Treatment with nasal CPAP decreases automobile accidents in patients with sleep apnea. *American Journal of Respiratory Critical Care Medicine, 161*, 857–859.

Gilbert, S. C. (2002). Bell's palsy and herpes viruses. *Herpes, 9*(3), 70–73.

Gottlieb, D. J. (2002). Cardiac pacing: A novel therapy for sleep apnea? *New England Journal of Medicine, 346*(6), 444–445.

Hansell, R. (1995). The role of the general medical practitioner in the management of MS. *MS Management, 2*(2), 19–23.

Hayes, E. B., & Piesman, J. (2003). How can we prevent Lyme disease? *New England Journal of Medicine, 348*(24), 2424–2429.

Jankovic, J. (1999, July). New and emerging therapies for Parkinson's disease. *Archives of Neurology, 56*, 785–790.

Janson, C., Leone, P., & Freese, A. (2002). Parkinson's disease: Part I. Molecular pathology. *Science and Medicine, 9*, 328—338.

Janson, C., Leone, P., & Freese, A. (2003). Parkinson's disease: Part II. Cellular basis of medical treatment. *Science and Medicine, 9*(1), 24–35.

Johnson, K. P., & Baringer, J. R. (2001, April 15). Current therapy of multiple sclerosis. *Hospital Practice*, pp. 21–29.

Litvan, I. (1998). Parkinsonian features: When are they Parkinson disease? *Journal of the American Medical Association, 280*(19), 1654–1658.

Livneh, H., & Antonak, R. F. (1997). *Psychosocial adaptation to chronic illness and disability.* Gaithersburg, MD: Aspen.

Livneh, H. (2000). Psychosocial adaptation to spinal cord injury: The role of coping strategies. *Journal of Applied Rehabilitation Counseling, 1*(2), 3–10.

Lutton, J. D., Winston, R., & Rodman, T. C. (2004). Multiple sclerosis: Etiological mechanisms and future directions. *Experimental Biology and Medicine, 229*(1), 12–20.

McAweeney, J. G., Forchheimer, M., & Tate, D. G. (1996). Identifying the unmet independent living needs of persons with spinal cord injury. *Journal of Rehabilitation, 63*(3), 29–33.

McCabe, M. P., McDonald, E., Deeks, A. A., Vowels, L. M., & Cobain, M. J. (1996). The impact of multiple sclerosis on sexuality and relationships. *Journal of Sex Research, 33*(3), 241–252.

McDonald, W. I. (2000). Relapse, remission, and progression in multiple sclerosis. *New England Journal of Medicine, 343*(20), 1486–1487.

Nieto, F. J., Young, T. B., Lind, B. K., et al. (2000). Association of sleep-disordered breathing, sleep apnea, and hypertension in a large community-based study. Sleep Heart health study. *Journal of the American Medical Association, 238*, 1829–1836.

Noseworthy, J. H., Lucchinetti, C., Rodriguez, M., & Weinshenker, B. G. (2000). Multiple sclerosis. *New England Journal of Medicine, 343*, 938–952.

Nussbaum, R. L., & Ellis, C. E. (2003). Alzheimer's disease and Parkinson's disease. *New England Journal of Medicine, 348*(14), 1356–1364.

Phillips, P. (1999a). Keeping depression at bay helps patients with Parkinson disease. *Journal of the American Medical Association, 282*(12), 118–119.

Phillips, P. (1999b). New surgical approaches to Parkinson disease. *Journal of the American Medical Association, 282*(12), 1117–1118.

Pires, M., & Adkins, R. (1996). Pressure ulcers and spinal cord injury: Scope of the problem. *Topics: Spinal Cord Injury Rehabilitation, 2*(1), 1–8.

Rinala, D., Young, J., Hart, K., Clearman, R., & Fuhrer, M. (1992). Social support and the well-being of persons with spinal cord injury living in the community. *Rehabilitation Psychology, 37*, 155–163.

Roessler, R. T. (2001). Job retention services for employees with spinal cord injuries: A critical need in vocational rehabilitation. *Journal of Applied Rehabilitation Counseling, 32*(1), 3–8.

Roessler, R. T., Fitzgerald, S. M., Rumrill, P. D., & Koch, L. C. (2001). Determinants of employment status among people with multiple sclerosis. *Rehabilitation Counseling Bulletin, 45*(1), 31–39.

Roessler, R. T., Rumrill, P. D., & Fitzgerald, S. M. (2004). Predictors of employment status for people with multiple sclerosis. *Rehabilitation Counseling Bulletin, 47*(2), 96–102.

Roux, F., D'Ambrosio, C., & Mohsenin, V. (2000). Sleep-related breathing disorders and cardiovascular disease. *American Journal of Medicine, 108*, 396–402.

Rowland, L. P., & Shneider, N. A. (2001). Amyotrophic lateral sclerosis. *New England Journal of Medicine, 344*(22), 1688–1698.

Salcido, R. (2000). Rehabilitation of the post-polio patient. *Topics in Geriatric Rehabilitation, 15*(3), 95–97.

Salinas, R. (2002). Bell's palsy. *Clinical Evidence, 7*, 1140–1144.

Schapiro, R. T., Scheinberg, L., Weiner, H. L., & Wolinsky, J. S. (1997, January 15). Living with MS: The outlook improves. *Patient Care*, pp. 87, 88, 91, 92, 97, 102–104, 106–108, 119.

Shahar, E., Whitney, C. W., Redline, S., et al. (2001). Sleep-disordered breathing and cardiovascular disease: Cross-sectional results of the Sleep Heart health study. *American Journal of Respiratory Critical Care Medicine, 163*, 19–25.

Siegel, J. M. (2000). Narcolepsy. *Scientific American, 282*, 76–81.

Stansberry, T. T. (2001). Narcolepsy: Unveiling a mystery. *American Journal of Nursing, 101*(8), 50–53.

Veale, D., Chaileux, E., Hoorelbeke-Ramon, A., et al. (2000). Mortality of sleep apnea patients treated by nasal continuous positive airway pressure registered in the ANTADIR observatory. *European Respiratory Journal, 15*, 326–331.

Walling, A. D. (1999). Amyotrophic lateral sclerosis: Lou Gehrig's disease. *American Family Physician, 59*(6), 1489–1496.

Wekerle, H., & Hohlfeld, R. (2003). Molecular mimicry in multiple sclerosis. *New England Journal of Medicine, 349*(2), 185–186.

Woolsey, R. M., & McGarry, J. D. (1991). The cause, prevention, and treatment of pressure sores. *Neurology Clinics, 9*, 797–808.

Yamamoto, H., Akashiba, T., Kosaka, N., Ito, D., & Horie, T. (2000). Long term effects of nasal continuous positive airway pressure on daytime sleepiness, mood, and traffic accidents in patients with obstructive sleep apnea. *Respiratory Medicine, 94*, 87–90.

# CHAPTER 4

# Conditions of the Eye and Blindness

## NORMAL STRUCTURE AND FUNCTION OF THE EYE

The eyeballs are spherical organs encased in the orbital cavities of the skull. Muscles located on the top, bottom, and side of each eye enable it to rotate in different directions (Figure 4–1). The eyelid serves a protective function. Through frequent blinking, the eyelid helps keep the eye moist, preventing irritation. The *lacrimal glands*, which lie in the upper outer side of the eye behind the eyelid, secrete tears to keep the eyeball moist and help rid the eye of foreign material.

In front of the eye lies a transparent curved structure called the *cornea*, which admits light and protects the inner eye from foreign particles and organisms. Although the cornea contains no blood vessels, it is richly supplied with nerve cells. Connected to the cornea and completely covering the eyeball except for the part covered by the cornea is a fibrous membrane called the *sclera*. The sclera forms the white part of the eye and has the primary function of supporting and protecting the eye and maintaining eye shape. Lining the exposed area of the sclera and inner eyelid is a sensitive membrane called the *conjunctiva*. Lying underneath the sclera and also surround-

ing the eyeball is the *choroid coat*, which contains most of the blood vessels that nourish the eye.

The colored part of the eye is called the *iris*. At the center of the iris is a round opening called the pupil, which admits light to the inner part of the eye. The cornea covers both the iris and the pupil. Smooth muscle fibers on either side of the pupil cause it to contract or dilate, thereby automatically regulating the amount of light that enters the eye. In bright light the pupil contracts to reduce the amount of light admitted. In the dark, the pupil dilates to admit as much light as possible.

Directly behind the iris is a space called the *posterior chamber*. Contained in the posterior chamber is a structure called the *ciliary process*, which produces a transparent fluid called the *aqueous humor*. The aqueous humor escapes from the posterior chamber through the pupil into a space lying between the iris and cornea called the *anterior chamber*, which lies between the iris and the cornea. The aqueous humor then drains from the eye into lymph channels and into the venous system through a sievelike structure called the *canal of Schlemm (trabecular network)*, which is located at the junction of the iris and the sclera. The balance between the amount of aqueous humor produced and

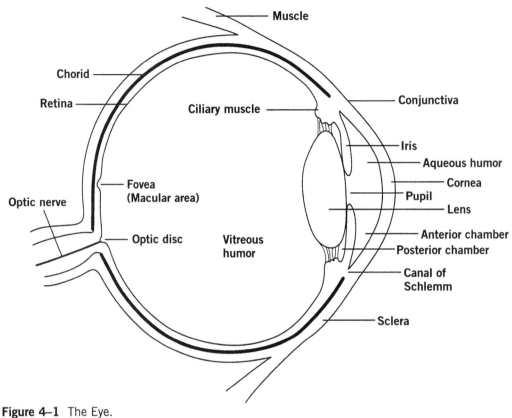

**Figure 4–1**  The Eye.

the amount drained helps to maintain normal *intraocular pressure* (pressure within the eyeball).

The aqueous humor nourishes both the cornea and a structure located directly behind the iris called the *lens*. The lens is a small transparent disk enclosed in a transparent capsule. Attachments around the circumference of the lens, called *ciliary muscles*, automatically contract or expand, changing the shape of the lens from fat to thin or vice versa in response to the proximity or distance of an object being visualized. The changing shape of the lens permits the eye to focus for near or far vision, a process called **accommodation**. To focus on objects in the distance, the ciliary muscles relax, thinning and flattening the lens. To focus on objects close by,

the ciliary muscles contract so that the lenses becomes more rounded. Behind the lens is a larger cavity known as the *vitreous space*. This space is filled with a jelly-like, translucent substance called the *vitreous humor*, which helps to maintain the form and shape of the eyeball.

At the very back of the eye is the innermost coat of the eye, the *retina*. The retina contains two layers, a pigmented layer that is fixed to the choroid and an inner layer that contains special light-sensitive cells called *rods* and *cones*.

*Rods* are involved with detecting light and dark as well as shape and movement and are primarily necessary for night vision and peripheral vision. Rods contain a derivative of vitamin A, *rhodopsin*, a highly light-sensitive substance that breaks down rapidly when exposed to light. This chemical process causes a reaction that activates the rods so that the eye adjusts, enabling individuals to see in the dark. This process is called adaptation.

*Cones* are involved primarily in daylight and color vision as well as in the perception of sharp visual detail. Most of the cones are located in a spot on the retina called the *macula*. The macula is the area of clearest central vision. The center of the macula, the *fovea*, contains no rods and is the area where vision is clearest in good light.

The *optic nerve* enters the back of the eye through an area called the *optic disk*. This area is sometimes called the *blind spot* because it does not contain light-sensitive cells. Light rays pass through the cornea, enter the pupil, pass through the lens, and register on the retina. Sensory cells of the retina receive light stimuli and convert them into electrical impulses. These electrical impulses are then transmitted to the optic nerve, which carries them to the *occipital lobe* of the brain, where they are interpreted.

After exiting the optic disk, the optic nerves from each eye combine at the base of the brain just in front of the brain stem to form the *optic chiasm*. At this point half of the nerve tracts from each eye cross over to the opposite side of the brain. Both eyes receive information from a combination of both visual fields. *Depth perception* requires that the brain receive input from both eyes. The portion of the visual field detected by both eyes is called the *binocular visual field* and is necessary for depth perception.

## MEASURING VISION

**Visual acuity** is defined as the sharpness of the visual image perceived. Visual acuity tests are used to measure the level of best vision and to measure the need for corrective lenses. A standard test of visual acuity is the *Snellen test*. The chart used for the test contains a series of letters on nine lines of decreasing size. Lines are identified according to the distance from which they can be read by individuals with unimpaired vision. For example, individuals with normal visual acuity can read the top line of the chart at 200 feet and the last line at 20 feet. When taking the Snellen test, individuals view the Snellen chart at the equivalent of 20 feet and read the lines on the chart from the largest to the smallest. Results of the test are expressed as a fraction, the numerator denoting the equivalent distance from the chart at which the individual being tested views the chart (20 feet) and the denominator denoting the distance from the chart at which a person with normal vision would be able to read the same line. Consequently, a visual acuity of 20/100 means that the individual being tested can see at 20 feet what a person with normal visual acuity could see at 100 feet, indicating that the individual has a visual impairment. On the other hand, a result of 20/10 would indicate that the individual being tested has better-than-normal visual acuity, since he or she can see at 20 feet what individuals with normal visual acuity can only see at 10 feet.

**Visual field** is defined as the size of the area that individuals can see without turning the head or moving the eyes. **Peripheral vision** (side vision) is measured by a curved device called a *perimeter*. Individuals look into the perimeter, and a test object is systematically moved from outside the peripheral field of vision toward the center until the individual indicates visualization of the object. **Central vision** (vision in the center of the visual field) is tested with the individual looking at a *tangent screen* on which a test object is systematically moved across the screen. Individuals' ability to see the object at certain points is then mapped, outlining their central field of vision.

## TYPES OF VISUAL IMPAIRMENTS

When any deviation from normal vision exists, individuals are considered to have a **visual impairment**. Visual impairments range from mild impairment to total loss of vision. In general, conditions involving the eye that result in visual impairment can be categorized as follows:

- Refractive errors
- Difficulty with coordination of the eyes
- Opacities of the eye
- Injuries to the eye
- Damage secondary to other conditions
- Degenerative changes of the eye

Visual impairments may be temporary, reversible, progressive, or permanent and may involve the following:

- Central field of vision: Individuals are able to see images in the periphery of the visual field but not images in the center.
- Peripheral field of vision: Individuals are able to see images in the center of the field of vision but not in the periphery (*tunnel vision*).
- Night vision: Individuals have difficulty seeing at night (*night blindness*).
- Color vision: Individuals have difficulty distinguishing colors, especially red and green. Rarely, individuals have complete lack of color vision with associated low visual acuity (**achromatopsia**).
- Binocular vision: Individuals have difficulty with the coordinated use of both eyes to produce a single image. As a result, they may have double vision (**diplopia**).

Severe visual impairment can be defined as the inability to read ordinary newsprint even with the aid of glasses (Lighthouse, 1990). When deviations of vision are great enough to cause total loss of light perception, the term *blindness* is used. Many individuals, however, have some usable vision if they use special aids or devices to perform most tasks. When ordinary glasses, contact lenses, medical treatment, and/or surgery is unable to correct sight to the normal range, individuals are said to have *low vision* or to be *partially sighted* (Butler, 1997). The term *legal blindness* describes both those who have total loss of vision and those who have some remaining visual function but are severely handicapped by visual impairment. In the United States, legal blindness has been defined as follows:

1. Visual acuity not exceeding 20/200 or worse in the better eye with correcting lenses
2. Central field of vision limited to an angle of 20 degrees or less

## CONDITIONS CAUSING VISUAL IMPAIRMENT OR BLINDNESS

### Refractive Errors

Refractive errors make up the most common type of eye disorder and occur when changes in the cornea, aqueous humor, lens, or vitreous humor prevent proper bending of light rays to converge on the retina. One type of refractive error, **myopia** (nearsightedness), results from elongation of the eyeball so that light rays focus on a point in front of the retina. Individuals with this condition have good visual acuity for close objects but difficulty seeing objects in the distance. The opposite type of refractive error is **hyperopia** (farsightedness), in which the eyeball is shorter than normal so that light rays focus on a point beyond the retina. Individuals with hyperopia have good visual acuity for objects in the distance but have difficulty focusing on things at close range. Another type of refractive error, **astigmatism**, results from irregularity of the shape of the cornea or at times the lens so that vision is distorted. Myopia, hyperopia, and astigmatism can occur at any age.

**Presbyopia** is a condition usually associated with aging in which there is gradual loss of accommodation due to loss of elasticity of the lens and weakening of the ciliary muscle. Individuals with presbyopia must hold small objects and printed material farther and farther away to see clearly because the eye can no longer adjust the shape of the lens to allow clear vision of close objects.

Refractive errors are usually remedied with corrective lenses. A surgical procedure called *radial keratotomy* (discussed later in the chapter) is now often performed to correct myopia. The procedure attempts to correct nearsightedness by altering the shape of the cornea, causing it to flatten.

## Difficulty with Coordination of the Eyes

To achieve good vision, both eyes must work together so that images from each eye can fuse into one single image. When this does not occur, vision may be impeded to some degree. Uncoordination of the eyes can be the result of heredity, disease, or damage to the brain.

**Nystagmus** is a condition in which the eyes move involuntarily even though the gaze is fixed in one direction. The movement may be in any direction, but most often movement is horizontal. Nystagmus may be congenital or may develop late as a result of a neurological disease or other disorder. Although the condition may cause little visual disturbance and be unnoticeable to the individual, it may be distracting and noticeable to others.

**Strabismus** is a condition in which the eyes cannot be directed to the same object or in which the eyes are crossed, turning inward. It may result from unequal ocular muscle tone or from a neurological condition. It can often be corrected by surgery, corrective lenses, medications, or a combination of the three.

**Suppression amblyopia** (lazy eye) is a condition in which one eye does not develop good vision, usually because of strabismus. The condition is usually treated at an early age by placing a patch over the eye. The eye usually responds to early treatment and the condition is corrected. If, however, the condition is not treated early, the condition can persist for life.

## Opacities of the Eye

### Opacities of the Cornea

Any condition, including injuries, inflammation, or disease of the cornea, that causes scarring or clouding of the cornea can cause permanent partial or total loss of vision. Because of its rich nerve supply, inflammation or injury to the cornea can cause severe pain. Prompt treatment of a corneal inflammation can prevent subsequent formation of scar tissue, which can interfere with vision. When clouding or scarring of the cornea causes permanent visual loss, a *corneal transplant* (discussed later in the chapter) may be performed. When a corneal transplant is successful, vision may be restored with few, if any, restrictions.

### Cataract

A **cataract** is a clouding or opacity of the lens of the eye. Although cataracts are a common cause of visual impairment in older adults, they may also be congenital, hereditary, the result of ocular trauma or inflammation, or associated with a variety of other conditions, such as diabetes. They can also be drug induced, such as from the use of high levels of certain types of steroids. Individuals with cataracts often describe their vision as looking through a cloudy pane of glass, or through a fog.

Although cataracts are generally bilateral, they may form at different rates in each eye. As the lenses become more opaque, vision gradually diminishes. If cataracts are the result of injury, such as from radiation or a foreign object striking the lens, loss of vision occurs more rapidly. Cataracts associated with aging progress more slowly over time.

Because there is no way to return the lens to its normal transparency, treatment of cataracts involves removing the lens and then replacing it with an implant, with glasses, or with both. There are two major methods of cataract removal. One method, *extracapsular cataract extraction*, is a surgical procedure in which the lens is removed but the posterior portion of its capsule is left in position. An intraocular prosthetic lens is generally inserted into the eye at the time of surgery. The second method, *intracapsular cataract extraction*, is a surgical procedure in which the lens and its capsule are completely removed. Both types of surgeries are usually performed on an outpatient basis. Any implanted lens has a fixed focal length, so that vision is clear at only one distance. Thus, individuals who have undergone cataract surgery may continue to need corrective lenses, such as bifocals.

## Injuries to the Eyes

Eye injuries are common and also preventable. The most common type of eye injury is an injury to the cornea caused by a foreign body in the eye. Although often considered minor injuries, these types of injuries can become serious if there is a scratch or abrasion to the cornea that becomes infected or causes scarring, which can impede vision. When the cornea becomes so scarred that vision is severely compromised, a surgical procedure, *corneal transplant* (**keratoplasty**), may be performed. Corneal transplantation may also be performed when the shape of the cornea is distorted. Donor eyes for corneal transplantation come from individuals who have recently died. During the surgical procedure, the opaque area of cornea from the recipient's eye is replaced with the clear donor cornea, which is sutured into place. Because the cornea has no blood vessels, the healing process is slow. Although a corneal transplant can restore vision, there is also the chance of graft rejection or the need for a second operation.

More serious injuries are chemical burns, corneal laceration, or bleeding into the anterior chamber (**hyphema**), all of which can threaten vision. Chemical agents with an *alkaline base*, such as cleansing agents, fertilizers, plaster, or refrigerants, can penetrate the eye rapidly, leading to cell disruption and tissue death. Chemical agents with an *acid base* cause protein coagulation in the eye so that penetration is not as rapid but scarring of tissue can still result in visual loss. In both instances immediate irrigation of the eye can decrease the amount of damage; however, emergency medical treatment should also be sought immediately.

Some injuries involve puncture or laceration of the eye. Common causes are work-related injuries, such as from chopping or sawing wood, or chiseling or hammering metal on metal, in which a stray fragment of material causes the laceration. In some instances, the puncture is so small that it may not be immediately detected.

Puncture or laceration of the eye warrants immediate medical attention.

Deep penetration or laceration of the eye can cause bleeding into the anterior chamber (**hyphema**). Blows to the head or the eye can also cause damage to the internal structures of the eye, causing hemorrhage, retinal damage, or other injury. When bleeding causes increased intraocular pressure, surgical intervention may be needed to relieve the pressure and prevent further damage.

Any injury to the eye necessitates a consultation with an **ophthalmologist** (a physician who specializes in diseases and treatment of the eye). The degree of visual loss that results from an eye injury is a function not only of the extent and type of injury but also frequently of the delay or promptness of emergency treatment.

Most eye injuries are preventable. Using appropriate eye protection for work, home, and sports activities that carry a risk of eye injury is one of the major forms of prevention.

### Inflammation and Infections of the Eye

The most common eye disease is **conjunctivitis** (inflammation of the membrane that lines the eye, the *conjunctiva*. It may be caused by infectious organisms, allergy, or chemicals. In most instances, conjunctivitis is easily treated, is self-limiting, and has no permanent effects. Some types of infectious conjunctivitis, such as *gonococcal conjunctivitis*, or *trachoma*, however, can cause ulceration of the cornea and subsequent blindness.

**Uveitis** is an inflammation of the *uveal tract* (*iris, ciliary body, choroid*). It may be associated with an autoimmune disease such as *ankylosing spondylitis* (see Chapter 14), *inflammatory bowel disease* (see Chapter 10), or local or systemic infection, such as human immunodeficiency virus (HIV).

Symptoms may include decreased vision and sensitivity to light (**photophobia**). It is usually treated with topical medication.

**Keratitis** is an inflammation of the cornea that can be associated with a number of infectious conditions, including herpes simplex (**herpetic keratitis**); it can also be a complication of HIV. Another common cause of keratitis is use of contacts. *Microbial keratitis* is associated with the use of contact lenses and is usually caused by improper handling of contact lens equipment and solutions (Bienfang, Kelly, Nicholson, & Nussenblatt, 1990). One decreases the risk of infection by washing hands and using the appropriate technique for cleaning and applying contact lenses.

### Glaucoma

**Glaucoma** is a condition involving increased intraocular pressure. If left untreated, permanent damage to the optic nerve can result, causing blindness. Glaucoma can occur as a primary condition or secondary to other conditions, such as diabetes, trauma, infection, or prolonged use of medications such as steroids. Glaucoma occurs when the amount of aqueous humor produced exceeds the amount being drained from the eye, much like a sink into which water continues to flow even though the drainage pipe is blocked, resulting in overaccumulation of water in the sink.

#### Types of Glaucoma

There are several types of glaucoma. Broad categories are based on the reason for the problem with the aqueous flow.

##### Chronic Open-Angle Glaucoma

The most common type of glaucoma, *chronic open-angle (simple) glaucoma*, occurs when the outflow of aqueous humor from the eye is reduced. Because the outflow no longer equals the inflow, the amount of aqueous humor builds and pressure in the eye increases. Open-angle glaucoma generally progresses slowly over many years, producing no symptoms until the optic nerve is sufficiently damaged to reduce visual acuity and visual field. At this point, the damage is irreversible. Vision loss generally begins with the loss of *peripheral* (side) vision so that individuals can see only straight ahead, as if looking through a tunnel (*tunnel vision*). Because loss of peripheral vision is often gradual, individuals may be unaware of the problem until advanced stages of the condition. If untreated, the field of vision continues to narrow until all vision is lost. There is no cure for chronic open-angle glaucoma. However, if the condition is detected early, appropriate medical treatment can control it for many years. Consequently, early detection is important.

### Acute Closed-Angle Glaucoma

*Acute closed-angle glaucoma* develops much more rapidly than chronic open-angle glaucoma and is a medical emergency. Symptoms include sudden severe pain, sharply decreased vision, nausea and vomiting, and rapid damage to the optic nerve with associated vision loss. Acute closed-angle glaucoma results from an abrupt blockage and obstruction of the *canal of Schlemm* so that aqueous humor rapidly accumulates in the *anterior chamber* of the eye. Although acute closed-angle glaucoma is much less common than chronic open-angle glaucoma, it is a medical emergency and must be treated immediately to prevent blindness. Initially it may be treated with medications, but surgical intervention is also often necessary.

### Treatment of Glaucoma

Treatment of glaucoma is directed toward reducing the intraocular pressure by decreasing the amount of aqueous humor produced or by increasing its outflow. This can be accomplished with medication or through surgically creating a new pathway for drainage.

Medication for the treatment of glaucoma, whether eye drops or oral medication, must be used daily throughout life to control eye pressure and prevent further damage to vision. In either type of glaucoma, early detection and treatment are critical to prevent irreversible damage to the optic nerve and subsequent blindness. Regardless of the type of glaucoma, lifetime medical supervision is required. Most people with glaucoma can lead normal, unrestricted lives without blindness if the condition is identified early and the medical regimen is followed as prescribed.

### Treatment of Chronic Open-Angle Glaucoma

Chronic open-angle glaucoma may be controlled with medication in the form of eye drops alone to decrease production of aqueous humor or in combination with oral medication that reduces pressure in the eye, thus halting progression of the disease. Because eye drops are absorbed into the bloodstream, they may affect other body functions and cause systemic side effects ranging from generalized weakness to central nervous system, cardiovascular, or gastrointestinal symptoms. Oral medications for the treatment of glaucoma work by decreasing the production of aqueous humor. Like eye drops, oral medications can also affect other body functions and cause systemic side effects. Consequently, individuals who use eye drops or oral medication for treatment of glaucoma should be under continuing medical supervision, not only to monitor the condition itself but also to identify any side effects of the medication.

When intraocular pressure cannot be successfully controlled with medication, individuals with chronic open-angle glaucoma may have a surgical procedure called *trabeculectomy* that relieves pressure by creating a passageway for the aqueous humor to drain. Individuals may also need to continue using eye drops or oral medication after surgery to control pressure; however, in some instances surgery may eliminate the need for medication.

### Treatment of Acute Closed-Angle Glaucoma

Acute closed-angle glaucoma results from the forward displacement of the iris, which narrows or obstructs the path for aqueous humor outflow. Eye drops called *miotics* constrict the pupil, thus enlarging the drainage passageway and facilitating the outflow of aqueous humor. Because of the emergency nature of acute closed-angle glaucoma, oral or intravenous medication is given immediately to relieve pressure on the optic nerve temporarily. Once the pressure level has dropped to a safe level, a surgical procedure called *iridotomy* may be performed. Iridotomy involves the removal of a small section of the iris so that the aqueous humor can flow freely from the posterior to the anterior chamber of the eye, thus preventing further eye damage by relieving built-up pressure. This procedure is often performed with a laser. At times iridotomy may also be performed prophylactically in the unaffected eye after an acute attack.

## Retinopathy

Any disease or disorder of the retina is a *retinopathy*. Retinopathies are often named for their cause. For example, *arteriosclerotic retinopathy* is due to changes that occur in blood vessels in the retina because of arteriosclerosis. *Hypertensive retinopathy* is due to changes that occur in blood vessels in the retina because of high blood pressure. In both instances, treatment of the primary underlying condition can control the progress of retinopathy.

The most common type of retinopathy, and the most common cause of blindness, is *diabetic retinopathy*. Diabetic retinopathy is the result of damage to the retina and is a complication of *diabetes mellitus* (see Chapter 9). Usually there are no symptoms in early stages of diabetic retinopathy. Consequently, regular comprehensive eye examinations by a physician are important in helping to prevent visual loss.

There are two categories of diabetic retinopathy:

1. *Nonproliferative diabetic retinopathy*
2. *Proliferative diabetic retinopathy*

*Nonproliferative diabetic retinopathy* is caused by changes in blood vessel walls that allow fluids to leak into retinal tissue. At the same time, small blood vessels in the retina may become occluded, disturbing circulation in the retina so that some retinal tissue receives too little oxygen and dies (**necrosis**).

*Proliferative diabetic retinopathy* results from extensive areas of closure of the small blood vessels in the retina. As a result, retinal tissues receive too little oxygen (**ischemia**) and growth of new vessels is stimulated. These new blood vessels are abnormally fragile and prone to bleed, causing hemorrhage into the *vitreous humor*. The degree of vision loss depends on the amount of hemorrhage. Vessels may burst, filling the back of the eye with blood and resulting in significant visual loss. In some instances, scar tissue associated with new vessels can pull on the retina so that it detaches from underlying tissue. (See "Retinal Detachment" below.)

Surgery may be performed to remove *vitreous gel* and hemorrhage (**vitrectomy**), or laser treatment may be performed to stop the bleeding. *Laser photocoagulation* is a procedure in which an intense beam of light from a laser is used to seal leaking blood vessels of the retina. The laser beam passes through the lens of the eye and vitreous fluid without harming the structures. It then is directed to a very precisely defined area to destroy fragile vessels prone to hemorrhage or diseased areas of the retina in which there may be additional proliferative vessel changes. Laser photocoagulation may help reduce the risk of visual loss, but it does not stop the progression of diabetic retinopathy. Laser treatment is usually performed on an outpatient basis.

### Retinal Detachment

With detached retina, the sensory layer of the retina becomes separated from the pigmented (choroid) layer, depriving the sensory layer of blood supply. Detached retina may result from a sudden blow to the head, a tumor in the choroid layer, retinal degeneration caused from conditions such as arteriosclerosis, or hemorrhage with conditions such as diabetic retinopathy.

Symptoms may develop suddenly or slowly over time. Individuals may notice flashes of light or a loss of vision in different areas of the visual field, or they may experience a complete loss of vision in the affected eye. Usually there is no pain accompanying symptoms. Retinal detachment in one eye may indicate an increased risk of detachment in the other eye. Prompt diagnosis and surgical treatment are essential to prevent permanent vision loss. A surgical procedure called *scleral buckling* is sometimes used to treat retinal detachment. Scleral buckling mechanically restores contact of the retina with the choroid. The area of the sclera that lies over the retinal defect is depressed with an implant so that the choroid and retina are pressed together.

### Retinitis Pigmentosa

A hereditary condition, **retinitis pigmentosa**, involves the slowly progressive loss of peripheral vision. Although there is progressive restriction of the visual field due to loss of peripheral vision, the remaining central visual acuity is often good. Frequently the first symptom of retinitis pigmentosa is difficulty with night vision (*night blindness*), which usually begins in late youth or early adulthood. Total bilateral loss of vision can occur in later stages of the disease. There is no cure or treatment for the condition; however, a number of assistive devices may be utilized to enhance function. (See "Assistive Devices and Low-Vision Aids" later in the chapter.)

### Macular Degeneration

Degenerative changes in the macula, the part of the eye needed for seeing fine detail and central vision, results in a condition known as *macular degeneration*.

Macular degeneration usually occurs after the age of 50, from no apparent cause. Painless loss of central visual acuity is usually slow, with visual distortion or blurring of vision being the first symptom. Eventually individuals may develop a blind spot in the center of their field of vision that gradually increases in size as the condition progresses. Since warning signs of macular degeneration are absent until central vision is affected, regular eye examinations are important for early identification of the condition and so treatment to its progress can be implemented.

Macular degeneration does not result in complete blindness, but it destroys some or all of the sight in the center of the field of vision. There are two types of macular degeneration: dry form and wet form. Most cases of macular degeneration are *dry form*, in which there is **atrophy** (shrinkage) and thinning of the macula, causing mild to moderate vision loss. The type of macular degeneration called *wet form* is characterized by significant loss of vision due to abnormal blood vessel formation and hemorrhage.

Both types of macular degeneration are characterized by loss of central vision while peripheral vision remains intact. There is no treatment or cure for macular degeneration, but the use of assistive devices may increase visual function (see "Assistive Devices and Low-Vision Aids" below). Activities such as reading may become difficult because of distortion of letters or parts of words or sentences in the center of the reading material that appear to be missing. Large print with black type and white background may make reading easier, as well as assistive devices such as a magnifying glass.

## DIAGNOSTIC PROCEDURES FOR CONDITIONS OF THE EYE

### Comprehensive Eye Exam

Eye examinations usually include an external eye exam that measures eye movements and the size of the pupils and their ability to react to light. It also includes testing visual acuity and visual field as described earlier in the chapter. This part of the exam may be performed by an **optometrist** (nonphysician who specializes in correcting refractive errors). An **ophthalmologist** (physician who spe-

cializes in evaluation and treatment of conditions of the eye) may also conduct tests of visual acuity, but he or she also checks ocular movement, the function of the optic nerve, and light reflexes of the pupils, as well as identifying any optic nerve pathology.

Individuals may also be asked to view a chart through an instrument called a refractor. The physician then shines a light through the refractor onto the retina to estimate the eye's ability to focus on distant objects. Also included in a comprehensive eye exam is a *tonometry* (described below) and a *slit-lamp exam*, which evaluates the eye's structures, including the cornea and iris, and screens for cataracts. A *retinal examination* to check for retinal disease may also be included. This requires that the pupil of the eye be dilated.

### Tonometry

*Tonometry* is used to measure pressure in the eye in order to detect glaucoma. An instrument called a *tonometer* is placed directly on the cornea after the cornea has been anesthetized with drops of a local anesthetic. The tonometer measures the amount of pressure within the eye, thus making it possible to detect glaucoma.

### Gonioscopy

For *gonioscopy*, a special contact lens that contains a mirror is gently placed on the eye. The ophthalmologist uses the lens like the periscope of a submarine to examine structures inside the eye. The test is especially helpful in detecting glaucoma.

### Ophthalmoscopic Examination

A direct *ophthalmoscopic examination* is a procedure used to examine the internal structures of the eye. It is performed with an instrument called an *ophthalmoscope* that is placed close to the eye. The ophthalmoscope contains a light that shines into the eye and magnifies internal structures so that the physician can note any pathologic changes.

The internal structures of the eye may also be observed with a *slit lamp*, a type of microscope that is placed in front of the eye. The physician shines a finely focused slit of brilliant light onto the eye to magnify details of the cornea, iris, and lens. A slit lamp is especially useful in identifying foreign bodies in the eye, evaluating corneal ulcers, and diagnosing cataracts.

### Fluorescein Angiography

The purpose of *fluorescein angiography* is to detect changes in the blood vessels of the retina. A fluorescein dye is either taken orally or injected into the bloodstream. When the dye reaches the blood vessels of the eye, special ultraviolet lights enable the physician to photograph the vessels for later study. Any swelling or leakage of the vessels of the retina is apparent on the photograph.

### TREATMENT AND MANAGEMENT OF CONDITIONS OF THE EYE AND BLINDNESS

### Eyeglasses and Contact Lenses

*Corrective lenses* may be in the form of eyeglasses or contact lenses. Because there are so many different types of eye disorders that interfere with visual acuity corrective lenses must be prescribed individually. They are prescribed by an **ophthalmologist** (a physician who specializes in the diagnosis and treatment of disorders of the eye, including surgery and prescription of medications and optical corrections) or an **optometrist** (an individual who does not have a medical degree but is trained to measure refractive errors and perceptual dysfunctions of the eye, as well as to diagnose visual conditions and prescribe optical corrections). Optometrists do not prescribe medications or perform surgery. Lenses for glasses are made by **opticians**, technicians who have been trained to fill optical prescriptions. They grind and construct the lens according to the prescribed specifications.

When visual acuity at several different distances must be corrected, *bifocal* or *trifocal* lenses may be prescribed. Individuals with *bifocal lenses* use the lower portion of the lens for near vision and the upper portion for far vision. *Trifocal lenses* have three different divisions: one for near vision, one for intermediate vision, and one for far vision.

There are several different types of contact lenses; however, the most common are hard and soft corneal lenses. Hard lenses cover the central area of the cornea and are generally more durable. Soft lenses cover the entire cornea and are generally more fragile. Regardless of the type, contact lenses must be individually prescribed and constructed. They are helpful for a variety of visual conditions, but they do not correct astigmatism.

Generally, there are no complications associated with wearing eyeglasses. Contact lenses, however, can damage the eye if they are not worn and cared for properly. Not all people can or should wear contact lenses. Overwearing of hard lenses can cause corneal abrasions and associated complications. Individuals who do not use good hygienic practices when inserting the contact lens may develop an infection of the eye, in which case contact lenses should not be worn.

### Refractive Eye Surgery

Growing numbers of individuals, hoping to discard corrective lenses, have refractive surgery to correct their vision. Refractive surgery may be used to treat **myopia** (nearsightedness), **hyperopia** (farsightedness), or **astigmatism** (irregularity in the shape of the cornea or lens resulting in distortion of the visual image). Three primary surgical techniques are used in refractory eye surgery: *radial keratotomy, photorefractive keratectomy*, and *laser-assisted in situ keratomileusis*. Although refractive eye surgery is often effective in correcting the visual problem, there is also the potential for complications (Buckingham, 2000).

## Prosthetic Devices and Eye Replacement

When injury or disease necessitates removal of the eyeball, or when there is a congenital absence of the eye (**anophthalmia**), a prosthetic eye may be constructed and worn by the individual. The prosthetic eye, while not contributing to vision, serves a cosmetic purpose and can enhance the individual's body image and self-concept.

Visual impairment due to conditions in which there is interruption of electrical stimulation somewhere along the visual pathway or to the retina, where photoreceptors are located, has spurred research into the use of electrical stimulation to overcome visual loss. *Optical prostheses*, which emulate functions of photoreceptors located in the retina, are an example of devices that have the potential for restoring rudimentary vision (Scarlatis, 2000). Although still in experimental stages, the development of optical prostheses is an important advance that may make it possible for individuals with retinal damage to have partial vision restored.

## Assistive Devices and Low-Vision Aids

Assistive devices and low-vision aids should be part of an overall program to en-hance the life of the individual, not just to enhance the visual system. The types of devices used should be based on individual needs as well as the willingness and ability to use them. The overall goal is to recapture, strengthen, and maintain individuals' self-confidence for safe, independent functioning. These aids enhance remaining visual abilities through the use of individually prescribed adaptive equipment appropriate to individuals' specific lifestyle.

Adaptive equipment for activities of daily living may include optical devices, such as high-powered lenses and telescopic spectacles, or nonoptical devices that are readily available and require no special training, such as large-print reading material or large-button telephones. Low-technology devices such as talking watches, raised dot markings for oven dials, or templates for check signing require little training and may require only simple adaptations. Additional devices, such as talking clocks and timers, writing guides, talking books, and audiocassettes, also help to meet the communication needs of individuals with visual impairments.

High-technology devices are more sophisticated electronically and may require specialized training. Examples are video magnifiers and computer systems. Video magnifiers use closed-circuit television and can magnify a printed page on a television screen for reading. Numerous computer software programs and adaptive devices can be used to enlarge printed materials or to convert print into synthetic speech output. These devices include large-print computer monitors, programs that enlarge print size on the screen, printers that modify font size, synthetic speech software programs with external audio units, and typewriters equipped with synthetic speech output that interface with personal computer units. Speech packages allow for adjustments in the rate of speech and the tone of voice to meet the needs of the individual user.

One of the best-known tactile aids is *Braille*. Hard-copy Braille uses the familiar raised dot method, whereas soft-copy Braille is stored on electromagnetic tape and presented as patterns by a set of pins that represent a Braille dot. Individuals place their fingers on display units through which the pins protrude. Another type of tactile aid is an *electromechanical vibratory system*. A small camera is passed over a line of print, and each printed letter is then displayed as a pattern of vibration that the individual can feel with the finger.

A number of professionals recommend and provide training in the use of optical, nonoptical, low-technology, and high-technology aids. These include *occupational therapists, low-vision specialists, orientation and mobility instructors, rehabilitation teachers*, and *adaptive technology specialists*.

The key to the successful use of any assistive or adaptive device is making sure that the individual using the device is involved in selecting it so that the device meets his or her requirements, capabilities, and needs. This customization helps individuals view the device positively and use it to best enhance their own functional capacity (Lacey & MacNamara, 2000).

## Orientation and Mobility Training

The goal of *orientation and mobility training* is to enable individuals with a visual impairment to achieve as much mobility as possible according to their capabilities and desires and to recapture, strengthen, and maintain self-reliance for safe and independent function. *Orientation and mobility (O&M) specialists* provide training that helps individuals know where they are in relation to their surroundings and how to safely navigate within their environment (Turnbull, Turnbull, Shank, Smith, & Leal,

2002). O&M specialists help individuals move independently indoors and outdoors and in familiar or unfamiliar environments and also provide training in the use of public transportation, use of the cane, and use of mobility lights or electronic travel aids. Through individualized training, individuals with visual impairments learn to orient themselves to their environment by using compensatory strategies, including illumination techniques and the use of contrast, magnification, memorization of location, and auditory and tactile feedback. Compensatory strategies may involve such things as listening for the direction of traffic, arm and hand positioning for guidance along walls and railings, and systematic search techniques for dropped or lost objects.

### Mobility Aids

Various types of mobility aids, such as sighted guides, guide dogs, canes, and electronic devices, are available to help individuals with a visual impairment move about the environment more freely (Cox & Dykes, 2001). Orientation and mobility specialists can help the individual find the best system.

Guide dogs not only increase the mobility of the individual with a visual impairment but can also provide protection and companionship. Guide dogs undergo intensive training before being matched with the individual to whom they are assigned. They are taught how to respond to various commands as well as how to respond to curbs, traffic, and other potential hazards in the environment. The individual and dog train together for a number of weeks to become an effective team. Not all individuals are able to use a guide dog, and some individuals prefer to use other forms of mobility aids, such as a long cane.

The most common mobility aid is the prescription or long cane, which is usually made of aluminum or fiberglass. An orientation and mobility specialist prescribes the cane according to the individual's height, length of stride, and comfort. The cane is used by those with visual impairments in a systematic way. The individual moves the cane rhythmically in an arc in front of the body to ensure a safe space for the next step. Although this provides some protection, it does not account for objects above the waist that are in the individual's path. In an attempt to compensate for this type of obstacle, some canes have tone-emitting radar units that give a differential pitch for the direction and height of obstacles in front of the individual. Some individuals prefer collapsible, folding, or telescopic canes, which are less obtrusive and can be collapsed and slipped into a purse or under a chair when not in use.

Electronic travel aids may also be used. These devices emit light beams or ultrasound waves. When the light beam or ultrasound wave hits an object in the individual's path, the device vibrates or emits a sound.

## PSYCHOSOCIAL ISSUES IN CONDITIONS OF THE EYE AND BLINDNESS

### Special Issues for Individuals Who Are Partially Sighted

Individuals with low vision or who are partially sighted do not quite fit into the category of either the blind or sighted population. Consequently, they often have special needs that are overlooked. The social community often lacks understanding of the true nature of vision impairment, so that individuals with low vision are ridiculed in public for appearing to see more than would be expected by a person with visual impairment (Vance, 2000). Individuals with partial sight may be viewed as malingerers by their families and acquaintances because they can see some things but not others. Even when they attempt to function with appropriate assistive devices, they may be suspected of denying their condition by those who expect individuals with visual impairments to be dependent and isolated.

Adjustment to vision loss is not necessarily correlated with the degree of remaining vision. Individuals with partial sight do not have fewer adjustment issues than those who are totally blind, and in fact may have more adaptation difficulties because their partial sight presents an ambiguous situation for others. In addition, individuals with partial sight may exhibit high levels of anxiety because they may be unsure about whether or when they will lose more of their residual vision.

Even when individuals with severe visual impairments function independently for the most part, there may be some activities for which they are more dependent on assistance from others. The greater dependence associated with many severe visual impairments may be a source of conflict and may have a negative impact on formerly close relationships, especially if others have misperceptions or misunderstandings about the nature of the impairment. In other instances individuals, in an attempt to demonstrate self-reliance and independence, may reject help from family and friends, causing alienation and social isolation. Counseling individuals to understand sighted people's reactions may facilitate social interactions and enhance the development of constructive and realistic interactions. At times, individuals with visual impairment may find it helpful to share their experiences and problems with others who also have low vision.

Because partially sighted individuals have some remaining sight, they may attempt to "pass" as a sighted person to avoid potential rejection or avoidance by others. They may deny their disability altogether and associate only with sighted persons in an attempt to be accepted by the mainstream of society. They may make excuses for awkward behavior or attempt in other ways to conceal the fact that they have low vision. They may refuse to use low-vision aids, such as a cane, for mobility or reject suitable orientation and mobility training. In extreme cases they may engage in dangerous activities such as illegal driving. People often view the ability to drive as very important to the maintenance of independence. This makes it extremely difficult for individuals who are losing their vision to give up this activity. Furthermore, by its very nature, the gradual loss of vision creates a time period in which the decision to stop driving is particularly difficult. The emphasis on self-care and independence for individuals with partial vision must be tempered with judgment and concern for the welfare of the individual as well as for that of others.

## Psychological Issues in Conditions of the Eye and Blindness

Vision loss often precipitates a sense of fear and reduced personal competence, which may result in isolation and social withdrawal. Visual impairments may be present at birth, or they may develop suddenly or slowly at any time in an individual's life. Often visual loss follows an unpredictable and uncontrollable progression. Adjustment to loss of vision depends on many factors, including the degree of loss and the age at which the individual becomes visually impaired. Those who are congenitally blind, for example, have not had the opportunity to learn concepts such as distance, depth, proportion, and color. Because of their lack of visual experiences in their environment, such as the observation of others' tasks or behaviors, concepts that sighted individuals often take for granted must be learned by other means. This adaptive learning of tasks then becomes a natural part of their development, so that adjustment to visual limitations is incorporated into their self-perception and daily activities as a normal part of growing up.

Individuals with loss of vision later in life have the advantage of being able to draw on visual experiences in the environment as a frame of reference for physical concepts, but they may find it more difficult to accept blindness than those who have never had vision. Individuals who lose vision later in life must modify their self-perception as a result of physical changes and the subsequent need to restructure daily activities. Individuals who are newly blind may experience grief and despair over their loss of visual function. They may become dependent, feel insecure in new situations, and perceive a marked loss of autonomy. Some may become reluctant to interact in social situations because they want to avoid the awkwardness of initial attempts at social interactions. Loss of control over standard methods of initiating conversations (e.g., eye contact and other nonverbal cues), the noticeable discomfort or overhelpfulness of sighted persons, and often prolonged gaps in conversations may lead newly blind individuals to believe that they are being watched or ignored.

Accommodation to visual loss or blindness is multifaceted. Individuals with a visual loss must adjust their self-concept and personal goals to take into account the realistic limits imposed by vision loss. They must develop adaptive skills and new abilities, and they must draw on personal resources to adjust. Individuals who have lost vision because of traumatic blindness (conditions in which there has been a sudden loss of partial or total vision because of an internal or external event, such as a head injury, direct injury to the eye, or chemical burn) may have to cope not only with sudden loss of vision but also with insurance company representatives, attorneys, and other legal and bureaucratic aspects surrounding the circumstance of their disability. In these situations, family members may also react to the situation, showing anger, revenge, or overprotectiveness.

## Lifestyle Issues in Conditions of the Eye and Blindness

Vision is crucial for many activities of daily living. Individuals with little or no vision must learn new techniques for carrying out routine activities of self-care and mobility. They must orient themselves to the home environment so that they may move freely from room to room without risk of injury. Family members can contribute to their sense of mobility by never moving furniture within a room without informing them and by leaving doors either completely open or completely closed after informing them of the plan so that they do not bump into a partially open door.

At first, tasks such as pouring water into a glass without spilling it, buttering bread, or cutting meat may seem insurmountable for the individual with visual impairment. However, most people learn to prepare their meals and dine independently once they have been oriented to the location of food, tableware, and cooking utensils. Cooking can be learned through techniques such as the systematic placement of cooking equipment and utensils and

special labeling on cans, frozen foods, oven dials, and other items.

Through training, individuals with visual impairments are gradually able to assume personal responsibility for self-care. *Rehabilitation teachers* provide in-home training in skills of daily living. Activities such as bathing, combing the hair, shaving, applying makeup, and dressing in a coordinated fashion can all be performed independently through skills training and systematic organization and labeling of personal items.

Although individuals with a moderate to mild visual impairment may carry on much of their personal business with low-vision aids, those with a severe visual impairment or blindness may need someone else's help to read a bill, a check, an invoice, or a personal letter. Some individuals have difficulty adjusting to this loss of privacy. In other instances, documents or forms must be translated into Braille or read to the individual, perhaps reducing the efficiency of action or response to the document.

Outside the home, individuals with severe visual impairments can learn techniques of mobility in new environments with the use of a cane or guide dog. Through these techniques, even those who are severely impaired or blind are able to travel to work or other destinations of their choice. They can also learn methods of carrying money so as to discriminate between bills and between different coins. Individuals can continue to enjoy a number of leisure activities, including outdoor activities such as swimming, hiking, and fishing. With special adaptive procedures, even bicycling is still possible.

Although visual loss does not affect sexual activity directly, the impact of loss of vision on self-esteem may be substantial. In addition, individuals with severe visual impairment are unable to see the facial expressions and other nonverbal forms of communication that are an integral part of sexual relationships. Information about relationships that is normally developed through visual modeling may not be available if they have been without sight since an early age. Consequently, visually impaired teenagers or young adults may need to be taught appropriate social behaviors that others generally learn by observation.

## Social Issues for Individuals with Visual Conditions or Blindness

Major obstacles to the effective functioning of individuals with visual impairment in social environments are social stereotyping and the attitudes of sighted people toward those individuals. Many sighted people view individuals who have severe visual impairments or are blind as helpless and dependent. Others believe the myth that people with severe visual impairments or blindness develop extraordinary powers of hearing and touch to compensate for the loss of vision, rather than recognizing that they learn to make more effective use of other senses in their effort to interpret their environment. Negative attitudes or stereotypical views held by friends, employers, and casual acquaintances can have a major impact on individuals with visual impairment. Unfortunately, many people with visual impairment tend to conform to social expectations, thus limiting their own potential. Understanding and accepting that others may be uncomfortable with them because of lack of previous interactions with people with visual impairments or because of misinformation provide the basis for formulating proactive strategies for solving problems, understanding perspectives, and making social inferences that can result in fuller social integration.

The inability of individuals with visual impairment to see the social behavior of others affects their social interactions. Much social interaction and communication are mediated by watching the nonverbal actions and reactions of others, such as posture, facial expression, or movement. Absence of these visual cues can place individuals with visual impairment at a disadvantage in a social setting, unless all concerned have developed increased awareness and sensitivity to the individual's inability to observe nonverbal cues.

Although the attitudes of family members are important factors in adjustment to most disabilities, they appear to have an especially powerful influence on the adjustment of those with visual impairment. How families react depends on their patterns of belief, feelings, and resources. When family members believe that the demands being placed on them exceed their available resources, stress and strain may develop. If, on the other hand, families are able to meet the major needs of their members so that they can pursue realistic goals, they will be better able to cope successfully.

Family attitudes during rehabilitation may determine individuals' motivation to learn and accept major changes in lifestyle. Overprotective or overly anxious families who encourage dependency may prevent or impede rehabilitation. On the other hand, families that foster positive attitudes and demonstrate respect and recognition of the individual with visual impairment can contribute greatly to rehabilitation.

## VOCATIONAL ISSUES FOR INDIVIDUALS WITH CONDITIONS OF THE EYE OR BLINDNESS

Person who are blind or who have low vision are underrepresented in the competitive labor market (Crudden & McBroom, 1999). The degree of the vocational impact of a visual disorder depends on the nature of the employment, the type of visual impairment, and the life stage at which the visual impairment occurs. Many individuals with partial vision are able to continue in their field of employment with special adaptive or low-vision aids. Others must learn new job skills. When visual loss is progressive, ongoing evaluation and planning for decreasing visual acuity should be part of the rehabilitation plan.

Barriers to employment may include deficits in skills or education, lack of work experience, lack of job preparation skills, or lack of motivation or information. Paid reader support may be necessary to gain information about job openings or training opportunities. In other instances, lack of direction by family and friends or lack of expectation that individuals with visual impairments can be competitive in the workplace may make it more difficult to continue looking for work or preparing for employment.

Not only on-the-job activity, but also the ability to get to and from work may be a barrier to employment. If individuals are no longer able to drive and no public transportation is available, suitable alternatives for transportation to and from work must be devised. Unreliable transportation can be a major barrier to obtaining and maintaining employment.

For individuals with low vision, the level of visual acuity, and thus the individual's ability to resolve visual detail, must be considered in any position in which reading or seeing fine visual detail is required. Accommodations may involve making the image larger through some form of magnification or using an optical device to make the object appear larger. Individuals with low vision may need additional lighting to enhance vision; however, lighting that produces glare can be detrimental to their visual acuity and comfort. Those with visual field deficits may have difficulty with peripheral or central vision. Those with peripheral vision problems have difficulty detecting objects around them. In addition, peripheral field deficiency can interfere with mobility and with performing near tasks such as reading or writing. Central vision loss affects individuals' straight-ahead vision and probably also reduces visual acuity. Consequently, reading and tasks requiring visualization of detail will be affected. The degree of functional impairment is dependent on the size and location of the loss of vision.

## CASE STUDIES

### Case I

Ms. A. is a 32-year-old female who recently got married. Her husband is a landscaper. They have no children. Shortly after their marriage Ms. A. became totally blind from proliferative diabetic retinopathy. She has no light perception. Ms. A. has a bachelor of science degree in retail management and has been working for the past 10 years as a buyer for a major retail firm. Her job involves determining which products to buy for distribution based on her projection of their ability to sell, the sales activities of other retail firms, and the general economic conditions and buyer trends. She uses a computer for many of her activities.

#### Questions

1. With regard to Ms. A.'s blindness, are there special adaptive devices or special accommodations that might assist her at her current job?

2. What adaptive devices or accommodations might Ms. A. need in other aspects of her life because of her blindness?
3. Are there issues in Ms. A.'s personal life that could affect her rehabilitation potential?
4. What additional types of services would help Ms. A. reach her highest level of independence?

## Case II

Mr. J. is a 25-year-old man with progressive vision loss from retinitis pigmentosa. He currently has moderate visual loss but refuses to use adaptive devices or special aids. He did not complete high school, but he did obtain a GED. He has a scattered work history, working for a time in his late teens as a worker on a river barge, as a personal attendant for an individual with a disability, and most recently as a freight mover at a local factory. He states he has lost contact with his family and appears to have no close friends or relatives in the area.

### Questions

1. What additional information about the personal and work characteristics of Mr. J. would you need to help him to develop a rehabilitation plan?
2. What specific characteristics about his visual impairment would you consider?
3. If Mr. J. would use adaptive devices, which types would be most helpful to him given his specific type of visual impairment?

## REFERENCES

Bienfang, D. C., Kelly, L. D., Nicholson, D. H., & Nussenblatt, R. B. (1990). Ophthalmology. *New England Journal of Medicine, 325*(14), 956–967.

Buckingham, B. K. (2000). Refractive eye surgery: Focusing on risks. *Trial, 35*(5), 18–27.

Butler, R. N. (1997). Keeping an eye on vision: New tools to preserve sight and quality of life. *Geriatrics, 52*(9), 48–55.

Cox, P. R., & Dykes, M. K. (2001). Effective classroom adaptations for students with visual impairments. *Teaching Exceptional Children, 33*(6), 68–74.

Crudden, A., & McBroom, L. W. (1999, June). Barriers to employment: A survey of employed persons who are visually impaired. *Journal of Visual Impairment and Blindness*, 341–350.

Lacey, G., & MacNamara, S. (2000). User involvement in the design and evaluation of a smart mobility aid. *Journal of Rehabilitation Research and Development, 37*(6), 709–723.

Lighthouse. (1990). *Statistics on blindness and vision impairment: A resource manual.* New York: Lighthouse.

Scarlatis, G. (2000). Optical prostheses: Visions of the future. *Journal of the American Medical Association, 283*(17), 2297.

Turnbull, A., Turnbull, R., Shank, M., Smith, S., & Leal, D. (2002). *Exceptional lives: Special education in today's schools* (3rd ed.). Upper Saddle River, NJ: Merrill.

Vance, J. C. (2000). A degree of vision. *Lancet, 356* (i9240), 1517–1519.

# CHAPTER 5

# Hearing Loss and Deafness

## NORMAL STRUCTURE AND FUNCTION OF THE EAR

The ear is made up of two systems, each with a specific function:

- The **auditory system** is involved with the detection of sound waves, and consequently hearing.
- The **vestibular system** is involved with body equilibrium, orientation, and balance.

The ear consists of three divisions: the outer, middle, and inner ear (Figure 5–1).

### The Outer Ear

The outer ear includes the *pinna (auricle)* and the *external ear canal (external auditory meatus)*. The *pinna*, the visible portion of the ear, is made up of elastic cartilage covered with skin. The *external ear canal* is a little longer than one inch and extends from the opening of the ear to the eardrum. It contains special glands that produce **cerumen** (earwax), which protects the ear against the entry of foreign material. The function of the pinna is to collect sound waves and conduct them to the eardrum (*tympanic membrane*).

### The Middle Ear

The tympanic membrane separates the outer ear from the middle ear (*tympanic cavity*). The tympanic cavity is an air-filled cavity connected to the throat by the *eustachian tube*, which helps equalize air pressure on both sides of the tympanic membrane. Changes in atmospheric pressure, such as with change in altitude, necessitate equalization of air pressure in the middle ear. When the ears "pop" during altitude changes, the eustachian tube has allowed air in the middle ear to equalize with the pressure outside the head. When this does not occur, considerable discomfort can result. The eustachian tube, which is normally collapsed in adults, opens with yawning or swallowing, allowing air pressure on both sides of the tympanic membrane to equalize. Another pathway connects the tympanic cavity to the *mastoidal air cells* within the *mastoid process* of the temporal bone.

The middle ear lies between the eardrum and the inner ear. It contains three small movable bones called *ossicles* that transfer sound vibrations from the eardrum to the inner ear. These small bones, the *malleus*, the *incus*, and the *stapes*, are

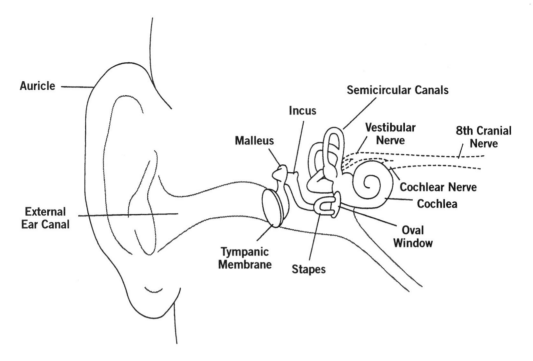

**Figure 5–1**  The Outer, Middle, and Inner Ear.

connected by small ligaments and are attached to the tympanic membrane by the handle of the malleus. The footplate of the stapes connects to a thin membrane called the *oval window,* which connects to the inner ear. Also connecting the middle ear with the inner ear is an opening called the *round window.*

## The Inner Ear

The inner ear (*labyrinth*) is a fluid-filled cavity that lies deep within the *temporal bone* of the skull. The inner ear is important not only for hearing (as part of the *auditory system*), but also for maintaining body balance and equilibrium (as part of the *vestibular system*). Contained within the inner ear is the *cochlea,* which is part of the *auditory system,* and the *semicircular canals,* which are part of the *vestibular system.* The cochlea has a snail-like ap-

pearance and contains tiny hair cells within a structure called the *organ of Corti,* the end organ of hearing. Movement of fluid within the inner ear stimulates nerve endings in both the auditory and vestibular systems. Impulses from both systems are converted into nerve impulses and transmitted from the inner ear to the brain by the *eighth cranial nerve,* sometimes called the *acoustic* or *auditory nerve,* which contains two branches: the *cochlear nerve branch,* which conducts sensory information about sound, and the *vestibular nerve branch,* which conducts impulses regarding body balance and movement.

Sound waves enter the external ear and move through the external ear canal, striking the eardrum and causing it to vibrate. The chained movement of the malleus, incus, and stapes conducts sound waves from the eardrum to a thin membrane called the *oval window,* which connects to the inner ear. The vibration of the eardrum first moves the malleus, which transmits the vibration to the incus; in turn, the incus transmits the vibration to the stapes. The stapes vibration in the oval window stimulates the fluid in the inner ear, which stimulates the tiny hair cells in the organ of Corti. The movement of the hair cells stimulates the nerve endings located around their bases to transmit impulses to the *cochlear nerve*, which carries the impulses to the *auditory center* of the brain, where they are interpreted as sound.

The *vestibular structures* in the ear, concerned with maintaining equilibrium, include the *semicircular canals* and a small rounded chamber at their base called the *vestibule*. The *semicircular canals* contain the nerve endings through which balance is controlled. Like the organ of Corti, they contain numerous hair cells that project into the fluid of the inner ear. The movement of the head sets the fluid in motion and moves the hair cells, stimulating the nerve endings, which then transmit the impulses to the *vestibular nerve*. These impulses are carried to the portion of the brain involved with maintaining equilibrium and coordinating movement.

## HEARING LOSS AND DEAFNESS

### Frequency and Intensity of Sound

The sense of hearing is the neural perception of *sound energy* and is based on transmission of external sound to the structure of the outer, middle, and inner ear, the nerves to the brain, and portions of the brain involved in processing acoustic information. Sound is characterized by *pitch* (*tone*) and by *intensity* (*loudness*). Traveling vibrations known as sound waves produces sound. Pitch or tone is determined by the *frequency* of vibrations of sound waves. The faster the vibrations or

frequency, the higher the pitch. Frequencies are measured in *Hertz* or cycles per second. Intensity, or loudness, depends on the *amplitude* of sound waves. The greater the amplitude, the louder the sound. Loudness is measured in *decibels*.

Individuals with hearing loss can have diminished hearing with regard to frequency, intensity, or both. Hearing loss related to frequency results in a *distortion of sound* so that individuals may be unable to differentiate between many of the sounds of speech. For example, words with similar sounds such as *cat* and *rat* may be easily confused. Increasing the volume does not improve the quality of sound or make the words more clear if this type of hearing loss exists. Hearing loss related to intensity or loudness involves more difficulty in hearing because of reduction in sound volume. With this type of hearing loss, amplification of sound may improve hearing. In instances where individuals have hearing loss related to both frequency and intensity, increasing volume alone will not improve overall hearing.

### Definition and Classification of Hearing Loss

Disruption of any part of the hearing system can result in hearing loss. Any degree or type of hearing loss is classified as a *hearing impairment*. The greater the degree of hearing impairment, the more difficulty individuals have hearing in a number of situations.

Hearing loss may be partial or total, temporary or permanent, mild to profound. Hearing loss can affect both the volume and clarity of sound. Some individuals have hearing loss that results in reduced *hearing sensitivity*. Individuals with sensitivity loss may be unable to hear soft speech or may have difficulty hearing speech when there is background noise.

Other individuals have difficulty with *speech discrimination*. Individuals with discrimination deficit may, even though volume is adequate, be unable to clearly hear certain phonetic elements of speech (for example, consonants such as *f* and *s*) because they occur at frequencies where hearing loss is present. Individuals can have both sensitivity loss and discrimination deficit at different degrees.

Hearing loss is classified through a number of different criteria:

- Cause and location of hearing loss
- Duration of loss or age of onset
- Degree of hearing loss

### Cause and Location

Cause and location of the loss are classified as:

- conductive
- sensorineural
- mixed

**Conductive hearing loss** occurs when there is damage, obstruction, or malformation in the *external* or *middle ear* that prevents sound waves from reaching the cochlea in the inner ear. In many cases, correction of the underlying problem can restore diminished hearing. Conductive loss may result from buildup of earwax in the ear canal, a foreign object in the ear, infection of the middle ear (**otitis media**), or hardening of the small bones in the ear (**otosclerosis**) that are important for conducting sound. Conductive hearing loss is a mechanical problem that alters the loudness of sound but does not reduce its clarity because the inner ear, where sound is "processed," is not compromised. Sometimes conductive hearing impairments cannot be corrected and hearing aids may be used to amplify sound and restore normal loudness. Conductive hearing losses are generally of mild to moderate degree. Individuals with mild to moderate conductive hearing loss usually have good success with hearing aids if hearing aids are necessary.

**Sensorineural hearing loss** results from damage or malformation of the *inner ear* and/or the *auditory nerve* and can lead to total deafness. Sensorineural loss involves damage to the hair cells of the inner ear, which in turn interferes with the reception of nerve impulses. In some cases, the hair cell function of the cochlea is unaffected; rather, the cause of hearing loss is related to the nerve transmission pathway to the brain. With sensorineural loss, hearing is affected in terms of not only loudness but also pitch or clarity. Individuals may perceive no sound, or sound when perceived may be distorted. Sensorineural hearing loss can be caused by a number of factors, including heredity, acute infection such as meningitis or mumps, *ototoxic drugs* (drugs that damage nerves of the central nervous system that are associated with hearing), tumors, or exposure to loud noise. The problem may also be due to a disorder of the *auditory centers of the brain*, such as from head injury or stroke. When this type of hearing loss occurs, the individual is said to have **central deafness**. In this type of deafness, there is a disruption of the ability of the sound stimulus to reach the hearing centers of the brain, or the hearing center in the brain incorrectly receives and processes signals. Sensorineural hearing impairments are almost exclusively irreversible. Because sensorineural hearing loss involves damage to the hair cells of the cochlea and/or nerve cell damage, and because the nerve function cannot be restored, associated hearing loss is usually permanent. Although the cause of sensorineural loss should be evaluated medically, individuals with sensorineural hearing loss should also consult with a licensed audiologist for evaluation and potential fitting of hearing aids as well as for training in communication strategies.

When individuals have **mixed hearing loss**, there is a combination of *conductive hearing loss* and *sensorineural hearing loss.* The conductive component may lend itself to medical treatment while the sensorineural component remains. Individuals in some instances may benefit from amplification. The extent of the hearing loss experienced with mixed impairments and the success of intervention depend on the degree and type of sensorineural damage.

### Duration of Loss or Age of Onset

Another classification of hearing loss is based on when the hearing loss occurred:

- **Prelingual hearing loss** occurs before the individual acquires language, usually before the age of 3.
- **Postlingual hearing loss** occurs after verbal language is obtained.
- **Prevocational hearing loss** occurs after an individual acquires language but before entering the work force, usually before the age of 19.
- **Postvocational hearing loss** refers to hearing loss that has occurred after the individual has started to work.

### Degree of Hearing Loss

Hearing loss can also be classified according to the *degree* of hearing loss:

- *Hard of hearing* refers to individuals with *mild* to *moderate* hearing loss. Individuals who are hard of hearing usually have difficulty understanding conversational speech through the ear *with* or *without* a hearing aid.
- *Deaf* refers to individuals with *severe to profound* hearing loss. Deafness is

the most severe type of hearing loss. Individuals with severe or profound hearing loss have an extreme inability to understand conversational speech through the ear that precludes their ability to use hearing for communication.

The degree of hearing loss is commonly defined on the basis of the audiogram, described later in the chapter. The audiogram is a method of recording the softest sounds individuals can hear. Normal hearing sensitivity ranges from –10 to +20 decibels. A general guide for describing the degrees of hearing loss associated with decibel losses is found in Table 5–1.

**Table 5–1** Functional Implications of Degrees of Decibel Loss

| | |
|---|---|
| 26–40 | Mild hearing loss. In ideal listening conditions, hearing is minimally affected;  there may be difficulty hearing faint, distant speech even in ideal conditions; background noise may interfere with hearing. |
| 41–55 | Moderate hearing loss. Hears conversational speech but only at close distances; understanding speech is more difficult with background noises. |
| 56–70 | Moderately severe hearing loss. Hears loud conversational speech that is close by. Has difficulty hearing in group situations. |
| 71–90 | Severe hearing loss. Conversational speech severely affected. Perception of sound is usually distorted. |
| Greater than 90 | Profound. May hear (or feel from vibrations) only very loud sounds. Hearing is not the primary communication channel. |

*Source*: Moore, D. F., 2001.

## Causes of Hearing Loss

Hearing loss may be *congenital* or *acquired*. *Congenital hearing loss* is present at birth. The major causes of congenital hearing loss are *genetic transmission* (*inherited hearing loss*), caused by the mother's prenatal ingestion of drugs that are harmful to the developing auditory system of the fetus or prenatal exposure to infections, such as measles (*rubella*).

*Inherited hearing loss* may be part of specific genetically linked conditions that involve a variety of other abnormalities, or it may occur by itself. The degree, progression, and age of onset of inherited hearing loss vary widely, depending on the specific condition or syndrome. In some instances, genetics may not cause deafness per se but rather predispose individuals to hearing loss induced by noise, drugs, or infection (Steel, 2000). In many instances hearing loss is multifactorial, caused by both genetic and environmental factors (Williams, 2000).

*Acquired hearing loss* occurs after birth or later in life. There are a number of causes of acquired hearing loss. Premature birth can be a cause of very early hearing loss, and recurrent ear infections (e.g., otitis media) with complications often cause conductive hearing loss in young children. *Noise-induced hearing loss* is a common but preventable type of acquired hearing loss. Avoiding loud noises or wearing ear protectors when exposed to loud noise could drastically reduce the incidence of noise-induced hearing loss. Acquired hearing loss can also result from injury or disease, such as from traumatic brain injury or from multiple sclerosis affecting the auditory pathway. **Presbycusis** (hearing loss associated with aging) is an acquired hearing loss. The extent to which degeneration of portions of the auditory system is due to the aging process or to cumulative noise trauma throughout life may be difficult to determine.

The type and degree of hearing loss experienced by individuals, regardless of the cause, are varied. Hearing loss usually involves more than a reduction in the loudness of sound. Some hearing losses also result in a distortion of sound so that words may be heard but are difficult to understand or are garbled. In this case, increasing the loudness is unlikely to enhance individuals' ability to understand what is being said.

Some individuals with hearing loss may develop **recruitment**, a symptom characterized by an abnormally rapid increase in the perception of loudness with small changes in signal energy. Individuals with recruitment have a narrow range between a level of sound loud enough to be understood and a level of sound that causes discomfort or pain. Unexpected sounds may startle individuals with recruitment and distract them from interpretating the sound's meaning. Therefore, increasing the loudness of sound does not correct the hearing problem and can actually increase the discomfort.

## Conditions of the Ear Contributing to Hearing Loss

### Conditions of the Outer Ear

Conditions of the outer ear can contribute to hearing loss when there is an obstruction that disrupts the mechanical transmission of auditory stimuli, decreasing hearing acuity. Although conditions of the outer ear may not have a major impact on hearing or may be correctable, they may also be disfiguring, causing cosmetic concerns. Deformities or abnormalities of the outer ear can result from congenital conditions or from trauma. Other conditions of the outer ear that may impede hearing are buildup of earwax (**cerumen**), foreign bodies in the ears, or growths (e.g., polyps) that cause obstruction.

For the most part, partial occlusion of the external ear canal has no influence on the efficiency of sound transmission and causes no significant hearing loss. Complete occlusion, however, generally results in a low to moderate conductive loss. Conditions of the outer ear that cause temporary conductive hearing impairments can usually be corrected or alleviated by surgical or mechanical intervention.

### Conditions of the Middle Ear

Conditions of the middle ear may cause temporary or permanent hearing loss.

#### Perforated Tympanic Membrane

A thickened or *perforated tympanic membrane* (ruptured eardrum) may or may not impair hearing. Rupture of the eardrum may result from an injury (e.g., a blow to the ear or head, or an explosion) or infection or inflammation.

#### Otitis Media

**Otitis media** (inflammation and fluid buildup in the middle ear) can cause conductive hearing losses because of collection of fluid in the middle ear or because of damage to the *tympanic membrane* (eardrum) as a result of infection or rupture. Usually, with appropriate treatment, permanent hearing loss will not result. If not treated promptly, however, otitis media can lead to *mastoiditis* (Hendley, 2002).

#### Mastoiditis

**Mastoiditis** is an infection of the *mastoid cells* within the *mastoid process* located in the temporal bone of the skull. Because of the proximity of the mastoid cells to other important structures in the head, mastoiditis may lead to a number of complications, including paralysis of the facial muscles and infection or abscess of the brain. Mastoiditis is not as prevalent as it once was because of the earlier detection of otitis media and treatment with antibiotics; however, chronic mastoiditis and associated complications can result if previous ear infections are left untreated.

#### Otosclerosis

**Otosclerosis** is a hardening of the ossicles (*incus, stapes,* and *malleus* of the middle ear), which transmit sound impulses to the inner ear. Early symptoms may include trouble hearing on the telephone but not in crowds. The condition appears to be partly hereditary. It causes conductive hearing loss because hardening of the *ossicles* reduces the efficiency of the transfer of sound impulses to the inner ear. Otosclerosis produces progressive hearing loss accompanied by **tinnitus** (ringing or noise in the ear). Some individuals may also have *vestibular symptoms* such as **vertigo** (dizziness) or impaired equilibrium.

Individuals with otosclerosis often hear amplified speech well and without distortions; consequently, they are usually good candidates for hearing aids. Hearing can also often be restored or improved with surgical intervention; however, surgery does not fully remedy the loss. When determining if surgery is appropriate, individuals' lifestyle and occupation are considered. Since surgery may affect vestibular function, individuals who require fine balance for employment may find amplification through hearing aids a better choice than surgery. If individuals' hobbies or occupations expose them to large and rapid changes in barometric pressure, or if heavy lifting is required, hearing aids may also be a better choice because of the chance of postoperative complications or vestibular disturbances.

### Conditions of the Inner Ear

Many conditions of the inner ear cause permanent hearing loss.

#### Labyrinthitis

**Labyrinthitis** (inflammation of the labyrinth of the inner ear) may be acute without resulting in permanent hearing loss. Labyrinthitis may occur as a complication of otitis media, influenza, or upper respiratory infections. Because the inner ear is involved, symptoms of **vertigo** (dizziness), nausea, and vomiting frequently accompany the condition.

#### Tinnitus

**Tinnitus** (ringing or noise in the ears) may or may not be accompanied by hearing loss. It can result from overexposure to loud noise or can be a symptom of a more serious condition, such as tumor, high blood pressure, or head injury. It can also result from side effects or toxic effects of some medications. In some instances, tinnitus may be a separate entity, not associated with a specific disorder and with no identifiable cause. Treatment of tinnitus is dependent on the cause. If the cause can be identified and treated, the ringing can sometimes be eliminated. In other instances, even though the cause is identified, damage may be permanent and tinnitus cannot be cured.

Most people with tinnitus adjust to its presence and experience no severe residual effects; however, some individuals have difficulty adjusting and experience disabling effects, including severe emotional distress. Some individuals complain of problems sleeping because of the constant noise and may need background noise, as from a radio, to mask the sound. A number of therapies, including group cognitive therapy, have been used to help people cope with tinnitus. Adjustment to tinnitus does not appear to be related to the severity of the disorder, but rather to the coping styles of those affected.

#### Meniere's Disease

**Meniere's disease** is a disorder of the inner ear that encompasses the triad of recurrent severe *vertigo*, *sensorineural hearing loss*, and *tinnitus* (noise or ringing in the ears). The cause of Meniere's disease is unknown. One or both ears may be affected. Meniere's attacks are episodic, and the disease is characterized by remissions and relapses. When attacks do occur, they are dramatic, often debilitating individuals during the episode.

*Vertigo* usually appears suddenly and is often accompanied by nausea and vomiting. *Tinnitus* may be intermittent or may be constant between attacks, becoming worse during an attack. The hearing loss associated with Meniere's disease is variable. Typically, hearing loss becomes progressively greater with repeated active attacks. Lower tones may be affected first, but all tones are affected as the disease progresses.

#### Trauma or Disease

Hearing loss may also result from damage to the inner ear or to the *acoustic nerve*. Among causes of *sensorineural deafness* are traumatic head injury or stroke; hypertension and arteriosclerosis, which produce vascular changes in the central nervous system; exposure to high levels of noise, which can damage the hair cells in the inner ear; the ingestion of *ototoxic agents* (drugs or other chemicals that destroy the hair cells of the inner ear or damage the eighth cranial nerve); and infections, such as meningitis. Growths or tumors inside the head may cause hearing loss by mechanically impinging on the acoustic nerve or by involving it directly. Other neurological conditions such as multiple sclerosis may produce changes in the auditory pathway that contribute to hearing loss.

### Presbycusis

**Presbycusis** is caused by degenerative changes in the inner ear, neural pathways, or both; however, the reason that presbycusis occurs is unknown. It has become a catchall term to include many types of auditory deterioration, but it is commonly thought to accompany structural changes in the ear due to aging. Most often presbycusis occurs in both ears equally. Onset is slow, and hearing loss can vary in degree from mild to severe. Ability to hear higher tonal frequencies is usually affected first, but the ability to hear lower frequencies is gradually affected as well. Hearing loss experienced as a result of presbycusis most often is accompanied by word discrimination difficulties, especially if the hearing loss has greatly affected individuals' perception of the higher-pitched consonants.

## CONDITIONS OF THE VESTIBULAR SYSTEM

The vestibular system in the ear contributes to the sense of balance and equilibrium. Although conditions of the vestibular system can be associated with conditions that affect hearing, such as *Meniere's disease*, symptoms related to the vestibular system can also exist with other conditions such as stroke or can result from the side effects of certain medications. Regardless of the cause, conditions

of the vestibular system can cause symptoms that interfere with individuals' functional capacity.

One of the classic symptoms associated with vestibular dysfunction is vertigo. **Vertigo** is an illusory sense of motion, usually described as a spinning sensation, and often thought of in terms of *dizziness*. Although vertigo can be associated with many conditions, it is always related to the body's vestibular system.

Episodes of vertigo can last from a few seconds to days. **Vestibular neuronitis** (inflammation of the vestibular nerve), a disorder of the inner ear, can cause vertigo that lasts for days or weeks and is extremely disabling during that time. During the episode, individuals become nauseous with vomiting and feel a violent spinning of their surroundings. The cause of vestibular neuronitis is unknown.

Vertigo is also associated with Meniere's disease, as discussed above. It can also be associated with head injury or other neurological conditions, such as brain tumor or multiple sclerosis.

## DIAGNOSTIC PROCEDURES

### Identification of Hearing Loss

Before hearing loss can be evaluated or treated, it must be identified. Individuals with hearing impairments may not be aware of the degree of loss, or they may deny that hearing loss exists. An important tool in the diagnosis of hearing loss may be simple observation of behaviors that may indicate such an impairment.

Indications of possible hearing loss in infants and small children include unresponsiveness to sound, delayed development of speech, and behavior problems (e.g., tantrums, inattention, and hyperactivity). School-age children with undiagnosed hearing loss may have speech impairments, may demonstrate attention disorders, or may demonstrate below-average ability in school.

Adults with undiagnosed hearing loss may be irritable, hostile, or hypersensitive. They may deny their inability to understand or respond appropriately by blaming others for not enunciating distinctly. They often avoid situations in which hearing is more difficult, such as large crowds or large groups. Individuals with undiagnosed hearing loss may speak too loudly and may require increased volume to hear the television and radio.

Heightened sensitivity and patience are often necessary when encouraging individuals with suspected hearing loss to obtain evaluation and treatment. Initial resistance to these recommendations is not unusual.

### Physical Examination

Physicians may be the first to recognize or be consulted about a potential hearing loss. Although often omitted, screening for hearing loss should be part of every physical exam. Various check sheets and questionnaires may be used initially to elicit the signs and symptoms associated with hearing loss. During physical examination physicians may also examine the ear canal for obstruction and visualize the tympanic membrane with an instrument called an *otoscope*. Rudimentary auditory screening may also be performed in the physician's office.

Physicians sometimes use *tuning forks* in routine physical examinations in their offices as an initial screening method for hearing impairments. This method can help differentiate between conductive or sensorineural hearing loss; however, it does not quantify the degree of impairment, if one exists. Because of the gross nature of this screening method, it has been widely replaced by other methods.

Tuning forks can be used as a screening method to detect problems in both air conduction and bone conduction of sound. The ability to hear by air conduction is tested by placing a vibrating tuning fork in the air near the ear but out of the individual's sight. The inability to hear the sound is an indication of hearing loss that requires further evaluation. Hearing by bone conduction is evaluated by placing a vibrating tuning fork in different positions on the individual's skull, which causes vibration throughout the skull, including the inner ear. Both conductive and sensorineural impairments can be detected in this manner. Abnormal test results warrant further testing and evaluation.

When problems with hearing are identified, referral for additional testing may be made. For further testing and evaluation, individuals may be referred to an **audiologist**, a person with a master's or doctoral degree in *audiology* who specializes in the evaluation and rehabilitation of individuals with hearing disorders. If testing by the audiologist reveals that medical intervention is necessary, referral is made to an **otolaryngologist** (physician who specializes in diagnosis and treatment of conditions of the ear and related structures).

### Audiometric Testing

*Audiometric testing* measures the degree of hearing loss with an electronic device called an *audiometer*. An *audiologist* usually performs the test. Tests routinely used by audiologists attempt to define three major aspects of hearing:

- The degree of hearing
- The type of hearing loss
- The ability to understand speech under various conditions

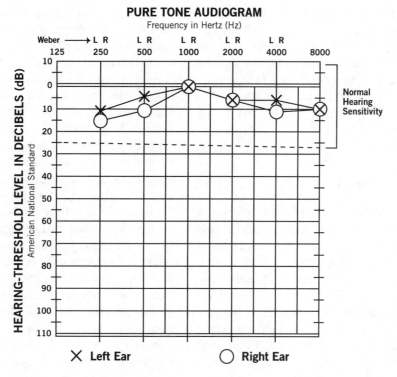

**Figure 5–2** Pure-Tone Audiogram.

A complete audiometric evaluation usually includes *pure-tone air audiometry, bone conduction audiometry, speech audiometry,* and *acoustic immittance measurement.* From audiometric results the type and degree of hearing loss can be determined as well as the degree of speech understanding.

*Pure-Tone Air Audiometry*

The accurate measurement of sound is an important component of a hearing test. Changes in sound intensity are measured in *decibels* and heard as changes in loudness. Changes in sound frequency are measured in *Hertz* and are heard as changes in pitch. Individuals' ability to detect sound and pitch in each ear is plotted on the *audiogram* (see Figure 5–2). A *pure-tone audiogram* is a graph on which an individual's responses to calibrated tones are plotted as *thresholds*. Numbers across the top of the audiogram represent pure-tone frequencies ranging form 125 to 8,000 Hertz. Along the side of the audiogram are numbers ranging from –10 to 110. These numbers represent measurement of decibels.

The *audiogram* illustrates the degree of hearing loss. The *audometric exam* takes place in a sound chamber (booth) to eliminate distracting sounds. An *audiometer* emits sounds (*pure tones*) or words through earphones worn by the individual being tested (*air conduction audiometry*). As the tones are transmitted through the earphones, the individual indicates when sound is first heard. Results of the test are then plotted on the audiogram. The hearing level scale is constructed so that average normal hearing equals 0 decibel;

normal hearing sensitivity ranges from –10 to +25 decibels. The higher the number on the decibel scale, the greater the degree of hearing loss. The audiogram tests speech frequencies that range from 250 to 8,000 Hertz. The inability to discriminate frequencies within this range may interfere with everyday communication.

### Bone Conduction Audiometry

When audiometric testing reveals a hearing loss, the audiologist conducts further testing to determine whether hearing loss is sensorineural, conductive, or mixed. Tests used for this purpose include *bone conduction tests*. The procedure for *bone conduction audiometry* consists of placing a vibrator on the individual's mastoid process or on the forehead. Calibrated tones from the vibrator go directly into the inner ear, bypassing the external and middle ear systems. The individual's responses to the thresholds are plotted on the audiogram and contrasted with the air conduction test results.

To determine the type of hearing loss, thresholds for air and bone conduction are compared. Depending on the differences between the two thresholds, hearing loss is classified as *sensorineural, conductive*, or *mixed*.

### Speech Audiometry

Whereas *pure-tone audiometry* is used to determine individuals' ability to hear specific tones, *speech audiometry* may indicate individuals' ability to understand speech in everyday situations. Two measures are *speech reception threshold* and *speech discrimination threshold*. In both tests individuals wear headphones and listen to words being transmitted through the headphones without any visual cues.

Tests of *speech reception threshold* help identify the lowest intensity, or softest sound level (*decibels*), at which an individual first understands speech. Words from a standardized list with two syllables, such as *baseball*, *ice cream*, or *cowboy*, are presented to the individual through the earphones. Individuals demonstrate acuity by repeating the words they have heard. The speech reception threshold should correspond closely to average pure-tone air conduction thresholds and provides a check for the accuracy of the pure-tone measurements. The higher the decibel level required for either threshold, the greater the hearing loss. A speech reception threshold or average pure-tone threshold of 25 decibels (dBHL) (HL = hearing level), for instance, is considered borderline normal hearing for adults. Limits for children are reduced to 15 to 20 decibels (dBHL). A threshold of 26 to 40 decibels is considered a mild hearing loss.

In addition to measuring how loud speech has to be to be heard, testing also determines how well individuals understand speech once it is loud enough to hear. *Speech discrimination tests* (sometimes called *word recognition tests*) help to provide this information. During the test, words from standardized lists of phonetically balanced one-syllable words are presented to the individual through earphones without visual cues. Words are presented at a suprathreshold level, and the individual must identify and repeat words back to the examiner. The test is scored as the percentage of correctly repeated words. The lower the percentage, the greater the problem in understanding. Individuals with speech discrimination hearing loss may be able to recognize speech but be unable to understand it. The speech discrimination score provides a measure of the ability to understand words at a comfortable volume. It assesses the ability to judge acoustic information and to distinguish between similar speech sounds, such as the letters *p* and *b* or the letters *t* and *d*.

### Acoustic Immittance or Impedance Audiometry

*Acoustic immittance measurement* includes a battery of tests that evaluate middle ear status. *Tympanometry* is a test of *acoustic immittance* in which the mobility or flexibility of the tympanic membrane is assessed by measuring how much sound energy is admitted into the ear as air pressure is varied in the external auditory canal. The status of the eardrum is assessed by altering the air pressure in the ear canal and measuring the response of the eardrum to sound transmissions under these varying conditions and different stimuli. As sound energy strikes the eardrum, some is transmitted to the middle and inner ear, but some is reflected back into the ear canal. If the tympanic membrane is stiff, much of the sound energy is reflected back into the external ear canal. The less impedance, the more sound energy is admitted to the middle and inner ear. An increased level of resistance is diagnostic of middle ear pathology. The results are plotted on a graph called a *tympanogram*. The ear's response is plotted on the vertical dimension of the graph, and air pressures are plotted on the horizontal dimension. Acoustic immittance testing may also be used to measure the *acoustic reflex*, the movement of the muscles attached to the *malleus* and *stapes* as a response to intense sound. It should occur in both ears in response to a loud sound, even if only one ear is stimulated. Acoustic reflex testing may be helpful in diagnosing conditions or problems that involve the cochlea or auditory nervous system.

Acoustic immittance testing requires no voluntary responses from the individual. Consequently, tympanometry is frequently used to detect or rule out conductive hearing loss in children or in adults who are unable to cooperate fully during pure-tone testing.

### Electrocochleography

*Electrocochleography* is a procedure in which stimulus-related electrical activity generated in the cochlea and auditory nerve is recorded. For the test, the individual reclines with electrodes placed in the external auditory canal. Sound stimulus is then delivered through earphones. The test is useful in evaluating inner ear fluid disorders such as *Meniere's syndrome*.

### Auditory Brain Stem Response (ABR) Testing

The ABR records electrical activity generated as sound travels from the auditory nerve through the auditory brain stem pathway. The individual reclines with electrodes placed on the mastoid or on the ear lobe. A stimulus is then presented through earphones, and electroencephalogram activity is evaluated and the auditory brain stem response assessed. The ABR is useful in ruling out auditory diseases such as diseases of the cochlea; degenerative or demyelinating diseases of the auditory system, such as multiple sclerosis; or tumors of the auditory system.

### Otoacoustic Emissions Testing

*Otoacoustic emissions* are measured reflections in the outer ear of mechanical activity in the cochlea. Otoacoustic emissions testing allows one to measure hearing in infants, young children, and difficult-to-test persons such as those with dementia or mental retardation. The technology has enhanced the ability to detect hearing impairment early in life.

## Evaluation of the Vestibular System (Disorders of Balance)

Individuals who experience **vertigo** (dizziness) or who have problems with balance are frequently tested for inner ear and sensorineural disorders related to vestibular function. These tests are performed either by an audiologist or physician. In one test of vestibular nerve function, the *caloric test*, either cold or hot water is introduced into the external auditory canal. The water stimulates the fluids within the inner ear, thus stimulating the vestibular nerve. The introduction of the water into the ear creates a reflex response of the eye called **nystagmus** (involuntary horizontal eye movement). By monitoring the direction of eye movements, the audiologist or physician can determine the origin of the dizziness and whether there may be nerve damage. Eye movement may be monitored visually or with *electronystagmography*, a procedure in which electrodes are placed near the eye to record eye muscle activity.

## TREATMENT OF HEARING LOSS AND DEAFNESS

Both medical and nonmedical interventions may be used in the treatment of hearing loss. *Medical interventions* may involve surgery or medications, and *nonmedical interventions* may include use of hearing aids or other assistive listening devices and special training programs. Treatment in most cases involves a variety of professionals. An **otolaryngologist** (a physician who specializes in disorders of the ear and relat-

ed structures) provides medical evaluation and treatment of hearing loss. **Audiologists**, in addition to conducting evaluations of hearing function, manage the nonmedical treatment of hearing loss, including selecting and fitting amplification devices. The audiologist reviews hearing test results and consults with individuals about their listening needs before recommending which style or type of hearing aid would be most beneficial. Children with hearing loss may also have speech production difficulties because of lack of auditory feedback. *Speech and language pathologists* often work with individuals to help them with particular aspects of speech, language, or both in order to increase intelligibility.

Auditory training is often helpful for individuals with special problems in communication. Such training may be included in hearing aid orientation and/or special programs on listening for the sounds of speech and other environmental sounds.

## Surgical Procedures

Surgical procedures may be performed to eliminate pathological conditions and to restore or improve hearing.

### *Myringotomy*

When the middle ear is infected, as in *otitis media*, or when there is a fluid buildup in the middle ear, surgical intervention may be necessary to drain pus or fluid, thus relieving pressure and preventing rupture of the eardrum (t*ympanic membrane*). A **myringotomy** is a procedure in which an incision is made into the eardrum for this purpose. Because the procedure is performed under controlled conditions, it seldom leaves enough scar tissue to have a negative effect on hearing. If fluid has accumulated in the middle ear, the physician may perform a needle aspiration to remove it. Needle aspiration may not remove fluid that has invaded the *mastoid air cell system*, however, and additional intervention may be necessary if the mastoid system is to be rendered dry. A common procedure performed during myringotomy is placing *ventilation- or pressure-equalizing tubes* in the tympanic membrane. The pressure-equalizing tubes act as an artificial *eustachian tube*, equalizing middle ear pressure. Abnormal eustachian tube function is the most common cause of middle ear problems. The ventilation tubes usually extrude on their own within 3 to 18 months with few complications. When the ventilation tube is in place and operating properly, *conductive hearing loss* due to middle ear disease is usually completely eliminated.

### Mastoidectomy

Since the advent of antibiotics for treatment of *mastoiditis*, mastoidectomy is performed less frequently. **Mastoidectomy** is a surgical procedure for removal of infected *mastoid air cells*, which are located in the mastoid process. Because the mastoid is a portion of the acoustic system of the middle ear, there may be permanent hearing loss after surgery, depending on the nature of the surgery. For example, individuals who have had a **radical mastoidectomy**, in which other structures in addition to the mastoid cells are removed, may have a greater degree of hearing loss or permanent hearing loss. Individuals having a **simple mastoidectomy**, in which only mastoid cells are removed, may have unaffected hearing.

### Tympanoplasty

Surgical procedures involving the middle ear are referred to generally as **tympanoplasty** (repair of the *tympanic membrane*). **Myringoplasty** is a specific type of tympanoplasty in which the damaged eardrum is repaired. Other types of tympanoplasty may be performed for the surgical repair or reconstruction of the *ossicles* of the middle ear. Repairing or reconstructing the conductive mechanisms of the middle ear may improve or restore the conductive component of individuals' hearing.

### Stapedectomy

The most common surgical treatment for *otosclerosis* is **stapedectomy**, a surgical replacement of an immobile or fixed stapes with a prosthesis. The surgery reestablishes a more normal sound pathway between the middle and inner ear; it usually improves hearing but does not totally restore it.

## Devices and Aids for Hearing Loss

### Cochlear Implant

Currently, cochlear implants are the standard treatment for individuals with severe to profound hearing loss who are unable to have effective oral communication even with the benefit of a hearing aid (Gates & Miyamoto, 2003). A **cochlear implant** is an *auditory prosthesis*. The implant is an inner ear device that helps individuals detect medium to loud environmental sounds. Cochlear implants translate sounds into digital impulses that are fed directly to the auditory nerve, bypassing hair cells of the inner ear. This electronic device consists of a *microphone* that picks up sound; a *battery-powered processor*, either at ear level or typically worn on a belt, that converts sound into digital impulses; and a *receiver* implanted into the *temporal bone* that transmits digital impulses down the electrode that has been surgically placed in the cochlea and that stimulates the auditory nerve directly.

The microphone is mounted on the ear-level processor and picks up sounds in the environment. The processor converts sound into digital impulses and sends it to the receiver (the internal component, about the size of a quarter, that is surgically implanted in the temporal bone behind the ear under the skin). The receiver is connected to electrodes in the cochlea that receive impulses and stimulate the auditory nerve with these digital impulses, permitting perception of the digitally processed information as speech.

Cochlear implants can be life-changing for many individuals with severe to profound hearing loss. With the addition of speech reading, these individuals may be able to engage in more effective verbal communication because the implants enable them to distinguish the beginnings and endings of words, as well as the intonation and rhythm patterns being used. Individuals can typically hear moderate sounds, although they may have difficulty perceiving speech clearly in noisy environments and may also have difficulty clearly hearing music. Implants can also have a positive impact in work environments. In addition to being able to hear verbal communication, individuals with cochlear implants are also better able to hear and identify warning signals (Saxon, Holmes, & Spitznagel, 2001).

Although cochlear implants do not restore normal hearing and the sound heard is not like an acoustic signal, individuals with implants become accustomed to hearing via this electrical stimulation. Not all deaf individuals are candidates for cochlear implants. For adults, the following criteria should be met before receiving a cochlear implant:

- Severe to profound sensorineural deafness
- Little or no benefit from hearing instruments
- Postlingually deafened
- Motivated and psychologically suitable for the implant

The chief predictor of success for a cochlear implant is a short duration of deafness (Fischetti, 2003; Gates and Miyamoto, 2003). Age does not appear to be relevant, although children who are prelingually deafened may benefit from early implantation to facilitate speech development. Individuals receiving a cochlear implant should have realistic expectations for hearing ability after the implantation. Optimal use of cochlear implants requires a commitment to rehabilitation, training, and daily practice. Although the cost of a cochlear implant is typically covered by many insurances, reimbursement for auditory rehabilitation, a key to successful use of implants, may be minimal or nonexistent.

Before being treated with cochlear implants, individuals are carefully screened with an audiological assessment as well as a thorough hearing history, physical examination, and psychosocial assessment. Individuals who are prelingually deafened and have strong ties to the Deaf community may be unprepared for the social ramifications of a cochlear implant, since some individuals in the Deaf culture (discussed later in the chapter) are strongly opposed to cochlear implants for cultural reasons. Consequently, in some instances a cochlear implant can socially isolate individuals from other friends who are Deaf (Tucker, 1998).

### Hearing Aids

A hearing aid is any mechanical or electronic device that improves hearing. Hearing aids come in different shapes and sizes and are prescribed and fitted according to individual need. Common styles of hearing aids are as follows:

- Behind-the-ear style, which curves around the back side of the ear
- In-the-ear style, which fits in the ear canal and outer ear bowl
- Canal style, which fits entirely within the ear canal so it is barely visible

All hearing aids, regardless of type or shape, magnify sound and have:

- a micophone to pick up sound
- an amplifier that makes sound louder
- a receiver that conveys sound to the ear
- a battery that provides power for the hearing aid to work

Some hearing aids have special features called *telecoil circuitry* or *tone control*.

Hearing aids with *telecoil circuitry* have a special switch or push button (*T-switch*) located on the hearing aid case that activates the telecoil. A *telecoil* is a very small coil of wire that acts as an antenna, picking up electromagnetic energy that is then delivered to the receiver of the hearing aid and converted into sound. Also available is a plug called a *boot* or *shoe* that is designed to fit over the end of a behind-the-ear type of hearing aid and that is equipped with direct auditory input. This device enables individuals to be connected to an external sound source, such as a radio signal or microphone. It improves the signal-to-noise ratio, improving sound quality. Telecoil circuitry enables individuals to use other assistive listening devices discussed later in the chapter.

*Tone control* is a feature on conventional analog hearing aids (discussed shortly) that allows the audiologist to modify the frequency sensitivity of the hearing aid amplifier to best frequency-shape the hearing aid response to the individual's

hearing loss. For instance, individuals with hearing loss at higher frequencies have difficulty hearing some higher-pitched tones of speech. Tone control is an attempt to amplify the high frequencies without amplifying the lower frequencies.

The most up-to-date technology includes *digital hearing aids*, which change acoustic signals to a discrete series of digital signals so the audiologist can most appropriately frequency-shape the hearing aid response to the individual's hearing loss. As a result, digital hearing aids can theoretically be programmed for each individual hearing loss and provide more precision and clarity of sound. Many contain special "noise-reduction circuits" that aid in reducing background noise. Digital hearing aids have become much more affordable in recent years, with technology options from basic digital to premium digital with directional microphones.

Conventional amplification with older technology is still available in *analog hearing aids*. These original amplification devices make all sounds louder with the exception of the soft speech sounds so necessary for good speech intelligibility. There are limited adjustments available, and therefore sound quality is often lacking.

Hearing aid units are dispensed and fitted by *audiologists* and/or *hearing aid dispensers*. They may be fitted to one or both ears. *Monaural* refers to one hearing aid, and *binaural* refers to two. Recent trends show that binaural fittings are becoming the norm for a variety of reasons, including improved localization skills, safety, and ease of hearing in noise. Most individuals are given a written contract that provides them with a 30-day trial evaluation period, after which, if they are not satisfied, they can receive a refund for the cost of the hearing aid, less any service charges. Although the hearing aid industry has become more regulated, in order to prevent potential misuse it is highly recommended that individuals seeking amplification consult with a licensed audiologist who specializes in hearing aid dispensing. As always, a referral from a friend, family member, or trusted medical professional is the best way to ensure that the individual is working with a skilled and reputable professional.

Although hearing aids may improve hearing and may be beneficial for many individuals, they do not correct hearing in the way that glasses can improve vision to 20/20 (Desselle & Proctor, 2000). Hearing aids can improve volume but not always clarity of speech. Because they work as amplifiers, they make speech louder but not always more clear. In addition, hearing aids amplify not only speech but other sounds in the environment as well, which can interfere with the individual's ability to decipher speech. Individuals with hearing aids may need speech reading to help fill in the gaps in comprehension that still exist. Digital hearing aids have a unique advantage in that they can provide more volume to the soft sounds of speech and less volume to the louder, background sounds that can interfere with understanding.

Hearing aids should be carefully prescribed to meet individual needs. It is recommended after purchase of hearing aids that individuals are provided with a 30-day trial and evaluation period. For best practice, hearing aids should be dispensed with appropriate verification and orientation regarding proper care and use. Orientation is vital to the success of hearing aid use because it helps establish realistic expectations. Additional audiological rehabilitation training or counseling will also help individuals learn ways to enhance communication and to minimize communication obstacles. One of the barriers to effective hearing aid use is the attitude of the individual. Some individuals may be resistant to using a hearing aid because they believe society will view them as less capable. Although smaller, less conspicuous hearing aids have improved acceptance, negative attitudes are still one factor that may prevent many from benefiting from hearing aids.

Hearing aids are delicate devices that need routine care and maintenance to ensure maximum function. Batteries must be replaced regularly. Individuals using hearing aids must also be careful to avoid damaging the internal components. They should refrain from dropping them and from subjecting them to extremes in temperature, excess moisture, or exposure to other substances, such as hairspray, that could damage the microphone or receiver.

### Telephone Devices

There are many different types of telephone devices to assist with telephone communication. Some of them are compatible with hearing aids and work in conjunction with the hearing aid *telecoil*. These telephones enable the hearing aid user to utilize the *telecoil circuitry* and therefore receive a clearer signal without annoying acoustic feedback or squeal. The telecoil circuitry allows the hearing aid user to tap the electromagnetic signal from the telephone. Electromagnetic energy is transferred to the receiver of the hearing aid and converted into sound. At present not all phones are compatible with telecoil; however, the Federal Communication Commission has made changes in statutes that now require all new phones, including cell phones, to be hearing aid compatible.

There are also other telephone devices that may be used without a hearing aid. *Portable telephone amplifiers* can be slipped over a telephone receiver and may be useful for hard-of-hearing individuals who travel and need a louder signal. Other telephone amplification devices may be wired to the *telephone handset* so that volume is increased, giving the user more control. Public telephones equipped with amplifier handsets, although not always readily available, are becoming more common. These telephones are usually identified with an access sign.

### Telecommunication Display Devices (TDDs)

*Telecommunication display devices* (*TDDs*), also called *teletypewriters* or *TTYs*, are used to transmit conversations in printed format over regular telephone lines. Individuals on both ends of the line must have compatible devices with which to type their messages and visualize the printed message on a screen or paper. If one individual does not have a TDD, a third-party system may be used or a *relay operator* can transmit the message to the other individual. Telecommunication relay services allow a person using TDD to communicate with another person using a voice telephone, with the relay operator acting as an interpreter. Special software is also available that allows a personal computer to interact with a TDD and provide a synthesized speech signal. Computers are also allowing greater access for deaf and hard-of-hearing individuals with e-mail.

### Assistive Listening Devices

*Assistive listening devices* include a wide variety of equipment other than hearing aids that can be used by persons with hearing loss. Some may be used independently, and others supplement the hearing aid. Since individuals with hearing loss may have more difficulty perceiving the high-pitched sounds common in speech, or hearing in background noise, assistive

listening devices help to improve the signal-to-noise ratio by facilitating listening and reducing background noise and reverberation.

### Hard-Wired Systems (Personal Listening Systems)

*Hard-wired systems* are individual devices that amplify speech and minimize outside noise so that speech can be more easily understood. The systems must have a direct connection to the sound source using either a microphone or a direct plug-in wire to convey amplified speech signal directly to the receiver (a hearing aid, earphone headset, or neck loop) worn by the individual. When a microphone is used, the speaker speaks into the microphone, speech travels through a cord, and then directly reaches the receiver worn by the listener. When a plug-in is used, a wire is plugged into the sound source (such as a television or radio) and the sound travels through the wire directly to the individual's personal receiver. Using hard-wired systems with television or radio enables individuals with hearing loss to increase the volume on their personal receiver without altering the volume for others in the room.

Hard-wired systems are considered personal listening systems and are more useful in one-to-one communication than in group settings. The systems are small, with the amplifier being contained in a pocket.

### Large Area Systems

Background noise competes with speech sounds, creating a more challenging listening environment for individuals with hearing loss. Additional reverberation affects sound quality in large groups and brings a more distorted signal to hard-of-hearing individuals. Finally, distance is the third factor that has a negative effect for those with hearing loss. A number of *large area devices* to enhance hearing in group settings are available:

- Audio loop systems
- FM systems
- Infrared systems

*Audio Loop.* **Audio loop systems** are made up of a microphone, amplifier, and coil of wire (also called induction coil) that loops around the seating area. Electricity flows through the coil, creating an electromagnetic field that can be picked up by the telecoil of a hearing aid that has been activated through the T-switch or push button. The telecoil acts as an antenna and picks up the electromagnetic energy, delivering it to the user's hearing aid. Individuals using the audio loop must sit within or near the loop for it to operate effectively. Audio loop systems can be permanently installed in public meeting rooms, churches, or theaters or can be set up as needed.

*FM Systems.* **FM systems** are wireless and work much the same as listening to FM radios. Sound is picked up and transmitted through a frequency-modulated band directly to a receiver worn by the individual with hearing loss. Wireless FM systems have greatly reduced the hardware needed, especially with regard to hearing and compatibility. FM systems enhance listening in noisy environments by improving the signal-to-noise ratio.

*Infrared Systems.* **Infrared systems** require the installation of an infrared light emitter that is usually piggybacked onto an existing public address system. Sound is transmitted by invisible, harmless infrared light waves and picked up by a receiver, which can be a headset for use without a hearing aid or a receiver that can be used with hearing aids equipped with a T-

switch. These systems are best suited in rooms or meeting areas without windows, since sunlight affects the signal.

### Caption Services and Telecaption Adapters

*Closed captioning* may be used for television or movies in which printed dialogue appears on a corner or at the bottom of the screen. Real-time caption services display the text on the video monitor immediately. All televisions manufactured after July 1993 that are 13 inches or larger must be equipped with a closed caption option. Older models can utilize a decoder that is connected to the television. Captioned feature and educational films are also available through various distribution services.

### Alerting Devices

Hearing enables individuals to respond to sounds such as sirens, the horn of an approaching car, the doorbell, or a baby's cry. Hearing loss can hamper individuals' ability to respond to everyday environmental sounds, potentially increasing the risk of accidents and possibly increasing feelings of insecurity. Various devices and systems are available commercially to alert individuals with hearing loss to these cues. They may use *visual cues*, such as flashing lights; *auditory cues*, such as increased amplification of sound; or *tactile cues*, such as a vibrator. *Certified Hearing Guide Dogs* (International Dogs, Inc.) are dogs that are trained to react to certain environmental sounds (a telephone ringing, etc.). The dog does not bark but rather makes physical contact with the individual and then runs to the source of the sound.

### Speech Reading (Lip Reading)

*Speech reading* is a communication skill in which individuals with hearing loss watch for clues from the lips, tongue, and facial expression of the speaker. Only one-third of the English language is visible on the lips; therefore, individuals who speech-read often supplement meaning by observing the facial expressions of the speaker and gathering conceptual cues (Myers & Thyer, 1997). Speech reading may also be supplemented with a manual communication system such as *cued speech*.

Speech reading requires good lighting. The speaker must face the individual who is speech reading and must be close enough to enable the individual to see the speaker's lip formation. The speaker should use a natural speaking voice and expression, avoiding distortions of the mouth through movements such as grimacing. Speech reading is more difficult when the speaker speaks very rapidly or enunciates poorly, or when distracting hand movements, a beard, or a mustache obstructs view of the lips. Speakers should avoid chewing, turning away from the listener, or moving about while talking. The speaker should obtain the listener's attention before beginning to speak and clarify statements as necessary. Considerable concentration is required for most people with hearing loss to grasp the spoken word. It is a complex process that can be very tiring when conversation is extended.

### Sign Language

*Language* is a set of symbols combined in a certain way to convey concepts, ideas, and emotions. There are many ways of transmitting language. *Speech* is the verbal expression of language concepts. *Sign language* is a means of communication in which specific hand configurations symbolize language concepts.

There are several types of sign language, the two most common being American Sign Language (ASL) and Signed English.

*American Sign Language* is a distinct and complete language that contains linguistic components that constitute a sophisticated, independent language. It is the native language of Deaf culture. ASL has its own grammar and syntax, idioms and metaphors. It has no written form. Moreover, it is conceptual in nature, rather than word oriented. The signs of ASL are abstract symbols that are capable of expressing multiple elements simultaneously. *Signed English*, in contrast, follows the syntax and linguistic structure of English. Often, people who use Signed English also mouth the words that they sign. This process is called *simultaneous communication. Cued speech*, another system of communication, is phonetically based and uses hand shapes to represent speech sounds.

### Interpreters

*Certified interpreters* can provide an important communication link between the deaf or hard-of-hearing individual and the hearing world. In both group settings and one-to-one interactions, the interpreter is able to translate information so that accurate communication can take place. In situations where it is important for the translation to be precise and accurate, such as professional medical or counseling situations, it is crucial that the interpreter be properly trained and be certified by the *Registry of Interpreters for the Deaf*. In particular situations, such as medical or counseling interactions, it is beneficial to use a professional interpreter with experience in mental health or medical paradigms who can properly assist with complex communication needs. Although family members sometimes serve as interpreters for deaf or hard-of-hearing individuals in more informal situations, in professional situations, their use may obscure objective information and therefore should be avoided if possible.

The presence of an interpreter can be intrusive and alter the dynamics of the medical or counseling interaction. Use of interpreters means that a third party will be present, reducing the sense of privacy that is normally expected in a number of professional situations. Certified interpreters, however, practice under a stringent Code of Ethics that requires that all transactions must be strictly confidential. It takes some adjustment for the employer, counselor, physician, or other person working with the deaf or hard-of-hearing individual to become accustomed to having a third party present in situations that normally take place on a one-to-one basis.

## PSYCHOSOCIAL ISSUES IN HEARING LOSS

### Deafness and Deaf Culture

The needs of people who are deaf or hard of hearing are different from those of individuals with other disabilities. Hearing is vital to verbal communication and to perception of environmental cues; thus all hearing loss interferes with daily function to some degree. The ability of individuals to cope with hearing loss depends on the type and degree of loss, the age of onset, and the extent to which it interferes with daily communication and activity.

Deafness pervades every aspect and activity of an individual's life. It affects speech intelligibility and other basic aspects of hearing, such as localization, recognition, or identification of sound. Severe hearing loss or deafness experienced congenitally or in early childhood also has developmental implications. Hearing loss occurring prior to language development affects individuals' experience and opportunity to gain concepts generally taken for granted in the hearing world. Children learn many concepts from overheard conversations, background information from radio or television, and a multiplicity of other sources. Through this peripheral, daily communication, children learn cultural norms and expectations, generate and shape ideas, and form and enhance values and beliefs. Children who have severe hearing loss or are deaf are not exposed to many elements of communication that enrich the language base, help to formulate concepts, and impart social norms.

Individuals with congenital deafness or with hearing loss acquired before speech development require special programs to help them learn to communicate. Unfortunately, hearing loss in the very young is not always recognized immediately and may be misinterpreted as intellectual deficits, mental retardation, or behavior disorders. Normal development and healthy adjustment of children with hearing loss are dependent to a large degree on early diagnosis and treatment, early social and cultural influences, and parental attitudes and acceptance.

The diagnosis of deafness in a child often results in parental guilt, overprotection, or rejection. Professional assistance for the family of a newly diagnosed deaf infant may be critical to their acceptance of the child's needs and to their competence in providing a nurturing environment for the child's emotional development.

Individuals who have acquired a hearing loss during adulthood have memories of sound, language, and previous function. Speech patterns have already been learned and can be maintained through speech and conversation therapy. Individuals who have acquired hearing loss in adulthood may, however, feel uncomfortable and fear that others will reject them if they admit their disability. They may deny that hearing loss exists or may develop strategies to hide it, such as dominating the conversation to minimize the necessity of understanding anyone else, or accusing others of not speaking clearly or mumbling. Some individuals exhibit aggressive and dominating behavior as a reaction to their hearing loss. Individuals with hearing loss may withdraw completely from situations in which they have difficulty hearing. Being unable to understand what is being said, individuals with hearing loss may believe that the laughter and talk of others are being directed toward them.

Hearing loss can lead to isolation, loneliness, and frustration, as well as to sensory deprivation. Hearing helps individuals communicate on a daily basis with family and friends, and in the social and work setting. At the most basic level, hearing helps individuals keep in touch with the environment. Background sounds, such as the wind in the trees, children playing down the street, or a train whistle in the distance, keep individuals aware of what is happening in the outside world. Hearing also acts as a signal to action. The sounds of a telephone ringing or a baby crying, the horn of an approaching car, or the sound of footsteps from behind are all cues for some type of action. Thus, not only must individuals with a loss of hearing alter activities for which hearing is vital, but also they carry a sense of vulnerability because of their inability to hear sounds that once served as cues to action or danger.

There is a distinction between Deaf culture and the Deaf people who are in it and those who are deaf. Using a capital *D* indicates individuals who are part of a Deaf culture and describe themselves as a *linguistic minority* sharing a culture, not a medical condition (Phillips, 1996; Porter, 1999). From the vantage point of Deaf cul-

ture, deafness is not a disability, not a deficiency, not a handicap, but rather a culture (Lane, 1995).

Culture influences knowledge, beliefs, attitudes, values, and perceptions. It underlies the meaning given to action and the means by which experiences in the world are organized and understood. One of the key components of culture is language, which is necessary for communication. Language is an important part of every cultural identity and determines to a great extent who talks with whom and what is discussed (Rendon, 1992). For those with hearing loss, there is no common language. Not all individuals with severe or profound hearing loss use the same language to communicate. Some use Signed English; some use ASL; some rely to a large extent on speech reading. Especially for prelingually deaf individuals who use ASL as their primary language, English may be viewed as a foreign language.

ASL is a source of pride for the Deaf community. It is a language with its own structure and syntax that has developed over time and that has no written form (Filer & Filer, 2000). Consequently, those who use ASL and especially those who are prelingually deaf frequently become part of the larger Deaf culture.

The Deaf community has its own theater, literature, and schools, along with social rules that are different from those of the hearing community (Barnett, 1999). These differences, especially in social norms, patterns, and traditions, can cause misunderstandings and misperceptions by those in the hearing world. Members of the Deaf culture have rules for behaviors such as getting the attention of individuals with whom they would like to communicate. Stomping a foot or tapping the hand of an individual to get his or her attention may be perfectly acceptable social behavior in the Deaf community but may be viewed as rude by those in the hearing world. Consequently, individuals in the Deaf community may tend to associate with others in the Deaf community rather than with those in the hearing world, may prefer state residential schools for educating the deaf rather than mainstreaming, and may reject efforts to incorporate them into the hearing world. In some instances, pride in the Deaf culture may even preclude procedures such as cochlear implant that could improve the ability to hear. Deaf individuals may believe that attempts to correct their hearing is an implication that they have a medical condition that needs a cure, perpetuating the view of the Deaf as disabled. Some may go as far as to view efforts to cure deafness as an attempt to obliterate Deaf culture (Tucker, 1998).

The Deaf culture does not exist in a vacuum. Individuals may be imbedded in the Deaf culture, but they are also imbued with values, attitudes, and behaviors that are part of a larger national culture as well as often part of ethnic minority cultures (Moore, 2001). This fact creates another layer of diversity.

## Psychological Issues in Hearing Loss

Hearing loss is often associated with isolation because of the very nature of the disability itself. Grief reactions are not uncommon for individuals with acquired hearing loss because they have memories of sounds. Their inability to hear cherished sounds, such as the voices of loved ones, music, or the chirping of birds, may be a difficult loss to accept.

Because hearing loss is an invisible disability, denial is common, especially for those who acquire a hearing loss later in life. They may react with increased sensitivity or irritability when they do not understand words. The increased social pressure to understand may cause anxiety and frustration, and they may avoid activities and interactions that they once enjoyed. Unwillingness to acknowledge hearing loss may result in individuals' refusal to participate in hearing evaluations or reluctance to wear hearing aids.

Individuals with an acquired hearing loss, especially if the onset is sudden, may experience depression. The suddenness of the loss does not give individuals the opportunity to adapt gradually as hearing diminishes; consequently, they are unlikely to have developed signing skills. Depression can also interfere with learning and using new communication skills. Its effects are circular; depression is a barrier to communication, thus intensifying feelings of isolation and making the individual more depressed. Counselors trained in sign language may not be readily available, and the use of an interpreter for counseling sessions may increase the reluctance to participate or to disclose feelings openly.

Any and all of the emotional states experienced by the adult with hearing loss may be experienced by the parents of children who have been identified as hard of hearing or deaf. Just as adults with hearing loss must work through their feelings to achieve a healthy adjustment, so must parents before they can be of optimal assistance to their child.

Individuals who have hearing loss depend heavily on visual channels and on manual means of communication. The development of additional medical conditions that threaten these resources is of increased concern. A visual impairment or conditions that affect the hands, such as rheumatoid arthritis, can seriously hamper individuals' accustomed means of communication if they are using ASL or Signed English, necessitating additional training in new ways of communicating.

## Lifestyle Issues in Hearing Loss

Many daily activities involve the sense of hearing. For individuals with hearing loss, simple transactions, such as purchasing items from a local store, communicating with a repair person, or obtaining directions, require additional means of communication. In some instances, use of a third party as an interpreter may be a solution; however, individuals who are hard of hearing or deaf may resent the loss of privacy or the sense of independence associated with the use of an interpreter.

Signal dogs trained to alert their deaf owners to environmental sounds or signals are increasing in popularity. Special devices are necessary to make daily environmental sounds, such as a knock on the door, known to individuals with hearing loss. Technology and special aids become, in many instances, a necessity.

Everyday activities with family members may require more effort on the part of all involved. For instance, without awareness and sensitivity of other family members, individuals with hearing loss may be unable to participate actively in family conversations at mealtime or engage in small talk while performing various tasks. They may also find themselves increasingly left out of family decision making and discussions.

Depending on the degree of hearing loss, special activities, such as watching television or attending movies, plays, and concerts, may also be affected. Special devices mentioned previously may help individuals participate more fully in such activities. In addition, television decoders that provide captioned programming may be available to enable individuals with hearing loss to enjoy television.

Although hearing loss does not directly affect sexual activity, verbal communication during lovemaking may no longer be possible, which may be viewed by some individuals as an emotional loss. Individuals who are single may have more difficulty meeting potential partners and establishing communication that could lead to a more intimate relationship.

## Social Issues in Hearing Loss

The social environment of individuals with hearing loss is profoundly altered because of the need for alternate means of communication. Individuals who have been deaf since birth or early childhood may integrate well with the Deaf community, where a common language is shared. Those who acquired hearing loss later in life, however, frequently do not join the Deaf community and may feel more isolated, feeling they fit neither into the Deaf community nor into the hearing world.

Language plays an important role in regulating social play interactions and is paramount for framing and setting up play activities. Children who are deaf or hard of hearing may have difficulty developing cooperative play with hearing playmates. Promoting socialization between children with hearing loss and hearing peers includes building on the strengths of the children and fostering a shared communication system that encourages social integration. Hearing loss at an early age also has implications for literacy. Individuals who have been deaf from an early age usually have a literacy level of fourth to fifth grade after high school (Barnett, 1999). Low literacy rates may be attributed to lack of consensus on educational methods. Emphasis is often placed on techniques of communication, with less emphasis on content matter. In addition, since English is often a second language to individuals who are deaf, children who are deaf may face the same educational barriers as those experienced by other minority groups whose primary language is not English.

People with acquired hearing loss in adulthood are more likely to maintain social and cultural contacts with the hearing world because they have grown up with the language and culture of the hearing world. Many people, however, who were deaf from an early age and use ASL as their primary language feel part of the Deaf community, which has established a culture in which there are, in addition to language, specific norms and characteristics. Individuals in this culture identify with the Deaf community and tend to view deafness not as a disability but rather as an alternative culture and associated lifestyle. Individuals who do not speak the language are frequently viewed as outsiders and are not readily integrated into the Deaf culture.

Individuals with hearing loss may limit social contacts to family members and a few close friends, or they may avoid social contacts altogether because of their inability to understand what is being said. Difficulty in understanding verbal communication can cause withdrawal from social situations to avoid the embarrassment of giving inappropriate responses to questions or statements. Lack of understanding by others can contribute to social isolation. New acquaintances, unfamiliar with hearing loss or unaware of the individual's inability to hear, may perceive them as aloof or even rude because of their failure to respond to a friendly statement that they did not hear.

Individuals may have more difficulty keeping up with conversations in group settings, especially if others in the group are unaware of or insensitive to their needs. Group settings with poor lighting make lip reading more difficult, and competing sounds, such as the rattling of dishes in a restaurant, may make communication difficult even for individuals with milder hearing loss.

Engaging in conversation requires cooperation from others. Some people may feel uncomfortable or impatient while attempting to communicate with individuals with hearing loss; consequently, they may avoid contact with them. Some may consider deafness a social stigma because of myths and misconceptions about hearing impairments. Such attitudes build a barrier to acceptance by others and to inclusion in the larger social community. Societal responses can create difficult and stressful situations for individuals with a hearing impairment, discouraging further participation in social functions. A number of support groups directed toward individuals with adult or late-onset hearing loss are available. One such group is Self Help for Hard of Hearing People (SHHH). Another example of such a group is the Association of Late Deafened Adults (ALDA). In addition to offering support to individuals who are hard of hearing or deaf, SHHH and ALDA strive to increase community understanding about the rights and needs of individuals with hearing loss, as well as to make social environments more accessible. Many communities also have other types of support groups for people with hearing loss.

Although family members serve as a support group for individuals with hearing loss, their attitudes may also impede individuals' acceptance of their condition and subsequent rehabilitation. Family members may perceive a hearing loss as feigned or may attribute the difficulty to inattention. As a result, they may become angry, ignore the individual, or exclude him or her from conversations rather than learn techniques to enhance the individual's ability to maintain an active role in conversation. Family members who serve as interpreters for those with hearing impairments may, on the other hand, begin to resent their role, feeling stifled in social interactions.

## VOCATIONAL ISSUES IN HEARING LOSS

Individuals with hearing loss face the same issues with regard to employment as others with disability; however, there are additional special vocational issues that must be considered. Many jobs require individuals to be alert to auditory cues in order to perform or maintain safety. Most jobs also require communication with coworkers and/or customers. People who are deaf or hard of hearing may have difficulty receiving instructions or supervision or participating in staff meetings or in-service training. In addition, they may have difficulty interacting in work-related social functions. Assistive devices may be needed to help them with basic communication, or there may be a need for job restructuring, redesigning procedures, or redelegation of assignment to accommodate their communication needs.

Just as there are myths and stereotypes about hearing loss in the social world, so there are myths and stereotypes in the world of work. Employers and fellow workers may not understand hearing loss and may be unaware of the special needs of deaf or hard-of-hearing individuals, or of the special techniques available to enhance communication with those who experience it. Since hearing loss is an invisible disability, coworkers or supervisors may not recognize the need for special accommodations or may feel that individuals with hearing loss are feigning their degree of disability. In some instances, individuals' lack of ability to hear may be interpreted as lack of intellectual ability, and those with hearing loss may be relegated to jobs requiring less cognitive ability.

In the work setting, individuals with a hearing loss may need special assistive devices, communication aids, and signaling devices. The use of such devices is often dependent on the availability and expense of the purchase and installation of the special items. Equipment may be prioritized according to need if funds are limited. For example, a signaling device that may be crucial for safety may be considered vital, while equipment that would enhance individuals' performance may not receive as high a priority.

Because visual cues are so important to communication for individuals with hearing loss, good lighting in the workplace is a necessity. Many individuals with hearing loss experience discomfort with loud noises; therefore, the noise level in the environment should be evaluated. In some instances, it may be necessary for individuals to wear ear protectors to prevent further hearing loss. Room acoustics must also be considered, because the reverberation of sound in an environment can interfere with hearing aid effectiveness.

Hearing aids can greatly enhance some individuals' performance in the work setting. Although technological advances have made hearing aids more durable, they are intricate devices that may be susceptible to damage from environmental factors. They are sensitive to extremes of temperature, especially extreme cold, and they require protection from perspiration in hot and humid environments.

Individuals with hearing loss are a heterogeneous group and should be considered as such. Although special needs associated with hearing loss should be considered, individuals' special talents and interests should also be considered in helping those with hearing loss adjust to the work environment. With the use of assistive devices, many job opportunities not previously available to individuals with hearing loss are now possibile. Central to success in vocational placement of individuals who are deaf or have hearing loss is employer familiarity with indi-viduals' accommodation needs (Schroedel & Geyer, 2001). In addition, some attitudinal barriers still exist that may preclude the individual with hearing loss from obtaining satisfactory employment.

## CASE STUDIES

### Case I

Mrs. G. is a 42-year-old woman who has worked as a public relations specialist at a major university for the past 10 years. In this position Mrs. G. handles community relations, establishes cooperative relationships with the community and local businesses, and keeps university administrators aware of public interests and concerns. She also is responsible for preparing written press releases and special interest stories that promote activities at the university. In addition, she is responsible for preparing reports and writing proposals for various projects. Over the past few years Mrs. G. has noted a significant decline in hearing in her left ear with moderate loss in her right ear. On evaluation by an audiologist she was found to have sensorineural deafness resulting from small strokes. Hearing loss in the left ear was at the 45-decibel range, and loss in the right ear was at 30 decibels. Mrs. G. has a master of science degree in public policy. She is married and lives with her husband in a small city of 50,000. She has two grown children.

### Questions

1. To what extent will Mrs. G.'s degree of hearing loss impair her ability to continue to function in her current occupation?
2. Given the type and extent of Mrs.G.'s hearing loss, what adaptive devices or reasonable accommodations may help her maintain her current employment?
3. Should Mrs. G. receive additional evaluation?
4. How do Mrs. G.'s current skills and work history affect her rehabilitation potential?
5. What additional information would you want to gain about Mrs. G.'s specific duties at her current job?

### Case II

Mr. M. is a 55-year-old male who works as a printing press operator for a large city newspaper. While printing presses are running, he monitors the printing process for paper jams and even ink distribution, and he attempts to keep the printing process running smoothly. There is considerable pressure on the job because the presses work under high printing speeds, and press machinery is potentially hazardous as well as noisy. Mr. M. has experienced increasing difficulty hearing and on evaluation is found to have mixed hearing loss, with moderate loss in both ears. He has a high school education. He has never been married and lives alone in a small apartment several blocks from work.

### Questions

1. What specific environmental issues would you address with Mr. M. and/ or his employer regarding his current job situation?
2. What specific issues about Mr. M.'s type and level of hearing loss would you address?
3. Are there issues regarding Mr. M.'s age that you would consider in working with him on his rehabilitation plan?

## REFERENCES

Barnett, S. (1999). Clinical and cultural issues in caring for deaf people. *Family Medicine, 31*(1), 17–22.

Desselle, D. D., & Proctor, T. K. (2000). Advocating for the elderly hard-of-hearing population: The deaf people we ignore. *Social Work, 45*(3), 277–281.

Filer, R. D., & Filer, P. A. (2000, Winter). Practical considerations for counselors working with hearing children of deaf parents. *Journal of Counseling and Development, 78*, 37–43.

Fischetti, M. (2003, June). Cochlear implants: To hear again. *Scientific American, 288*, 82–83.

Gates, G. A., & Miyamoto, R. T. (2003). Cochlear implants. *New England Journal of Medicine, 349*(5), 421–423.

Hendley, J. O. (2002). Otitis media. *New England Journal of Medicine, 347*(15), 1169–1174.

Lane, H. (1995). Constructions of deafness. *Disability and Society, 10*(2), 171–189.

Moore, C. L. (2001). Racial and ethnic members of under-represented groups with hearing loss and VR services: Explaining the disparity in closure success rates. *Journal of Applied Rehabilitation Counseling, 33*(1), 15–20.

Moore, D. F. (2001). *Educating the deaf: Psychology, principles, and practices* (5th ed.). Boston: Houghton Mifflin.

Myers, L. L., & Thyer, A. (1997). Social work practice with deaf clients: Issues in culturally competent assessment. *Social Work in Health Care, 26*(1), 61–74.

Phillips, B. A. (1996). Bringing culture to the forefront: Formulating diagnostic impressions of deaf and hard-of-hearing people at times of medical crisis. *Professional Psychology: Research and Practice, 27*(2), 137–144.

Porter, A. (1999). Sign-language interpretation is psychotherapy with deaf patients. *American Journal of Psychotherapy, 53*(2), 163–176.

Rendon, M. E. (1992). Deaf culture and alcohol and substance abuse. *Journal of Substance Abuse Treatment, 9*, 103–110.

Saxon, J. P., Holmes, A. E, & Spitznagel, R. J. (2001). Impact of a cochlear implant on job functioning. *Journal of Rehabilitation, 67*(3), 49–54.

Schroedel, J. G., & Geyer, P. D. (2001). Enhancing the career advancement of workers with hearing loss: Results from a national follow-up survey. *Journal of Applied Rehabilitation Counseling, 32*(3), 35–44.

Steel, K. P. (2000). New interventions in hearing impairment. *British Medical Journal, 320*(7235), 622–629.

Tucker, B. P. (1998). Deaf culture, cochlear implants, and elective disability. *Hastings Center Report,* July–August, pp. 6–14.

Williams, P. J. (2000). Genetic causes of hearing loss. *New England Journal of Medicine, 342*(15), 1101–1109.

# CHAPTER 6

# Psychiatric Disabilities

## DEFINING PSYCHIATRIC DISABILITY

Psychiatric disabilities encompass a broad range of conditions in which there are behavioral or psychological symptoms associated with distress and/or altered function. Effective mental functioning depends on a variety of social and environmental factors, as well as on the efficient functioning of structures within the brain. As with physical conditions, the degree of disability experienced with psychiatric conditions is variable.

Symptoms of psychiatric conditions vary widely, consisting of both behavioral manifestations and subjective feelings. Some psychiatric conditions are characterized by deficits in or loss of intellectual function, whereas others are associated with loss of contact with reality (**psychosis**). Some psychiatric conditions do not have symptoms of psychosis but rather changes in mood that cause distress or impaired function. In still other psychiatric conditions, intellectual function, sense of reality, or mood may be unimpaired, but symptoms are manifested by maladaptive behavior.

The extent of disability experienced as a result of a psychiatric condition is dependent, to a great extent, on the degree to which the condition interferes with in-

dividuals' ability to function within the environment, the degree to which their behavior disturbs others, and the degree to which the condition causes subjective distress. The goal of psychiatric rehabilitation is to help individuals develop skills and supports that will enable them to function at their highest capacity in the residential, educational, or vocational setting of their choice.

Psychiatric conditions are more difficult to define and diagnose than are physical conditions. Causes are not always identifiable, and there are no laboratory tests readily available to confirm the diagnosis. In many cases, the primary basis for diagnosis and prediction of functional capacity is the experienced judgment of the professionals conducting the evaluation. Moderating variables, such as the ethnic status, education, and/or socioeconomic status of both the client and the professional, may influence individuals' performance on evaluation as well as professionals' interpretation of the evaluation results.

## THE DIAGNOSTIC AND STATISTICAL MANUAL OF MENTAL DISORDERS

The need for a systematic, more standardized approach to the diagnosis of psychiatric conditions has been recognized for well over a century. Although initially psychiatric conditions were codified for the purpose of collecting statistical information, in 1952 the American Psychiatric Association Committee on Nomenclature and Statistics published the *Diagnostic and Statistical Manual of Mental Disorders* (*DSM-I*), a book that was the first official manual of mental disorders that had clinical utility. Since that time, there has been continued work to revise and refine the diagnostic manual.

As more empirical research and field trials are available, reliability, descriptive validity, and performance characteristics for diagnostic criteria have been established. Updated versions of the manual bear the number of the edition (DSM-II, DSM-III, and DSM-IV). The fourth edition of the manual, the DSM-IV, was published in 1994, and in 2000 the DSM-IV-TR (4th edition Text-Revision) was published, representing the latest effort in empirical documentation on which to base diagnostic decisions.

The manual is an attempt to establish objective criteria for the diagnosis of psychiatric conditions. In addition to providing specific criteria by which to diagnose, it provides consistency among professionals in communicating about psychiatric conditions. The use of the manual for diagnostic purposes requires specialized clinical training, since the criteria within the manual are meant to be guidelines and are not considered absolute. Professionals working with individuals with psychiatric conditions should be familiar with the manual; however, responsibility for the diagnosis most frequently lies with psychiatrists, psychologists, and, in some states, social workers.

The DSM-IV-TR, rather than taking a theoretical approach to defining psychiatric conditions, attempts to describe conditions by defining observable symptoms. It should be emphasized that diagnostic criteria should *not* be used to categorize or label people, but rather to assist in treatment planning.

The DSM-IV-TR uses a *multiaxial system* of diagnosis to increase specificity. Since psychiatric conditions, like physical conditions, rarely occur in a vacuum and vary from individual to individual, the multiaxial approach helps professionals avoid focusing only on specific symptoms. Rather, it enables professionals to take a comprehensive approach to identifying other variables that could impact on treatment and help to predict outcome.

The manual incorporated multiaxial diagnosis in 1980 to clarify the complexities and relationships of symptoms and, thus, assist professionals in more appropriate treatment planning. The DSM-IV-TR uses five axes:

- Axis I describes clinical syndromes.
- Axis II describes personality disorders and mental retardation.
- Axis III describes medical conditions that may also be present and relevant to individuals' treatment.
- Axis IV describes relevant psychosocial or environmental problems that may have contributed to the development of the condition or that may affect individuals' treatment or prognosis.
- Axis V is used for reporting individuals' overall level of functioning in the judgment of the clinician who has done the evaluation, in accordance with the Global Assessment of Functioning (GAF) scale.

Level of functioning is determined by using the *GAF scale*. The scale is a guideline for determining individuals' psychological, social, and occupational functioning on a hypothetical continuum of mental health and illness. Impairment in functioning due to physical or environmental limitations is not considered. Overall level of psychological functioning is rated on a scale of 1 to 100. The scale ranges from superior level of functioning at the level of 100 to persistent danger of hurting self or others at the level of 1.

---

**Table 6–1** Multiaxial Recording of Evaluation Results

---

*Case I*

| | | |
|---|---|---|
| Axis I | 309.81 | Posttraumatic Stress Disorder |
| | 305.0 | Alcohol Abuse |
| Axis II | V7.09 | No Diagnosis |
| Axis III | 491.20 | Bronchitis, Chronic Obstructive Pulmonary Disease (COPD), Without Acute Exacerbation |
| Axis IV | | Unemployment |
| Axis V | | GAF = 53 (current) |

*Case II*

| | | |
|---|---|---|
| Axis I | 295.30 | Schizophrenia, Paranoid Type |
| Axis II | V71.09 | No Diagnosis |
| Axis III | 250.01 | Diabetes Mellitus, Type I/ Insulin Dependent |
| Axis IV | | Abusive Caregiver |
| Axis V | GAF = 27 (on admission) | |
| | GAF = 52 (on discharge) | |

*Case III*

| | | |
|---|---|---|
| Axis I | 296.23 | Major Depressive Disorder, Single Episode, Severe Without Psychotic Features |
| Axis II | 317 | Mental Retardation |
| Axis III | None | |
| Axis IV | None | |
| Axis V | GAF = 60 (current) | |

---

Psychiatric conditions are coded according to the *International Classification of Diseases*, Ninth Revision, Clinical Modification (ICD-9-CM). In reporting evaluation results, the ICD-9-CM code precedes the name of the condition. Diagnostic codes are used for record-keeping purposes and for reimbursement. Examples of multiaxial recording of evaluation results with ICD-9-CM coding can be seen in Table 6–1.

## COMMON PSYCHIATRIC DISABILITIES

### Conditions Diagnosed in Infancy, Childhood, or Adolescence

A number of conditions are included in the DSM-IV-TR diagnostic class of *"Disorders Usually First Diagnosed in Infancy, Childhood, or Adolescence."* Some of the more common conditions in this category are mental retardation, autism, Asperger's disorder, and attention deficit disorder. The conditions are lifelong. Although usually diagnosed prior to the age of 18, at times these conditions are not diagnosed until adulthood.

#### *Mental Retardation*

The term *mental retardation* describes conditions in which:

- occurrence is *before* the age of 18
- intellectual functioning is below average
- adaptive behavior is deficient (American Psychiatric Association, 2000)

The American Association on Mental Retardation defines mental retardation as "a fundamental difficulty in learning and performing certain daily life skills" (1992).

Although many individuals still equate mental retardation with intelligence quotient (IQ), the condition clearly encompasses both intellectual functioning and adaptive behavior. Adaptive behavior encompasses individuals' social skills and performance in the social environment, including communication and management of tasks of daily living. In most instances adaptive behavior parallels intellectual capacity. In addition to limited intellectual or adaptive capacity, individuals with mental retardation may have other medical conditions or sensory or motor deficits that further affect their functional capacity. Any physical or behavioral problems must also be considered in determining the individual's ability to function within the environment.

Although the exact cause of mental retardation cannot always be identified, a number of factors are known to be associated. Prenatal causes of mental retardation can include maternal infections, maternal nutritional deficiency, trauma, exposure to toxic sources during fetal development, maternal oxygen deprivation, and compromise of the fetal blood supply. A variety of hereditary disorders, such as metabolic disorders (e.g., phenylketonuria), chromosomal abnormalities, or some familial syndromes, may also result in mental retardation. Other specific conditions that were acquired in childhood, such as meningitis, traumatic brain injury, or exposure to toxic substances, can also lead to mental retardation.

### Classification of Mental Retardation

There are varying degrees of mental retardation or developmental delay. Degrees of severity of intellectual disability can range from mild to profound. Individuals with mental retardation have a wide range of abilities as well as disabilities. The extent of support needed varies with the individual and with his or her circumstances. Some individuals with mental

retardation may also have delays in motor-skill development, speech and language problems, and vision or hearing impairments. In addition, there may be emotional challenges and vulnerabilities that can be caused by pathologic or environmental factors.

Mental retardation is generally categorized as mild, moderate, severe, or profound and is expressed in relation to the IQ (see Table 6–2). The IQ is obtained through administration of individualized standardized intelligence tests such as the *Wechsler Intelligence Scales for Children-Revised* or the *Stanford-Binet*. For a particular individual, the degree of retardation is classified according to evaluation and testing of both the individual's intellectual performance and adaptive behavior. Adaptive behavior refers to the individual's ability to cope with common life demands as would be expected of others in their age group.

---

**Table 6–2** Classification of Mental Retardation

| Classification | IQ |
| --- | --- |
| Mild | 50–55 to 70 |
| Moderate | 35–40 to 50–55 |
| Severe | 20–25 to 35–40 |
| Profound | Below 20–25 |

---

Although a number of scales were developed to measure adaptive functioning, assessment information is more useful if derived from a number of sources, such as teacher evaluation or educational development, in addition to adaptive scale scores. A variety of other factors, such as environment and stimulation, also help to determine intellectual functioning and adaptive capability, so test results are not always absolute. In all instances, not only intellectual capacity but also adaptive functioning must be considered.

### Functional Ability According to Classification of Mental Retardation

Mild Retardation. Generally, individuals with **mild mental retardation** are considered capable of attaining intellectual function up to a sixth-grade level. During their pre-school years, they are generally capable of attaining social and communication skills consistent with their peers; consequently, some individuals may not be distinguishable from other children in their age group. Individuals with mild retardation may be able to obtain employment and live independently or with minimal support and supervision, although they may need additional support and guidance when in particularly stressful or new situations. Generally, individuals in this category can live independently in the community.

Moderate Retardation. Individuals with **moderate mental retardation** often attain intellectual function at the second-grade level, but they may require more supervision in activities of daily living, although they can usually manage self-care. Processing abstract information is generally difficult. Individuals with moderate mental retardation are usually capable of learning some vocational skills, although they may function best in a supervised work environment, such as a sheltered workshop or supported employment situation. They may have differing degrees of expressive and receptive language skills. They are generally able to live in the community, but in supervised settings.

Severe Retardation. Individuals with **severe mental retardation** generally have limited communication skills and poorly developed motor skills. During school age, they may attain some elementary self-care skills and may learn to read some key words; however, for the most part, they will require close supervision for most tasks. In adulthood, they may live in community group homes or with their families. Many individuals in this category of mental retardation have an associated central nervous system disorder, visual and/or hearing impairment, severe motor and physical disabilities, and lack of expressive language skills. Because of the severity of the condition, most individuals require close supervision and provision of most daily care. They generally respond best to a consistent caretaker and to a low-stimulus environment.

### Psychosocial Issues in Mental Retardation

The opinions and expectations most people have about themselves are influenced to a great degree by the behavior of those around them. When minimum expectations or lack of belief in individuals' ability to achieve are communicated, the chances for individuals to progress in attaining goals are diminished. Because a number of inaccurate and stereotypical ideas about individuals with mental retardation still exist, barriers to reaching optimal function and independence continue to be present. Although societal and employer attitudes are changing slowly, there is continued need for education and integration of individuals with mental retardation into society and into the workplace.

Although all individuals with mental retardation can experience stresses due to societal stereotypes and attitudes, individuals with mild retardation may confront specific stresses because they may appear normal to others and consequently limitations may not be recognized as a disability. Lack of acceptance and devaluation can resultant in low self-esteem and isolation, which in turn can lead to deviant behaviors or acting out. In more severe cases, a psychiatric disorder may be developed as a means of coping.

### Vocational Issues in Mental Retardation

The level of occupational functioning for individuals with mental retardation depends to some extent on the degree of disability. Because mental retardation is often accompanied by other medical conditions, the physical limitations associated with any medical condition must also be considered. Individuals with mental retardation usually perform better in a structured environment. Many individuals may need to be taught how to function independently and may need accompanying social skills training.

As with other disabilities, the largest barrier to the individual reaching full potential may be societal stereotypes and prejudice. Although there has been heightened effort and interest toward increasing integrated employment opportunities for individuals with mental retardation, rehabilitation outcomes, especially for individuals of racial and ethnic under-represented groups, have been less than ideal (Moore, 2001). Consequently, continued equality in service delivery and assurance and education of potential employers may be crucial factors in successful occupational placement.

### Pervasive Developmental Disorders

Pervasive developmental disorders are conditions in which there is *stereotypical behavior* or impairment in several areas of development, including *social interaction* and *verbal and nonverbal communication*. Although a number of conditions are in-cluded in this category, two of the most common are autism and Asperger's disorder.

### Autism

Autism has shown a steady increase in incidence since it was first described in 1943 (Merrick, Kandel, & Morad, 2004). Considered one of a family of developmental disabilities, autism (autistic disorder) is a disorder of brain function that has a broad range of behavioral consequences, including impairment in reciprocal social interaction and impairment in verbal and nonverbal communication (American Psychiatric Association, 2000). Other symptoms may include repetitive and stereotyped mannerisms, intense preoccupation with a specific and restricted area of interest, lack of spontaneous play or shared enjoyment with others, hyperactivity, aggressiveness, or self-injurious behaviors. Hypersensitivity to sensory stimuli may also be present. Often there is also impairment in cognitive skills and intellectual capacity (Yeung-Courchesne & Courchesne, 1997). Many individuals with autistic disorder have an associated diagnosis of mental retardation. The severity of symptoms varies.

Individuals usually exhibit symptoms of autism from birth; however, because of the subtlety of early symptoms, the condition may not be diagnosed until symptoms are more noticeable later in development. By definition, onset occurs prior to the age of 3.

Treatment of Autism. There is no cure for autism. Medications are usually used to control specific symptoms, such as attention deficit, aggression, or self-abusive or other stereotypic behaviors. The most important intervention for individuals with autism is remedial education directed toward improving communication skills and assisting with behavioral disorders.

Functional Implications of Autism. Each individual with autism has unique strengths and interests that should be accommodated to help him or her achieve the maximal degree of functional capacity (Olney, 2000). Although symptoms may improve as the child develops, most individuals with autism maintain a degree of dependence in their adult years. Those with mild manifestations of symptoms may, with support, function independently to some degree; however, social interaction and communication skills may still be problematic. Supported work environments and group homes may help individuals function with less dependence on their family.

### Asperger's Disorder

Asperger's disorder is characterized by the DSM-IV-TR as "severe and sustained impairment in social interaction and development of restricted, repetitive patterns of behavior, interest, and activities" (American Psychiatric Association, 2000). Controversy continues, however, regarding the extent to which Asperger's disorder differs from autism (Macintosh & Dissanayake, 2004; Mayes, Calhoun, & Crites, 2001). Individuals with Asperger's disorder show core symptoms of autism in the presence of high verbal intelligence (Frith, 2004), and some question whether the disorder (sometimes called "high-functioning" autism) necessarily leads to disability (Baron-Cohen, 2000).

Individuals with Asperger's disorder usually have no significant language delays or delays in cognitive development, age-appropriate self-help skills, or adaptive behavior (American Psychiatric Association, 2000). Diagnosis is often not made until children enter school and have difficulties with social interaction. Although cognitive function is normal, adults with Asperger's disorder may continue to have difficulty with social interaction.

### Attention Deficit/Hyperactivity Disorder

Attention deficit/hyperactivity disorder (ADHD) is a condition characterized by inattention, hyperactivity, and impulsivity, with symptoms appearing prior to the age of 7 (American Psychiatric Association, 2000). Symptoms appearing in childhood can persist into adulthood, causing adjustment problems at work as well as at home and in other social settings. The cause of ADHD is unknown. Parents may first observe symptoms during the toddler years, when the child seems to be constantly "on the go" and has difficulty sitting still during "quiet" activities. The condition is more likely to be diagnosed, however, during the school years, when the need for sustained attention in a more structured environment brings symptoms under closer attention.

Individuals with the disorder have difficulty paying attention or giving attention to details. They may have difficulty with organizational skills and may be easily distracted. In social situations, they may appear to not be listening to what others say, changing the subject of conversation frequently. Individuals may have difficulty sitting still, with frequent fidgeting and squirming, and difficulty remaining seated. They may also have difficulty remaining quiet when appropriate, instead talking excessively, blurting out responses at inappropriate times, and interrupting others frequently. Individuals with ADHD may appear impatient, careless, and disorganized. As they reach adulthood, symptoms may become less conspicuous.

## Delirium and Dementia

Delirium and dementia have in common symptoms in which there is a decrease in cognitive ability or memory from a prior level of functioning. These conditions are characterized by alteration of brain function and are often caused by an identifiable organic factor.

These disorders can occur at any age and can be secondary to another medical condition (e.g., heart disease, in which circulation and consequently oxygen to the brain are diminished) or can be caused by a systemic disease (e.g., thyroid disease), by injury to the brain itself (e.g., ministrokes), or by toxic substances (e.g., poisons, alcohol, or other drugs); several causes may be present simultaneously. Manifestations of these conditions may affect psychological, cognitive, or behavioral function. In previous editions of the DSM, these conditions were classified as *organic mental disorders*. The DSM-IV-TR no longer uses this term because it implies that other mental disorders may not have a biological basis.

The diagnosis of mental conditions in this category is usually based on a detailed history of symptoms, findings on physical and neurological evaluation, and clinical studies and laboratory studies, as well as neuropsychological assessments.

These conditions affect a variety of cognitive abilities, such as:

- memory
- orientation judgment
- attention
- computational and organizational skills

There may also be associated *psychomotor* or *language impairments, sleep disturbances,* and *other behavioral manifestations.* Although some of these conditions remain stable, others are associated with progressive deterioration and decline of function.

Conditions classified in this DSM category can be acute or chronic. Symptoms of acute disorders are sudden in onset, such as symptoms caused by generalized infection or intoxication. Symptoms of chronic disorders generally occur more slowly and are characterized by the deterioration

of cognitive processes over time, such as symptoms occurring with arteriosclerosis or Alzheimer's disease.

Mental conditions in this category may be reversible or irreversible. If the underlying cause of the symptoms can be corrected and the brain has not been permanently damaged, the condition is said to be *reversible*. If the underlying cause cannot be corrected or treated, or if the damage to the brain is permanent, the condition is *irreversible*.

### Delirium

Delirium is characterized by difficulty in sustaining attention to external stimuli, difficulty in shifting attention to new stimuli, and difficulty in maintaining a coherent thought process. Symptoms of delirium characteristically develop over a short period of time and include:

- a clouded state of consciousness
- confusion or disorientation

Symptoms of delirium may be caused by:

- infection
- the consequences of another medical condition
- medication side effects or drug interaction effects
- substance intoxication or substance withdrawal
- a combination of causes

If the cause of delirium can be identified and is appropriately treated, and if no permanent brain damage has resulted, the condition is reversible.

### Dementia

Dementia is a global deterioration of multiple intellectual abilities, including memory. There are also impairments in other higher intellectual functions, such as the ability to abstract or make judgments, and personality variables. There are many causes of dementia, some of which are listed in Table 6–3.

**Table 6–3** Potential Causes of Dementia

Alzheimer's disease
Anemia
Anoxia
Binswanger's disease
Brain tumor
Chronic alcohol/drug use/abuse
Chronic liver disease
Chronic lung disease
Communicating hydrocephalus
Creutzfeld-Jakob disease
Depression
HIV infection
Huntington's disease
Infections of the central nervous system
Metabolic disorders
Multicerebral infarcts
Multiple demyelinating lesions
Parkinson's disease
Pick's disease
Subdural hematoma
Syphilis
Systemic lupus erythematosus
Thyroid disorders
Uremia
Vitamin B12 deficiency

**Table 6–4** Potential Reversible Causes of Dementia

Thyroid disorder
Anemia
Nutritional deficiencies
Depression

Some types of dementia are reversible, and some are not. Some potentially reversible dementias are listed in Table 6–4.

Dementias such as those in Alzheimer's disease, multi-infarct dementia, or arteriosclerosis are not reversible. Some conditions responsible for *irreversible dementia* are described below.

### Alzheimer's Disease

Alzheimer's disease is a progressive, degenerative type of dementia. Onset is generally insidious, with gradual deterioration of cognitive function, eventually resulting in death. Alzheimer's disease accounts for 50 to 75 percent of all cases of dementia (Kawas, 2003). Although it has commonly been thought of as a condition that occurs in older age groups, it may occur as early as middle life.

Although there are identifiable, structural changes of the brain characteristic of Alzheimer's disease, there is currently no definitive way to make the diagnosis except by direct examination of the brain itself at autopsy. Diagnosis is based on documentation of memory impairment, thorough cognitive testing, a detailed personal and social history, a description of the progression of symptoms, drug evaluation, and elimination of other causes of symptoms through laboratory, physical, and neurological examinations.

The progression of the condition and the severity of symptoms at different stages vary from individual to individual. Although several drugs to help symptoms are currently on the market, there is no cure for the disease. Treatment is directed to helping individuals maintain their general health, well-being, and functional capacity as long as possible and to supporting the family responsible for their care.

### Multi-Infarct Dementia

Multi-infarct dementia refers to conditions in which deficits in cognitive function result from small strokes in various locations of the brain. Areas of damage can be identified through a computed tomography scan or magnetic resonance imaging. Once permanent damage to the brain occurs, functional loss of affected areas of the brain is not reversible. Treatment is directed to controlling the underlying condition responsible for the small strokes so as to prevent further damage from occurring.

### Dementia Due to Other Causes

Arteriosclerosis can contribute to dementia when vessels supplying blood to the brain become narrowed or occluded, diminishing blood flow and subsequent oxygen to the brain. Larger vessels, such as the carotid arteries in the neck, are often affected. Arteriosclerosis is a chronic condition (see Chapter 11). Consequently, treatment of dementia caused by arteriosclerosis is directed toward controlling the underlying disease.

Dementia due to human immunodeficiency virus (HIV) disease is experienced by some individuals with HIV (see Chapter 8). In this type of dementia, there is destruction of brain tissue, resulting in symptoms of forgetfulness, difficulty with concentration and problem solving, and general slowness. There may also be behavioral symptoms of apathy and social withdrawal, as well as motor symptoms such as tremor or difficulty walking.

Dementia due to brain trauma from a single injury is not progressive, but damage to the brain and consequent associated symptoms are permanent (see Chapter 2). Individuals who are exposed to repeated head trauma may have increased symptoms as additional trauma occurs. The degree and severity of symptoms will depend on the extent and location of injury in the brain. Symptoms may range from severe cognitive, motor, and sensory deficits to mild concentration and memory difficulties.

## Schizophrenia

Schizophrenia is a chronic, lifelong mental condition characterized by distortion of reality and disturbances of thought, speech, and behavior. Symptoms of the condition cause impairment in work or education, interpersonal relations, and self-care.

Symptoms are categorized as either positive or negative. *Positive symptoms* refer to what has been added to the individual's state because of the condition; they include symptoms such as distortions or exaggerations of thought, language, or behavior. *Negative symptoms* refer to what has been diminished for the individual, such as social ability, the ability to experience pleasure (**anhedonia**), or movement ability.

Specific symptoms of schizophrenia include:

- psychotic symptoms, including delusions and/or hallucinations
- disorders of thought
- flattening of affect
- disorganized speech and/or behavior (American Psychiatric Association, 2000)

No specific cause of schizophrenia has been found, but it appears that multiple genetic and environmental factors contribute to disturbances in brain function (Tsuang, 2000), and there is some evidence of structural or chemical disturbances in the brains of individuals with schizophrenia (Freedman, 2003).

The first episode of schizophrenia occurs most commonly in adolescence or young adulthood. The active form of schizophrenia is characterized by the presence of **psychosis** (loss of contact with reality). Prior to the appearance of psychosis, individuals' daily level of functioning has usually begun to deteriorate over several months. Decline in function may be marked by difficulty in concentrating or in expressing ideas logically.

Individuals with schizophrenia may demonstrate emotional responses inappropriate to the situation, or they may display general apathy and indifference. They may also experience **delusions** (false beliefs), such as believing that their thoughts are being controlled from outside sources. Delusions may also include ideas of reference in which personal significance is attached to events that are unrelated, such as believing that a presidential address on television contains special coded messages directed to them personally.

Persons with schizophrenia may also experience **hallucinations** (sensory experiences even though there are no stimuli from the environment); for example, they may hear voices, see visions, smell odors, and feel sensations even though there are no sources for these sensations. Individuals may experience *loosening of associations*, in which there is no logical progression of thought and rapid shifting from one unrelated idea to the other. There may be *poverty of speech*, in which words spoken convey little meaning. Individuals may have *flat affect*, showing little emotional responsiveness. They may *withdraw from involvement* with the outside world and *exhibit little motivation*, having *difficulty with self-initiated activity* and *decision making*. Grooming and hygiene are also often neglected, and psychomotor activity may be slowed.

### Subtypes of Schizophrenia

Five subtypes of schizophrenia are described in the DSM-IV-TR (American Psychiatric Association, 2000):

- Paranoid type
- Disorganized type
- Catatonic type
- Undifferentiated type
- Residual type

Each subtype shares common symptoms of schizophrenia but is differentiated by specific symptoms. The *disorganized type* is characterized by incoherence of speech, loosening of associations, grossly disorganized behavior, and flat or inappropriate affect. The *catatonic type* of schizophrenia includes psychomotor behavior that is either agitated or so retarded that the individual appears to be in a stupor. The *paranoid type* of schizophrenia is characterized by persecutory or grandiose delusions that are often supported by hallucinations. Individuals with the *undifferentiated type* have prominent psychotic symptoms, but the symptoms do not fall into any specific category of schizophrenia. In the *residual type* of schizophrenia, individuals have experienced at least one schizophrenic episode in the past but show no current prominent psychotic symptoms, although some residual signs may remain.

### Functional Issues in Schizophrenia

The acute or active phase of schizophrenia severely impairs personal and social functioning. During this phase, individuals require supervision and direction in order to meet basic needs and to prevent self-injury. Depending on individual circumstances and the degree of available support, many individuals are able to function independently and obtain employment after the psychosis has been resolved. The degree of independent function possible depends on the success of the chemotherapeutic management of the disorder, the extent of the individuals' insight into the disorder, and the extent to which they continue the treatment protocol. Some individuals need continued assistance because of repeated exacerbation of symptoms, residual symptoms, or impairment.

### Treatment of Schizophrenia

There is currently no cure for schizophrenia. Long-term antipsychotic therapy is the cornerstone of management of schizophrenia (Ray, Daugherty, & Meador, 2003). Treatment is directed toward reducing and/or controlling symptoms through antipsychotic medications, which reduce the psychotic symptoms and help individuals function more effectively and appropriately. The type of medication and the dose are individually determined. Medications are usually needed throughout life. Individuals taking antipsychotic medications should be carefully monitored to determine the effectiveness of the medication in controlling symptoms and to identify any side effects or problems.

Although antipsychotic drugs help reduce the risk of future psychotic episodes and help individuals function independently, they are not a guarantee against relapse. Moreover, the medications used to treat schizophrenia are not without potential side effects. Individuals may experience restlessness, decreased energy, weight gain, muscle spasms or tremors, dry mouth, difficulty with urination, or constipation. Individuals with schizophrenia who experience side effects, who fear that side effects may occur, or who deny their need for medication may discontinue the medication on their own. However, abrupt discontinuation of antipsychotic medication may not only be potentially dangerous, but also can cause relapse. Individuals expressing concerns about their medication should be referred to their physician for advice and monitoring.

In addition to medication, individuals are treated with a variety of psychosocial treatments to improve their functioning. Counseling and individual and/or group therapy can help them understand and accept their condition as well as to build self-esteem. Case management, behavioral interventions, social skills training, family groups, and support groups are other interventions that have been used successfully.

### Psychosocial Issues in Schizophrenia

The severity of the symptoms and the chronicity of schizophrenia have a profound impact on individuals and their families (Rhoades, 2000). Individuals and families can experience social stigma and isolation, disruption of activities of daily life, interruption of future goals, financial burden, and other stressors that have effects on health and well-being.

Substance dependence and abuse are also a risk for individuals with schizophrenia and are associated with poor outcome (Swofford, Scheller-Gilkey, Miller, Woolwine, & Mance, 2000). Other risks include suicide attempts and homelessness. Individual and family therapy can help individuals and their family develop the resources necessary to cope with a chronic lifelong condition and can also facilitate communication and enhance problem solving, increasing the chances of a positive outcome. Although medical treatment remains the key in helping individuals with schizophrenia achieve their maximum functional capacity, psychosocial interventions are the key to helping individuals and families achieve acceptance and ultimate successful outcomes.

### Vocational Issues in Schizophrenia

Because individuals with schizophrenia generally have their first symptoms in adolescence or young adulthood when job and career choices and skill building are major tasks, individuals may have limited work skills. Likewise, they may also have difficulty with social skills. They may need extensive job training and training in problem solving, money management, the use of public transportation, and social skills. Individuals with schizophrenia may have difficulty coping with stress. Consequently, the amount of physical and emotional stress in the workplace and individuals' ability to cope with stress should be considered.

## Mood Disorders

Mood disorders consist of conditions in which the characteristic symptom is disturbance in mood. Symptoms of mood disorders usually occur when individuals are in their twenties; however, depressive disorders may be experienced as early as infancy. Hospitalization is frequently necessary during the acute phase of mood disorders because of the severity of the disturbance that the disorder creates in interpersonal and/or occupational functioning. Disturbances in mood can be subdivided into *depressive disorders* and *bipolar disorders*.

### Major Depressive Disorder

Major depression is defined by depressed mood or loss of interest in nearly all activities (or both for at least 2 weeks) that is accompanied by three or more of the following symptoms:

- insomnia or **hypersomnia** (sleeping too much)
- feelings of worthlessness or excessive guilt
- fatigue or loss of energy
- diminished ability to think or concentrate
- substantial change in appetite or weight
- psychomotor agitation or retardation

- recurrent thoughts of death or suicide (American Psychiatric Association, 2004)

Depression can be an enormous individual and societal burden in terms of economic cost, disability days, and pervasive effects on physical, mental, and social well-being (Kroenke, 2001). Not only does it exist as a primary disability, but it also has the potential to coexist with any chronic illness or disability (Bishop & Sweet, 2000). It is frequently underdiagnosed because symptoms can be confused with symptoms of other medical conditions (Whooley & Simon, 2000).

Individuals with a major depressive episode experience feelings of hopelessness and discouragement, loss of interest in activities previously found pleasurable, decreased energy, and difficulty with memory. They may also express feelings of worthlessness or guilt and have impaired cognitive functions, expressing the inability to concentrate or to make decisions. Other symptoms, such as sleep and appetite disturbances (too much or too little sleep; weight gain or weight loss), are called *vegetative signs*.

The degree of impairment due to major depression varies, although social and occupational activities are usually affected to some degree. Chronic depression causes marked impairment in psychosocial function and work performance (Keller et al., 2000; Scott, 2000). With severe depression, incapacitation can be so great that individuals are unable to attend to their own daily needs, such as basic hygiene and nutritional needs.

### Bipolar Disorders

The diagnostic category of bipolar disorder is broken down into several subcategories, including *bipolar I disorder* and *bipolar II disorder*.

*Bipolar I Disorder*

Bipolar I disorders are characterized by the occurrence of at least one *manic episode* or *mixed episode*. During manic episodes, mood becomes distinctly elevated and behavior hyperactive. Individuals in a manic episode appear flamboyant and overly enthusiastic, often engaging in excessive activity and needing little sleep. Speech becomes rapid, loud, and difficult to follow because of rapid changes from one unrelated topic to another. A *mixed episode* is characterized by symptoms involving rapidly changing moods alternating between elation and sadness.

Manic episodes impair social and occupational functioning considerably. During a manic episode, individuals may be easily distracted. Their attention shifts rapidly from one activity to another unrelated activity with little provocation. They may have grandiose delusions in which they believe that they have special skills, knowledge, or relationships. Hallucinations may occur during a manic episode and often relate to individuals' mood or delusions. Poor judgment during the manic phase can lead to catastrophic financial losses or illegal activities.

*Bipolar II Disorders*

Bipolar II disorders are characterized by the occurrence of at least one major depressive episode and at least one *hypomanic episode*. The presence of the hypomanic episode distinguishes bipolar II disorders from major depressive disorders (American Psychiatric Association, 2000). As already described, a major depressive episode is characterized by loss of interest in activities, sadness, and depressed mood. A hypomanic episode is characterized by elevated or irritable mood over a period of time that is not quite as severe as a manic state. If indi-

viduals experience a manic or mixed episode, they are then categorized as having a bipolar I rather than bipolar II disorder.

### Dysthymia and Cyclothymia

**Dysthymia** is a mood disorder characterized by symptoms similar to those experienced in major depression, but to a lesser degree. Although symptoms are not so severe, the chronic nature of the condition may impair social and occupational functioning. The essential distinction between major depressive disorder and dysthymia is the severity and duration of the symptoms. Major depression generally has a more acute onset, whereas individuals with dysthymia may be in a depressed mood most of the time for months or years.

**Cyclothymia** is a mood disorder characterized by symptoms similar to those of bipolar disorders, with both hypomanic symptoms and depressive symptoms. Because symptoms are usually milder, cyclothymia causes less impairment in function than does a bipolar disorder. The distinction between bipolar disorders and cyclothymia is not clearly demarcated, and the diagnosis often depends on the judgment of the evaluator. Because the condition is chronic, individuals with cyclothymia can experience symptoms for months or years.

## Anxiety Disorders

There are several different types of anxiety disorders. Their common features include not only anxiety but also increased arousal and avoidance of situations that the individual perceives as anxiety provoking.

### Panic Disorders

*Panic disorders* are types of anxiety disorders in which individuals experience feelings of intense fear or discomfort; they are characterized by *panic attacks*, episodes in which the individual has feelings of intense anxiety or terror, accompanied by a sense of impending doom (American Psychiatric Association, 2000). During a panic attack, individuals experience shortness of breath, increased heart rate and palpitations, sweating, and, at times, nausea or other physical discomfort. Panic attacks are not triggered by a certain event and, at least initially, are unpredictable. Attacks usually last from a few minutes to a few hours. In themselves, they may be only mildly debilitating.

Panic disorder is distinguished from generalized anxiety in that individuals with panic disorders become preoccupied with the physical symptoms associated with a panic attack (Mahoney, 2000). Treatment focuses on amelioration of symptoms through medication and counseling.

### Agoraphobia

Panic disorders are sometimes accompanied by *agoraphobia*, the fear of being in a situation or place in which it might be difficult or embarrassing to escape or in which there may be no help available if the individual experiences a panic attack. Although not all individuals who have panic attacks experience agoraphobia, those who do may severely restrict their activity, hampering both social and occupational functioning. They may refuse to venture outside their home alone, or they may be reluctant to travel by car, bus, or other common means of transportation.

### Phobias

The term *phobia* refers to fear and anxiety related to specific situations, persons, or objects. Different types of phobias are categorized on the basis of the object of fear. For example, social phobia is a condition in which individuals fear situations that may potentially result in ridicule or humiliation.

Impairments resulting from phobias may vary from mild to severe. A phobia may be more of a nuisance than a disability. On the other hand, a phobia may be so disabling that individuals are unable to function effectively in their day-to-day activities if the phobia causes them to avoid particular objects or situations or causes such anxiety that they are unable or unwilling to engage in necessary activities.

### Obsessive-Compulsive Disorder

*Obsessive-compulsive disorder* is a chronic disorder that can cause significant disability if not treated, with symptoms following a waxing and waning course (Maj, Sartorius, Okasha, & Zohar, 2002). Individuals with an obsessive-compulsive disorder have recurrent **obsessions** (persistent thoughts) or **compulsions** (persistent actions) that they are unable to control. For instance, they may have recurrent thoughts of the death of a loved one, or they may have an irresistible urge to perform repetitively some behavior that seems purposeless, such as turning a light on and off three times before retiring for the night. Attempts by individuals to ignore the compulsions only increase anxiety, discomfort, and distress.

Cognitive-behavioral therapy is a major treatment for obsessive-compulsive disorder (Foa, Franklin, & Moser, 2002). Medication is often used in combination with cognitive-behavioral therapy, especially for individuals who are unable to function in their job or in social situations because of their symptoms (Jenike, 2004).

### Posttraumatic Stress Disorder

Posttraumatic stress disorder (PTSD) was initially thought to be primarily a disorder experienced by individuals who had been in military combat; however, it is now recognized as a condition that affects people in all walks of life (Khouzam & Donnelly, 2001). PTSD is an anxiety disorder that develops after an individual has experienced or observed a traumatic or life-threatening event, such as violence, fire, natural disaster, or plane crash. It is one of the few psychiatric conditions whose symptoms are attributed to situational causes alone (Hodges, 2003). The symptoms of the disorder may include persistent recollection of the event, sleep difficulties and recurrent nightmares, difficulty in concentrating, and a feeling of hypervigilance or increased arousal (Khouzam & Donnelly, 2001). Individuals may persistently reexperience the event in distressing images, nightmares, or flashbacks; they may avoid reminders of the event, including persons or places; or they may have hyperarousal symptoms, such as insomnia, irritability, impaired concentration, or hypervigilance (Yehuda, 2002). Individuals may demonstrate little emotion or appear detached and lose interest in previously enjoyed activities or in important close relationships.

PTSD, which may occur at any age, causes varying degrees of impairment. Although many individuals experience acute forms of PTSD at some time during their life, most recover. When PTSD persists, it can be debilitating and require psychological and pharmacologic intervention (Ursano, 2002). Education and counseling can help individuals understand the nature of their condition and can facilitate recovery. Cognitive therapy and anxiety management therapies can also be helpful. Group therapy has been found to reduce isolation and stigma (Foa, Keane, & Friedman, 2000).

## Somatoform Disorders

Somatoform disorders are conditions in which individuals experience physical symptoms for which no organic cause can be found. Symptoms can cause significant distress and impairment in social, occupational, and interpersonal functioning (American Psychiatric Association, 2000).

There are a number of somatoform disorders, several of which are discussed below.

### Somatization Disorder

Somatization disorder is a type of somatoform disorder that is characterized by recurrent, multiple physical complaints for which a medical cause cannot be found. Physical symptoms can be so distressing that they impair social or occupational function. Because physical symptoms are often similar to symptoms of a variety of medical conditions, individuals may receive medical treatment for their symptoms even though no organic cause can be found.

Individuals with somatization disorder do not consciously produce the symptoms but truly experience them, even though there is no organic cause of symptoms readily identifiable.

### Conversion Disorder

Another type of somatoform disorder is conversion disorder, in which individuals lose a physical function, often related to a neurological function (e.g., paralysis, blindness, or numbness of a body part). Symptoms do not typically follow a pattern that would correspond to a specific disease or injury. Again, the individual does not intentionally produce the symptoms.

### Hypochondriasis

Hypochondriasis, another type of somatoform disorder, is characterized by preoccupation with physical illness. Individuals with this condition may fear or believe they have a serious physical illness or perceive the symptoms of a coexisting disease or condition in an exaggerated way. For example, they may perceive a cough associated with a common cold as a sign of tuberculosis or lung cancer.

### Pain Disorder

Pain disorder is a preoccupation with pain that is severe enough to cause impairment in function at home, school, or work, although no organic cause can be found to explain the pain symptom. Individuals with pain disorder do not consciously produce the symptoms of a pain and actually experience the pain reported. This disorder can be extremely incapacitating, often severely limiting social and work activities.

## Factitious Disorders

Although not severely disabling, a variety of other types of mental disorders may interfere with effective functioning. Factitious disorders are conditions in which individuals *voluntarily* produce psychological or physical symptoms, feigning illness because of a seemingly compulsive need to assume the sick role (American Psychiatric Association, 2000). A factitious disorder differs from **malingering** (in which individuals also produce symptoms intentionally), in that the goal of a malingerer is usually obvious, such as a desire to receive an insurance settlement or to collect disability payments.

## Dissociative Disorders

Conditions in which individuals experience an alteration in memory, consciousness, or identity for no organic reason are called *dissociative disorders*. *Dissociative fugue* is a condition in which individuals leave their environment and assume a new identity without being able to recall their previous identity. *Dissociative amnesia* is the inability to recall events that occurred within a certain period of time or the inability to recall information regarding one's own identity. *Dissociative identity disorder*, formerly known as *multiple personality disorder*, is a condition in which at least two personalities exist within the same individual and control the individual's behavior.

## Personality Disorders

Everyone has personality traits or characteristics. If these traits are maladaptive, they can interfere with the ability to function, especially during times of crisis. *Personality disorders* describe disorders characterized by inflexible or maladaptive behaviors that have usually lasted a long time and that impair interpersonal or occupational functioning or cause subjective distress (American Psychiatric Association, 2000).

Individuals with personality disorders may have no insight into the role that their own behavior plays in creating problems within their environment. They may rationalize their actions, blaming others for their situation or misfortune without examining their own responsibility for the situation at hand.

There are many types of personality disorders (e.g., paranoid, antisocial, and borderline), which cause varying degrees of impairment. When a personality disorder exists in combination with other mental disorders, the prognosis is more guarded, and treatment and management of the personality disorder are more difficult. At times, these individuals may not have a full-blown personality disorder but rather maladaptive personality traits that may interfere with the treatment or diagnosis of the concomitant disorder.

## DIAGNOSTIC PROCEDURES IN PSYCHIATRIC DISABILITY

The diagnosis of mental conditions is often an art as well as a science. It requires skill and experience on the part of those evaluating individuals' symptoms and interpreting the results of the various tests designed to measure psychological or intellectual function. Many professionals may be involved in testing and evaluation; *psychiatrists* and *clinical psychologists* are frequently involved in the diagnosis of mental disorders. Diagnosis is usually based on information from a variety of different sources.

### Uses of Diagnostic Psychological Testing

Systematic samples of certain types of verbal, perceptual, intellectual, and motor behavior under standardized conditions can be obtained through psychological testing. Psychological tests may be used to evaluate intelligence, personality, or behavior.

The results of psychological tests provide partial information needed for the accurate diagnosis of a mental condition. No single test is adequate to offer a definitive diagnosis in all situations. Often, because mental disorders affect a variety of functions, several psychological tests that measure different functions may be necessary.

### Intelligence Tests

The term *intelligence* is difficult to define. Theoretically, intelligence consists of a number of skills and abilities, some of which cannot be measured. Intelligence is a combination of individuals' own unique mental structure and processes along with cultural and educational experiences.

Psychological science has developed a number of tests to define intelligence operationally for a variety of capacities. The most commonly used intelligence tests are the Wechsler Intelligence Scale for Children-Revised, the Wechsler Preschool and Primary Scale of Intelligence, the Stanford-Binet, and the Wechsler Adult Intelligence Scale-Revised.

The limitations of intelligence testing originate from:

- the difficulty of tapping all aspects of intellectual ability
- the individual's ability to take the test
- the degree to which the test measures aptitude rather than prior learning and experience
- the impact of cultural variation on test results

One way of classifying levels of intelligence is through a numerical value known as the IQ. There is considerable individual variability in abilities, however, and results of intelligence tests, like results of other forms of psychological tests, must be evaluated within the context of the individual's culture and environment. Much intelligence testing involves sampling individuals' intellectual capacity in a variety of different spheres. Many tests focus on cognitive processes, including problem solving, adaptive thinking, and other aspects of performance. Tests alone should not determine a definitive diagnosis.

### Mental Status Examination and Assessment Through Interviews

The structured interview is one way in which the mental functioning of individuals with a suspected mental disorder may be assessed during the initial evaluation. Information obtained in this way may aid in determining the diagnosis, as well as in making plans for future treatment.

Structured interviews provide information regarding individuals' orientation, form and content of thought, speech, affect, and degree of insight. Observations made during the interview of individuals' general appearance, behavior, and emotional state are also relevant.

The *mental status examination* is a specific type of structured interview used as a screening instrument in assessing intellectual impairment. Such an examination may be used to detect dementia or impaired intellectual function, as well as to determine the severity of the impairment. There are several mental status examinations of varying lengths. Although some mental status instruments are part of other instruments that measure functional status, a number of short screening instruments have been devised especially for the purpose of evaluating mental status. One widely used mental status test is the *Short Portable Mental Status Questionnaire*, which is used to assess orientation, personal history, remote memory, and calculation. Another short mental status examination is the *Mini-Mental State Examination*, which is used to assess orientation, memory, and attention, as well as the ability to write, name objects, copy a design, and follow verbal and written commands.

## Personality Assessment

Personality may be assessed by either *objective* or *projective* means. Objective personality assessment instruments are structured, standardized tests for which clear and concise criteria have been established. These tests have undergone research and scientific scrutiny to establish their reliability and validity. Although numerous *objective personality tests* are available, one of the most commonly used is the *Minnesota Multiphasic Personality Inventory* (*MMPI*). The MMPI has a number of clinical scales that can be useful in the diagnosis of a variety of mental disorders, ranging from schizophrenia to depression, social introversion, and substance abuse.

*Projective personality tests*, such as the *Rorschach Inkblot Test* and the *Thematic Apperception Test*, also have criteria on which interpretations are based, but they are generally more subjective in nature. Projective testing usually consists of asking individuals to describe vague and ambiguous pictures. There are no right or wrong answers. The assumption is that the way in which individuals interpret the pictures is a reflection of their personality.

Projective tests may be more time consuming than are objective tests, and professionals who administer them require special training. As with all other clinical data, the results of personality assessment tests are only part of the total information needed for an accurate diagnosis of a particular mental disorder. No matter what type of test is used, the accuracy of the results is dependent on individuals' honesty and care in answering test questions. If individuals answer questions in a socially desirable way rather than as an expression of their true feelings, test results can be invalid.

## Neuropsychological Testing

Standardized neuropsychological test batteries may be used to assess major functional areas of the brain. These tests make it possible to assess a variety of cognitive, perceptual, and motor skills.

Traditionally, neuropsychological testing has been used to identify or localize brain damage that has behavioral consequences; however, with newer technological advances such as computed tomography and magnetic resonance imaging, this function is now not widely promoted. Neuropsychological tests have become increasingly popular to rule out and/or monitor the progression of symptoms of mental disorders that have an identified organic basis. Because individual performance on neuropsychological tests changes with brain function, test results provide a baseline against which future impairment of brain function can be measured and also provide information that can be incorporated into the diagnosis.

A variety of comprehensive standard neuropsychological test batteries are available for adults; two of the more widely recognized tests are the *Halstead-Reitan Battery* and the *Luria-Nebraska Neuropsychological Battery*.

### Behavioral Assessment

Some methods of assessing mental function involve direct, systematic observation of individuals' behavior. Trained observers, family members, or even individuals themselves may monitor and record individuals' behavior. Observation and measurement of behavior may take place in individuals' own environment or in a controlled environment. Behavioral assessment methods are being applied to an increasing number of conditions because they offer not only information that can be used in diagnosis but also a method of monitoring improvements in behavior once treatment has been initiated.

### GENERAL TREATMENT OF PSYCHIATRIC DISABILITY

Treatment of mental disorders is based on a comprehensive assessment of the individual's problems and needs. It is usually a collaborative effort involving the individual, the family, and professionals from a variety of disciplines, such as *psychiatrists*, *psychologists*, *social workers*, *nurses*, and *rehabilitation counselors*. Treatment

may be provided in a variety of settings, depending on the individuals' particular condition and specific needs.

Levels of treatment range from the *least restrictive*, such as that provided in an outpatient setting, to the *most restrictive*, such as that provided in an institutional setting. Levels of treatment in between include intensive outpatient treatment, residential care, and halfway houses.

Acute episodes of mental disorders may initially be treated by attempts to alleviate symptoms. Ongoing treatment is directed toward preventing recurrence of symptoms and/or helping individuals attain maximal functional capacity. Many mental conditions require ongoing treatment or periodic evaluations of the effectiveness of the treatment prescribed. Some mental conditions, like many physical conditions, require daily medication to control symptoms and have periods of remission and exacerbation. In many instances, individuals' willingness and ability to adhere to the prescribed treatment can determine the success of treatment. A variety of treatment modalities, including both nonpharmacologic and pharmacologic methods, may be used in the treatment of mental illness. More intensive levels of care may include, in addition to psychotherapy and pharmacologic treatment, *occupational therapy*, *art* and *music therapy*, or *recreational therapy*. Often different types of treatment are used simultaneously.

### Psychiatric Rehabilitation

The purpose of psychiatric rehabilitation is to help individuals with psychiatric disabilities increase their functional capacity so they can be successful and satisfied in the environment of their choice with the least amount of ongoing professional intervention (Anthony, Cohen, Farkas, & Gagne, 2001). Psychiatric rehabilitation is a multidisciplined approach to assisting individuals with chronic psychiatric disability; it is correlated closely with treatment and is often offered simultaneously. The basic goals of psychiatric rehabilitation include recovery, community integration, and improved quality of life (Pratt, Gill, Barrett, & Roberts, 1999). Psychiatric rehabilitation is community based, client centered, and empowerment oriented (Leech & Holcomb, 2000). It helps individuals identify and obtain the resources and support needed to attain their goals (Garske, 1999).

In the 1950s the clubhouse model of psychosocial rehabilitation was created at Fountain House in New York City. This model provides integrated mental health, employment, and peer support services and has become mandated as a mental health service under managed care in several states (Macias, Jackson, Schroeder, & Wang, 1999). In the 1990s many states shifted to a case management approach, and by the end of the decade independent employment models were being created within clubhouses to help members achieve employment with higher wages and more advancement potential (Reed & Merz, 2000). The effectiveness of each of these programs has been evaluated, and the results are mixed (Pratt et al., 1999; Reed & Merz, 2000). Continued research to assess the efficacy of psychiatric rehabilitation programs in integrating individuals into both society and the workplace is essential to effective rehabilitation (Accordino, Porter, & Morse, 2001).

## Nonpharmacologic Approaches to Treatment of Psychiatric Disability

### Psychotherapy and Counseling

Psychotherapy and counseling are conversational approaches to treatment in which a close relationship between the individual and the therapist is established and used as a therapeutic tool. This approach is used to help individuals explore and modify their behavior in order to decrease their discomfort and/or increase their satisfaction and productivity.

There are numerous schools of thought regarding psychotherapy and counseling, each having a different approach and theoretical framework. Examples of some approaches are psychoanalysis, rational-emotive therapy, Gestalt therapy, reality therapy, behavior therapy, and transactional analysis. Although therapists may use a specific theoretical framework predominantly in their treatment approach, many use a variety of therapeutic approaches, depending on which type seems most appropriate for a specific individual.

Psychotherapy may be conducted on an individual basis, in a group, with a family, or between marital partners. Depending on individual need, a combination of therapies may be included in the treatment plan. Individual therapy is directed toward effecting changes in individuals' behavior, and group therapy is directed toward helping individuals develop more satisfying modes of interaction with others. Group therapy may also be educative if the content is fixed and the goal of the group is to relay information, or supportive if group members receive and give mutual support and encouragement. Family therapy is directed toward improving family function as an interdependent group, and marital therapy focuses on the marital relationship and the impact of both parties' behaviors on the relationship.

### Behavioral Approaches

Behavior is a reflection of inner drives, traits, or patterns of thinking, as well as environmental influences. A number of treatments designed to help individuals modify their learned responses and learn new patterns of more adaptive behavior have been used in the treatment of mental illness.

Several different forms of behavior therapy have been derived from different theoretical models, including the *respondent* (*classical*) *model*, the *instrumental* (*operant*) *model*, the *observational model*, and the *cognitive learning model*. There are countless applications of behavioral approaches in the treatment of mental illness. Behavior therapy may be used alone or in conjunction with other treatments.

### Social-Skills Training

The purpose of social-skills training is to identify specific social-skills deficits and the circumstances under which these deficits occur. Educational interventions are then directed toward correcting these deficits. Interventions usually begin with targeting small elements of behavior and then gradually adding other elements of behavior, always working toward the ideal behavior. Through social-skills training groups, individuals learn to make specific responses to specific social situations, as well as to recognize relevant social cues and to determine appropriate action by using the cues. Social-skills training may involve specific interventions, such as role modeling, feedback and reinforcement, and practice, in helping individuals to perform specified behaviors reliably and to generalize the behavior to other situations.

### Specialized Groups

Individuals with some types of mental illness may neglect their own needs of daily living, including personal hygiene, money management, or housing needs. Special groups (e.g., activities of daily living groups) may help individuals with these disorders learn the specific skills needed for day-to-day functioning.

Individuals with some types of mental illness may require ongoing supervision, and many require a period of transition from the inpatient to the outpatient setting. A variety of therapeutic living arrangements may be used to meet these needs, including group homes, therapeutic communities, and transitional living centers. Day programs provide a structured environment in which individuals may participate in the program during the day and return to the community setting at night. The goal of day programs is to facilitate the adjustment of these individuals to the community setting, to maintain their optimal level of functioning, and to prevent hospitalization.

## Pharmacologic Approaches to Treatment of Psychiatric Disability

### Antipsychotic Medications

Treatment of psychosis may require the use of *antipsychotic medications* (see Table 6–5). Antipsychotic medications, sometimes called *neuroleptic medications* or *major tranquilizers*, do not cure psychosis but rather control the symptoms. The first antipsychotic drug, *chlorpromazine* (*Thorazine*), was developed in the 1950s. Since that time, numerous other antipsychotic medications have been developed. These drugs are classified into different chemical groups. Drugs in each group have varying potency, and individual responses to any of the medications vary.

Duration of treatment with antipsychotic medications is determined individually and based on individuals' life situation and condition. They may be prescribed for up to a year as a prophylactic measure after psychosis is controlled. All individuals should have their medications reviewed annually by a psychiatrist to evaluate the possibility of gradual discontinuation.

**Table 6–5** Common Antipsychotic Agents

| Trade Name | Generic Name |
| --- | --- |
| Clozaril | Clozapine |
| Compazine | Prochlorperazine |
| Haldol | Haloperidol |
| Loxitane | Loxapine |
| Mellaril | Thioridazine |
| Navane | Thiothixene |
| Prolixin | Fluphenazine |
| Stelazine | Trioridazine |

It is believed that the symptoms of psychosis may be due to excessive levels of the neurotransmitter *dopamine*. Consequently, it has been postulated that antipsychotic medications reduce symptoms by blocking the action or transmission of dopamine. Because of this blocking, however, one of the side effects of antipsychotic medications may be psychomotor symptoms similar to those seen in Parkinson's disease (see Chapter 3). These are called *extrapyramidal effects*, because changes take place in the extrapyramidal tracts of the central nervous system. The possible extrapyramidal effects of antipsychotic medications include **dystonia**, characterized by severe contractions of the muscles of the jaw, neck, and eye so that the head is turned to one side and the eyes look upward; **akinesia**, characterized by decreased motor activity and apathy; and **akathisia**, characterized by extreme restlessness so that the individual cannot sit still or remain in one place for any length of time. The most severe extrapyramidal side effect of antipsychotic medications is **tardive dyskinesia**, which consists of abnormal movements of the mouth, such as chewing motions or thrusting movements of the tongue. Tardive dyskinesia often indicates irreversible damage to the brain.

*Antiparkinsonian medications*, such as *benztropine* (*Cogentin*) and *trihexphenidyl* (*Artane*), are often prescribed along with antipsychotics to prevent extrapyramidal side effects. Tardive dyskinesia is best treated through prevention, since the occurrence of the symptom is frequently related to drug dosage. Individuals on antipsychotic medication must be carefully monitored by a physician so that the early symptoms of tardive dyskinesia may be identified and dosage of the medication adjusted to avoid permanent damage.

Individuals on antipsychotic medications may also develop *photosensitivity*, which makes them more sensitive to the effects of the sun and predisposes them to sunburn. Some medications that have potent sedating effects may decrease alertness and produce drowsiness. These symptoms usually subside within 2 weeks after the individual begins to take the medication; if they persist, alteration in medication may be necessary. Individuals may also experience **orthostatic hypotension**, in which their blood pressure drops when they move from a seated or prone position to a standing position, resulting in dizziness or lightheadedness. Individuals may complain of other uncomfortable side effects, such as dry mouth, after beginning antipsychotic medications. These symptoms generally subside within 2 weeks, however. Men on antipsychotic medication may become impotent or unable to ejaculate. Reducing the dosage or changing the medication may alleviate this side effect. Any medication change should always be conducted under the direction of a physician.

### Antidepressants

Conditions in which depression is a symptom may be treated with *antidepres-*

*sants*. Although the exact way antidepressants work has not been determined, they are classified according to their presumed mode of action. The most widely used antidepressants, *tricyclic antidepressants*, are thought to act by blocking the uptake of the neurotransmitters *norepinephrine* and *serotonin*, thus increasing their concentration. Levels of both of these neurotransmitters appear to be reduced in depression.

*Monoamine oxidase (MAO) inhibitors*, less frequently used antidepressants, are thought to act by blocking the action of the enzyme monoamine oxidase, which usually breaks down norepinephrine and serotonin, so that the concentration of the neurotransmitters increases.

The type of depression and the symptoms experienced, as well as other individual factors, determine the type of antidepressant used. As with all medications, some side effects may be experienced. Individuals on tricyclic antidepressants may experience symptoms such as *orthostatic hypotension* (described previously), *dry mouth*, or *urinary retention*. A more serious possible side effect is the development of *cardiac arrhythmia*, which can result in myocardial infarction or, in the case of overdose, death.

The use of MAO inhibitors has been limited because of their potential side effects; however, their use is gaining popularity. Individuals with chronic alcoholism or liver damage are not good candidates for treatment with MAO inhibitors. In addition, there are a number of dietary restrictions associated with their use, and individuals who use these medications must follow these restrictions carefully to prevent potentially serious side effects. Monoamine oxidase is essential for the metabolism of a substance called *tyramine*, which is present in a number of foods, including aged cheese, wine, beer, chocolate, coffee, and raisins. If individuals tak-ing MAO inhibitors ingest tyramine-containing foods, they may experience a *hypertensive crisis* in which there is sudden and extreme elevation in blood pressure, which could result in stroke.

Suicide is always a possibility with individuals who are depressed. The availability of antidepressant medication that could be used in a suicide attempt is a risk to be considered. The risk of attempted suicide may be higher when the antidepressant begins to take effect because suicidal impulses are still present and as individuals' energy returns so does their motivation to attempt suicide. Although antidepressants are an important aspect of treatment for depressive disorders, psychotherapeutic modes of treatment should be used in combination with the pharmacologic approach.

### Mood Stabilizers

*Lithium* is an antimanic agent used to treat the manic symptoms in bipolar disorder. It is an element that occurs naturally as a salt. Use of lithium for treatment of mental disorders in the United States began in the 1970s, and lithium is now widely used in bipolar disorders, both in the treatment of symptoms and in the prevention of recurring symptoms. In some instances, lithium has been used alone or in combination with antidepressants to treat depressive disorders. Because not all individuals respond to lithium in the same way, lithium use is decided on an individual basis.

The way in which lithium works is unclear. It may produce some side effects, including *endocrine effects* (e.g., hyperthyroidism), *muscle weakness*, or *weight gain*. Other common side effects include **polyuria** (excessive urination) and **polydipsia** (excessive thirst). Individuals who use lithium should have regular blood tests to measure levels of the medication in the blood and must be monitored by a physician on a regular basis.

### Antianxiety Medications

Formerly called *minor tranquilizers, antianxiety medications* are generally used for mental disorders in which anxiety is the predominant symptom. These medications are commonly classified as *benzodiazepines* (e.g., diazepam [Valium], oxazepam [Serax], or lorazepam [Ativan]), *barbiturates* (e.g., phenobarbital), or *antihistamines* (e.g., hydroxyzine [Vistaril or Atarax]). Antianxiety medications are used mainly for time-limited, short-term treatment of anxiety. These medications should not be regarded as the mainstay or sole treatment of anxiety disorders, but rather should be used in combination with other types of treatment, such as psychotherapeutic approaches. Because many antianxiety agents also have the risk of abuse or physical dependence, their use should be carefully monitored. Side effects can include drowsiness and sedation or motor difficulty.

## Electroconvulsive Therapy

Before psychopharmacologic preparations were readily available, electroconvulsive therapy (shock therapy) was a major mode of treating some types of mental illness. Its use has diminished with the advent of a variety of psychotherapeutic drugs, but some centers continue to use it for treatment. It may be especially useful when the long-term administration of medication is contraindicated (Fink, 2000). Although electroconvulsive therapy does not cure mental disorders, it can bring about a remission of symptoms. It may be used in conjunction with psychotherapeutic medications or alone.

## PSYCHOSOCIAL AND VOCATIONAL ISSUES IN PSYCHIATRIC DISABILITY

### Psychological Issues

Individuals with psychiatric disability experience a wide range of symptoms that affect psychological and cognitive function, and their needs are multifaceted and complex (Kress-Shull & Leech, 2000). Although the benefits of medication in the treatment of psychiatric disability are substantial, medication usually does not cure the condition but rather controls the symptoms. Individuals often have residual symptoms, deficits, and impairments as a result of their condition, and many are subject to periodic relapses with recurrence of symptoms.

Individuals with psychiatric disability may be particularly vulnerable to stress and may lack the ability to withstand pressure or to cope with the normal stresses of everyday life. They may have limited problem-solving ability or find it difficult to engage in self-directed activity. Some individuals may become passive, apathetic, or oversubmissive as a direct result of repeated hospitalizations or as a result of the condition itself.

Symptoms experienced vary with the condition, causing varying degrees of impairment. Although fear and anger are normal emotional responses, these responses may be acutely disproportionate to the stimuli in some psychiatric disabilities. Some individuals' responses are covert, whereas others' responses are more pronounced. Some individuals manifest their condition through patterns of behavior rather than in emotional manifestations. Others experience subjective distress, such as an inner sense of weakness, jealousy, or anxiety, although function in most of their life is minimally disturbed. Some psychiatric disabilities are characterized by disorganization of mental capacities, which can affect individuals' ability to function in an unstructured environment. Disorders of memory and perception can severely limit independent function. Individuals may fail to carry out age-appropriate role functions and have varying degrees of dependence on others.

Symptoms of the psychiatric disability may cause psychic stress and anxiety, further compounding the disabling component of the condition. Individuals' own anguish over their impoverished life can be devastating. Awareness of their own impaired function and the impact of their condition both on others and on their future may cause considerable pain and discomfort. In some instances, individuals with psychiatric disability may be reluctant to seek appropriate help because of their fear of the stigma associated with psychiatric conditions that require professional help. In other instances, individuals may not be aware of their symptoms and the effect of their symptoms on function, which also hinders them from using appropriate treatment.

### Lifestyle Issues

The degree to which psychiatric disability affects individuals' lifestyle depends to a great extent on the nature of the condition. Some psychiatric disabilities so severely impair individuals' ability to carry on the activities of daily living that constant supervision or hospitalization is necessary. In other instances, individuals are able to carry on these activities, but in an altered manner.

At times, the treatment itself requires lifestyle changes. Individuals may need to rearrange their schedules so that they can attend therapy sessions. Some medications used in the treatment of psychiatric disability may require special lifestyle consid-

erations. For example, the use of MAO inhibitors in the treatment of depression requires careful monitoring of diet. Other medications have side effects, such as drowsiness and sedation, that also affect daily function.

Either the psychiatric disability or its treatment may alter sexual function. Individuals with a depressive disorder may lose interest in sexual activity, whereas individuals with a bipolar depression may have excessive sexual interests. The side effects of some medications can alter sexual function as well. In addition, subjective manifestations of lowered self-esteem and self-confidence may make it more difficult for individuals to form intimate relationships.

### Social Issues

The impact of a psychiatric disability on social function also depends on the nature of the condition. Individuals who experience mania as a part of their disability may enjoy the euphoria and feel that it contributes to their social well-being.

Even though attitudes of society have become more accepting of individuals with mental illness, family members may continue to be resistant to recognizing the problem and pursuing appropriate treatment (Hall & Purdy, 2000). If, however, individuals manifest bizarre, abusive, or socially offensive behavior, family members or others within a social group may avoid the individual altogether, leaving him or her socially isolated.

Other psychiatric disabilities may lead to social withdrawal. Families of individuals with psychiatric disability may experience a variety of stresses engendered by the condition. These stresses may be caused by their objective problems in dealing with the individuals and their condition, as well as by more subjective psychological distress (Hall & Purdy, 2000).

Psychiatric disabilities, especially those in which individuals need close supervision or long-term care and treatment, may place financial hardships on their family because of medical bills, the individual's economic dependency, and special needs related to household functioning. In some instances, the demands of caregiving may require family members to curtail their social activities or alter their relationships with friends and acquaintances. The time commitments of caregiving may lead to neglect of other family members' needs, further disrupting the family as a unit.

Social barriers are frequently erected against individuals with a mental disorder and against their families. Social stigma may be the result of fear of individuals' behavior, ignorance about psychiatric disability, or feelings of inadequacy in interacting with those who have psychiatric disability. Regardless of the cause, the results can be a source of continuing stress for individuals and their families, as well as a barrier to social activity and interaction. Social stigma and stereotypes can also have an effect on the extent of the deficits individuals experience. Deficits sometimes occur not only because of the psychiatric condition, but also because of the public's reaction to it (Corrigan & Calabrese, 2001).

## Vocational Issues

Individuals with psychiatric disability have a condition that limits their capacity to perform certain tasks and functions and their ability to perform certain roles (Farkas & Anthony, 2001). The ability to work depends on the type of disability, the type of work in which they are involved, and the attitudes of those within the work setting. Although work is important to increase self-esteem for those with a number of disabilities, it can be an especially strong therapeutic tool for those with a

psychiatric disability (Tschopp, Bishop, & Mulvihill, 2001). The skills, aptitude, motivation, and objective symptoms of individuals with psychiatric disability are important, and their ability to endure and cope with stress and to engage in active problem solving also determines their ability to work. Job restrictions may be related to job pressure or the ability to work with others, regardless of the individual's level of skill or physical and cognitive ability to perform work-related tasks.

Other considerations may relate to individuals' treatment. It may be necessary to arrange scheduled absences so that individuals can attend therapy sessions. Some medications used in treatment may produce side effects, such as drowsiness or sedation, that could adversely affect work performances. In addition, individuals' level of adherence to the therapeutic regimen is especially important if failure to do so means possible relapse and recurrence of symptoms.

Individuals' reaction to the work environment, including noise and distractions, should be taken into account, as should their level of personal responsibility and ability for self-direction and decision making. Limited interpersonal and coping skills may make it difficult for some individuals to adjust to unforeseen circumstances. Individuals' flexibility to take advantage of chance occurrences and their degree of flexibility in the workplace must also be taken into consideration (Szymanski, 2000). Some individuals may need a more structured work environment; in some instances, a workshop environment may be preferable. Some individuals' expectations of work or of their own capabilities may be unrealistic. Unless these unrealistic notions are identified and dealt with before they enter or reenter the work setting, discouragement, disappointment, or even relapse may occur.

Individuals with significant mental retardation may need specialized training and other assistance in job placement, job site training, and long-term support. A *job coach* may be utilized to provide individualized assistance and to act as an advocate. The job coach provides specific assistance by helping individuals fill out an application, going with them for the job interview, and participating in travel training and skill training at the job site. The job coach gradually reduces involvement over time as the individual adjusts to the work environment.

*Supported employment* may be successful for a number of individuals with psychiatric disability. In supported employment, individuals work in integrated settings with monitoring, support, and follow-up provided on a regular basis. Supported employment provides permanent jobs that are based on individuals' skills and abilities. This model is useful for individuals with intellectual disabilities and other types of psychiatric disabilities.

Social skills, aptitude, and the ability to work are not necessarily concurrent in individuals with psychiatric disability. Employment for each individual must be considered in the context of his or her particular symptoms and feelings and the nature of the work environment. The role that social stigma plays in individuals' perceptions of their own condition and their willingness to accept and follow up with treatment are crucial aspects in their total rehabilitation.

The unemployment rate for individuals with psychiatric disabilities continues to be high (Fabian & Coppola, 2001; Kress-Shull, 2000). Although it is believed that people with psychiatric disabilities have been significantly discriminated against in the workplace, the extent to which discrimination exists is difficult to determine because of lack of relevant data (Spirito

Dalgin, 2001). Continued advocacy that includes educating not only employers but also individuals with psychiatric disability is necessary in the ongoing process of reducing employment discrimination.

## CASE STUDIES

### Case I

Mr. B. is a 27-year-old individual with mild mental retardation that has been established through testing. He is a third-generation individual of Chinese descent. He has never been employed and lived with his widowed mother until several months ago, when she died and he moved to a group home. Mr. B. was very protected by his mother, and although he went to special education, he did not build relationships with individuals outside his close family. Since coming to the group home, he has become increasingly more animated and social and expresses the desire to be employed. He states he is particularly interested in a job like that of one of his roommates, who is a dining room attendant who keeps the serving areas stocked, cleans tables, and removes dirty dishes.

### Questions

1. What specific issues in assessment would you consider when working with Mr. B. to establish a rehabilitation plan?
2. Given Mr. B.'s level of mental retardation, what level of function might you expect him to attain?
3. What personal and/or social factors might you consider when working with Mr. B. that may be a factor in his rehabilitation potential?
4. How would you approach a potential employer in attempting to find a placement opportunity for Mr. B.?

5. Given Mr. B.'s level of mental retardation, how realistic is his desired occupational goal of becoming a dining room attendant?

## Case II

Ms. S. is a 37-year-old female who was diagnosed with schizophrenia at the age of 20 when she was hospitalized in an acute psychotic state. At the time of her diagnosis, she had completed 2 years of college, where she was studying accounting. After hospitalization she did not return to college and has had a series of part-time jobs since that time. Her symptoms have been fairly well controlled on medication; however, she tells you that she is concerned about side effects and has considered going off her medication. Since her original diagnosis, she has been hospitalized twice, and on each occasion she had stopped taking her medication. Over the past 17 years she has had a scattered work history and has held jobs as a library assistant and as an order clerk. Her current employment is as a file clerk at an insurance company, where she stores and retrieves information as needed and updates files. She feels her current job places considerable stress on her that at times she has difficulty coping with, and she requests assistance in finding other employment. She currently lives alone. She is unmarried and her family lives several hours away.

### Questions

1. What factors might you consider in helping Ms. S. develop a rehabilitation plan?
2. How would you handle Ms. S.'s comment that she has considered going off her medication because of her concern about side effects?
3. Given Ms. S.'s diagnosis, are there any occupations that may not be suitable for her? Why or why not?
4. Are there other support strategies that may be helpful to Ms. S. to enhance her overall rehabilitation potential?

## REFERENCES

Accordino, M. P., Porter, D. F., & Morse, T. (2001). Deinstutionalization of persons with severe mental illness: Context and consequences. *Journal of Rehabilitation, 67*(2), 16–20.

American Association on Mental Retardation. (1992). *Mental retardation: Definitions, classification, and systems of support* (9th ed). Washington, DC: Author.

American Psychiatric Association. (2000). *Diagnostic and statistical manual of mental disorders* (4th ed., Text Revision). Washington, DC: Author.

Anthony, W. A., Cohen, M. R., Farkas, M., & Gagne, C. (2001). *Psychiatric rehabilitation* (2nd ed.). Boston: Boston University, Center for Psychiatric Rehabilitation.

Baron-Cohen, S. (2000). Is Asperger syndrome/high-functioning autism necessarily a disability? *Developmental Psychopathology, 12*(3), 489–500.

Bishop, M., & Sweet, E. A. (2000). Depression: A primer for rehabilitation counselors. *Journal of Applied Rehabilitation Counseling, 31*(3), 38–45.

Corrigan, P. W., & Calabrese, J. D. (2001). Practical considerations for cognitive rehabilitation of people with psychiatric disabilities. *Rehabilitation Education, 15*(2), 143–153.

Fabian, E. S., & Coppola, J. (2001). Vocational rehabilitation competencies in psychiatric rehabilitation education. *Rehabilitation Education, 15*(2), 133–142.

Farkas, M., & Anthony, W. A. (2001). Overview of psychiatric rehabilitation education: Concepts of training and skill development. *Rehabilitation Education, 15*(2), 119–132.

Fink, M. (2000). Electroshock revisited. *American Scientist, 88*, 162–167.

Foa, E. B., Franklin, M. E., & Moser, J. (2002). Context in the clinic: How well do cognitive-behavioral therapies and medications work in combination? *Biological Psychiatry, 52,* 987–997.

Foa, E. B., Keane, T. M., & Friedman, M. J. (2000). *Effective treatments for PTSD: Practice guidelines from the International Society for Traumatic Stress Studies.* New York: Guilford Press.

Freedman, R. (2003). Schizophrenia. *New England Journal of Medicine, 349*(18), 1738–1749.

Frith, U. (2004). Emanuel Miller lecture: Confusions and controversies about Asperger syndrome. *Journal of Child Psychology and Psychiatry. 45*(4), 672–686.

Garske, G. G. (1999). The challenge of rehabilitation counselors: Working with people with psychiatric disabilities. *Journal of Rehabilitation, 65,* 21–25.

Hall, L. L., & Purdy, R. (2000). Recovery and serious brain disorders: The central role of families in nurturing roots and wings. *Community Mental Health Journal, 36*(4), 427–441.

Hodges, S. (2003). Borderline personality disorder and posttraumatic stress disorder: Time for integration? *Journal of Counseling and Development, 81*(4), 409–417.

Jenike, M. A. (2004). Obsessive-compulsive disorder. *New England Journal of Medicine, 350*(3), 259–265.

Kawas, C. H. (2003). Early Alzheimer's disease. *New England Journal of Medicine, 349*(11), 1056–1063.

Keller, M. B., McCullough, J. P., Klein, D. N., Arnow, B., Dunner, D. L., Gelenberg, A. J., Markowitz, J. C., Nemeroff, C. B., Russell, J. M., Thase, M. E., Trivedi, M. G., & Zajecka, J. (2000). A comparison of Nefazodone, the cognitive behavioral analysis system of psychotherapy, and their combination for the treatment of chronic depression. *New England Journal of Medicine, 342*(20), 1462–1470.

Khouzam, H. R., & Donnelly, N. J. (2001). Posttraumatic stress disorder. *Postgraduate Medicine, 110*(5), 60–62, 67–70, 77–78.

Kress-Shull, M.K. (2000). Continuing challenges to the vocational rehabilitation of individuals with severe long-term mental illness. *Journal of Applied Rehabilitation Counseling. 31*(4), 5–10.

Kress-Shull, M. K., & Leech, L. L. (2000). Effective psychiatric rehabilitation: A collaborative challenge [Editorial]. *Journal of Applied Rehabilitation Counseling, 31*(4), 3–4.

Kroenke, K. (2001). Depression screening is not enough. *Annals of Internal Medicine, 134*(5), 418–419.

Leech, L. L., & Holcomb, J. M. (2000). The nature of psychiatric rehabilitation and implications for collaborative efforts. *Journal of Applied Rehabilitation Counseling, 31*(4), 54–60.

Macias, C., Jackson, R., Schroeder, C., & Wang, Q. (1999). Brief report: What is a clubhouse? ICCD 1996 survey of USA clubhouses. *Community Mental Health Journal, 35*(2), 181–190.

Macintosh, K. E., & Dissanayake, C. (2004). The similarities and differences between autistic disorder and Asperger's disorder: A review of the empirical evidence [Annotation]. *Journal of Child Psychology and Psychiatry, 45*(3), 421–434.

Mahoney, D. M. (2000). Panic disorder and self states: Clinical and research illustrations. *Clinical Social Work Journal, 28*(2), 197–212.

Maj, M., Sartorius, N., Okasha, A., & Zohar, J. (Eds.). (2002). *Obsessive-compulsive disorder* (2nd ed.). Chichester, England: John Wiley.

Mayes, S. D., Calhoun, S. L., & Crites, D. L. (2001). Does DSM-IV Asperger's disorder exist? *Journal of Abnormal Child Psychology, 29*(3), 263–271.

Merrick, J., Kandel, I., & Morad, M. (2004). Trends in autism. *International Journal of Adolescent Medical Health, 16*(1), 75–78.

Moore, C. L. (2001). Disparities in closure success rates for African Americans with mental retardation: An ex-post-facto research design. *Journal of Applied Rehabilitation Counseling, 32*(2), 31–36.

Olney, M. F. (2000). Working with autism and other social-communication disorders. *Journal of Rehabilitation, 66*(4), 51–56.

Pratt, C. W., Gill, K. J., Barrett, N. M., & Roberts, M. M. (1999). *Psychiatric rehabilitation.* San Diego: Academic Press.

Ray, W. A., Daugherty, J. R., & Meador, K. G. (2003). Effect of a mental health "carve-out" program on the continuity of antipsychotic therapy. *New England Journal of Medicine, 348*(19), 1885–1894.

Reed, S. J., & Merz, M. A. (2000). Integrated service teams in psychiatric rehabilitation: A strategy for improving employment outcomes and increasing funding. *Journal of Applied Rehabilitation Counseling, 31*(4), 40–46.

Rhoades, D. R. (2000). Schizophrenia: A review for family counselors. *Family Journal: Counseling and Therapy for Couples and Families, 8*(3), 258–266.

Scott, J. (2000). Treatment of chronic depression. *New England Journal of Medicine, 342*(20), 1518–1520.

Spirito Dalgin, R. (2001). Impact of Title I of the Americans With Disabilities Act on people with psychiatric disabilities. *Journal of Applied Rehabilitation Counseling, 32*(1), 45–50.

Swofford, C. D., Scheller-Gilkey, G., Miller, A. H., Woolwine, B., & Mance, R. (2000). Double jeopardy: Schizophrenia and substance use. *American Journal of Drug and Alcohol Abuse, 26*(13), 343–358.

Szymanski, E. M. (2000). Disability and vocational behavior. In R. Frank & T. Elliot (Eds.), *Handbook of rehabilitation psychology* (pp. 499–517). Washington, DC: American Psychological Association.

Tschopp, M. K., Bishop, M., & Mulvihill, M. (2001). Career development of individuals with psychiatric disabilities: An ecological perspective of barriers and interventions. *Journal of Applied Rehabilitation Counseling, 32*(2), 25–30.

Tsuang, M. (2000). Schizophrenia: Genes and environment. *Biological Psychiatry, 47*, 210–220.

Ursano, R. J. (2002). Post-traumatic stress disorder. *New England Journal of Medicine, 346*(2), 130–132.

Whooley, M. A., & Simon, G. E. (2000). Managing depression in medical outpatients. *New England Journal of Medicine, 343*(26), 1942–1950.

Yehuda, R. (2002). Post-traumatic stress disorder. *New England Journal of Medicine, 346*(2), 108–114.

Yeung-Courchesne, R., & Courchesne, E. (1997). From impasse to insight in autism research: From behavioral symptoms to biological explanations. *Development and Psychopathology, 9*, 389–419.

# CHAPTER 7

# Conditions Related to Substance Use

## DEFINING SUBSTANCE USE DISORDERS

For much of human history a wide array of substances, including plants or plant derivatives, alcohol, nicotine, caffeine, inhalants, and tonics, have been condoned and used by different cultures for therapeutic, ritualistic, religious, or recreational purposes. When society becomes ambivalent toward the use of a substance or determines it to be inappropriate, or when substance use becomes uncontrolled, hazardous, or disruptive to individuals or to others, it is considered to be pathological and in some instances becomes illegal. Conditions related to maladaptive changes in behavior or health that occur as a result of the more or less regular use of a substance in this way constitute *substance use disorders*.

Substance use disorders reflect a combination of biological, psychological, social, and environmental factors and may involve substances that are *licit, illicit, prescribed*, or *not prescribed*. The etiology and treatment of substance use disorders entail a complex interface among all these factors. No one factor explains the development of substance use disorders.

Just as all chronic illness and disability affect physical, social, psychological, and

vocational aspects of individuals' lives, so do substance use disorders. Like other chronic, relapsing conditions, substance use disorders produce a variety of impairments. The implications of these disorders must be evaluated in the context of individuals' specific situations. Substance use disorders can occur alone or in combination with one or more other physical or psychiatric disabilities. The effects of substance use combined with manifestation of another disability can cause additional physical, psychological, and social complications, adding to the disabling effects of both.

## SUBSTANCE ABUSE AND DEPENDENCE

A variety of substances are included in substance use disorders, including both legal and illegal substances. **Substance use disorders** are classified either as *abuse* or as *dependence*. Essential features of each are as follows:

- **Substance abuse** is a maladaptive pattern of substance use resulting in recurrent and significant consequences of substance use, such as neglect of work or family obligations, repeatedly driving under the influence, recur-

rent disorderly conduct or legal problems, or interpersonal problems related to use of the substance.

- **Substance dependence** refers to substance use resulting in physical or psychological symptoms related to substance tolerance, symptoms of withdrawal, and a pattern of compulsive
substance-taking behavior, in which
individuals become so preoccupied
with the substance that much of their
daily activity revolves around obtaining it, despite recurrent negative consequences (American Psychiatric Association, 2000).

Substances of abuse or dependence may
be taken simultaneously or sequentially.
With continued substance use, individuals experience diminished effects with the
same amount so that the amount taken
must be increased to achieve the same
effects. This is called **tolerance**. The degree
of tolerance experienced varies from individual to individual and with the specific substance being used.

Individuals using substances chronically may behaviorally adapt so that they are
able to continue functioning at work, at
home, or in social situations, even though
they are under the influence of a substance.
Although tolerance is not always an indication of dependence, tolerance is a common symptom in individuals with substance use disorders. Furthermore, individuals who develop a tolerance for one
substance may also develop higher tolerance for related substances. This condition
is known as **cross-tolerance**.

The toxic effects of large concentrations
of a substance cause physical disturbances
to occur when the amount is decreased or
suspended. As a result, individuals experience physical symptoms known as **withdrawal**. Symptoms of withdrawal depend
on the substance.

## Intoxication

**Intoxication** refers to a reversible syndrome caused by intake of a specific substance and characterized by behavioral or
psychological changes related to the effect
of the substance on the nervous system
(American Psychiatric Association, 2000).
The level of drug or alcohol intoxication
is determined by the concentration of the
substance in the blood. The rate at which
substances are absorbed is dependent on
the route. Substances that are injected directly into a vein have an immediate effect. The rate at which substances ingested
orally, such as alcohol, are absorbed into
the bloodstream is dependent on the
amount ingested, the presence or absence
of food in the stomach, and the rate of
gastric emptying. Concentration of substances in the blood is also dependent on
body size. For instance, blood alcohol levels are proportionately less in large individuals than in small individuals, even
though they consume equal amounts of
alcohol under similar conditions.

## Withdrawal

Consumption of large amounts of alcohol or other drugs at frequent intervals for
prolonged periods creates a state of physical dependence so that cessation of drug
or alcohol intake or reduction in the
amount consumed produces distressful
and incapacitating symptoms, known as
substance **withdrawal**. Symptoms experienced during withdrawal vary in severity.
Initial symptoms, regardless of the substance, may consist of **dysphoria** (exaggerated feelings of depression and unrest),
insomnia, anxiety, irritability, nausea, agitation, **tachycardia** (fast heartbeat), and
**hypertension** (high blood pressure).

Individuals with mild to moderate withdrawal symptoms with no preexisting con-

ditions and who have social support may have withdrawal managed on an outpatient basis. It is important for health professionals treating withdrawal to know the type of substance abused, since there are substantial differences in complications as well as management of withdrawal from different substances. Individuals with more serious withdrawal symptoms, such as the delirium tremens associated with alcohol (described later in the chapter) or the psychotic symptoms experienced with stimulants or opioids, or those who have co-existing psychiatric or medical conditions, usually require inpatient management of withdrawal (Kosten & O'Connor, 2003).

Detoxification is the first step in substance abuse treatment. The goal of detoxification is to initiate abstinence, reduce symptoms of withdrawal, prevent complications, and retain individuals in treatment (Kosten & O'Connor, 2003). After detoxification, medical treatment consists of giving medications that act as substitutes for the abused substances, with the dosage gradually being tapered off.

## Addiction

The American Psychiatric Association uses the term *dependence* rather than *addiction*; the term *addiction* emphasizes the behavioral component of a substance abuse disorder rather than physical dependence (Maddux & Desmond, 2000). *Addiction* refers to a chronic, relapsing disorder in which individuals exhibit compulsive drug-seeking and drug-taking behavior to induce pleasant states or to relieve stress (Camí & Farré, 2003). The physical and psychological craving for the drug becomes so consuming that individuals expend tremendous effort and energy, as well as financial resources, to obtain it, often at the expense of the safety and well-being of themselves as well as others.

In addiction, drug-taking behavior becomes more than merely "wanting" or "liking" the drug. The brains of individuals who are addicted become hypersensitized, which causes pathological craving of the drug, independent of physical signs of withdrawal (Robinson & Berridge, 2001). Compulsive drug-seeking and drug-taking behavior is facilitated by difficulties in decision making and the ability to judge the consequences of this behavior (Robinson & Berridge, 2003).

Several factors appear to predispose individuals to addiction. Personality traits such as a tendency to take risks or to seek novelty have been found to be more prevalent in individuals who abuse or are dependent on drugs (Helmus, Downey, Arfken, Henderson, & Schuster, 2001). Individuals with psychiatric disorders, especially schizophrenia, bipolar disorder, and depression, have an increased risk of abuse. A dual diagnosis also has been shown to have more unfavorable implications for treatment and outcome (Kavanagh, McGrath, Saunders, Dore, & Clark, 2002).

## SUBSTANCE USE AND CHRONIC ILLNESS AND DISABILITY

Individuals with chronic illness and disability can also manifest substance use disorders. Substance abuse can be a factor in the acquisition of a chronic illness or disability as well as an adjustment to it. Whether substance use was a precursor of the acquired chronic illness or disability or a coping mechanism after it, a diagnosis of two disabling conditions makes treatment of both conditions more complex.

A number of factors may place individuals with chronic illness or disability at higher risk for substance use disorders:

- Medical factors, such as easy access to prescription medication to alleviate symptoms such as chronic pain, mak-

ing it easier to use the medication excessively; or unnecessary or unwarranted prescription of medication for symptoms that could have been treated by alternative means
- Psychological factors such as depression, boredom, or frustration, so that substances are used as a means of escape from reality
- Social factors such as oppression and alienation, so that substances are used recreationally in an attempt to gain acceptance and normalization (Greer, Roberts, & Jenkins, 1990; Watson, Franklin, Ingram, & Eilenberg, 1998)

The coexistence of a substance use disorder with other chronic illness or disability can exacerbate and accentuate symptoms as well as increase individuals' vulnerability to medical complications, leading to the acquisition of additional disability. Although substance abuse can coexist with any disability, comorbidity between substance abuse and mental illness (*dual diagnosis*) is very common (Allen Doyle-Pita, 2001; Volkow, 2001). Whether a substance use disorder is the primary or secondary disability, appropriate intervention and treatment are necessary to enable individuals to reach their full rehabilitation potential.

## PHYSICAL EFFECTS OF ALCOHOL ABUSE AND DEPENDENCE

The effect of alcohol on the body, like the effect of any drug, depends on the interaction between properties of the specific pharmacologic agent and the characteristics of a specific individual. There is evidence to suggest that women tend to be more sensitive to the effects of alcohol and more susceptible to adverse effects of excessive alcohol consumption than men (Blume, Counts, & Turnbull, 1992; Harley,

1995; Kandall, 1996; Scott-Lennox, Rose, Bohlig, & Lennox, 2000). The medical complications of alcohol abuse and/or dependence result from the direct effects of alcohol (ethanol) on body tissues and from adaptive responses of the body to excessive exposure to alcohol.

Initially alcohol acts as a stimulant because it suppresses the central nervous system's inhibitory systems. As alcohol levels increase in the body, however, it has a sedative effect, causing motor incoordination, ataxia, and impaired psychomotor performance (Holdstock & deWit, 1998). Alcohol is rapidly absorbed into the bloodstream from the stomach and intestines and is rapidly metabolized, making it a fast-acting drug. Because it diffuses quickly into the water content of all body tissues, the blood concentration of alcohol is an accurate reflection of the concentration of alcohol in other body tissues.

Some alcohol is eliminated through the kidneys and lungs, but the liver metabolizes most. Although a moderate dose of alcohol normally clears from the blood in approximately 1 hour, only a fixed amount of alcohol can be metabolized at a time. When the rate of alcohol consumption exceeds the body's ability to metabolize it, alcohol accumulates in the bloodstream, elevating the blood alcohol concentration.

Alcohol has a direct pharmacologic effect on the nervous system. It is a powerful central nervous system depressant. The intoxicating effects of alcohol correlate roughly with the alcohol concentrations in the blood, which, in turn, reflect the alcohol concentration in the brain. At low levels of intoxication (0.05 percent), alcohol may produce a sense of relaxation and well-being. As the concentration of alcohol increases (0.11 to 0.20 percent), neurological signs of **ataxia** (defective coordination of muscles, especially with voluntary movement) occur. Judgment may also be impaired. Continued elevation of blood alcohol concentrations (0.31 to 0.41 percent) can produce confusion, mild stupor, and ultimately coma. Blood alcohol levels of 0.51 percent usually lead to death from depression of the respiratory center of the brain.

Another effect in the spectrum of neurological disturbances associated with intensive alcohol intoxication is the occurrence of *blackouts*, periods of amnesia characterized by an inability to remember events during the time of the blackout.

Alcohol withdrawal can be complicated by seizures and delirium. The most severe form of alcohol withdrawal is *delirium tremens*. Individuals with delirium tremens experience significant restlessness, gross disorientation, cognitive disruption, and elevation of temperature and pulse rate. Although delirium tremens can be fatal, the course is often self-limiting. The acute period of delirium tremens usually lasts from 2 to 10 days, but it can be more prolonged if withdrawal is severe. The withdrawal syndrome may be treated medically by the administration of a cross-tolerant drug, such as a sedative. Initially, sedatives are given in large doses to suppress the withdrawal symptoms. Then the dose is reduced or the interval between doses is increased, or both, so that the dosage is progressively tapered to zero. Because of wide variations in drug tolerance, treatment is individualized.

### Treatment of Alcohol Dependence

Alcohol dependence is a chronic, lifelong disorder. It requires long-term treatment that extends beyond the initial period of detoxification and generally involves a wide variety of services, including individual, group, and family therapy. In addition, self-help groups, such as

*Alcoholics Anonymous* for alcohol-dependent individuals, and *Alanon* and *Alateen* for their families, are widely recommended. Typically, the goal of treatment is abstinence from alcohol and other mood-altering substances. In some circumstances, drugs are used to discourage and inhibit the use of alcohol. One such drug, disulfiram (*Antabuse*), interferes with the normal metabolism of alcohol. Consequently, individuals who ingest alcohol after taking Antabuse have severe gastrointestinal distress. Thus, the drug acts as a deterrent to alcohol intake.

### Alcohol-Related Medical Illness

Medical conditions that can result from chronic alcohol abuse, other than those caused by trauma due to intoxication, are generally caused by dietary insufficiency, by the direct toxic effects of alcohol on body tissue, or both. These conditions can involve all organ systems. The prognosis of alcohol-related medical illness depends on the nature of the illness and its severity. Although some alcohol-related medical illnesses are reversible, almost no alcohol-related illness can be cured if the individual continues to abuse alcohol.

### *Nervous System*

#### Korsakoff's Syndrome

Associated with an excessive intake of alcohol, chronic malnutrition, and a deficiency of the B vitamins (thiamine in particular), *Korsakoff's syndrome* is characterized by gross disturbances in forming new memories and recalling past memories. The use of confabulation, in which individuals make up experiences to fill memory gaps, is a common characteristic of those with Korsakoff's syndrome. In addition to abstinence, treatment consists of the administration of thiamine. Some cognitive improvement is possible, but full recovery is unlikely. Several months may be required before improvement is noticeable.

### Wernicke's Encephalopathy (Wernicke's Disease)

Although *Wernicke's encephalopathy* can occur in other conditions, it is most commonly associated with chronic alcohol abuse. It is characterized by the sudden onset of confusion, double vision, and difficulty with balance. It often occurs in combination with Korsakoff's syndrome and, like Korsakoff's syndrome, is related to *thiamine* deficiency. Treatment consists of the replacement of thiamine. Early treatment is mandatory to prevent permanent deficits. Prompt treatment resolves many of the symptoms. When Korsakoff's syndrome accompanies Wernicke's encephalopathy, however, memory deficits remain.

### Peripheral Neuropathy

Although there are many causes of peripheral neuropathy, a number of individuals who chronically abuse alcohol develop disorders of the peripheral nerves (see Chapter 3). Peripheral neuropathy associated with chronic alcohol abuse is thought to be the result of inadequate nutrition, specifically inadequate amounts of *thiamine* and the other B vitamins. The condition affects the extremities and includes symptoms such as numbness, painful sensations, weakness, and muscle cramps. Burning pain of the feet may also occur. Good nutrition and the administration of supplemental B vitamins can bring about improvement, but the improvement may be slow.

### Cardiovascular System

### Cardiomyopathy

Alcoholic cardiomyopathy occurs after long-term chronic use of alcohol. It results from the direct toxic effects of alcohol on the heart muscle itself. The heart may become enlarged (**cardiomegaly**), and the heart muscle may become more fibrous. The heart's ability to pump effectively may be compromised so that symptoms of congestive heart failure, such as difficulty in breathing and swelling (see Chapter 11), may occur as the cardiac damage increases.

### Beriberi Heart Disease

A deficiency in *thiamine* is thought to contribute to the development of beriberi heart disease. Individuals with the condition have a high cardiac output, even at rest, because of the dilation of the peripheral small blood vessels. Beriberi heart disease responds well to the administration of supplemental thiamine.

### Alterations in Heart Rate and Rhythm

Alcohol can affect both the speed at which the heart beats and the rhythm that it maintains. The direct long-term effect on blood pressure is variable. Alcohol withdrawal can put a heavy load on the heart, sometimes compromising cardiac function so severely during detoxification that death can result. Consequently, detoxification should be conducted under careful medical supervision.

### Alterations in Blood

Alcohol can have a direct and adverse effect on the development of red blood cells, white blood cells, and platelets, resulting in subsequent anemia, lower resistance to infection, and interference with blood clotting. One of the mechanisms by which alcohol affects blood cell formation is by interfering with the use of folic acid, a nutritional substance that bone marrow requires to manufacture healthy cells effectively.

**Megaloblastic anemia** (the presence of large abnormal red blood cells) with **leukopenia** (an abnormal decrease in the number of white blood cells) and **thrombocytopenia** (an abnormal decrease in the number of platelets) occurs frequently in individuals with low folic acid intake. Treatment with the administration of supplemental *folate*, proper nutrition, and abstinence from alcohol can generally reverse these abnormalities.

### Respiratory System

Alcohol has a direct toxic effect on lung tissue. In combination with cigarette smoking, a higher incidence of chronic obstructive pulmonary disease (see Chapter 12) can result from chronic alcohol abuse. In addition, because chronic alcohol abuse affects some of the lungs' natural defenses, individuals who abuse alcohol have a greater tendency to develop lung infections.

### Musculoskeletal System

Regardless of the nutritional status, alcohol has a direct toxic effect on skeletal muscle; destruction of muscle fibers leads to weakness, pain, tenderness, and swelling of affected muscles. **Myopathy** (disease of muscle) due to alcohol abuse may be acute or chronic. The more common form is *chronic alcoholic myopathy*, which evolves over months to years. Pain may be less severe in chronic myopathy, although muscle cramps can occur. In addition, muscles may **atrophy** (shrink or become

smaller) and become weak. Most symptoms of myopathy improve with the cessation of alcohol abuse, but continued alcohol abuse leads to continued deterioration. Excessive alcohol consumption can also contribute to **osteoporosis** (reduction in bone mass), causing bones to become weakened, fragile, and easily broken; see Chapter 14). Osteoporosis occurs not only because calcium intake is insufficient but also because alcohol interferes with the absorption of calcium from the intestine.

In addition to the direct effect on the musculoskeletal system, alcohol can also contribute to major injury. Individuals under the influence of alcohol may have decreased balance and coordination and demonstrate impaired judgment. As a result, they may be injuried in falls, fires, or motor vehicle or pedestrian accidents.

### Gastrointestinal System

It is possible for alcohol to affect almost every organ of the gastrointestinal tract. Individuals who consume alcohol excessively have an increased incidence of cancer of the throat and esophagus (see Chapter 16). Whether the increased incidence of cancer is due to direct contact of alcohol with the tissues, the presence of carcinogenic substances in some alcoholic beverages, or a combination of the two is unknown. Despite the fact that alcohol is considered a **hepatotoxin** (substance that is harmful to the liver), individuals who chronically abuse alcohol differ widely in their susceptibility to liver disease.

#### Esophagitis and Gastritis

**Esophagitis** is inflammation of the esophagus. **Gastritis** is an inflammation of the stomach. Both can occur with the acute and chronic abuse of alcohol. The severity of these conditions depends on the individual. In some instances, the conditions produce only a mild discomfort, but in other instances, the irritation and inflammation produce ulcerations and bleeding. Treatment is directed toward reducing the inflammation. Obviously, abstinence from alcohol is a major treatment objective.

## Esophageal Varices

Some individuals who abuse alcohol develop *esophageal varices*, "varicose" veins of the esophagus, a condition in which the veins become dilated and tortuous. Esophageal varices are usually a complication of cirrhosis. They may cause no symptoms. If the varices become ulcerated due to irritation, however, or if there is increased strain from coughing or vomiting, the distended veins may rupture, causing serious hemorrhage.

Treatment is directed toward controlling hemorrhage, usually by inserting a special tube (*Sengstaken-Blakemore tube*) into the esophagus. A balloon on the tube is then inflated to exert pressure against the bleeding vein. Because the esophagus needs rest in order to heal, other types of feeding may be instituted until the esophagus is healed (see Chapter 10).

## Alcoholic Hepatitis

During alcohol metabolism, fat is deposited in the liver. When individuals consume excessive amounts of alcohol, the accumulation of fat enlarges the liver, a condition called *fatty liver*. If individuals continue to consume alcohol, liver cells may die, causing the liver to become inflamed. This inflammatory condition, in which the liver is usually enlarged and painful, is known as *alcoholic hepatitis*. Abstinence from alcohol can reverse the effects of both fatty liver and alcoholic hepatitis. Individuals who continue to abuse alcohol, however, have a high chance of developing cirrhosis.

## Cirrhosis

**Cirrhosis** is most frequently caused by either hepatitis C or alcoholism (Ginès, Cárdenas, Arroyo, & Rodés, 2004). It involves the reaction of the liver to injury by **hepatotoxins** (substances that are harmful to the liver), in this case, alcohol. When alcohol injures the liver repeatedly over a period of time, fibrous tissue replaces liver cells. Circulation within the liver becomes less efficient, resulting in obstructions and thus increasing pressure in the vessels.

All blood from the gastrointestinal tract, spleen, pancreas, and gallbladder is carried to the heart through the liver by the *portal system*. Because of the fibrous changes that occur in the liver with cirrhosis, there is increased pressure in the portal vein, a condition known as *portal hypertension*. Backflow of blood results in the enlargement of the spleen (**splenomegaly**), accumulation of fluid in the abdominal cavity (**ascites**), and development of *esophageal varices*.

Some individuals with cirrhosis experience no symptoms. Others experience weakness, nausea, loss of appetite (**anorexia**), and **jaundice** (yellow discoloration of the skin and whites of the eyes due to the accumulation of bile pigments in the blood). Treatment of cirrhosis is largely symptomatic, but abstinence from alcohol is a necessity for survival. Individuals with cirrhotic changes in the liver have an increased risk of cancer of the liver. Those who continue to abuse alcohol despite cirrhotic changes in the liver, or despite other complications, have a significantly decreased survival rate.

## Pancreatitis

A variety of conditions other than alcohol abuse may cause **pancreatitis** (inflammation of the pancreas). *Alcoholic pancreatitis*, however, is a form of pancreatitis that develops in susceptible individuals after chronic alcohol abuse. In this condition, the pancreatic ducts become obstructed. The enzymes that the pancreas normally secretes into the small intestine to aid in digestion become active while they are still in the pancreas (see Chapter 10). As a result, the pancreas essentially begins to digest itself, causing progressive degeneration with scarring and calcification of pancreatic tissues. Pancreatic function is often severely curtailed. Chronic pancreatitis can lead to severe disability from pain, malabsorption of nutrients resulting in weight loss, and diabetes mellitus secondary to the destruction of the *islets of Langerhans* (see Chapter 9).

Treatment of pancreatitis is directed toward halting destruction of tissue and alleviating the symptoms. As with other conditions of the gastrointestinal tract, effective treatment requires that individuals abstain from alcohol. If they no longer consume alcohol, many individuals recover from alcoholic pancreatitis to live a normal life. If they continue to drink, however, the prognosis is generally poor.

## Reproductive System Problems

Excessive alcohol use has been found to lower the level of the male hormone *testosterone*, which, in turn, has been related to decreased libido and, in some instances, impotence. Excessive alcohol intake also increases the level of *epinephrine* and other hormones. The toxic effects of alcohol on the developing fetus during pregnancy can result in a deformity of the infant called **fetal alcohol syndrome**. The amount of alcohol that pregnant women must consume before the fetus is injured is unknown and appears to vary with the individual. Fetal alcohol syndrome is characterized by prenatal and postnatal *growth retardation*, **microcephaly** (abnormal smallness of the head), *abnormalities of the nervous system*, and *facial disfiguration*. Other congenital anomalies may include *mental retardation*, as well as *musculoskeletal* and *cardiac abnormalities*.

# USE DISORDERS INVOLVING OTHER SUBSTANCES

## Caffeine and Nicotine

Tolerance and dependence have been established for both caffeine and nicotine, although these substances are not commonly thought of as substances of abuse. Caffeine is commonly obtained from coffee or tea, but it may also be consumed in soft drinks, chocolate, and many over-the-counter drugs. Caffeine is a powerful central nervous system stimulant (Ochs, Holmes, & Karst, 1992) that can also affect cardiac muscle, elevate blood pressure, increase gastric acid secretion, and have a diuretic effect. It can exacerbate existing disabling conditions as well as generate new symptoms.

Caffeine can produce both psychological and physical dependence. Headaches that are not relieved by regular analgesics are a manifestation of withdrawal from caffeine. Although caffeine abuse in itself is not usually disabling, it may aggravate preexisting conditions, such as ulcer disease, hypertension, or cardiac arrhythmia. The availability of a large number of decaffeinated products makes it possible to decrease caffeine consumption, if necessary.

*Nicotine* is a highly dependence-producing drug (Christen & Christen, 1994). The amount of dependence is proportional to the quantity of the drug used. Nicotine consumed through smoking, chewing, or snuffing tobacco is absorbed through the mucous membranes or surfaces of the lung. Taken into the body, nicotine produces initial stimulation, followed by sedation. Withdrawal effects of nicotine include restlessness, irritability, and tension.

The health consequences of tobacco use can be severe. Cancer of the lung or oral cavity and a variety of other lung diseases have been linked to tobacco use. In addition, tobacco use has been shown to aggravate other preexisting conditions, such as heart disease and hypertension. The addictive nature of nicotine can also interfere with treatment of smoking-related diseases. An early study reported that at least 50 percent of individuals recovering from surgery for a smoking-related condition such as lung cancer or cardiovascular disease continued to smoke while they were hospitalized or resumed smoking shortly after they were discharged (Burling, Stitzer, Bigelow, et al., 1985). Although smoking was once socially acceptable, pressure from various groups and public awareness of the health hazards of smoking have resulted in sanctions on public smoking behavior. Treatment of nicotine dependence varies widely, ranging from the use of nicotine-containing gum to hypnosis to behavioral and group programs. The success of most programs designed to stop tobacco use is directly related to the smoker's motivation to stop.

## Sedatives

Sedation implies calmness and tranquility. *Sedatives* are classified according to the pharmacologic action they produce, namely, *depression of the central nervous system*. Examples of sedative drugs are *alcohol, barbiturates, diazepam (Valium)*,

and *alprazolam* (*Xanax*). If taken in higher doses to produce sleep, they are called hypnotics. Sedatives are sometimes also called *minor tranquilizers* or *antianxiety agents*. Whether they have been prescribed for treatment of a specific condition or symptom or whether they have been obtained illegally, sedatives may be associated with abuse, tolerance, and dependence.

Individuals commonly abuse sedatives in combination with alcohol, and they often abuse opiates and stimulants concurrently. Commonly abused sedatives are *barbiturates* (e.g., phenobarbital, secobarbital, and amobarbital sodium), *benzodiazepines* (e.g., chlordiazepoxide hydrochloride [Librium], *diazepam* [Valium], and *chlorzepate dipotassium* [Tranzene]), and other *central nervous system depressants* (e.g., methaqualone [Quaalude], meprobamate, and ethchlorvynol [Placidyl]).

Withdrawal from sedatives is similar to withdrawal from alcohol. Some sedatives, such as benzodiazepines, may have a delayed withdrawal effect, beginning several days after ceasing to take the drug. If individuals have become sedative dependent on lower doses of the drug, withdrawal symptoms may consist only of irritability, sleep disturbance, and generalized anxiety. If, however, individuals became dependent on higher doses, withdrawal can be life-threatening. Sudden withdrawal, especially from barbiturates, can result in acute psychosis and seizures. Therapeutic withdrawal from a sedative, like the therapeutic withdrawal from alcohol, usually involves the administration of a cross-tolerant drug to suppress withdrawal symptoms with gradual tapering of the dosage. The drug being withdrawn determines the length of time required for tapering. For some sedatives, 7 to 10 days is sufficient for detoxification. Longer-acting drugs that have been used at high dosages may require 14 or more days for detoxification.

## Opioids

Because *opioids* (narcotic drugs such as morphine, meperidine [Demerol], propoxyphene [Darvon], oxycodone [Percodan], and codeine) are frequently prescribed for pain, addiction can occur through regular prescription use. In other instances, these medications are obtained illegally. A commonly used illegal opioid is heroin.

In addition to producing pain relief, narcotics produce euphoria, sedation, and a feeling of tranquility. At first, individuals may take illegal narcotics primarily for the feeling of euphoria. Repeated administration rapidly produces tolerance and intense physical dependence. Eventually, as the dosage and/or frequency of drug administration increases, individuals need to continue to take the drug regularly to avoid symptoms of physical withdrawal.

There are numerous negative health consequences related to opiate use, especially to long-term use of heroin (Fiellin & O'Connor, 2002; Gonzalez, Oliveto, & Kosten, 2002), including lethal respiratory depression with overdose. Drugs that are injected increase individuals' risk of contracting *HIV infection* or *hepatitis C* if needles are shared. Adding adulterants to substances or using nonsterile techniques of injection may also produce medical complications. Skin abscesses, **cellulitis** (inflammation of tissues), **thrombophlebitis** (inflammation of a vein with associated clot formation), **septicemia** (presence of toxins in the blood), and bacterial **endocarditis** (inflammation of the inner lining of the heart) are frequent complications.

Withdrawal symptoms vary in severity and duration, depending on the particular drug abused. Withdrawal from narcotics is generally not life-threatening. Many symptoms of withdrawal are flulike, although they may include anxiety, irritability, and restlessness.

Opiate substitution drugs are sometimes used in treatment of opiate addiction and may be used for either detoxification or maintenance. Methadone and another opiate-substitute, levomethadyl acetate, may be used to reduce the use of illicit opiates and the high-risk behaviors associated with drug use (Fudala et al., 2003; O'Connor, 2000), as well as to provide medical assistance with withdrawal of opiates. When used for detoxification, the drug dosage is gradually tapered during the withdrawal period. Some individuals may be enrolled in a *maintenance program* in which they do not undergo detoxification but rather receive maintenance doses of an opiate substitute along with counseling. The goal of such programs is first to help individuals return to a socially rehabilitated state and then to help them achieve a drug-free state.

Opiate substitution therapy is provided only in a strictly regulated environment in which medication is taken under clinical observation and supervision (Clark, 2003).

## Stimulants

Acting directly on the central nervous system, *stimulants* create an increased state of arousal and concentration and speed up mental and motor activity. Individuals may take stimulants for such effects as increased alertness and increased sense of well-being, increased confidence, reduction of fatigue, or decrease in appetite. *Amphetamines* (Benzedrine or Dexedrine), *methylphenidate* (Ritalin), *cocaine*, and *caffeine* are all stimulants. They can be taken *orally*, *topically*, *intravenously*, or by *inhalation*. In addition to central nervous system effects, stimulants have generalized systemic effects, including an *increase in heart rate*, an *increase in blood pressure*, a *rise in body temperature*, and the *constriction of peripheral blood vessels* (Sarnyai, Shaham, & Heinrichs, 2001). Cocaine can also cause **cardiac arrhythmia** (irregular heartbeat) and can *increase the respiratory rate* (Kloner & Rezkalla, 2003). Long-term use of stimulants can cause irritability, aggressive behavior, and paranoid psychosis (Camí & Farré, 2003).

In recent years, cocaine has become one of the most widely abused stimulants. It may be taken orally, used intranasally (snorted), smoked, or injected intravenously. The technique of *free-basing* cocaine, which gained popularity in the 1980s, involves heating a flammable solvent such as petroleum or ether, and then using it to heat cocaine. The process "frees" cocaine hydrochloride from its salts and adulterants, converting it to a form of cocaine that will vaporize. The free-base cocaine can be inhaled or smoked, usually with a water pipe, for direct absorption through the alveoli in the lungs. The technique rapidly delivers high concentrations of cocaine to the brain and results in blood levels as high as those for self-injection.

The free-basing technique can cause additional disability caused by the burns from fires started during the free-basing process. The level of tolerance for cocaine rapidly increases, and the need for additional cocaine to function normally can rapidly lead to the use of *crack*. Crack, a solid form of cocaine free base, is thought to be one of the most addictive substances yet encountered. Dependence is produced very rapidly. Crack is smoked rather than sniffed. Its concentrated form and its route of administration make its potency many times greater than that of cocaine alone. The euphoric effect produced by crack lasts only a matter of minutes, however, and is often followed by irritability, restlessness, and depression. The aftereffects of crack can be so intense that individuals continue to smoke it, despite obvious adverse consequences.

Individuals using cocaine, especially at higher dosages, may use depressant drugs to counterbalance the stimulant effects. For example, alcohol and cocaine are commonly combined for this purpose. The simultaneous injection of cocaine and heroin (*speedballing*) is also common. Aside from its psychological, social, and vocational consequences, cocaine use can have serious medical consequences. Freebasing or smoking crack can lead to *pulmonary complications*. Chronic use of intranasal cocaine may cause *ulceration* or *perforation* of the nasal septum. Cocaine intoxication can produce *neurologic effects*, such as confusion, anxiety, hyperexcitability, agitation, and violence. More serious effects are the result of acute *cocaine toxicity*, which is dose related, in which individuals can experience *stroke* or *seizures*, severe **hyperthermia** (increased body temperature), **arrhythmia** (irregular heartbeat), **myocardial infarction** (heart attack), and, in some instances, *sudden death*. *Cocaine psychosis*, another side effect of cocaine use, is manifested by paranoia, panic, hallucinations, insomnia, and picking at the skin. The psychotic episode can last from 24 to 36 hours. Individuals with this condition are usually hospitalized and treated with antipsychotic medication.

Substances added to adulterate cocaine to increase its weight, thereby increasing profit on its sale, may cause additional medical complications. Problems can result from the nature of the substance used to cut the cocaine or from the dosage taken. Adulterants such as talc or cornstarch can cause complications ranging from *inflammation* to **embolus** (undissolved matter in the blood).

*Procaine, PCP,* or *heroin,* which also may be added to cocaine, may potentiate the effects. Because the user can never be certain of cocaine's potency, the effects are not always predictable. The withdrawal syndrome from cocaine consists of a craving for more cocaine, depression, irritability, sleep disturbances, gastrointestinal disturbances, headaches, and possibly suicidal ideation. Because it is not unusual for individuals who are cocaine dependent to also be dependent on other drugs, a withdrawal reaction from other substances may be experienced as well.

A newer street drug classified as an amphetamine is *crystalline methamphetamine ("ice"),* which is highly addictive physically and psychologically (Lukas, 1997). Like crack, it can be heated and inhaled. The technique is similar to that of smoking free-base cocaine. Ice has greater strength and more enduring effects, lasting from 8 to 24 hours. Greater stimulation to the brain makes it more dangerous mentally because it creates a craving that can continue years after cessation of use (Wermuth, 2000). Toxic levels can produce severe paranoid thinking with hallucinations. There is also greater risk of suicidal depression. Chronic use of methamphetamine in any form can result in serious psychiatric, cardiovascular, metabolic, and neuromuscular changes.

## Cannabis

When cannabis (*marijuana*) is smoked, the active compound (THC) that it contains produces euphoria, relaxation, dreamlike states, and sleepiness. It also impairs cognitive function and performance of psychomotor tasks (Camí & Farré, 2003). Some individuals report enhanced perceptions of colors, tastes, and textures. The

psychoactive responses to the drug depend to a great extent on the dose, the personality and the experience of the user, and the environment in which the drug is used. Often, users report a sense of time slowing and an impairment in their ability to learn new facts while they are under the influence of the drug.

Overdose can produce anxiety, panic states, and psychosis (Hall & Solowij, 1998). Systemically, cannabis produces an increase in heart rate, dilation of the bronchioles, and dilation of the peripheral blood vessels. Because of the stimulatory effect on the heart, cannabis use may lead to cardiac complications in individuals with heart disease. Chronic smoking of cannabis produces inflammatory changes in the lungs that contribute to the development of chronic conditions such as emphysema (see Chapter 12). Furthermore, the use of other drugs, including alcohol and tobacco, may compound the adverse effects of cannabis. For example, the combination of tobacco and cannabis use is thought to increase the risk of lung cancer.

Although cannabis may be ingested orally, oral consumption can delay its effects for up to an hour, and the effects are less potent. *Hashish,* the concentrated form of THC, is also smoked and has considerably more potency than does cannabis.

Some individuals use cannabis only on special occasions, but others become compulsively preoccupied with daily use. The long-term effects of cannabis use remain controversial. The degree to which cannabis creates physical dependence has not been established; however, it may be possible to develop psychological dependence on cannabis (Hall & Solowij, 1998). Symptoms of withdrawal including restlessness, irritability, and insomnia have been noted in heavy users (Budney, Hughes, Moore, & Novy, 2001).

There is no specific medical treatment for cannabis abuse. When cannabis use severely hampers individuals' functioning, treatment most often involves psycho-therapeutic techniques directed at under-lying problems. Because cannabis may be abused in combination with other drugs, treatment may occasionally be multifocal in nature.

## Hallucinogens

Sometimes called *psychedelics, hallu-cinogens* are drugs that, at some dosage, produce *hallucinations* or *distortions in per-ceptions or thinking*. Individuals under the influence of hallucinogens report in-creased awareness of sensory input and a subjective feeling of enhanced mental activity. Common hallucinogens are *LSD, PCP* (*angel dust*), and *mescaline.*

Controlled substance analogues, or *designer drugs*, can have dangerous, perma-nent effects. Users of one class of these drugs, the *methamphetamines* such as MDMA (*ecstasy*) or MDA (*street name Adam*), may be especially susceptible to permanent brain damage because the amount that produces psychological ef-fects is not far from the dosage that pro-duces neural damage. Designer derivatives of amphetamines (MDMA) produce eu-phoria but can also have hallucinogenic effects; they may also cause **cerebral hem-orrhage** (stroke), **hyperthermia** (elevated body temperature), altered mental status, panic, and psychosis.

Hallucinogens are usually taken orally. Although the use of hallucinogens has declined somewhat, patterns of use vary widely. Their use is now often concurrent with the use of other drugs. One of the most powerful hallucinogens is *LSD*. Its effects vary with the individual, the dose, and the environment in which the drug is used. Generally, the effects develop within several hours and last up to 12 hours. Individuals may report height-ened sensitivity and clarity, increased insights, a sense of time moving more slowly, and distortions of visual images. Some individuals experience adverse effects from LSD, such as a panic state with severe anxiety.

The physical consequences of hallucino-gen abuse in and of themselves are not sig-nificant. The psychological consequences, however, can be severe. Adverse effects of hallucinogens vary from *acute psychosis* to *self-mutilation* or *suicide*. Accidents can result from misjudgment or impairment. Some individuals experience "flashbacks" in which hallucinations reappear briefly even months after the last drug dose. An overdose of hallucinogens can result in exceedingly high body temperatures, seizures, and shock.

Because hallucinogens produce no physical dependence, there is no specific medical regimen for treatment. Adverse effects such as panic episodes are usually treated with a supportive environment and observation.

## Inhalants

Substances that cause perceptible changes in brain function through inhala-tion are called *inhalants*. Inhalants are gen-erally classified into four categories:

- Aerosols
- Gases
- Solvents
- Nitrites
  (Ballard, 1998)

A wide variety of substances are abused in this way, often because they are readily accessible and inexpensive. For example, commonly used inhalants are *airplane glue, typewriter correction fluid, marking pen-cils, industrial and household chemicals, gasoline, nitrites (poppers, snappers,* or *rush),* and *nitrous oxide.* Although individuals of all age groups practice inhalant abuse, it is especially prevalent among adolescents and preadolescents.

Although the effects of inhalants are brief, they can be serious, especially with prolonged or long-term use. Adverse effects of inhalants vary according to the type of substance inhaled. Organic solvents such as airplane glue can produce *cardiac arrhythmia, bone marrow depression, damage to the kidney and liver,* and, in some instances, *death.*

Prolonged use of *nitrites* is thought to *suppress the immune system,* increasing the individual's susceptibility to infection. Nitrites are frequently used to enhance sexual pleasure; consequently, individuals who use nitrites in this way and are also exposed to human immunodeficiency virus (HIV) may be at greater risk for developing HIV infection because of their suppressed immune system and subsequent increased vulnerability to infection. Chronic abuse of *nitrous oxide* can result in *nerve damage, seizures, bone marrow changes, respiratory depression,* or *death.* Because nitrous oxide distorts special senses, driving during intoxication is hazardous. Even though the effects of inhalants are brief, their use can result in dependence. No specific medical treatment is usually indicated for inhalant abuse, but specific psychotherapeutic measures may be used to prevent relapse and to help individuals discontinue inhalant use.

# MEDICAL CONSEQUENCES OF ABUSE OF OTHER DRUGS AND SUBSTANCES

Substance abuse leads to psychological, social, and vocational impairments and of-

ten to crimes committed to obtain drugs or to obtain money for additional drugs. Substance abuse also has medical consequences.

## Drug-Related Illness

### Dermatologic Complications

Many of the medical complications related to drug abuse result from nonsterile injections or from adulterants, rather than from the drug itself.

### Abscess

Bacterial infection may cause pus to collect in the tissues, forming an abscess. In association with drug use, improper cleansing of the skin before injection or the use of a nonsterile needle may lead to an abscess. Skin at the site becomes warm, red, swollen, and painful with a **purulent** (pus) discharge. Skin around the area frequently becomes **necrotic** (dies). If the abscess goes untreated, individuals may develop systemic symptoms of fever, loss of appetite, and fatigue. Infection may spread to the bloodstream, creating a generalized systemic infection (**bacteremia**). Treatment of an abscess consists of draining the purulent material and **debriding** (removing) the area of dead tissue. Antibiotics are usually prescribed, especially if individuals demonstrate systemic symptoms.

### Cellulitis

An acute inflammation of the tissues without **necrosis** (tissue death) is called cellulitis. When associated with intravenous drug abuse, cellulitis is caused by the invasion of a variety of organisms or by irritation of the tissues from the drug itself. The tissue becomes red and tender, and there may be **adenopathy** (swelling of lymph nodes). Treatment of cellulitis depends on the cause. Occasionally, cellulitis progresses to abscess formation.

### Other Dermatologic Complications

Injections with nonsterile needles or injections of drugs that have been contaminated by adulterants may leave *needle track scars*. Injections cause a mild inflammatory reaction and, with subsequent injections, produce scarring at the injection site. Injection of a drug into an artery instead of a vein can cause an extreme reaction of intense pain, swelling, and coldness of an extremity. If not treated properly, *gangrene* may develop, necessitating amputation.

### Cardiovascular Complications

Other than direct effects on the heart from the drug itself, most cardiovascular complications that result from drug use are related to the use of nonsterile injection techniques or to contamination of the drug with adulterants. A common complication is **endocarditis** (inflammation of the inner lining of the heart), which affects the valves of the heart and can lead to potentially serious consequences (see Chapter 11).

Some drugs have a direct toxic effect on the heart muscle or may directly affect heart rhythm. In some instances, inflammation of the veins with clot formation (**thrombophlebitis**) may occur because of the toxic effects of the drug.

### Respiratory Complications

The intravenous injection of drugs to which adulterants such as talc, starch, or baking soda have been added may result in pulmonary complications. Because these substances do not dissolve, they circulate in the blood and may become lodged in lung tissue. The lodged particles cause an inflammatory reaction in the lungs, resulting in *fibrosis* of the lung tissue. If the fibrous changes are extensive, they affect the oxygen-exchanging ability of the lungs. Symptoms similar to those of emphysema may develop. Changes in lung elasticity can eventually result in *pulmonary hypertension* and subsequent *heart failure*. (See Chapter 12 for a discussion of the symptoms of emphysema and Chapter 11 for a discussion of pulmonary hypertension and heart failure.)

Lung infections or lung abscesses may occur if organisms localize in the lung after the nonsterile injection of a substance. *Aspiration pneumonia*, an inflammation of the lung, may result from the inhalation of foreign substances or chemical irritants. Aspiration of gastric contents is also a common cause of aspiration pneumonia. Individuals who become unconscious because of a drug overdose may, in their unconscious state, vomit and subsequently inhale the vomitus. If they inhale a large quantity, the results can be fatal.

Individuals who abuse drugs, including alcohol, may also develop *tuberculosis* (see Chapter 12). Rather than being a direct result of drug use, tuberculosis is more likely the consequence of the general lifestyle and living conditions of individuals who abuse drugs. Malnourishment, poor hygiene, and overcrowding all contribute to development of the disease. In addition, because some drugs have an immunosuppressant effect, individuals may be more susceptible to the infection. An overdose of narcotics or sedative/hypnotics can severely depress the respiratory center, causing cessation of breathing and consequent death. Overdoses of narcotics have also been associated with development of severe **pulmonary edema** (collection of fluid in the lungs), which, without treatment, can also result in death.

## Gastrointestinal Complications

Because the liver acts as the detoxification center for the body, individuals who chronically abuse drugs may damage their liver. Some substances appear to be more directly harmful to the liver than others. Chronic, excessive abuse of solvents, for example, can cause liver **necrosis** (tissue death). Other substances may cause liver abnormalities such as inflammation or fibrosis.

*Hepatitis* is a common complication of drug abuse. Hepatitis A may be related to poor hygiene habits and poor environmental conditions. More commonly, *hepatitis B* (*serum hepatitis*) occurs as the result of nonsterile or contaminated intravenous injections. (See Chapter 10 for a discussion of hepatitis A and hepatitis B.) *Hepatitis C* is caused by the hepatitis C virus (HCV). HCV causes what was previously called *non-A, non-B hepatitis* and is transmitted through infected blood. Consequently, individuals who use intravenous drugs and share needles are at high risk for developing the disease. Hepatitis C generally becomes a chronic disease and can predispose the individual to cirrhosis (Ginès et al., 2004). The only treatment currently used for hepatitis C consists of injections of *interferon*; however, about half of people treated relapse.

## Neurological Complications

Seizures may result from an overdose of drugs or a hypersensitivity to adulterants. Seizures are especially prevalent after an overdose of amphetamines, heroin, or hallucinogens. In some instances, stroke may also accompany an overdose. The toxic effects of adulterants on the nervous system can lead to blindness and peripheral nerve damage.

## Other Complications

The chronic use of some drugs may result in **nystagmus** (involuntary eye movement). Use of solvents can produce *bone marrow changes* and *aplastic anemia*. An overdose of drugs can result in *acute renal failure*, which can progress to permanent kidney damage (see Chapter 13). Individuals who abuse drugs also have a higher incidence of *venereal disease*, such as gonorrhea and syphilis, related to their general lifestyle and sexual practices. One of the most serious and hazardous complications of drug use in the past few years has been infection with HIV (see Chapter 8), which is related to both intravenous drug use and unsafe sexual practices.

Drug abuse during pregnancy has serious implications for the offspring. Some fetal hazards are related to the lifestyle of the mother, which results in poor prenatal care, poor nutrition, and a generally poor health status. The direct toxic effects of drugs on the developing fetus (*tetratogenic* effects) can include neurological and/or physical abnormalities, as well as the dangers of the withdrawal syndrome to the infant after birth.

## DIAGNOSTIC PROCEDURES

Diagnosis of substance use disorders is often delayed or symptoms overlooked. The result is continued disabling effects, further development of medical complications, and progression of dependence. Denial and resistance to acknowledging the problem are universal symptoms of substance abuse and dependence. Consequently, even if family members or associates have identified a substance use problem, the individual who abuses substances may deny the condition and refuse to seek treatment.

Substance use disorders are frequently associated with other health and personal concerns. Consequently, many individuals presenting at health or counseling facilities may have coexisting or secondary substance use problems that are not identified or diagnosed. Some professionals may feel uncomfortable questioning or confronting individuals about substance use disorders, in which cases diagnosis or treatment of the problem is further delayed. Undetected substance use problems have significant effects on the health and well-being of individuals as well as their family and others.

## Screening Instruments

Routine screening of individuals presenting for health care or counseling helps professionals determine whether a problem exists and whether there is need for more in-depth assessment. Several types of screening instruments are available. One of the best-known and most widely used instrument is the *Michigan Alcoholism Screening Test*. Others include the *CAGE*, the *T-ACE*, the *TWEAK*, the *Alcohol Use Disorders Identification Test*, the *Substance Abuse Life Circumstances Evaluation*, the *MacAndrew Scale* and *MacAndrew Scale-Revised*, and the *Substance Abuse Subtle Screening Inventory* (Piazza, Martin, & Dildine, 2000). Each screening test has its own assets and limitations. The type of screening test chosen should be based on the circumstances under which the test is used as well as on specific factors related to the individual.

## Direct Drug Screening

Direct testing for the presence of the substance in the body may involve breath analyzers and blood alcohol tests. Both tests serve as a measurement of intoxica-tion, but they do not reveal the extent of abuse or dependence. Screening of blood or urine samples is also used to verify suspected substance use. As with any laboratory test, there is a possibility of false-negative or false-positive results. Newer screening methods are designed to be more sensitive and produce more accurate results. Two common methods of urine testing available in most laboratories are thin-layer chromatography and gas chromatography. Drug testing is valid, however, only if accomplished under strictly controlled conditions. Many individuals who abuse or are dependent on drugs are aware of a variety of methods to invalidate test results, such as substituting specimens from a drug-free individual for their own specimen. The appropriate methods and times of drug screening are highly controversial. Routine screening for drugs without the individual's knowledge and consent evokes a variety of legal and ethical concerns.

## Medical Evaluation

Medical diagnosis of substance use may be attained from several sources. The physical manifestations of substance abuse and/or dependence may include a variety of disorders. Questions about substance use practices should be routinely asked in the examination of individuals with gastrointestinal disturbances, hypertension or heart disease, liver disease, neurological changes, or a history of traumatic injuries. Blood cell abnormalities, such as decreased number of platelets or signs of bone marrow depression (see Chapter 8), or other indirect clinical laboratory signs, such as elevated levels of gamma-glutamyltransferase or gamma-glutamyltranspeptidase, or an elevated red blood cell mean corpuscular volume, may suggest problems with substance abuse. Elevated levels of enzymes such as serum glutamic-oxaloacetic transaminase (SGOT) and serum glutamate pyruvate transaminase ( SGPT), may also be associated with substance abuse; however, increased concentrations of enzymes such as SGOT and SGPT can also be associated with other conditions (e.g., myocardial infarction).

## Behavioral and Psychological Screening

Investigation of subtle psychological or behavioral symptoms is also important in the diagnosis of a substance use disorder. Depression, hyperactivity, sleep disturbances, anxiety, sexual problems, or personality changes are common manifestations of substance use disorders. In addition, the incidence of accidents and injury is often increased.

## TREATMENT OF SUBSTANCE USE DISORDERS

The first step in the treatment of substance-related disorders is identifying and acknowledging the problem. Screening may be hampered by several barriers, including:

- denial of the problem by individuals or family members
- reluctance of medical and counseling personnel to confront or discuss the problem

Once the problem is identified and confronted, individuals should be assessed for medical and psychosocial problems that typically accompany it as well as for their motivation for change (O'Connor, 2000). Successful treatment of substance use disorders generally requires more than one level of care during the long recovery process. Treatment may involve outpatient or inpatient care and continued aftercare. Most individuals in treatment for substance

use consider themselves as "recovering," denoting the long-term and chronic nature of the recovery process. Relapse is a common part of recovery and, rather than being thought of as failure, can be viewed as an opportunity for learning and growth (American Academy of Pediatrics, 2000).

Many individuals with substance use disorders eventually experience physical, social, or psychological crises that require inpatient or residential treatment. The type of treatment received varies greatly from facility to facility and depends on the particular type of crisis experienced. Some facilities provide treatment for substance use disorders solely on an outpatient basis. Others provide a combination of inpatient or residential and outpatient treatment.

Treatment usually begins with detoxification, which may or may not involve inpatient or residential treatment, depending on the individual, the specific substance, and the presence of additional complications. Detoxification is only an initial step in the treatment of substance use disorders, however. Ongoing therapy that includes a variety of rehabilitation strategies, such as psychotherapy, family therapy, and self-help programs (e.g., Alcoholics Anonymous or Narcotics Anonymous), is necessary to prevent relapse. Several psychotherapeutic approaches to the treatment of substance abuse exist. The specific type of therapy used is often dependent on the facility in which the individual is being treated and the overall philosophy of professionals conducting the treatment. In almost all instances, abstinence is a treatment goal.

In some instances, drugs are prescribed in the ongoing treatment of substance dependence. *Antabuse* and *methadone* (or other opiate substitute), which were discussed earlier, are drugs commonly used in the treatment of alcohol and opiate dependence, respectively.

Individuals with a substance use disorder may also require ongoing medical treatment for any medical complications that have resulted from the substance use. Because nutritional deficiencies frequently accompany substance use disorders, most detoxification centers and residential facilities provide nutrition therapy as a part of the treatment. Educational programs that stress the importance of nutrition, as well as other aspects of a healthy lifestyle, are often incorporated into the general treatment program.

## PSYCHOSOCIAL AND VOCATIONAL ISSUES IN SUBSTANCE ABUSE

### Psychological Issues

The extent to which psychological disability is the direct result of a substance-related disorder or the cause of the disorder is not easily determined. Individuals with substance use disorders frequently have low self-esteem and experience depression. They may have feelings of inadequacy, loneliness, and isolation that lead to increased substance use. Influenced and controlled by the substance, they may rely on it rather than on their own resources. Doubt that they will be able to cope without the substance may erode their self-confidence and self-esteem even more.

Individuals who are psychologically dependent on a substance feel a need and longing for the substance and become irritable, depressed, anxious, and resentful when the substance is not available. Individuals with a psychological craving for a substance may attribute their need to a personal flaw in their character or may consider their need as a negative reflection on themselves. Either interpretation further contributes to lowered self-esteem and self-deprecation.

Individuals may use denial or rationalization as a form of self-protection and as a way to minimize substance use problems. They deny that a substance use problem exists or may rationalize their behavior by redefining their substance use so that it appears to be acceptable. Some individuals become aggressive or perform violent acts when they are under the influence of certain substances. Those who are predisposed to this type of reaction may become involved in criminal acts, such as brawls, homicide, rape, or child abuse.

As individuals become increasingly dependent on the substance, the concept of living without it produces fear and dread. Individuals interpret removal of the substance as removal of all joy and excitement from life. As with all types of perceived loss, individuals may experience grief and bereavement.

Recovery from a substance use disorder involves restoration of self-esteem and confidence, as well as willingness to accept responsibility for personal behavior. Individuals need assistance to accept the losses they have experienced and to develop skills for coping in the future. Recovery is a continuing process that includes long-term vigilance and a continuing commitment to remain drug-free.

### Lifestyle Issues

A substance-related disorder affects every aspect of individuals' daily life. As dependence on the substance becomes more pronounced, individuals may lose interest in self-care, may show a decreased desire for food, and may have a variety of sleep disturbances, resulting in sleep deprivation. Daily activities may become focused on obtaining more of the substance. Activities once enjoyed may offer little joy or stimulate little interest.

Substance use can affect individuals' ability to drive. Poor driving performance can result in accidents or arrests, which can lead to the loss of a driver's license. Therefore, transportation may become a problem, so that individuals must depend on others for their transportation needs.

Sexual dysfunction is common in individuals with substance use disorders. Women may experience decreased libido or may become promiscuous. Men may experience not only decreased libido but also adverse effects on sexual performance, including impotence, a common side effect of chronic alcohol abuse. Individuals recovering from a substance use disorder may need to learn or relearn the components of a healthy lifestyle, such as good hygiene and grooming, proper diet, and the importance of exercise. These aspects of daily living may be a vital part of an individual's rehabilitation.

## Social Issues

The social effects of substance-related disorders are widespread, touching family relationships, relationships with friends and associates, and general functioning as a member of society. Individuals' ability to function as a member of a social group may gradually deteriorate as substance use increases. To some extent, social factors may determine the social implications of substance use. For example, the availability of substances within a group or as part of a social event may determine whether or not individuals participate in that group or event.

The extent of the social tolerance of individuals' behavior while intoxicated may either curtail or enhance substance use at first. As individuals become increasingly substance-dependent, however, the substance becomes more important and social contacts and activities become less important.

Individuals with a substance use disorder may be unable to function within their social network. Repeated, heavy use of the substance often leads to upheavals in relationships. Social and family relationships are strained and often destroyed if individuals become abusive and violent or if they engage in socially unacceptable behavior while under the influence of the substance. Their behavior often alienates others, leading to social isolation. Decreasing reliability in performing social roles and continued inability to maintain commitments cause those affected by the individual's deterioration to feel disappointed and angry. Others in the social environment may have to alter their own roles to incorporate duties the individual once had. This places additional burdens on all concerned and may eventually lead to resentment or even banishment from the group. Family members and associates may begin to withdraw from the individual emotionally. As individuals become increasingly more isolated, feelings of self-loathing, guilt, and shame may develop. Feeling rejected by family and associates, they may limit their social contacts to relationships with others who also focus on substance use.

The broader social consequences of substance use disorders may have legal and even criminal implications. There is a strong relationship between substance use disorders and a variety of accidents; motor vehicle accidents, for example, can lead to physical disability not only for the individual with the substance use disorder, but also for others. Thus, the loss of a driver's license and more serious criminal charges are potential effects of substance abuse and/or dependence. Furthermore, individuals who become dependent on illegal substances may engage in illegal activities to gain money for the purchase of additional drugs. Even if they do not face criminal charges, they can become focused on obtaining the drug rather than on functioning in a productive social role.

In some cases, family and social relationships can be salvaged in the recovery process. In other instances, the loss of these relationships is permanent. Depending on individual circumstances, therapeutic recovery may involve the development of new social roles and relationships or the reestablishment of old ones.

## Vocational Issues

In the early stages of a substance-related disorder, individuals may be concerned that the use of the substance will interfere with their work. If substance use progresses to abuse or dependence, however, concern may be reversed so that individuals become more concerned that their work will interfere with the use of the substance. The substance becomes ultimately important, thus drastically affecting work performance.

Although early identification of and intervention with workers with a substance use disorder are most desirable, the problem may not be recognized until there is a progressive deterioration of work performance, increased absenteeism, or an increase in job-related accidents. Fear that they will lose their jobs if their employers become aware of these indicators may motivate individuals with a substance use disorder to seek treatment.

The ability of individuals to return to their former employment after treatment for substance abuse and/or dependence depends on the circumstances. In some instances, the stress and tension imposed by the job may be beyond individuals' tolerance and coping ability. It may be beneficial to find a less stressful work setting, especially in the early stages of recovery, until their tolerance for stress gradually

increases. Physical disability resulting from substance abuse and/or dependence must also be considered when evaluating vocational potential.

It is essential to identify past work problems that may extend beyond issues of substance abuse and/or dependence. Some individuals may need to learn social skills, work-appropriate behaviors, or good hygiene or grooming practices; some need to improve their work skills. Individuals who began abusing substances at an early age may not have developed sufficient work skills or work history to obtain employment and may require additional education or job training. If they return to the same work setting that originally precipitated feelings of inadequacy and that contributed to the development of substance abuse and/or dependence, return to work may increase the risk of relapse. In some cases, learning new skills or coping strategies may enable individuals to return successfully to the work setting. In other instances, however, a new work environment may be necessary.

Loss of a driver's license because of a substance use disorder may make transportation to and from work more difficult. In addition, if driving a motor vehicle had been part of the former employment, job restructuring or job change may be necessary. Some occupations require professional licensure. Therefore, revocation of individuals' licenses may limit their ability to work in their former occupation. Many professional licensing boards have provisions for the reinstatement of licensure after documented rehabilitation. If the professional license is reinstated, there may be a probationary period in which individuals' work performance is closely observed and monitored.

Conviction of criminal charges, especially felony charges, may prohibit employment in some occupations. Although decisions may be made on a case-by-case basis, such charges and their impact on employment in different fields and in different locations must be considered. As with most disabilities, the attitudes and concerns of employers must be addressed, especially since social stigma is often attached to substance use disorders. Employers may require particular encouragement to reinstate or hire individuals who have been convicted of criminal charges. Knowing the potential for rejection by employers based on these attitudes, recovering individuals may be reluctant to share their complete history with employers or may become defensive when asked questions about substance use. Fear of rejection because of prejudice must be considered when the individual returns to work. With increasing awareness of substance abuse and dependence and with educational efforts directed toward employers, however, individuals may encounter decreasing levels of prejudice.

Many individuals who are recovering from substance abuse and/or dependence return to their employment and lead full productive lives. In all instances, however, abstinence is a prerequisite for continuing productivity. Ongoing long-term treatment or involvement with self-help groups may also be necessary to prevent relapse.

## CASE STUDIES

### Case I

Ms. S. is a 35-year-old unmarried mother of an 18-month-old son. She began using cocaine when she was 20 while still in college, where she majored in business management. Her use continued after college and intensified after she obtained a position at a major real estate firm. She lost her job after 2 years because of her addiction, which by then had gone on to include heroin. She has been in and out of treatment for the past 10 years, and she has been drug-free since she became pregnant with her son; however, during her drug use she also developed hepatitis C, which is currently in remission. Ms. S. has been uneasy about returning to work but knows she needs to support her son. Her parents live nearby and have offered to care for her son while she works or goes back to school.

### Questions

1. What factors would you consider when working with Ms. S. to develop a rehabilitation plan?
2. How does the diagnosis of hepatitis C affect Ms. S.'s rehabilitation potential?
3. What social factors are important to consider when helping Ms. S. develop her plan for rehabilitation?
4. Given Ms. S.'s disability, education, social situation, and work history, what might be some appropriate occupations to consider?
5. How would you discuss Ms. S.'s disability with a prospective employer?

### Case II

Mr. W. is a 45-year-old white male who began drinking alcohol at age 16. He completed high school and obtained a job as a yard laborer at a railroad. He married at the age of 30, and he and his wife had four children who are now ages 14, 12, 8, and 5. Mr. W. was promoted to the position of brake operator at the time of his marriage and later became a rail yard engineer whose responsibility was to move cars within the yard, where they were then repaired. His alcohol use did not interfere with his work performance initially, although he drank heavily after work every day and was a binge drinker with his wife on days off. Five years ago his wife stopped drinking, and 3 years ago she filed for divorce. Mr. W.'s drinking intensified, and after several accidents that occurred at work because of his drinking he was fired. He has spent 3 months in a residential treatment facility, where he was treated for Wernicke's encephalopathy; however, Korsakoff's syndrome was not present. He is now in outpatient treatment and says his goal is to return to his former job. He also expresses a desire to reunite with his former wife, although he is concerned that she has begun drinking again.

## Questions

1. When working with Mr. W. to develop a rehabilitation plan, what significant factors would you consider about Mr. W.'s situation?
2. What ramifications does the diagnosis of Wernicke's encephalopathy have for Mr. W.'s rehabilitation?
3. How do social factors influence Mr. W.'s effective rehabilitation?
4. What types of services might be helpful for Mr. W. in his rehabilitation?
5. To what extent is Mr. W.'s desire to return to his former employment realistic?

## REFERENCES

Allen Doyle-Pita, D. (2001). Dual disorders in psychiatric rehabilitation: Teaching considerations. *Rehabilitation Education, 15*(2), 155–165.

American Academy of Pediatrics. (2000). Indications for management and referral of patients involved in substance abuse. *Pediatrics, 106*(1), 143.

American Psychiatric Association. (2000). *Diagnostic and statistical manual of mental disorders* (4th ed., text revision: DSM-IV-TR). Washington, DC: Author.

Ballard, M. B. (1998). Inhalant abuse: A call for attention. *Journal of Addictions and Offender Counseling, 19*, 28–32.

Blume, S. B., Counts, S. J., & Turnbull, J. M. (1992, July 15). Women and substance abuse. *Patient Care*, pp. 141–145, 148–151, 154–156.

Budney, A. J., Hughes, J. R., Moore, B. A., & Novy, P. L. (2001). Marijuana abstinence effects in marijuana smokers maintained in their home environment. *Archives of General Psychiatry, 58*, 917–924.

Burling, T. A., Stitzer, M. L., Bigelow, G. E., et al. (1985). Smoking topography and carbon monoxide levels in smokers. *Addictive Behavior, 10*, 319–323.

Camí, J., & Farré, M. (2003). Drug addiction. *New England Journal of Medicine, 349*(10), 975–986.

Christen, A. G., & Christen, J. A. (1994). Why is cigarette smoking so addicting? An overview of smoking as a chemical and process addiction. *Health Values, 18*(1), 17–24.

Clark, H. W. (2003). Office-based practice and opioid use disorders. *New England Journal of Medicine, 349*(10), 928–930.

Fiellin, D. A., & O'Connor, P. G. (2002). Office-based treatment of opioid-dependent patients. *New England Journal of Medicine, 347*, 817–823.

Fudala, P. J., Bridge, P., Herbert, S., Williford, W. O., Chaing, C. N., Jones, K., Collins, J., Raisch, D., Casadonte, P., Goldsmith, R. J., Ling, W., Malkerneker, U., McNicholas, L., Renner, J., Stine, S., & Tusel, D. (2003). Office-based treatment of opiate addiction with a sublingual-tablet formulation of buphernorphine and naloxone. *New England Journal of Medicine, 349*(10), 949–958.

Ginès, P., Cárdenas, A., Arroyo, V., & Rodés, J. (2004). Management of cirrhosis and ascites. *New England Journal of Medicine, 350*(16), 1646–1654.

Gonzalez, G., Oliveto, A., & Kosten, T. R. (2002). Treatment of heroin (diamorphine) addiction: Current approaches and future prospects. *Drugs, 62*, 1331–1343.

Greer, B. G., Roberts, R., & Jenkins, W. M. (1990). Substance abuse among clients with other primary disabilities: Curricular implications for rehabilitation education. *Rehabilitation Education, 4*(1), 33–44.

Hall, W., & Solowij, N. (1998). Adverse effects of cannabis. *Lancet, 352*, 1611–1616.

Harley, D. A. (1995). Alcohol and other drug use among women: Implications for rehabilitation counseling. *Journal of Applied Rehabilitation Counseling, 26*(4), 38–41.

Helmus, T. C., Downey, K. K., Arfken, C. L., Henderson, M. J., & Schuster, C. R. (2001). Novelty seeking as a predictor of treatment retention for heroin dependent cocaine users. *Drug and Alcohol Dependence, 61*, 287–295.

Holdstock, L., & deWit, H. (1998). Individual differences in the biphasic effects of ethanol. *Alcoholism, Clinical and Experimental Research, 22*, 1903–1911.

Kandall, S. R. (1996). *Substance and shadow: Women and addiction in the United States*. Cambridge, MA: Harvard University Press.

Kavanagh, D. J., McGrath, J., Saunders, J. B., Dore, G., & Clark, D. (2002). Substance misuse in patients with schizophrenia: Epidemiology and management. *Drugs, 62*, 743–755.

Kloner, R. A., & Rezkalla, S. H. (2003). Cocaine and the heart. *New England Journal of Medicine, 348*(6), 487–488.

Kosten, T. R., & O'Connor, P. G. (2003). Management of drug and alcohol withdrawal. *New England Journal of Medicine, 348*(18), 1786–1795.

Lukas, S. E. (1997). *Proceedings of the national consensus meeting on the use, abuse, and sequelae of abuse of methamphetamine with implications for prevention, treatment, and research*. Substance Abuse and Mental Health Services Administration and Center for Substance Abuse Treatment, DHHS Pub. No. (SMA) 96-8013.

Maddux, J. F., & Desmond, D. P. (2000). Addiction or dependence. *Addiction, 95*, 661–665.

Ochs, L. A., Holmes, G. E., & Karst, R. H. (1992). Caffeine consumption and disability: Clinical issues in rehabilitation. *Journal of Rehabilitation, 58*(3), 44–49.

O'Connor, P. G. (2000). Treating opioid dependence: New data and new opportunities. *New England Journal of Medicine, 343*(18), 1332–1333.

Piazza, N. J., Martin, N., & Dildine, R. J. (2000). Screening instruments for alcohol and other drug problems. *Journal of Mental Health Counseling, 22*(3), 218–228.

Robinson, T. E., & Berridge, K. C. (2001). Incentive-sensitization and addiction. *Addiction, 96,* 103–114.

Robinson, T. E., & Berridge, K. C. (2003). *Annual Review of Psychology, 54,* 25–53.

Sarnyai, Z., Shaham, Y., & Heinrichs, S. C. (2001). The role of corticotrophin-releasing factor in drug addiction. *Pharmacological Reviews, 53,* 209–243.

Scott-Lennox, J., Rose, R., Bohlig, A., & Lennox, R. (2000). The impact of women's family status on completion of substance abuse treatment. *The Journal of Behavioral Health Services and Research, 27*(4), 366–379.

Volkow, N. D. (2001). Drug abuse and mental illness: Progress in understanding comorbidity. *American Journal of Psychiatry, 158*(8), 1181–1183.

Watson, A. L., Franklin, M. E., Ingram, M. A., & Eilenberg, L. B. (1998). Alcohol and other drug abuse among persons with disabilities. *Journal of Applied Rehabilitation Counseling, 29*(2), 22–29.

Wermuth, L. (2000). Methamphetamine use: Hazards and social influences. *Journal of Drug Education, 30*(4), 423–433.

# CHAPTER 8

# Conditions of the Blood and Immune System

## NORMAL STRUCTURE AND FUNCTION

Blood is a combination of different types of cells and liquid that circulates continuously through the body. The quantity of blood in the adult body remains constant under normal conditions. Blood cells are produced in the bone marrow, as well as in lymphoid tissue and organs. All blood cells are formed from special cells called *stem cells*. The bone marrow is especially rich in stem cells.

Blood has many important functions:

- It carries oxygen and nutrients to the body tissues.
- It facilitates communication between the endocrine glands and other body organs by transporting hormones.
- It carries waste products from the tissues to the organs of excretion, such as the lungs and the kidneys.
- It protects the body from dangerous organisms (immune function).
- It promotes clotting to minimize excessive bleeding.
- It helps regulate the body temperature.

Several different types of cells make up the blood. Approximately two-fifths of the total blood volume is composed of cells that are formed by a process called *hemopoiesis* or *hematopoiesis*. The types of cells contained within the blood are *red blood cells* (**erythrocytes**), *white blood cells* (**leukocytes**), and *platelets* (**thrombocytes**). More than 99 percent of the cells in blood are red blood cells.

The number of circulating white blood cells under normal circumstances is minimal. When infection or other foreign stimuli are present, white blood cells proliferate so that there are large numbers of them circulating in the bloodstream. This condition is called **leukocytosis**.

The number of platelets circulating in the blood normally does not change. If there should be a decrease in the number of platelets, however, the condition is called **thrombocytopenia**; an increase in the number of platelets is called **thrombocytosis**. The liquid portion of the blood is a watery, colorless fluid called *plasma*. It contains no blood cells but is essential for carrying blood cells and nutrients through the circulation and for transporting wastes from the tissues. Approximately three-fifths of the total blood volume is plasma.

### Normal Structure and Function of Red Blood Cells

**Erythrocytes** (red blood cells) carry oxygen to the tissues. When mature, they are devoid of a nucleus. They are normally

231

disk shaped, with a thin center and thicker edges. Their flexible shape allows them to fit through blood vessels of differing sizes. **Hemoglobin** is the red-pigmented protein contained within the erythrocytes and is the specific part of the red blood cell that carries oxygen. Hemoglobin also contains iron.

Special cells in the bone marrow produce erythrocytes. Several vitamins, such as *vitamin B12* and *folic acid* (which is part of the vitamin B complex), are necessary for the formation of erythrocytes. They are obtained from the diet. Iron, which is also obtained from the diet, is important for the formation of hemoglobin. Excess amounts of iron and vitamin B12 are stored in the liver.

New red blood cells are constantly being formed. Although most erythrocytes are released into the blood, some are taken up by the spleen to be stored for emergency use when the red blood cell count drops significantly below normal levels, such as during *hemorrhage*. Newly formed red blood cells enter the bloodstream before they are totally mature. At this stage, they are called *reticulocytes*. Within several days, the cells mature to become *erythrocytes*. The life cycle of erythrocytes is approximately 120 days. As the erythrocytes reach the end of their life cycle, they become more fragile and rupture. Some of the old erythrocytes are destroyed in the *spleen*. Special cells within the spleen and liver absorb the old erythrocytes, making room for more new cells.

A decrease in the quantity of oxygen supplied to the tissues results in an increase in the number of red blood cells produced. For example, at higher altitudes, where less oxygen is available in the air, the bone marrow reacts by producing more red blood cells, even if there is an adequate number of red blood cells in the circulation.

## Normal Structure and Function of White Blood Cells and Immunity

The immune system is a complex organization of specialized cells and organs that distinguishes between self and nonself, defending the body against "foreign" invaders. Although the body is exposed to a number of microorganisms each day, the immune system helps it fight off bacteria, viruses, and other microbes. Although constantly bombarded by microorganisms or trauma that can result in infection, disease, or injury, the body has specific defenses to protect it against such invasions.

The immune system has traditionally been divided into *innate* and *adaptive* components, each with a different role and function (Medzhitov & Janeway, 2000). The body's first line of defense against foreign material is called *nonspecific* or *innate immunity*. This type of immunity includes the protection provided by the skin, which acts as a barrier to organisms, and by the mucous membranes, gastric secretions, and tears, which contain special chemicals that destroy potentially harmful organisms. Innate immunity requires no previous exposure to the foreign substance or recognition of any specific properties of the foreign material. When, despite external and chemical barriers, an organism or other foreign material gains entry into the body, an inflammatory response results (the *adaptive component*). The main purpose of the inflammatory response is to bring *phagocytes* (cells that destroy and ingest foreign material) to the area to destroy or inactivate the foreign substances so that the repair of tissue can begin.

Also important to the body's defense is a circulatory system called the *lymphatic system*. The lymphatic system is a circulatory system separate from the general circulation and consists of *lymph vessels*, *circulating lymph fluid* (clear fluid that bathes the body's tissues), and *lymph nodes* (small glands of the immune system that are located throughout the body and act as filters). Lymph nodes also serve as temporary storage reservoirs for **lymphocytes** (white blood cells that fight infection) and, with appropriate stimulus, as manufacturers of lymphocytes.

The lymphatic system is crucial to the body's defense against invading organisms and other foreign substances. It depends on muscle movement to circulate the fluid within it. Other organs and tissues important to the body's defense are the *spleen*, *thymus*, and *bone marrow*. Located in the upper left quadrant of the abdomen, the spleen is an organ composed of tissue that disposes of worn-out blood cells and lymphatic tissue that filters blood and helps to trap and destroy microorganisms. The thymus, which lies in the upper portion of the chest, is a lymphoid organ that produces a hormone important in controlling the development of lymphocytes. Bone marrow also produces lymphocytes and, consequently, is also classified as a lymphoid organ.

White blood cells (**leukocytes**), formed in the bone marrow, have the predominant role in the body's defense system. Leukocytes take action when body tissues have been damaged or invaded by organisms or other foreign material. Any infection or invasion by foreign substances causes a dramatic increase in the number of white blood cells in the blood. A type of leukocyte called a *phagocyte* is a scavenger that ingests bacteria and foreign particles. Phagocytes consist of *microphages*, which ingest bacteria, and *macrophages*, which ingest dead tissue. The process of ingesting cells and foreign objects is called *phagocytosis*.

In addition to phagocytosis activity, white blood cells fight infection through a process called *acquired immunity* (the ability of cells to recognize an organism to which there has been previous exposure and to neutralize or destroy the invading organism). This is part of the *adaptive component* of the immune system. Lymphocytes are white blood cells formed by the lymph nodes, spleen, thymus, and sometimes the bone marrow. They circulate throughout the bloodstream and the lymphatic system and are important to acquired immunity. The two major types of lymphocytes are B lymphocytes and T lymphocytes. B lymphocytes migrate to lymphoid tissue, such as the lymph nodes and spleen. When they are exposed to a foreign substance (**antigen**), they produce special substances called **antibodies** (immunoglobulins) that enter the bloodstream to lock with the antigen and destroy it. This type of immune response is called *humoral immunity*. Antibodies do not penetrate cells, but rather interact with circulating antigens. T lymphocytes are the regulators and controllers of the immune system. When T lymphocytes are exposed to an antigen, rather than producing antibodies, they react to the antigen directly, attacking body cells that have been invaded by the foreign substance or malignancy. This response is called *cellular immunity*.

T cells have different subsets of cells that behave differently. Regulatory T cells (*helper/inducer cells*) help to coordinate the immune response, helping activate B cells to make antibodies against antigens and activating other T cells, *natural killer cells*, and *macrophages*. These helper cells contain *markers* (T4/CD4) that recognize specific types of antigens. Other types of T cells deactivate or suppress B-lymphocyte and other cell activity when appropriate antibody levels have been reached. Normally, helper cells outnumber suppressor cells 2:1. Some T lymphocytes become memory cells so that if the specific organism invades the body again, it is "remembered" and the immune response is more intense. Another type of T cell, the *killer cell* or cytotoxic T cell, carries the T8 marker. Killer cells, in addition to working to rid the body of infected cells, are also responsible for the rejection of grafts or transplants. Lymphocytes called *natural killer cells* target tumor cells as well as other infectious organisms.

Cells carry markers (*allogens*) to ensure that the body recognizes its own tissue as self and not foreign. Sometimes the immune system becomes unable to recognize the body's own tissue and begins to produce antibodies and T cells that attack the body's own cells as if they were foreign substances; in these cases individuals are said to have an *autoimmune disease*. Examples of autoimmune diseases are *systemic lupus erythematosus* and *rheumatoid arthritis* (see Chapter 14).

A variety of conditions can alter the body's immune response and leave individuals more susceptible to disease. Because it is necessary to suppress the immune system of individuals who are about to receive an organ transplant to prevent rejection of the donor tissue, these individuals are more prone to infections. Individuals with certain types of cancers, such as lymphoma and leukemia (see Chapter 16), may become *immunodeficient* and develop serious infections. Overuse or abuse of narcotics or steroid drugs can also alter the immune response.

### Normal Structure and Function of Platelets and Coagulation

The term **hemostasis** refers to a series of events that stop bleeding from damaged vessels. *Platelets* are involved in the important first step in preventing excessive bleeding after an injury. Formed by special cells in the bone marrow, platelets are the smallest of the cells in the blood.

They are disk-shaped and contain no hemoglobin but are concerned with the clotting of blood. When injury occurs, the walls of the blood vessels contract, and platelets adhere to the site of the injury. They release a special substance that causes other platelets to collect at the site; thus, they "plug" injured blood vessels to stop the bleeding momentarily.

Platelets alone cannot stop the bleeding indefinitely. The formation of the plug activates *clotting factors* (coagulation factors from the liver, plasma, and other sources) so that a clot forms to control the bleeding. There are *intrinsic* and *extrinsic blood clotting factors*, most named by Roman numerals designated from I to XIII, in which different sets of substances play major roles. *Vitamin K* is necessary for the formation of some clotting factors. To prevent excessive clotting, other body mechanisms are also activated. For example, *basophils* (a type of white blood cell) are thought to have some role in stopping the coagulation process once the bleeding is under control.

## CONDITIONS AFFECTING THE BLOOD OR IMMUNE SYSTEM

The term **blood dyscrasias** is used to describe a large group of disorders that affect the blood. Disorders of the blood or blood-forming organs may arise from a number of different sources; may be manifest in a number of different ways; and may involve abnormalities of erythrocytes, leukocytes, platelets, or clotting mechanisms. These disorders may be characterized by the *overproduction of cells*, the *underproduction of cells*, or *defects in the clotting mechanism*.

### Anemia

Although not thought of as a disability per se, anemia is associated with a number of chronic illnesses and disabilities and also is a side effect of many conditions and their treatment. Anemia may be a complication associated with cancer or cancer treatment (Bokemeyer & Foubert, 2004), a symptom of dietary deficiency (Stabler & Allen, 2004), a symptom of gastrointestinal disorders, or a side effect of treatment of gastrointestinal disorders (Andres, Loukili, Ben, & Noel, 2004; Bodemar, Kechagias, Almer, & Danielson, 2004). Fatigue is a major symptom of anemia and can be debilitating, reducing individuals' ability to work, decreasing their physical and emotional well-being, and interfering with their cognitive ability, all of which can lead to anxiety and depression (Bokemeyer & Foubert, 2004).

Conditions that fall under the general term *anemia* are characterized by a *reduction* in the amount of *hemoglobin* or the *number of red blood cells*. Anemias are sometimes classified by the size and color of the red blood cell. For example, healthy, normal-sized cells are called *normocytic*; normal cells that are of normal color are called *normochromic*. Anemias in which the color of the red blood cells is paler than usual are called *hypochromic anemias*. Anemias in which the red blood cells are larger than usual are called *macrocytic anemias*, and those with cells smaller than usual are called *microcytic anemias*.

Anemias may also be classified according to their causative mechanisms. For example, anemias may result from an excessive blood loss, from decreased or abnormal red blood cell formation, or from the destruction of red blood cells. Destruction of red blood cells is called **hemolysis**. Anemias caused by excessive and/or premature destruction of red blood cells are called *hemolytic anemias*. A variety of abnormal conditions can cause red blood cell destruction. Hemolytic anemia

may occur in association with some infectious diseases or with certain inherited red blood cell disorders, or it may develop as a response to drugs or other foreign or toxic agents. Anemia results when the rate of destruction is greater than the ability of the body to produce red cells. The degree of anemia reflects the ability of the bone marrow to increase the production of red blood cells. The spleen usually becomes enlarged (**splenomegaly**) in chronic hemolytic conditions because of the need to remove an excessive number of damaged red cells.

*Aplastic anemia* (sometimes called *pancytopenia*) is caused by inadequate functioning of the bone marrow in manufacturing red blood cells. Aplastic anemia can occur spontaneously, or it can result from damage to the bone marrow through drugs, chemicals, or ionizing radiation.

*Iron deficiency anemia*, one of the most common types of anemia (Shah, 2004), is often caused by a deficiency of iron in the diet. It can also result from the body's failure to absorb iron, excessive or chronic blood loss, or increases in the body's iron requirements.

*Pernicious anemia* is a chronic condition caused by the inadequate secretion by the stomach of a substance (*intrinsic factor*) that is necessary for the intestine to absorb vitamin B12. It may also be caused by dietary deficiency of vitamin B12, especially in vegetarians (Stabler & Allen, 2004). The deficiency of vitamin B12 impairs production and maturation of blood cells. Consequently, the body is unable to produce adequate numbers of red blood cells, resulting in anemia.

Regardless of the cause, anemia disrupts the transport of oxygen to tissues throughout the body. Severe anemia increases the workload of the heart. Common symptoms of anemia are pale skin (**pallor**), weakness, fatigue, difficulty in breathing (**dyspnea**), and fast heart rate (**tachycardia**). Other possible symptoms of anemia include the inability to concentrate, irritability, and susceptibility to infection.

Treatment must be specific to the cause. If anemia is the result of blood loss, blood replacement through transfusion may be necessary. In other instances, dietary, vitamin, or iron supplements may be necessary.

## Thalassemia

The thalassemias are inherited *hemolytic anemias* common in individuals from the Mediterranean region, Africa, the Middle East, India, and Southeast Asia (Olivieri, 1999). Thalassemias are characterized by the production of thin, fragile red blood cells and defective hemoglobin synthesis. As a result, the hemoglobin content of the red blood cells is inadequate. In addition, there is often some interference with erythrocyte metabolism that causes the red blood cells to be deformed and decreases their survival time. Thus, the anemia associated with thalassemia can result both from the increased destruction of red blood cells and from the impaired production of hemoglobin.

Symptoms of thalassemia are similar to those of other types of anemias. Individuals whose symptoms are severe and consequently diagnosed early in life may require regular transfusions to survive (Olivieri, 1999). Even individuals with a mild form of the condition may experience complications, such as **osteopenia** (decreased bone density) in later age. In addition to transfusion therapy, iron chelation therapy is often necessary to prevent iron overload (Rodgers, 2000), and in some instances bone marrow transplantation may be indicated (Giardini, 1997).

## Polycythemia

In polycythemia, there is an increase in the number of red blood cells and in the concentration of hemoglobin within the blood. There are several types of polycythemia. One type, *polycythemia vera*, is associated with an overproduction of both red and white blood cells. The cause of polycythemia vera is unknown. Because of the increased number of cells in the blood, individuals with this condition may experience hypertension, congestive heart failure, stroke, or heart attack (see Chapter 11), or they may experience a hemorrhage because the congestion in the blood vessels may cause the vessels to rupture.

*Secondary polycythemia* occurs in conjunction with another disease. When the body's demand for oxygen increases, the bone marrow produces additional red blood cells to meet the increased demand. Chronic obstructive pulmonary disease is a condition in which secondary polycythemia may occur (see Chapter 12). Treatment focuses on the underlying condition.

Individuals with conditions in which there has been a loss of plasma without a loss of red blood cells, such as burns, may develop a state similar to polycythemia. Although there is no actual increase in the number of red blood cells, loss of fluid increases the proportion of red blood cells in the blood. In these cases, treatment involves fluid replacement to decrease the viscosity of the blood.

## Agranulocytosis (Neutropenia)

**Agranulocytosis** is the marked reduction in the level of a specific type of leukocyte. This reduction in leukocytes is called **leukopenia**. A common cause of agranulocytosis is *toxic reaction* to certain medications used in the treatment of chronic disorders, such as medications used to treat *epilepsy* or medications used to treat certain *mental disorders*. Agranulocytosis may also result from *exposure to certain chemicals* or to *ionizing radiation*.

Because white blood cells are important in fighting infection, a reduction in the number of these cells increases individuals' susceptibility to infection. Agranulocytosis is a potentially serious condition and, without prompt treatment, can result in death. Treatment is directed toward removing the toxic agent responsible and providing medications (e.g., antibiotics) to treat resulting infections.

## Purpura

**Purpura** is a condition characterized by hemorrhage of small blood vessels into the skin. Small amounts of blood leak into various tissues of the body. It can be caused by an allergic response or a deficiency in platelets, or it can be associated with other disorders in the body.

## Leukemia

The leukemias are caused by the cancerous production of lymph cells or white blood cells. They are discussed in greater detail in Chapter 16.

## Hemophilia

Hemophilia is an inherited, potentially disabling condition associated with high financial costs (Beeton, 2002). Several inherited blood disorders make up the condition known as *hemophilia*, a chronic bleeding disorder in which there is a deficiency in or absence of one of the clotting factors (Bolton-Maggs & Pasi, 2003). Individuals with hemophilia have a bleeding tendency. Although they do not initially bleed faster, the normal clotting mechanism is disturbed so that bleeding is prolonged or the oozing of blood may persist after injury. Because the platelet count is normal in hemophilia, bleeding from a small cut or scratch does not pose a severe problem. However, the deficiency in clotting factors does pose the danger of bleeding into the internal organs, joints, or the brain.

Hemophilia is transmitted from mother to son. Women do not develop the disease, but they can inherit the trait and pass it to their sons. If a woman is a carrier, each of her sons has a 50 percent chance of developing hemophilia; each of her daughters has a 50 percent chance of becoming a carrier. None of the sons of a man with hemophilia will have hemophilia; however, all of his daughters will be carriers.

There are several different types of hemophilia, which are differentiated by the specific clotting factor that is deficient. The most common type is *hemophilia A*, also known as *classical hemophilia*. In this type of hemophilia, a protein in *clotting Factor VIII* is deficient. The next most common type is *hemophilia B*, also called *Christmas disease*, in which *clotting Factor IX* is defective. The rarest type of hemophilia is *von Willebrand's disease*, in which *Factor VIII* manifests platelet dysfunction (Bolton-Maggs & Pasi, 2003).

The severity of hemophilia varies along a continuum from a tendency toward slow, prolonged, persistent bleeding to a tendency toward severe hemorrhage, and it is categorized as *mild, moderate,* or *severe* depending on the level of clotting factor present. Individuals with *mild hemophilia* will probably experience abnormal bleeding only after major injuries or minor surgery, such as a tooth extraction. Individuals with *moderate hemophilia* may have prolonged bleeding after major trauma or surgery. Individuals with severe disease may bleed spontaneously and have hemorrhages into deep muscles and joints.

Bleeding into the joint (**hemarthrosis**) is extremely painful and can cause significant joint destruction (Elander & Barry, 2003; Shapiro & Hoots, 2000). Knees and ankles are affected most frequently, although elbows may become involved later. Joint deformity and crippling may result from damage to the joint structure and from **atrophy** (wasting) of surrounding muscles. Bleeding into the muscle, if severe, may exert pressure on nerves and cause a temporary sensory loss. If the hemorrhage damages muscle tissue, fibrous tissue may form, causing varying degrees of functional loss.

### Treatment for Hemophilia

Hemophilia is not curable and requires treatment for bleeding problems throughout the individual's life. With proper care and treatment, however, individuals with hemophilia can manage their chronic disease, and their life expectancy approaches normal (Teitel et al., 2004).

To prevent damage from abnormal bleeding, significant blood loss, and chronic joint disease, all bleeding must be detected early and treated promptly. There are over 100 comprehensive hemophilia treatment centers throughout the country that help individuals with hemophilia manage their condition physically and psychologically. These care centers emphasize early intervention for bleeding episodes and train individuals to administer replacement therapy at home, thus markedly improving both school attendance and the amount of absences from work (Teitel et al., 2004).

Because there is no cure for hemophilia, treatment is directed toward preventing any injury that could precipitate bleeding and toward controlling bleeding episodes when they do occur. The mainstay of treatment for hemophilia is replacement therapy with plasma or plasma concentrates that contain the clotting factors in which the individual's blood is deficient. Because of the higher concentrations of clotting factors, plasma concentrates are given more frequently than is fresh plasma. Clotting factors are usually replaced through intravenous infusion (infusing substance directly into a vein). The amount, type, and duration of the infusion depend on the individual's clotting deficiency and the size and severity of the bleeding problem. Treatment may be instituted prior to surgery to prevent excessive bleeding.

Early treatment of bleeding helps to prevent complications. Consequently, learning to administer clotting factor concentrates at home is beneficial. To do so, however, individuals must be able to calculate the appropriate dose and mix and administer the concentrate intravenously. Home therapy is appropriate for mild bleeding but is not sufficient when major bleeding occurs. Major bleeding requires medical evaluation.

There are possible complications associated with replacement therapy. As with all therapies that involve intravenous infusion, there is the chance of the transmission of infection such as hepatitis and human immunodeficiency virus (HIV) (Parish, 2002). Needles and equipment should always be sterile and never shared. Although most blood products are now carefully screened for disease, individuals who received replacement therapy before 1985 may already have been exposed to HIV, which can be a persistent source of anxiety and concern. Individuals who receive blood products intravenously can also develop an allergic reaction to the infusion. Such reactions should be reported to a physician promptly.

Individuals with bleeding into a joint may require joint immobilization for several days in addition to replacement therapy. Joint pain may be treated with anti-inflammatory medications and analgesics. Medications that contain aspirin should be avoided, however, because aspirin interferes with platelet function and can cause increased susceptibility to bleeding. Physical therapy or prescribed exercise carried out at home may be necessary to maintain the range of motion of the affected joints. If the joints undergo severe degeneration, reconstructive orthopedic surgery, such as joint replacement, may also be necessary (see Chapter 14). Individuals with hemophilia should always wear a Medic Alert identification bracelet or necklace to alert others to their condition in case of an emergency.

### Psychosocial Issues in Hemophilia

How individuals respond to having hemophilia as adults is dependent to a great extent on their experiences with the disease during childhood. Because hemophilia is present from birth, the attitudes displayed by parents and significant others during individuals' development have a significant impact on their self-view and view of their condition. If parents are overprotective, individuals' social and psychological development may be stunted and dependency may result. Likewise, individuals may not have had the opportunity to participate in sports or other activities in which physical and motor skills are learned and mastered. If many hospitalizations are required because of the condition and individuals have had multiple school absences, their educational achievement may also be lower than that of others of the same age.

In some instances, the inability to predict when bleeding may occur or fear of being unable to control bleeding may result in passivity and inactivity. At other times, if individuals have had difficulty adjusting to the condition, are uncertain about the future, or deny the seriousness of hemophilia or the precautions that need to be taken to control it, they may indulge in excessive risk taking.

Although replacement therapy and home treatment have done much to improve the lives of individuals with hemophilia and to decrease the disability resulting from the condition, treatments are very expensive. This expense may be an additional source of stress.

Individuals with hemophilia may experience both acute and chronic pain if there has been bleeding into the joints. Consequently, pain medications are frequently used. If medications are not carefully used and monitored, drug dependence may result, sometimes necessitating drug rehabilitation. Individuals who have not adjusted well to their condition and may self-medicate to alleviate emotional discomfort may be at particular risk.

Sexual issues may also be of concern for individuals with hemophilia. The most serious complication of replacement therapy is the possibility of being exposed to HIV through contaminated concentrates. Although precautions have now been taken in the preparation of concentrates to make infection with HIV rare, individuals who were infused prior to 1985 had much greater chances of being exposed to HIV. For those individuals who have HIV as a result of replacement therapy, not only the stress and anxiety produced by having the disease, but also the anger, resentment, and depression because of being exposed to HIV may complicate individuals' ability to cope with the disease, as well as their ability to establish or maintain sexual relationships. Some individuals may feel stigmatized by their condition, especially the public's awareness of the link to HIV, and attempt to hide their condition. Even in the absence of HIV concerns, complications of hemophilia may affect sexual activity. Joint disability, medication side effects, and other complications can interfere with sexual function (Parish, 2002).

Hemophilia is a hereditary condition. The potential impact on long-term relationships and the decision of whether to have children may be troublesome for individuals with hemophilia. In some instances, they may avoid developing close, meaningful relationships because of their discomfort with having a hereditary condition.

### Vocational Issues in Hemophilia

Improved medical technology and the availability of self-infused coagulation factors have greatly increased the ability of individuals with hemophilia to decrease their disability and maintain employment in a variety of settings (Teitel et al., 2004). Individuals with severe hemophilia may also be able to perform a variety of job tasks without limitations; however, in severe disease, there is the increased unpredictability of when the bleeding will occur.

When bleeding does occur, individuals should be able to self-infuse the concentrates in 15 to 30 minutes; however, they will need to take a break from work to perform the replacement therapy. A semiprivate place to perform the infusion, as well as a place to store the equipment and concentrate, will also be needed.

Usually, individuals with hemophilia have few functional limitations in the vocational setting, unless they experience joint complications. Especially those with moderate to severe disease should avoid employment in which there is a direct threat of physical injury. Injuries that may

be minimal by most standards can have serious implications for individuals with more severe forms of hemophilia. Joint damage and/or subsequent joint replacement due to complications of hemophilia may impose the same limitations as do joint disorders from other causes. In some instances, surgical correction of damaged joints may be indicated (see Chapter 14). For the most part, however, the vocational functioning of individuals with hemophilia is determined primarily by their abilities and interests.

One barrier to employment may be lack of understanding on the part of the employer about the few limitations that are actually associated with hemophilia. Because the public has now connected hemophilia and the potential for HIV contamination, there may be fear and anxiety from coworkers when working with individuals with hemophilia, especially if bleeding occurs. Likewise, coworkers who observe individuals administering self-infusing concentrates and who do not understand replacement therapy may draw false conclusions about the activity, causing further discrimination. Educating employers and coworkers about hemophilia and its treatment may be one of the most crucial links to vocational success for the individual with hemophilia.

### Sickle Cell Disease

**Sickle cell disease** is a heredity condition that occurs primary in individuals of black African descent, but it can also occur in those with Mediterranean ancestry. Sickle cell disease occurs because of a genetic mutation of hemoglobin. Normal hemoglobin is called *hemoglobin A*. Individuals with sickle cell disease have an abnormal hemoglobin called *hemoglobin S*, and the disease gets its name from the shape that the red blood cell assumes when hemoglobin S is present. Hemoglobin S is protective against malaria and so is more prevalent in areas of the world where there is malaria (Lewing & Woods, 2000).

When hemoglobin S is present, individuals are said to have *sickle cell trait*. Individuals may only be *carriers* of the abnormal gene that causes the hemoglobin abnormality. Although carriers have no symptoms, they may pass the abnormal gene to their offspring. The offspring of an individual with sickle cell trait and an individual with normal genes have a 50 percent chance of being carriers of the abnormal gene. When *both* parents have the sickle cell trait, the chances with each pregnancy are 1 in 4 that the baby will have normal hemoglobin, 2 in 4 that the baby will have sickle cell trait, and 1 in 4 that the baby will have sickle cell anemia (Wang, Grover, & Gallagher, 1993). Children of one parent with sickle cell anemia and one with normal hemoglobin will all have sickle cell trait. If one parent has sickle cell trait and one has sickle cell anemia, there is a 50 percent chance with each pregnancy that the child will have sickle cell trait and a 50 percent chance that the child will have sickle cell anemia. When both parents have sickle cell anemia, so will all of their children (Lukens, 1993).

### Sickle Cell Anemia

*Sickle cell anemia* is the most severe form of sickle cell disease. It is characterized by lifelong hemolytic anemia and a wide variety of painful and debilitating vaso-occlusive events (Mentzer & Kan, 2001). When hemoglobin S molecules interact with each other, they become stacked up, especially when the oxygen concentration in the blood is low. The red blood cells become deformed so that, instead of being disk-shaped, they assume the abnormal shape of a crescent or sickle. Because of this distortion, the red blood cell becomes rigid and is unable to adapt its shape to fit through tiny blood vessels. The abnormal sickled cell becomes very fragile and is easily destroyed, which severely curtails its normal life span. As a result, the bone marrow drastically increases its production of red blood cells to keep up with the rate of destruction. Because the rate of production cannot keep up with the rate of destruction, however, individuals with sickle cell disease can become severely anemic, thus developing *sickle cell anemia*.

### Manifestations of Sickle Cell Disease

Individuals with sickle cell disease have an unpredictable course that can range from mild to severe (Cooper-Effa, Blount, Kaslow, Rothenberg, & Eckman, 2001). There may be varying physical limitations from sickle cell disease at each developmental stage (Westerdale & Jegede, 2004). The growth and development of individuals with sickle cell anemia are significantly impaired, although the exact way the disease contributes to delayed growth is still unclear. Although there is delay in physical and sexual maturation, individuals do reach full maturity (Scott & Scott, 1999).

*Sickle cell crisis* is a manifestation of sickle cell disease that occurs when blood flow to a body part becomes obstructed by rigid, sickled red cells. This is called a *vaso-occlusive crisis*. The affected body part does not receive adequate oxygen, resulting in severe pain. If blood flow is severely diminished, the affected tissue may undergo **necrosis** (tissue death). Any part of the body, including organs, may be affected; the resulting damage may be mild to severe, depending on the degree and length of blockage. The most common body parts affected are the chest, legs, arms, back, and abdomen. Sickle cell crisis can result in stroke (Gebreyohanns & Adams, 2004);

cardiovascular dysfunction, including myocardial infarction (heart attack) (Assanasen, Quinton, & Buchanan, 2003); chronic lung disease; or kidney failure (Lewing & Woods, 2000).

Individuals with sickle cell disease have multiple bouts of sickle cell crisis during their lives, which lead to chronic organ damage. If the spleen is repeatedly involved in crisis, it may become significantly enlarged and removal of the spleen (**splenectomy**) may be indicated. A condition called *aplastic crisis*, or *megaloblastic* crisis, may also be a manifestation of sickle cell disease. In this condition, there is a rapid onset of anemia so that blood transfusions are also indicated.

Because of the lowered resistance due to anemia, as well as the altered spleen function, serious infections may also become problems. Associated chronic anemia causes the heart to pump faster in an attempt to supply additional oxygen to the tissues. Increased heart action can contribute to enlargement of the heart (**cardiomegaly**) and decreased cardiac efficiency. Decreased oxygen supply caused by the chronic anemia can also produce symptoms of fatigue and difficulty in breathing on exertion (**exertional dyspnea**).

Occlusion of blood flow during a sickle cell crisis can damage bones and joints, leading to pain, swelling, and limited mobility of the joints, as well as resulting deformity. Occlusion of vessels in the brain can cause a stroke (see Chapter 2). Increased blood **viscosity** (thickness) may also cause sickle cell **retinopathy** in which there is damage to the vessels in the retina of the eye, which results in diminished vision and, possibly, retinal detachment (see Chapter 4).

Some individuals develop leg ulcers because of the interruption of circulation during sickle cell crisis. Ulcers may not heal and may become infected, necessi-

tating bedrest and, in some instances, skin grafts.

The specific causes of sickle cell crisis are unknown; however, certain factors, such as heavy exertional stress (Assanasen et al., 2003), mental stress, infection, dehydration, or extremes in temperature, may precipitate a crisis (Lewing & Woods, 2000).

The prognosis of individuals with sickle cell anemia is dependent on the individual and the degree of organ damage. In the past, many individuals with sickle cell anemia did not live to adulthood, but many now reach midlife and beyond, living productive lives (Cooper-Effa et al., 2001; McKerrell, Cohen, & Billett, 2004). The prediction of outcome is individually determined.

### Diagnosis of Sickle Cell Disease

Definitive diagnosis of sickle cell disease or sickle cell trait is based on a blood test called *hemoglobin electrophoresis*. Blood tests such as *sickle cell prep* are screening tests that can detect the presence of abnormal hemoglobin but cannot distinguish between sickle cell disease and sickle cell trait.

### Treatment for Sickle Cell Disease

For the most part, sickle cell disease is a chronic, lifelong disease without cure. Treatment is directed toward controlling its symptoms. Good nutrition is essential to combat anemia and to maintain the body's resistance to infection. Because of the propensity of those who have sickle cell anemia to develop infections, prophylactic antibiotics may be given on occasion.

Maintaining adequate fluid intake is also important for individuals with sickle cell disease, because adequate hydration can minimize the sickling of red blood cells and decrease the blood viscosity. The anemia associated with this condition sometimes necessitates transfusion therapy. A medication used to treat cancer, hydroxyurea, has recently been tested for use in the treatment of sickle cell anemia and has been found to prevent sickling of red blood cells in some individuals (Lewing & Woods, 2000). Other therapies, including the use of antisickling agents and bone marrow transplantation, may also be used in some instances.

Individuals with sickle cell disease who experience sickle cell crisis often require hospitalization. During the crisis, treatment focuses on restoring fluids if dehydration has occurred, and relieving the pain associated with the crisis, which usually requires the administration of narcotics. If another condition, such as an infection, has precipitated the crisis, treatment of that condition may also be instituted. Organ damage as a result of sickle cell disease is treated in a similar fashion to chronic organ disease from other causes.

Comprehensive medical care, preventative care, and health maintenance have been shown to increase the life expectancy of individuals with sickle cell disease. Care should be taken to avoid any factors that precipitate a sickle cell crisis.

## Psychosocial Issues in Sickle Cell Disease

Like hemophilia, sickle cell disease usually manifests itself in childhood, necessitating medical attention and, possibly, frequent hospitalizations, which can disrupt social development and educational progress. Psychological coping patterns are relevant both to the experience of pain and to broader adjustment issues (Anie, Steptoe, & Bevan, 2002). Coping with sickle cell disease may be especially difficult during adolescence as individuals struggle

to maintain a "normal" life and minimize their difference from peers (Atkin & Ahmad, 2001). Adherence to prophylactic measures may be especially difficult and require significant support (While & Mullen, 2004).

Because it is a hereditary disease, parents of children with sickle cell disease may experience guilt or fear of the loss of their child. As a result, they may become overly protective, promoting abnormal dependence in the child. At the same time, the child may learn manipulative behaviors to gain attention. These maladaptive means of coping may persist throughout life, creating a greater barrier than the condition itself.

Sickle cell disease carries the additional stress of unpredictability. Although some of the factors that provoke a sickle cell crisis may be identifiable, crises are often unpredictable and beyond individuals' control. Not only are the crises painful and debilitating, but there is also the potential for organ damage each time a crisis occurs. The lack of control over the frequency or severity of sickle cell crises can lead to feelings of hopelessness and depression.

Individuals with sickle cell disease can usually maintain regular schedules; however, the onset of sickle cell crises is unpredictable and may necessitate hospitalization. In most instances, individuals with sickle cell disease do not need to alter activities, unless activities appear to provoke a sickle cell crisis. Most activities, if performed in moderation, can be tolerated. The unpredictability of sickle cell crises can alter social functioning for individuals with sickle cell disease, who may have to cancel or alter plans at the last minute if a crisis should occur. The role of stress as a precipitating factor in sickle cell crisis must also be considered. Although stress is frequently associated with negative events, stress can also be associated with positive events, such as a graduation celebration or a wedding.

### Vocational Issues in Sickle Cell Disease

Individuals with sickle cell disease must consider not only the physical demands of the job as related to stamina, but also the role that strenuous exertion has in precipitating sickle cell crises. Because sickle cell disease is a lifelong condition, most individuals learn, over the years, which type of activity and how much activity they can usually tolerate. Despite the potential relationship of overexertion and sickle cell crisis, most individuals with sickle cell disease are capable of performing moderate and, in some instances, even heavy work.

Individuals who have experienced specific organ or joint damage as a result of repeated sickle cell crises have many of the same limitations as those who have similar conditions for other reasons. In addition, individuals with sickle cell disease should avoid extremes in temperature. Very hot weather places extra strain on the heart and predisposes to dehydration, which can precipitate a crisis. Very cold, damp environments can also precipitate a crisis. Consequently, it may be beneficial for individuals with sickle cell anemia to work in indoor or controlled environments.

Stress in the work environment and its contribution to the development of sickle cell crisis is another factor individuals with sickle cell anemia must consider. Not all individuals react to stress in the same way, nor are perceptions of stress always the same. Consequently, the importance of stress must be determined on an individual basis. The degree to which absences due to sickle cell crises become a hindrance to work performance is dependent on the individual, the frequency, and the seriousness of the crises when they occur.

### Human Immunodeficiency Virus (HIV) Infection

Not all viruses are harmful to humans, but some viruses can cause disease. Diseases that result from viruses range from the common cold and common childhood illness to more serious diseases, such as poliomyelitis and acquired immune deficiency syndrome (AIDS).

A virus can be defined as an infectious organism that cannot grow or reproduce outside living cells. In order to survive, a virus must enter a living cell and use the reproductive capacity of that cell for its own replication. Consequently, when a virus enters a cell, it instructs the cell to reproduce the virus. Normally, the body recognizes viruses as foreign and activates the immune system to attack and destroy the offending agent. Of those viruses that are not destroyed, some remain inactive (*dormant*) for long periods without causing problems; however, they remain integrated within the genetic material of the cell, and they are capable of replicating when triggered to do so. The direct damage the virus does to the cell itself may vary from slight damage to total destruction. Some cells are able to reproduce after being damaged, but others, especially those of the nervous system, are not able to reproduce and, consequently, are not replaced after invasion by a virus.

HIV infection is caused by a virus called the *human immunodeficiency virus*. It is called a *retrovirus* because it uses a complicated process called *reverse transcription*. This process uses a viral enzyme called *reverse transcriptase* to integrate its genetic material into the genetic material of other cells. In so doing, the HIV essentially takes over other cells and makes them produce other infected cells, each of which is slightly different.

There are two viruses that cause HIV infection: HIV-1 and HIV-2. HIV-1 is the most common and is responsible for most of the cases of HIV infection (Kilby & Eron, 2003). HIV-2 is confined largely to western Africa (Kalichman, 1998). HIV destroys a subset of helper T cells and impairs the ability of cells to recognize antigens. As a result, there is profound deterioration of the immune system so that the body has no defense against even the least aggressive organism. The virus reproduces within the T cell itself, producing additional HIV, which in turn, invades other T cells. The normal 2:1 ratio of helper cells to suppressor cells becomes reversed. The increased number of suppressor cells severely limits normal B-cell function, and they fail to respond to new antigens. The normal immune response becomes dysfunctional.

Most individuals with HIV infection exhibit no symptoms until the later stages of the disease. AIDS is the final stage of HIV infection and is characterized by symptoms of severe failure of the immune system.

### Transmission of HIV

HIV is found in the blood, as well as in body secretions such as sperm. Transmission can occur in a variety of ways. The virus can be transmitted through:

- infusion of infected blood or blood products
- an accidental stick with an infected needle
- intravenous drug use and sharing of equipment
- anal, oral, or genital intercourse
- contact with a cut or open wound on the skin

- fetal transmission from a woman with HIV infection to her unborn child

There is no evidence that transmission can occur in any way other than through direct blood-to-blood or sexual contact with an infected individual. The virus does not appear to be transmitted through coughing, sneezing, or casual contact. Moreover, because all viruses require living tissue to survive and multiply, the virus dies quickly once outside the body.

### Diagnosis of HIV/AIDS

The most common procedures for diagnosing HIV infection are blood tests that identify not the virus itself but the presence of antibodies that the body has produced against the virus. The enzyme-linked immunosorbent assay (*ELISA*), which is a blood test, is usually performed first because of its level of sensitivity to HIV antibodies. If the ELISA test is positive, it is repeated, since false-positive results are more common than false-negative results. If the ELISA is positive the second time, the test is confirmed by using a second procedure, the *Western blot*. A repeated positive ELISA and positive Western blot confirm the diagnosis of HIV infection. AIDS is usually diagnosed when HIV is present and the individual has developed an opportunistic infection and/or has a T-helper cell count that has fallen below a certain level (see below).

### Stages of HIV/AIDS

Infection with HIV can be separated roughly into several stages, although there are no firm guidelines that distinguish the different phases. During the early or acute phase, symptoms may be subtle or nonexistent. Initially, some individuals may experience mild flulike symptoms that subside, leaving them symptom-free, although the virus is still transmissible to others.

In the second stage, as the HIV infection progresses, the levels of circulating virus increase. At the same time, there is a decline in the number of helper T cells of the immune system. Infected individuals may experience some or all of the following symptoms.

- Weight loss of 10 or more pounds in less than 2 months for no apparent reason
- Loss of appetite
- Unexplained persistent fever
- Drenching night sweats
- Severe fatigue that is unrelated to exercise, stress, or drug use
- Persistent diarrhea
- Swollen lymph nodes (**lymphadenopathy**)

Stages of HIV infection can be characterized with greater precision by using T-helper lymphocyte cell counts. HIV infections can generally be classified according to three stages:

- Early-stage disease (generally asymptomatic) = T-helper cell counts above 500
- Middle-stage disease (swollen lymph nodes, fatigue, intermittent fever) = T-helper cell counts between 500 and 200
- Later-stage disease (presence of opportunistic infections such as pneumocystis carinii or tuberculosis) = T-helper cell counts less than 200 (Bartlett, 2000; Clement & Hollander, 1992)

### Symptoms of Advanced HIV Disease and AIDS

Many individuals with HIV infection remain **asymptomatic** (without symptoms) until they develop **opportunistic infections** (infections that would not occur in individuals with normal immune system function) and malignancies, or when the T-helper cell count falls below 200/mm. Many organisms commonly found in the environment pose no threat under normal circumstances because the functioning immune system resists them. When individuals have HIV infection, the immune system is no longer able to act as a defense, and individuals are susceptible to disease and infections that under normal circumstances would not become full-blown. These diseases and infections are called "opportunistic." Death in AIDS is not caused by the dysfunction of the immune system per se, but by complications of conditions that develop because of inadequate immune system function.

One common opportunistic infection associated with HIV infection is *Pneumocystis carinii pneumonia*, a parasitic infection of the lung. This condition is highly uncommon in healthy individuals, although it may be found in other immunocompromised individuals, such as in those who have cancer or those who have received immunosuppressants in association with organ transplantation. *Pneumocystis carinii* pneumonia is one of the most common manifestations of HIV infections. Symptoms usually begin with a dry cough and difficulty in breathing. Although some drugs are available to treat the disease, they can have toxic side effects that can further jeopardize the individual's condition.

Another type of opportunistic infection is *candidiasis* (yeast infection). The fungus *Candida* frequently invades the oral cavity of the HIV-infected individual, causing a superficial infection in the mouth and throat that is manifested by pain and white plaques. This condition, also known as *oral thrush*, may be the first clue that the individual is infected with HIV. Although it is uncomfortable and difficult to cure, infection with *Candida* is not likely to be fatal. Individuals with debilitating conditions other than HIV infections may also develop candidiasis.

In addition to opportunistic infections, an otherwise rare form of cancer called *Kaposi's sarcoma* is frequently associated with HIV infection; this is considered an opportunistic cancer. Kaposi's sarcoma causes pink, brown, or purplish blotches on the skin.

Many individuals with HIV infection develop neurological symptoms at some time during the course of the disease. These may be mild, such as a headache, or more severe, such as **aphasia** (inability to communicate through speech, writing, or signs due to brain dysfunction), seizures, gait disturbances, visual disturbances, and incontinence. Pain is a prevalent feature among individuals with HIV/AIDS (Marcus, Kerns, Rosenfeld, & Breitbart, 2000). This chronic pain often does not receive optimal treatment.

Individuals with HIV infection may also experience a type of dementia called *AIDS dementia complex*, which may include cognitive symptoms such as poor concentration or forgetfulness, motor symptoms such as loss of balance or clumsiness, and behavioral symptoms such as apathy and social withdrawal. The precise mechanism by which HIV causes dementia is unknown.

### Treatment for HIV/AIDS

Currently, there is no means of restoring the damaged immune function characteristic of HIV infections. However, advances in the medical management of HIV infection have improved the life expectancy of individuals living with HIV infection. *Antiretroviral drugs* directly inhibit HIV by disrupting its replication cycle or by interrupting the ability of HIV to bind with other cells. New antiviral treatments referred to as *highly aggressive antiretroviral therapy*, which includes a class of drugs called *protease inhibitors*, can be taken in combination with other antiviral drugs such as AZT. This *combination therapy* has offered dramatic improvements in the medical treatment of individuals with HIV/AIDS (Britton, 2000; Shernoff & Smith, 2001; Tashima & Carpenter, 2003).

Resistance to antiretroviral drugs, however, is a growing problem for individuals with HIV (Gerberding, 2003). Because of the toxicity of some of the medications, individuals may experience toxic side effects such as headache, nausea and vomiting, insomnia, diarrhea, and muscle pain. In addition, some individuals experience bone marrow suppression, which necessitates immediate discontinuation of the medication. Additional side effects of peripheral neuropathy, ulcerations of the mouth, and skin rashes may also be experienced.

The regimen of medications used in the treatment of HIV infection can be cumbersome as well as expensive, making the treatment not accessible to many individuals with HIV infection who are without insurance or who are underinsured. Newer antiviral drugs can cost up to $20,000 per year, which is more than twice that of the next most expensive antiretroviral drug (Steinbrook, 2003). In addition, the potentially serious side effects associated with the newer antiretroviral drugs can be of concern (Tashima & Carpenter, 2003).

In addition to medication, much of the treatment for individuals with HIV infection is geared toward supportive care and prevention of opportunistic infections. Individuals should have adequate rest, should engage in a program of moderate exercise, and should maintain adequate nutrition. As the condition progresses, individuals may need to modify their exercise program and allow for more frequent rest periods to conserve energy. As much as possible, individuals with HIV infection should attempt to prevent opportunistic infection. In addition to maintaining good health practices, they should avoid crowds and people with known infections such as colds and flu. If they develop symptoms of infection, they should consult a physician immediately.

In the later stages of HIV infection, when opportunistic and/or neurological symptoms occur, treatment is directed toward the specific infection or symptom manifestation. It is not unusual for individuals with later stages of HIV infection to experience a number of hospitalizations for acute opportunistic infections.

Individuals with HIV infection should take precautions not to transmit the virus. They should fully understand the importance of practicing safe sex; of informing sexual partners of their condition prior to sexual activity; and of not sharing needles, razors, toothbrushes, or any other item that could be contaminated with blood.

### Psychosocial Issues in HIV/AIDS

Distress and preoccupation with illness and imminent death may characterize individuals with any fatal disorder. Coping with a diagnosis of HIV and the changes the disease precipitates can be both physically and mentally exhausting (Bower & Collins, 2000). Individuals with HIV infection face an even more grim realization that, to date, no one with later stages of HIV infection has survived.

Individuals infected with HIV are confronted with ongoing stressful situations involving noxious symptoms, treatment with unpleasant side effects, periods of physical disability, potential loss of employment, possible rejection by family or friends, economic stress, and potential premature death (Fleishman, Donald-Sherbourne, Crystal, Collins, et al., 2000). Consequently, those who have tested HIV positive are likely to experience considerable anxiety.

In addition to the grave prognosis, there is much ambiguity associated with positive test results. It is impossible to predict when or how rapidly the infection will progress to the later stages. Individuals live with total unpredictability. Following periods of being very unwell, they may then recover and experience periods of well-being only to then develop another infection and return to an illness state (Cochrane, 2003). Living with the potential for progressing to the later stage and the uncertainty about the disease's progression often leads to additional stress and anxiety. Individuals may retreat from most of their former activities and may find it difficult to set goals for the future. They may put aside their personal aspirations and focus on the struggle to survive.

Individuals with HIV infection often bear the additional stress of the stigma and fear associated with the disease, both of which can lead to rejection and abandonment by others. Feelings of depression, despair, and hopelessness are common. Individuals may also experience considerable anger. There may be anger and resentment toward the society-imposed isolation that hampers HIV-infected individuals in their efforts to obtain social support and, at times, even the medical care afforded to individuals with other life-threatening conditions. Individuals who have become infected with HIV through medical treatment, such as blood transfusions, may experience additional anger at contracting the disease as "innocent victims." Those infected through contact with others may direct their anger against the individual or individuals from whom they contracted the disease.

If the HIV infection is the result of individuals' past behavior or lifestyle, they may also experience guilt and self-incrimination. Guilt, self-blame, fear of abandonment, and fear of imminent painful death can lead to self-destructive behaviors, including attempted suicide. For individuals whose families and friends had not been aware of their lifestyle, exposure may result in increased anxiety and fear of abandonment. In other instances, HIV-infected individuals may experience guilt because of the fear that they have been the source of contagion to others.

There may need to be a balance between periods of activity and rest to avoid becoming too fatigued. A moderate, regular program of exercise can help individuals with HIV infection maintain optimal emotional as well as physical health. As the condition progresses and stamina decreases, they may need to modify their activities. Individuals in the later stages of HIV infection often need assistance with everyday activities, including at first housekeeping chores and later extending to personal care.

The social effects of HIV infection are as varied as the symptoms associated with the condition. HIV infection is a disease that many fear and perceive as shrouded in mystery. Many social implications of HIV infection are related to this fear and misunderstanding.

Some segments of society believe that the illness is "deserved" because it has been associated with behavior that they consider unacceptable. Others avoid individuals with HIV infection because they fear contagion and are not aware of the actual modes of transmission. Such societal concepts can result in ostracism and discrimination against individuals with

HIV. They may find activities or social interactions at school, work, and social functions restricted because of social prejudice. The social stigma attached to the condition may be particularly overwhelming and traumatic if family and friends also express such reactions. Individuals with HIV infection are often left with little social support at a time when they need it most. Support groups, although beneficial in many chronic diseases, are even more important for individuals with HIV infection.

## Vocational Issues in HIV/AIDS

Maintaining vocational roles despite significant health issues is important in meeting individuals' emotional as well as economic needs (Lynch Fesko, 2001; McReynolds, 2001). With the advent of new therapies to treat HIV and the associated increase in life expectancy for some, individuals with HIV may also gain a more positive outlook. Despite increased functional capacity and longevity, however, many individuals living with HIV/AIDS remain unemployed or lose their jobs (Glenn, Ford, Moore, & Hollar, 2003). Barriers to returning to or maintaining employment are numerous and require motivation and commitment to overcome (Maticka-Tyndale, Adam, & Cohen, 2002).

Many psychosocial, financial, medical, and legal factors affect individuals' ability and willingness to maintain employment (Kohlenberg & Watts, 2003). Individuals are frequently confronted with conflicting pressures about whether or not they should continue to work (Nixon & Renwick, 2003). Contextual factors, such as disability and health insurance or drug plans, often influence individuals' decision (Ferrier & Lavis, 2003).

For individuals with HIV infection, the most serious impediments to successful functioning in the workplace are the fear, discrimination, and prejudice that they encounter. Many individuals who are HIV positive encounter discrimination at work, and as a result they may withdraw from the workplace altogether (Hunt, Jaques, Niles, & Wiezalis, 2003). Individuals with HIV frequently fear that they will lose their jobs as a result of their diagnosis, regardless of their continued mental and physical ability to work.

When individuals with HIV do maintain their employment, there are usually no special restrictions, especially in the early stages of the condition; however, because of the mode of transmission of the virus, they should avoid occupations in which their blood may contaminate the blood of others. Because infection can have such serious consequences for individuals with HIV infection, they should also avoid job situations in which they are likely to be exposed to infection. As the HIV infection progresses and individuals experience increasing fatigue, they may need to undertake less strenuous work or arrange for shorter work schedules or more frequent rest periods. In the later stages of the disease, mental changes may affect an individual's capacity to function in the work setting.

## DIAGNOSTIC PROCEDURES FOR CONDITIONS AFFECTING THE BLOOD OR IMMUNE SYSTEM

### Standard Blood Tests

The diagnosis of many blood disorders is dependent on laboratory analyses of the blood itself. *A complete blood count* is a test used to evaluate a number of different components in the blood. Sometimes these various components are also measured separately. The components of a complete blood count include the following:

- *Red blood cell count:* measurement of the total number of red blood cells in a cubic millimeter of blood
- *White blood cell count:* measurement of the total number of white blood cells in a cubic millimeter of blood
- *Differential:* measurement of the proportion of each type of white blood cell (i.e., neutrophils, eosinophils, basophils, lymphocytes, monocytes) in a sample of 100 white blood cells
- *Hemoglobin:* evaluation of the amount of hemoglobin content of erythrocytes in 100 milliliters of blood
- *Hematocrit:* measurement of the percentage or proportion of red blood cells in the plasma (based on the assumption that the volume of plasma is normal)

Other types of blood tests used to measure specific components of blood are as follows:

- *Reticulocyte count:* assessment of bone marrow function by measuring its production of immature red blood cells (*reticulocytes*)
- *Platelet count:* measurement of the number of platelets in a cubic millimeter of blood
- *Mean corpuscular volume (MCV):* calculation of the volume of a single red blood cell by dividing the hematocrit by the red blood cell count
- *Mean corpuscular hemoglobin concentration:* calculation of the amount of hemoglobin in each red blood cell by dividing the hemoglobin concentration by the hematocrit

### Bleeding Time Test

A *bleeding time* test measures the length of time it takes for bleeding to stop after a small puncture wound. The test determines how quickly a platelet clot forms. An abnormal bleeding time would indicate a tendency toward prolonged bleeding such as that found in conditions in which there is an abnormally low number of platelets circulating in the blood.

## Prothrombin Time (PT, Pro Time) Test

A *prothrombin time* test measures the length of time that a blood sample takes to clot when certain chemicals are added to it in the laboratory. It tests for very specific factors involved in clotting and may be used diagnostically to identify pathologic clotting disorders, such as may be found with liver dysfunction or in the absence of vitamin K. The test may also be used to monitor the effectiveness of certain anticoagulant medications used in the treatment of conditions in which clot formation is or has been a problem. Prolongation of clotting time indicates that individuals may be prone to abnormal bleeding. If the test indicates that clotting time is reduced, there may be blood hypercoagulability, which could contribute to the formation of blood clots.

## Partial Thromboplastin Time (PTT) Test

A *partial thromboplastin time* test is used to evaluate a special part of the clotting mechanism not evaluated by prothrombin time. As with the prothrombin time test, certain chemicals are added to a blood sample in the laboratory, and the amount of time it takes a clot to form is measured. Prolongation of time in which it takes a clot to form is indicative of a bleeding disorder, such as that found in *hemophilia*. Prolongation of clot formation may also be found with the use of the anticoagulant heparin, which affects a

specific part of the clotting mechanism that is not measured by the prothrombin time test.

## Bone Marrow Aspiration

*Bone marrow aspiration* involves removing a sample of bone marrow by inserting a special needle into the marrow space of the bone and then aspirating a small sample. The bone marrow is then examined microscopically for various abnormalities in the number, size, and shape of the precursors of red blood cells, white blood cells, and platelets.

## ELISA and Western Blot

Both the *ELISA* and *Western blot* are blood tests that screen for HIV antibodies. If the initial screening with the ELISA test produces positive results, a second ELISA test is performed. If the result of the second test is negative, the test result is considered negative. If the result of the second test is positive, the Western blot test is usually performed as a confirmatory test. If the result of the Western blot test is positive, it is highly suggestive that the HIV antibody is present and that the individual has been exposed to HIV.

## Hemoglobin Electrophoresis

*Hemoglobin electrophoresis* is a blood test by which a definitive diagnosis of sickle cell disease or sickle cell trait can be made.

## Sickle Cell Prep

*Sickle cell prep* is a blood test used in sickle cell screening. The test can detect the presence of abnormal hemoglobin but cannot distinguish between sickle cell disease and sickle cell trait.

## GENERAL TREATMENT FOR CONDITIONS AFFECTING THE BLOOD OR IMMUNE SYSTEM

For many disorders of the blood, treatment is directed toward symptoms and/or the underlying cause. If a blood disorder is caused by a toxic substance, the first line of treatment is to remove the offending agent. *Anemia* that is caused by a deficiency may be treated by supplementation or replacement therapy. For instance, *iron deficiency anemia* may be treated by the administration of oral or injectable iron preparations. *Pernicious anemia* may be treated with injections of vitamin B12. When there is an overproduction of red blood cells, as in *polycythemia*, treatment may involve the removal of blood. Venesection (**phlebotomy**) is a procedure in which quantities of blood are removed to reduce the volume of blood.

### Transfusion

Part of the treatment for a number of blood disorders may be the transfusion of whole blood or a blood component, such as packed red blood cells, plasma, or platelets. Because blood is living tissue, transfusion can be thought of as a form of transplantation, carrying the same risks of immune response as do other types of transplantation. For this reason, the exact matching of a number of factors in the blood between the donor and the recipient is crucial to prevent serious allergic reactions, which could be fatal. In addition to the risk of such a reaction, there is a risk that a blood transfusion will transmit a disease, such as hepatitis or HIV, although careful screening by blood banks has significantly reduced this risk.

### Bone Marrow Transplant

Bone marrow transplant is a procedure in which individuals' bone marrow is eradicated and healthy bone marrow is transplanted. Bone marrow transplants are used when the immune system is severely deficient or when certain types of cancers exist (see Chapter 16). Bone marrow cells are received from a donor, and a careful match is made to decrease the chances of rejection of the transplant and to prevent a reaction in which the transplanted cells attack the cells of the individual who has received the transplant.

## PSYCHOSOCIAL ISSUES IN CONDITIONS AFFECTING THE BLOOD OR IMMUNE SYSTEM

### Psychological Issues

Disorders of the blood and immune system have a variety of psychological implications. The specific implications for a particular individual are dependent on the condition. Some conditions may be controlled relatively easily, whereas others require constant vigilance. Although some conditions may be treated and, in some instances, cured, others require lifelong treatment and carry a more ominous prognosis.

Individuals with conditions affecting the blood and immune system generally have no visible reminders of their disability. Without external adaptive devices, such as wheelchairs, crutches, or canes, or any other signs of disability, individuals may react by denying the seriousness of their condition and resist medical directives. For example, individuals with *hemophilia* may engage in risk-taking behaviors, even though injury and subsequent bleeding could occur. Individuals with sickle cell anemia may engage in a flurry of activity, even though the associated stress and fatigue may precipitate a sickle cell crisis. Individuals with HIV infection may withhold their diagnosis from others with whom they engage in sexual activity, even though their behavior could put those others at risk.

Some disorders occur later in life, necessitating adjustment at the time the disability occurs. Disorders such as sickle cell anemia and hemophilia are lifelong disorders, however. Consequently, individuals with these disorders have had to cope with their condition in one way or another from childhood into adulthood, and most of them have experienced frequent illness and medical care throughout their childhood and adolescence. Although these experiences can build confidence in the ability to cope with adversity, they can also have a negative impact on development. Individuals may carry the coping behaviors and attitudes learned in childhood into the adult years, where they continue to affect their perception of themselves, their condition, and their abilities. Depending on the constructiveness of the coping strategy used, such behaviors may be an asset or a hindrance.

The possibility of early death, a source of anxiety and depression for those with any disorder, is a reality for individuals with hemophilia, sickle cell anemia, and HIV infection. Although hemophilia can be controlled to some degree, there is always the fear that an accident or traumatic event may occur in which bleeding may not be controlled. Individuals with sickle cell anemia are aware of the possibility that sudden death will occur as a result of a sickle cell crisis or complications. Individuals with HIV infection know that their progression to AIDS will probably result in death. Individuals may cope with the threat of early death in a variety of ways, ranging from the adoption of a philosophical view toward life to passivity and withdrawal.

The way in which individuals cope with a condition they have had since childhood depends on a wide variety of factors, some of which relate to the coping mechanisms learned in childhood. Individuals' reaction as an adult to their condition is dependent to some extent on how well their psychological adjustment was managed throughout development. Children who were encouraged to live as normal a life as possible, despite their condition, may exhibit a greater sense of self-esteem and autonomy as adults than do those who were kept in a dependent, overprotected state.

### Lifestyle Issues

Different conditions affecting the blood or immune system affect activities of daily living in varying degrees, depending on the associated symptoms. Symptoms of fatigue or difficulty in breathing with exertion may require individuals to pace their activities throughout the day to conserve energy. Individuals may need more frequent rest periods, or they may need to divide activities into smaller steps that they perform throughout the day, rather than completing a task all at once.

Good health practices are important to everyone; however, because of the increased susceptibility to infection that is part of many conditions affecting the blood or immune system (especially HIV infection), individuals must take extra care to have well-balanced diets and well-balanced regimens of rest and activity. Exercise is especially important to individuals with hemophilia. Regular, moderate exercise can build the muscles that protect joints and decrease the incidence of bleeding into the joints. However, activities that carry a higher probability of injury, such as contact sports, should be avoided.

The degree to which individuals can maintain their routine daily schedules depends on the specific condition, its progression, and its complications. For the most part, individuals with hemophilia need not interrupt their daily schedules. The use of home self-infusion therapy has greatly reduced their incapacity by providing prompt and early treatment of spontaneous bleeding.

Although neither hemophilia nor sickle cell anemia alters sexual function, both are inherited disorders, and individuals may wish to consider genetic counseling before deciding to have children. There is no direct effect on sexual function associated with HIV infection; however, because of the possibility of transmitting the virus to others, individuals with HIV infections should inform their sexual partners about their diagnosis prior to sexual contact and should engage only in safe sexual practices. When women with HIV infection become pregnant, the child may be born HIV infected.

## Social Issues

The social effects of conditions affecting the blood or immune system vary with the condition, the individual, and the particular circumstances. The fatigue and susceptibility to infection characteristic of many conditions affecting the blood or immune system may alter social functioning to some degree.

Because many conditions affecting the blood or immune system have no readily observable outward cues and signs, and because symptoms are often intermittent, others may not understand why individuals with these conditions must adhere to certain restrictions or why they are under continuing medical care. Because these individuals do not appear to be legitimately ill and, in many instances, have little physical impairment, they may receive less social support and understanding than individuals with more visible disabilities.

Conditions that are hereditary and those that occur in childhood can impair the socialization necessary for functioning in adulthood. Recurrent hospitalizations may affect children's school performance and, consequently, their sense of industry and achievement. In addition, frequent school absences, hospitalizations, or the inability to engage in some activities may affect children's interactions and relationships with peers, which, in turn, could affect their self-esteem and sense of self-worth.

Some children, as a means of dealing with the stress inherent in their condition, may learn to use their condition to manipulate and control the behaviors of others. The parents of a child with an inherited disorder, such as hemophilia or sickle cell anemia, may experience guilt, react with overprotectiveness, or foster a sense of dependency in the child. They may adopt a permissive or indulgent attitude rather than correcting the child when he or she misbehaves. They may also excuse the child from the normal responsibilities or the limits established for the child's siblings. Such parental reactions can impede the child's ability to function adequately as an adult in society.

## VOCATIONAL ISSUES IN CONDITIONS AFFECTING THE BLOOD OR IMMUNE SYSTEM

The cause and symptoms of a condition affecting the blood or immune system determine its vocational impact. If, for example, the condition has been caused in part by exposure to toxic substances within the environment, the hazards should be removed before individuals return to the workplace. If fatigue or dyspnea is a symptom of the condition, as in those conditions characterized by anemia, it may be necessary to consider the physical demands of the job and the need for more frequent rest periods. When infection is a potential complication of the disorder, individuals should avoid exposure to factors and environments that may precipitate infection. The functional impact of immune disorders is also dependent on the stage of the condition. With HIV infection, for example, prior to the development of severe immunodeficiency, no disability may be present. In the milder stages of the condition, individuals may be able to perform all but the most demanding tasks at work. As the immune system becomes more compromised, however, opportunistic infections may result in prolonged periods of illness and hospitalization, interfering with individuals' ability to work. In addition to the physical disability resulting from opportunistic infections, individuals with HIV infections may also develop central nervous system symptoms, which can affect their cognitive, motor, and behavioral abilities.

## CASE STUDIES

### Case I

Mr. G. is a 26-year-old male who is HIV positive. He contracted HIV from his partner, who died of the disease last year. Mr. G. has a high school education and is a certified nursing assistant working in a nursing home, where he performs routine care for nursing home residents, such as bathing, lifting, turning, and feeding. He has been employed at the nursing home for the past 10 years. He tells you he loves his work and very much wants to continue as long as possible, both for financial reasons and because his health insurance is tied to his employment. He also tells you that work has been therapeutic for him after the loss of his partner. Mr. G. states that his employer is unaware of his illness because it has not interfered with his job performance; however, lately he states he has had more difficulty keeping up with the physical demands at work because of fatigue and in the past few weeks he has developed lymphadenopathy. He has begun a new experimental medication that he also believes might have some side effects that could interfere with his ability to work. He has a strong support group of friends; however, his family has severed all ties with him.

### Questions

1. Is it appropriate for Mr. G. to not inform his current employer about his diagnosis and to continue to work in the current setting? Why or why not?
2. What is Mr. G.'s rehabilitation potential?
3. What factors will influence Mr. G.'s rehabilitation potential?
4. What medical factors related to Mr. G.'s condition would you consider when helping him develop a rehabilitation plan?

### Case II

Ms. S. is a 19-year-old African American female with sickle cell disease. She is a high school graduate and is currently enrolled in a junior college, where she is studying to be an X-ray technician. Since entering school at the junior college, she has had a number of sickle cell crises that have necessitated hospitalization. Ms. S. has developed severe damage to joints in her lower extremities as a result of her disease. Although her physician has recommended that Ms. S. reconsider her occupational goal given her series of sickle cell crises since being in school, she is determined to pursue her education and to become an X-ray technician. She continues to push herself even when she does not feel well.

### Questions

1. How would you approach Ms. S. about her vocational plans given her physician's recommendation?

2. How realistic is Ms. S.'s vocational choice?

3. What medical, physical, and psychological issues would you consider when working with Ms. S. to develop her rehabilitation plan?

4. What is the general prognosis for Ms. S.'s condition?

5. What general lifestyle issues might you address with Ms. S. that could contribute to her rehabilitation potential?

## REFERENCES

Andres, E., Loukili, N. H., Ben, A. M., & Noel, E. (2004). Pernicious anemia associated with interferon-alpha therapy and chronic hepatitis C infection. *Journal of Clinical Gastroenterology, 38*(4), 382.

Anie, K. A., Steptoe, A., & Bevan, D. H. (2002). Sickle cell disease: Pain, coping and quality of life in a study of adults in the UK. *British Journal of Health Psychology, 7*(Part 3), 331–344.

Assanasen, C., Quinton, R. A., & Buchanan, G. R. (2003). Acute myocardial infarction in sickle cell anemia. *Journal of Pediatric Hematology and Oncology, 25*(12), 978–981.

Atkin, K., & Ahmad, W. I. (2001). Living a "normal" life: Young people coping with thalassaemia major or sickle cell disorder. *Social Science and Medicine, 53*(5), 615–626.

Bartlett, J. A. (2000). Management and counseling for persons with HIV infection. In L. Goldman & L. C. Bennett (Eds.), *Cecil textbook of medicine* (21st ed., pp. 1942–1945). Philadelphia: W. B. Saunders.

Beeton, K. (2002). Evaluation of outcome of care in patients with haemophilia. *Haemophilia, 8*(3), 428–434.

Bodemar, G., Kechagias, S., Almer, S., & Danielson, B. G. (2004). Treatment of anaemia in inflammatory bowel disease with iron sucrose. *Scandinavian Journal of Gastroenterology, 39*(5), 454–458.

Bokemeyer, C., & Foubert, J. (2004). *Seminars in Oncology, 31*(3, Suppl. 8), 4–11.

Bolton-Maggs, P. H., & Pasi, K. J. (2003). Haemophilias A and B. *Lancet, 361*(9371), 1801–1809.

Bower, B. L., & Collins, K. (2000). Students living with HIV/AIDS: Exploring their psychosocial and moral development. *NASPA Journal, 37*(2), 428–438.

Britton, P. J. (2000). Staying on the roller coaster with clients: Implications of the new HIV/AIDS medical treatments for counseling. *Journal of Mental Health Counseling, 22*(1), 85–94.

Clement, M., & Hollander, H. (1992). Natural history and management of the seropositive patient. In M. A. Sande & P. A. Volberding (Eds.), *The medical management of AIDS* (3rd ed., pp. 87–96). Philadelphia: W. B. Saunders.

Cochrane, J. (2003). The experience of uncertainty for individuals with HIV/AIDS and the palliative care paradigm. *International Journal of Palliative Nursing, 9*(9), 382–388.

Cooper-Effa, M., Blount, W., Kaslow, N., Rothenberg, R., & Eckman, J. (2001). Role of spirituality in patients with sickle cell disease. *Journal of the American Board of Family Physicians, 14*(2), 116–122.

Elander, J., & Barry, T. (2003). Analgesic use and pain coping among patients with haemophilia. *Haemophilia, 9*(2), 202–213.

Ferrier, S. E., & Lavis, J. N. (2003). With health comes work? People living with HIV/AIDS consider returning to work. *AIDS Care, 15*(3), 423–435.

Fleishman, J. A., Donald-Sherbourne, C., Crystal, S., Collins, R. L., et al. (2000). Coping, conflictural social interactions, social support, and mood among HIV-infected persons. *American Journal of Community Psychology, 28*(4), 421–453.

Gebreyohanns, M., & Adams, R. J. (2004). Sickle cell disease: Primary stroke prevention. *CNS Spectrums, 9*(6), 445–449.

Gerberding, J. L. (2003). Occupational exposure to HIV in health care settings. *New England Journal of Medicine, 348*(9), 826–832.

Giardini, C. (1997). Treatment of B-thalassemia. *Current Opinions in Hematology, 4*, 79–87.

Glenn, M. K., Ford, J. A, Moore, D., & Hollar, D. (2003). Employment issues as related by individuals living with HIV or AIDS. *Journal of Rehabilitation, 69*, 30–36.

Hunt, B., Jaques, J., Niles, S. G., & Wiezalis, E. (2003). Career concerns for people living with HIV/AIDS. *Journal of Counseling and Development, 8*, 55–60.

Kalichman, S. C. (1998). *Understanding AIDS: Advances in research and treatment* (2nd ed.). Washington, DC: American Psychological Association.

Kilby, J. M., & Eron, J. J. (2003). Novel therapies based on mechanism of HIV-1 cell entry. *New England Journal of Medicine, 348*, 2228–2238.

Kohlenberg, B., & Watts, M. W. (2003). Considering work for people living with HIV/AIDS: Evaluation of a group employment counseling program. *Journal of Rehabilitation, 69*, 22–29.

Lewing, K. B., & Woods, G. M. (2000). Sickle cell disease. In R. Rakel (Ed.), *Conn's current therapy 2000* (52nd ed.). Philadelphia: W. B. Saunders.

Lukens, J. N. (1993). Hemoglobinopathies, S, C, D, E, and O and associated disease. In G. R. Lee, T. C. Bithell, & J. Foerster (Eds.), *Wintrobe's clinical hematology* (9th ed., pp. 1061–1101). Philadelphia: Lea & Febiger.

Lynch Fesko, S. (2001). Workplace experiences of individuals who are HIV+ and individuals with cancer. *Rehabilitation Counseling Bulletin, 45*(1), 2–11.

Marcus, K. S., Kerns, R. D., Rosenfeld, B., & Breitbart, W. (2000). HIV/AIDS-related pain as a chronic pain condition: Implications of a biopsychosocial model for comprehensive assessment and effective management. *Pain Medicine, 1*(3), 260–273.

Maticka-Tyndale, E., Adam, B. D., & Cohen, J. J. (2002). To work or not to work: Combination therapies and HIV. *Qualitative Health Research, 12*(10), 1353–1372.

McKerrel, T. D., Cohen, H. W., & Billett, H. H. (2004). The older sickle cell patient. *American Journal of Hematology, 76*(2), 101–106.

McReynolds, C. J. (2001). The meaning of work in the lives of people living with HIV disease and AIDS. *Rehabilitation Counseling Bulletin, 44*(2), 104–115.

Medzhitov, R., & Janeway, C. (2000). Innate immunity. *New England Journal of Medicine, 343*(5), 338–343.

Mentzer, W. C., & Kan, Y. W. (2001). Prospects for research in hematologic disorders: Sickle cell disease and thalassemia. *Journal of the American Medical Association, 285*(5), 640–642.

Nixon, S., & Renwick, R. (2003). Experiences of contemplating returning to work for people living with HIV/AIDS. *Qualitative Health Research, 13*(9), 1272–1290.

Olivieri, N. F. (1999). The B-thalassemias. *New England Journal of Medicine, 341*(2), 99–109.

Parish, K. L. (2002). Sexuality and haemophilia: Connections across the life-span. *Haemophilia, 8*(3), 353–359.

Rodgers, G. P. (2000). Hemoglobinopathies: The thalassemias. In L. Goldman & J. C. Bennett (Eds.), *Cecil textbook of medicine* (21st ed., pp. 884–889). Philadelphia: W. B. Saunders.

Scott, K. D., & Scott, A. A. (1999). Cultural therapeutic awareness and sickle cell anemia. *Journal of Black Psychology, 25*(3), 316–335.

Shah, A. (2004). Iron deficiency anemia—Part III. *Indian Journal of Medical Science, 58*(5), 214–216.

Shapiro, A. D., & Hoots, K. (2000). Hemophilia and related conditions. In R. Rakel (Ed.), *Conn's current therapy* (52nd ed.). Philadelphia: W. B. Saunders.

Shernoff, M., & Smith, R. A. (2001). HIV treatments: A history of scientific advance. *Body Positive, 14*(7), 16–21.

Stabler, S. P., & Allen, R. H. (2004). Vitamin B12 deficiency as a worldwide problem. *Annual Review of Nutrition, 24*, 299–326.

Steinbrook, R. (2003). HIV infection: A new drug and new costs. *New England Journal of Medicine, 348*(22), 2171–2172.

Tashima, K. T., & Carpenter, C. C. J. (2003). Fusion inhibition: A major but costly step forward in the treatment of HIV-1. *New England Journal of Medicine, 348*(22), 2249–2250.

Teitel, J. M., Barnard, D., Israels, S., Lillicrap, D., Poon, M.C., & Sek, J. (2004). Home management of haemophilia. *Haemophilia, 10*(2), 118–133.

Wang, W. C., Grover, R., & Gallagher, D. (1993). Developmental screening in young children with sickle cell disease. *American Journal of Pediatrics and Oncology, 15*, 87–91.

Westerdale, N., & Jegede, T. (2004). Managing the problem of pain in adolescents with sickle cell disease. *Professional Nurse, 19*(7), 402–405.

While, A. E., & Mullen, J. (2004). Living with sickle cell disease: The perspective of young people. *British Journal of Nursing, 13*(6), 320–325.

# CHAPTER 9

# Endocrine Conditions

## NORMAL STRUCTURE AND FUNCTION OF THE ENDOCRINE SYSTEM

The endocrine system works together with the other communication system, the *nervous system*, to regulate or direct various body functions. The endocrine system is composed of ductless glands (*endocrine glands*) scattered throughout the body (Figure 9–1). The endocrine glands produce chemical substances called *hormones* that are secreted directly into the bloodstream and act as messengers on target cells in other parts of the body. Endocrine glands include the:

- *thyroid gland*, located in the neck, in front of and on either side of the **trachea** (windpipe).
- *parathyroid glands*, small, bean-shaped glands buried within the thyroid gland.
- *adrenal glands*, small glands lying on top of the kidneys. Each adrenal gland has two parts, the *medulla* and the *cortex*. Each part has a different function.
- *pituitary gland*, located in the skull just above the roof of the mouth and connected to the brain by a slender stalk. It is divided into two parts, the *anterior* and the *posterior lobes*.

- *hypothalamus*, a area of the brain that coordinates functions of the nervous system and endocrine system.
- *islets of Langerhans*, special cells embedded in the pancreas.
- *testes* in males and *ovaries* in females.

The main function of the endocrine system is regulatory, with different hormones altering various body processes so that the body's internal balance (**homeostasis**) is maintained. Although each endocrine gland has its own unique and independent function, endocrine glands often work in concert. The hormones secreted by the endocrine system control and integrate a variety of body activities, establishing a delicate chain of communication between various body systems and influencing and regulating a number of physiologic processes:

- Growth and development of the body and brain
- Reproductive maturity and function
- Metabolism
- Adjustment to internal and external stress
- Water and electrolyte balance

Overproduction or underproduction of one hormone can affect a number of other endocrine glands and a variety of body functions. Some hormones have the sole function of regulating the production and secretion of another hormone.

The hormone *thyroxine*, which is secreted by the *thyroid gland*, regulates the rate of metabolism and also influences nervous system maturation. When the level of thyroxine in the blood is high, metabolism speeds up; when it is low, metabolism slows down.

*Parathyroid hormone*, which regulates the concentrations of calcium and phosphate in the body, is secreted by the *parathyroid glands*. Excessive amounts of the parathyroid hormone in the blood can result in the demineralization of bone, causing bones to become fragile so that they are easily bro-

ken. Insufficient amounts of the parathyroid hormone in the blood can cause spasm and involuntary contraction of the muscles (**tetany**). If parathyroid hormone is to be effective, vitamin D must be present.

The *inner* part of the *adrenal gland* (*medulla*) secretes the hormones *epinephrine* and, to a lesser extent, *norepinephrine* at times of stress to enable the body to prepare physiologically for emergencies. These hormones increase the heart rate, increase muscle tone, and constrict blood vessels in times of stress. The *outer* portion of the *adrenal glands* (*cortex*) secretes hormones called *steroids*, which regulate many essential functions, such as electrolyte and water balance, metabolism, immune re-

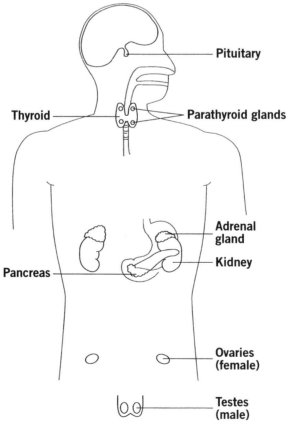

**Figure 9–1** Endocrine System.

sponses, and inflammatory reactions. The *adrenal cortex* is essential to life. If it is dysfunctional, death will occur within a few days unless the hormones that it normally secretes are replaced.

The *anterior lobe* of the *pituitary* secretes *thyroid-stimulating hormone* (TSH) (which is necessary for thyroid function), *growth hormone*, hormones that control reproductive function, and *corticotropin* (a hormone necessary for the function of the adrenal cortex). The *posterior lobe* of the *pituitary gland* stores hormones produced in the hypothalamus. *Antidiuretic hormone* (ADH), which increases water reabsorption by the kidneys, is produced by the hypothalamus but is stored in and secreted by the posterior lobe of the pituitary gland.

Special cells within the *islets of Langerhans* in the *pancreas* produce the hormones *insulin* and *glucagon*, which are necessary for the metabolism of carbohydrates, proteins, and fats. Hormones produced by the *testes* and *ovaries* are important not only to reproductive function, but also to normal growth and development.

## CONDITIONS OF THE ENDOCRINE SYSTEM

A number of medical conditions resulting from endocrine dysfunction constitute a major health problem (Wilson, 2001). Because symptoms of endocrine conditions are often similar to those associated with a number of mental disorders, some endocrine conditions may go unrecognized or misdiagnosed as psychiatric disorders. Likewise, administration of hormones in treatment of an endocrine deficiency may have side effects similar to those of some mental disorders. Clearly, the endocrine system, in addition to regulating internal body functions and maintaining homeostasis, has a role in human behavior and emotions.

## Hyperthyroidism (Graves' Disease, Thyrotoxicosis)

### Manifestations of Hyperthyroidism

**Hyperthyroidism** is the *overproduction* of thyroid hormone because of hyperfunction of the thyroid gland. Hyperthyroidism results in an *increased* metabolic rate. The term **thyrotoxicosis** is often used interchangeably with *hyperthyroidism*; however, thyrotoxicosis results from overingestion of the hormone or inflammation of the thyroid gland (**thyroiditis**) rather than from an overactive thyroid gland (Woeber, 2000).

The overactive thyroid gland may become so enlarged that there is a visible swelling in the neck, called a *goiter*. Other symptoms of hyperthyroidism include restlessness, irritability, nervousness, and weight loss. The increased rate of metabolism causes intolerance to heat; thus, environmental temperatures that seem comfortable to others seem unbearably warm to individuals with hyperthyroidism. **Exophthalmos** (abnormal protrusion of the eyeball) may also develop with hyperthyroidism. Once exophthalmos develops, the effects are permanent, giving individuals a wide-eyed and startled appearance. With early diagnosis and treatment, hyperthyroidism usually causes no permanent disability.

### Treatment and Management of Hyperthyroidism

In hyperthyroidism, treatment is directed toward curtailing the secretion of the thyroid hormone. Antithyroid medication that blocks the production of the hormone may be used. Symptoms usually subside within weeks or months after the treatment begins. Treatment does not, however, alleviate exophthalmos.

Some physicians recommend oral administration of 131I (radioactive iodine). Radioactive iodine destroys cells that produce thyroid hormone, and symptoms usually subside within weeks or months. This type of treatment causes some individuals to become *hypothyroid*, however, which requires that they take thyroid medication for life. Surgical treatment of hyperthyroidism is sometimes indicated. In these instances, a *subtotal thyroidectomy*, which involves the removal of most, but not all, of the thyroid gland, is performed. Because some of the thyroid gland is left in place, replacement therapy with thyroid hormone is not usually necessary.

## Hypothyroidism (Myxedema)

### Manifestations of Hypothyroidism

Hypothyroidism is the most common thyroid disorder in the adult population (Wu, 2000). Individuals with *hypothyroidism* have inadequate production of thyroid hormone. The symptoms of hypothyroidism are in many ways the opposite of those of hyperthyroidism. Individuals have a slowed metabolic rate, and may feel tired, lack energy, and gain weight. Their hair becomes dry, brittle, and thin, and their voice may be slow, low-pitched, and coarse. Emotional responses are subdued and mental processes slowed. Complications of hypothyroidism include the rapid development of atherosclerotic heart disease, including *angina pectoris, myocardial infarction*, and *congestive heart failure* (see Chapter 11). Individuals with severe hypothyroidism can also develop *psychosis*, with associated *paranoia* and *delusions*. Unless complications develop, however, appropriate treatment usually prevents any permanent disability.

### Treatment and Management of Hypothyroidism

The goal of treatment of hypothyroidism is to correct thyroid hormone deficiency. Consequently, a primary mode of treatment is replacement therapy. The medication of choice for thyroid hormone replacement is *levothyroxine (Synthroid)*, a synthetic thyroid preparation. Individuals with hypothyroidism need to remain on this medication for life. Appearance and level of physical and mental activity usually improve gradually as the level of thyroid hormone rises. Blood levels of thyroid hormone and TSH should be measured regularly when individuals are on thyroid hormone replacement therapy. They should not alter the medication regimen without consulting a physician.

## Cushing's Syndrome (Adrenal Cortex Hyperfunction)

### Manifestations of Cushing's Syndrome

Overproduction of hormones by the adrenal cortex leads to *Cushing's syndrome*, which is characterized by puffiness and a rounded moon face, obesity of the trunk of the body, fat pads at the back of the neck (*buffalo hump*), and weakness. The skin becomes thin and fragile, wound healing is poor, and bruising is frequent. Women with Cushing's syndrome may have menstrual irregularities and facial hair growth. Mood and mental acuity may also be altered.

### Treatment and Management of Cushing's Syndrome

Treatment involves prescribing medication to reduce the production of corticosteroids. Treatment may involve surgical intervention, pituitary irradiation, hormone replacement therapy, or other medications to suppress hormone production.

Despite treatment, Cushing's syndrome can have profound physical and emotional effects, requiring ongoing assessment of psychological well-being and functional capacity (Sonino, Boscaro, Fallo, & Fava, 2000). Full recovery may be slow, and there may be neuropsychological (cognitive and emotional) as well as physical (osteoporosis, hypertension) residual impairments (Boscaro, Barzon, Fallo, Sonino, 2001).

## Addison's Disease (Adrenocortical Insufficiency)

### Manifestations of Addison's Disease

In contrast to Cushing's syndrome, *Addison's disease* results from underproduction of hormones by the *adrenal cortex*. Weakness and fatigue are early symptoms; skin pigmentation may become darker. Individuals with Addison's disease may also experience weight loss, loss of appetite, and decreased cold tolerance. Because hormones secreted by the adrenal cortex play a prominent role in the body's adaptive response to stress, individuals with Addison's disease may have severe, potentially life-threatening reactions, such as extremely low blood pressure and severe electrolyte imbalance, in situations (e.g., uncomplicated surgical procedures) that do not normally elicit such a response.

### Treatment and Management of Addison's Disease

Although Addison's disease was once fatal, replacement therapy with synthetic corticosteroids now enables individuals to live full, normal lives. Replacement medication must be taken daily, however. Careful monitoring for the develop-

ment of the symptoms of excessive corticosteroid ingestion is necessary.

## Diabetes Insipidus

### Manifestations of Diabetes Insipidus

**Diabetes insipidus** is a condition in which there is inadequate secretion of ADH from the *hypothalamus*. Although there are a number of causes of diabetes insipidus, the most common cause is damage to the stalk connecting the hypothalamus to the posterior lobe of the pituitary gland (where ADH is stored), which prevents ADH from being secreted. As a result, excessive water is "lost" by the kidneys (**polyuria**). Individuals have excessive and constant thirst (**polydipsia**), consuming as much as 30 quarts of water per day. Diabetes insipidus may be a temporary condition or can become chronic. The condition is permanent, but symptoms can be controlled with medication, enabling individuals in most instances to live a normal life.

### Treatment and Management of Diabetes Insipidus

Depending on the cause, different hormonal preparations may be used to correct diabetes insipidus or to treat symptoms. If the condition has been caused by a pituitary tumor (a rare occurrence), surgical resection of the tumor may be indicated.

## Diabetes Mellitus

### Defining Diabetes Mellitus

A chronic, incurable disorder of carbohydrate metabolism, **diabetes mellitus** involves an imbalance of the supply of and demand for insulin and is the most common of all endocrine conditions (Olefsky, 2001). Every body system is affected by the condition. The impact of diabetes is immense. Over the last two decades the prevalence of diabetes in the United States has doubled (Centers for Disease Control, 2002). Over 18 million individuals (6.3 percent) of the population in the United States have diabetes (American Diabetes Association, 2004a). Diabetes mellitus is a leading cause of heart disease, stroke, hypertension, blindness, kidney disease, amputation, and nervous system damage (American Diabetes Association, 2004a; Taylor, 2004).

The cause of diabetes mellitus is unknown, but there may be a familial tendency to develop the disease. Obesity also greatly increases the risk of diabetes (Tataranni & Bogardus, 2001). Diabetes mellitus can also occur as a complication of other conditions, such as **pancreatitis** (inflammation of the pancreas) or tumors of the pancreas; as a side effect of medications that cause an abnormal tolerance to **glucose** (sugar); or as a result of specific conditions that increase the body's demand for insulin, such as **gestational diabetes** (diabetes that occurs during pregnancy). In these cases, the correction of the underlying cause may reverse the diabetes.

### Mechanisms of Diabetes Mellitus

Food that is ingested is eventually converted to **glucose** (sugar), where it is carried in the blood to nourish all cells of the body. Certain tissues, such as muscle and fat, need insulin to use glucose as a source of energy and to store glucose for future use. In diabetes mellitus, insufficient insulin is available to meet this need. The reason may be:

- failure of the *islets of Langerhans* to produce enough insulin

- destruction of insulin before it can be used

- inability of body tissues to use the insulin that is present

When there is insufficient insulin, cells are unable to utilize glucose, so large amounts accumulate in the blood. This condition is known as **hyperglycemia**.

As blood is filtered by the kidney, glucose is normally channeled back into the blood. Because individuals with diabetes mellitus have such a large amount of glucose in the blood, however, some glucose spills over into the urine (**glycosuria**). Because of the large concentration of glucose in the urine, the kidney excretes large quantities of water, a symptom called **polyuria**. As a result, individuals need to drink large quantities of water to replace the excess fluid lost (**polydipsia**). The body's inability to use glucose means that the food or energy available to body tissues is inadequate. To compensate, individuals with diabetes increase food intake dramatically (**polyphagia**). Despite this increased food intake, however, lack of insulin prevents the body from using food as an energy source. Consequently, individuals begin to lose weight and become increasingly weak. Unless supplemental insulin is available, they literally enter a state of starvation. Because the body's need for energy remains unmet, it metabolizes its own stores of fat and proteins for energy. As a result, *ketones*, the byproducts of fat metabolism, are formed. Normally, ketones are broken down and excreted. In individuals with diabetes mellitus, however, they accumulate more rapidly than they can be excreted. When ketone levels become toxic, a condition called **ketosis** or **ketoacidosis** (**diabetic coma**) occurs. Having too little or no insulin available for the amount of food ingested may also cause a diabetic coma.

### Types of Diabetes Mellitus

There are two types of diabetes mellitus, **Type I** (*insulin-dependent diabetes mellitus, or IDDM*) and **Type II** (*non-insulin-dependent diabetes mellitus, or NIDDM*). Type I accounts for about 10 percent of all diabetes, and Type II accounts for the remainder, or about 90 percent (American Diabetes Association, 2004a). In Type I the body produces little or no insulin, so that individuals require external sources of insulin for their survival. In Type II the body produces insulin, but the insulin produced is insufficient to meet the total body needs or the body is unable to use the existing insulin adequately. External sources of insulin may or may not be taken to control the symptoms of Type II, but survival does *not* depend on an external insulin source. Obesity is a major risk factor in development of Type II diabetes (Ludwig & Ebbeling, 2001; Tataranni & Bogardus, 2001).

### Treatment of Diabetes Mellitus

There is no cure for diabetes mellitus. Treatment is directed toward controlling the levels of glucose in the blood and preventing complications (Hoffman, 2001). A landmark study (The Diabetes Control and Complications Trial Research Group, 1993) demonstrated that strict control of blood glucose could significantly reduce the complications of diabetes. Regardless of the type of diabetes, diet is an important part of treatment (Chandalia et al., 2000; Rendell, 2000). Individuals with *Type II (non-insulin-dependent) diabetes* may be able to control their blood glucose level with diet alone or with a combination of diet and oral hypoglycemic agents and, at times, insulin. Individuals with *Type I (insulin-dependent) diabetes* control blood glucose levels through diet and the use of insulin

injections. Individuals with either type of diabetes must consider the amount of energy expended through exercise and balance it with calories available from food. All diabetic diets are designed to balance the number of proteins, carbohydrates, and fats ingested and to exclude foods that contain large amounts of sugar.

Pancreas transplantation has been used in some individuals with Type I diabetes who have poor glucose control and whose quality of life has been significantly impacted by their condition (Robertson, 2004). Transplantation of islets alone shows promise and can result in insulin independence and good glucose control (Shapiro et al., 2000), although it is still considered to be experimental (Robertson, 2000; Stevens, Matsumoto, & Marsh, 2001).

### Type I (Insulin-Dependent Diabetes Mellitus)

*Type I (IDDM)* is the most severe form of the disease. Insulin is the primary mode of therapy for all individuals with Type I diabetes. Gastric juices inactivate insulin. Consequently, insulin cannot be taken orally, so individuals who are insulin-dependent must inject insulin into the **subcutaneous** (fatty) layer of tissues.

The goal of insulin therapy is to maintain blood sugar levels as close to the normal range as possible and to delay or prevent complications. There are a number of different commercial insulin preparations from a number of different sources (beef, pork, beef-pork, or human synthetic insulin). Some are *rapid acting*, some intermediate acting, and others *long acting*. *Rapid-acting insulin* usually acts within 30 minutes to 1 hour after injection, and *intermediate* types work within 1 to 2 hours. *Long-acting insulin* works within 4 to 6 hours. Each type of insulin also has a different time of peak action and duration.

Because of body responses to insulin, absorption differences, and other factors, insulin absorption varies considerably from individual to individual, as well as in the same individual from day to day. Most individuals require more than one insulin injection per day. Some may be required to take several different types of insulin. Individuals must rotate the injection site to avoid a buildup of scar tissue, which can interfere with the absorption of insulin. They may use a regular syringe and needle for insulin injections, or some find it more convenient to use a device called an *insulin injector*, which resembles a pen. The device consists of a cylinder into which a cartridge filled with a predetermined dose of insulin and disposable needles is placed. The advantage of the device is that it is relatively reliable and accurate in delivering the amount of insulin injected, as well as convenient. These devices may be carried unobtrusively in a purse or pocket for use away from home. Individuals using the insulin injector do not need to carry extra syringes and insulin bottles. When at a social event, business meeting, or family outing, they can easily give themselves injections with minimal disruption.

Disposable syringes eliminate the need for cleaning and decrease the possibility of contamination and subsequent infection. For the most part, insulin no longer requires refrigeration for storage, but exposure to extremes in temperature and to intense light should be avoided. Other individuals may choose an *insulin pump*, which provides a slow, continuous subcutaneous infusion of insulin throughout the day, thus avoiding the need for numerous injections. Insulin is delivered to **subcutaneous** (fatty) tissue in the abdominal wall through a needle and an open loop delivery device consisting of a small insulin pump, about the size of a pager, that is worn 24 hours a day. Although more expensive than other methods, the pump provides more flexibility relative to meal timing.

Regardless of the method of insulin delivery, the amount and type of insulin are balanced with the number of calories consumed and the amount of physical activity performed daily. Because insulin injected into the body must be balanced with the amount of glucose available, individuals cannot, after receiving insulin, decide to "skip a meal." Likewise, since physical exercise burns glucose for energy, a drastic increase in activity, even though adequate amounts of food were consumed, may mean that the rapid consumption of glucose for energy will leave too much insulin in the body for the amount of glucose left.

Conditions that increase the metabolism rate or cause the body to consume more of the available glucose, such as stress, illness, infection, and pregnancy, all alter insulin requirements and, consequently, may necessitate an alteration in an individual's insulin dosage. Consequently, individuals with IDDM who become ill with flu, fever, or other types of illness should consult their physician regarding adjustments to their normal insulin dosage.

Dietary treatment is also an integral part of treatment. The primary goal of diet therapy is to optimize blood levels of glucose. Individuals with diabetes mellitus must consider, in addition to proper nutrition, the total number of calories ingested as well as the distribution of calories consumed throughout the day. Because those with IDDM take a predetermined amount of insulin, they must be especially careful to consume a specified number of calories at consistent times throughout the day to maintain a balance of insulin and glucose in the blood. For the most part, calories should be distributed evenly throughout the day so that there is not a large concentration of calories at any one time. Because the only source of insulin for individuals with IDDM is that which they administer externally, they must pay close attention to the timing of meals and must be sure that there is correct timing between the ingestion of food and the time course of action of the insulin they have injected. In addition to being cautious of the caloric value of food, individuals must also monitor the types of foods and their balance within the diet, since some types of foods affect the absorption and metabolism of others. Counseling by a **dietitian** or **nutritionist** (individuals who study and counsel individuals on the therapeutic use of food) is imperative in the treatment of diabetes. Diabetic diets are individualized based on many personal factors, such as weight, age, and type of daily activity (e.g., sedentary, moderately active, very active). Individuals who are overweight may be placed on a low-calorie reduction diet so that the body will need less insulin. Because of their growth needs, adolescents may be placed on a higher-calorie diet than an older individual of the same size. Individuals who engage in sedentary activities throughout the day do not require as many calories as do individuals who are very physically active in their job or at home. Compliance with the prescribed diet is usually better if lifestyle, religious, and cultural habits are considered as much as possible when dietary recommendations are made.

Exercise is important for the general health and well-being of all individuals. For individuals with diabetes mellitus, however, calories must be balanced with the amount of activity to be performed as well as with the amount of insulin taken. Unplanned exercise that is not coordinated with caloric intake can create an im-

balance between the amount of insulin previously taken and the amount of glucose remaining available in the blood. Individuals with IDDM must learn to balance exercise, insulin, and blood glucose levels to prevent **hypoglycemia (insulin shock)**. Considerable time and effort may be spent in learning how exercise of a given intensity and duration affects blood glucose levels, and what adjustments must be made in eating patterns and insulin dosages to compensate.

Self-monitoring of blood glucose levels is also important in the overall treatment of diabetes. Monitoring of blood glucose levels helps to determine the efficiency of the insulin dosage prescribed. Individuals who take insulin should monitor blood glucose levels at least several times a day. Many individuals monitor glucose levels before breakfast, lunch, and dinner, as well as at bedtime. Monitoring gives them information about the level of sugar in the blood and consequently changes in treatment that may be appropriate. For instance, if the blood sugar level is too low, they may need to ingest a "quick" sugar such as orange juice to prevent severe hypoglycemia. If the blood sugar level is too high, they may need to inject additional insulin.

There are a variety of different types of techniques available for testing blood sugar. Individuals may monitor their own blood glucose levels by lancing their finger and using a small portable machine called a *glucometer* to assess the glucose content of the blood. Blood glucose may also be monitored through a device for continuous monitoring that uses a tiny sensor inserted just beneath the skin, usually on the abdomen. The monitor records up to 288 readings per day for up to 3 days. At the end of 3 days the sensor is removed and the stored data are downloaded to a computer. The data enable physicians to make appropriate changes in insulin doses based on the glucose readings (Bode, Sabbah, & Davidson, 2001). During the time the continuous monitoring device is being used, individuals continue to use standard methods of measuring blood glucose, since the monitor does not display real-time glucose levels. Individuals may learn to alter their own insulin levels in accordance with their home blood glucose reading; however, such alterations should always be done with the advice and supervision of a physician.

### Type II (Non-Insulin-Dependent Diabetes Mellitus)

Although many of the same aspects of treatment for Type I diabetes also apply to individuals with NIDDM, some individuals with NIDDM may control blood sugar levels with diet alone. In other instances, weight loss may help to control the condition. When blood sugar levels are not controlled by following a carefully planned diet, individuals may need to take *hypoglycemic agents/oral agents* (oral medications that are effective in lowering blood sugar). There are several different types of oral medications available. When oral medications do not adequately control blood sugar, individuals with NIDDM may need to also take supplemental insulin.

### Diabetic Coma and Insulin Shock

Careful control of blood sugar is important to prevent complications, as discussed later in the chapter; however, another major concern is the potentially fatal acute conditions of *diabetic coma* or *insulin shock*. **Diabetic coma** occurs when there is too much circulating glucose in the blood. The onset of diabetic coma may be gradual. Few symptoms may appear until the blood sugar level becomes severe-

ly elevated. Individuals may become confused, drowsy, and then eventually slip into unconsciousness. They may have difficulty breathing or experience nausea, vomiting, and flushing of the skin, which remains dry. Water depletion and dehydration are common. Characteristically, the breath of individuals in diabetic coma has a fruity odor. Diabetic coma is a medical emergency that can result in death if appropriate treatment is not initiated. Medical treatment is directed toward lowering the level of blood sugar through the injection of insulin and correcting dehydration and electrolyte imbalance through the intravenous infusion of fluids.

**Insulin shock** is the opposite of diabetic coma, occurring when there is too much insulin in the blood for the amount of glucose present. Insulin shock may result from injecting too much insulin, from engaging in an unusual amount of exercise that burns up the glucose normally available, or from failing to take in sufficient amounts of food for the amount of insulin injected. Individuals going into insulin shock may feel hungry, weak, and nervous. They may perspire profusely, although their skin is cold to the touch. Confusion and personality changes may also occur. If insulin shock is untreated, individuals may lapse into unconsciousness. If it continues to go untreated, brain damage and eventual death can result. Treatment of insulin shock is directed toward raising blood sugar levels. If individuals are conscious, simple sugars such as candy, orange juice, or honey may be ingested orally; if individuals are unconscious, glucose must be infused intravenously.

### Complications of Diabetes Mellitus

Individuals with diabetes mellitus, whether Type I or Type II, are susceptible to a number of complications that can affect a number of different body systems and result in major disability (Stevens et al., 2001; Strauss, 2001). The exact reason individuals with diabetes mellitus develop these complications is unknown, although there does appear to be a link to the length of time they have had diabetes mellitus and the degree to which glucose has been controlled.

Some complications are related to the circulatory system. *Vascular changes* can contribute to **myocardial infarction** (heart attack; see Chapter 11) or **cerebrovascular accident** (stroke; see Chapter 2). They may also lead to poor circulation in the extremities (**peripheral vascular insufficiency**; see Chapter 11), so that even minor injuries are prone to become infected and may become so severely infected that **amputation** (see Chapter 14) is necessary. Vascular changes may also deprive the kidney of an adequate blood supply, causing *kidney failure* and requiring *dialysis* (see Chapter 13). Changes in blood vessels in the *retina* (**retinopathy**) can result in *blindness* (see Chapter 4). Other complications associated with diabetes mellitus may involve changes in the *nervous system*. Changes in the *peripheral nerves*, or **peripheral neuropathy**, may result in the loss of sensation in the extremities, so that the protective sensation of pain is absent, further making them prone to injury. Inappropriate footwear is the most common source of trauma to the feet of individuals with diabetes, resulting in foot ulcers that can lead to need for amputation (Boulton, Kirsner, & Vileikyte, 2004). Consequently, appropriate foot care is a necessity to prevent serious complications.

Other effects of neuropathy may be sexual impotence in men and decreased genital sensation in women. Individuals with diabetes mellitus have a higher incidence of surgery (such as cardiovascular surgery, amputation, or ophthalmological procedures) related to their complications and are also at higher risk for postsurgical complications because of poor wound healing, increased infection, and increased risk of acute renal failure (Plodkowski & Edelman, 2001).

The risk that individuals with diabetes mellitus will develop complications is variable. Factors such as the type of diabetes, the age of onset, the duration of the disease, and the degree to which individuals follow the prescribed protocol must be considered.

### Psychosocial Issues in Diabetes Mellitus

Diabetes mellitus not only involves lifelong multifaceted treatment, but it also significantly affects individuals' daily lives and futures, especially if complications develop. Psychological as well as physiological factors frequently determine the course of diabetes mellitus. Psychological factors may affect the management of diabetes directly by inducing metabolic changes that can affect individuals' ability to control blood glucose levels or indirectly by altering the degree to which individuals follow instructions related to medication, diet, and exercise. Motivation to follow the prescribed treatment is paramount in the control of diabetes mellitus.

Diabetes mellitus is a hidden disability, since its symptoms are not visible. Others may see no indication of chronic illness or disability that imposes restrictions, and therefore they may have no expectations that individuals may be restricted regarding some aspects of lifestyle or activity. If the individuals with diabetes have not adapted to their condition or if they fear social rejection because of their condition, they may attempt to hide their diagnosis from others, ignoring dietary restrictions or engaging in activities outside their treatment plan. Some individuals may believe that following a diabetic diet draws attention to the condition and, therefore, may neglect their diet.

In some instances, the benefit of careful adherence to the recommended regimen is not always apparent to individuals with diabetes mellitus. Even though instructions have been followed carefully, the blood glucose level may remain elevated, or complications may still develop. Such occurrences can result in discouragement and depression. If emphasis is placed on the restrictions associated with treatment of diabetes, individuals may feel depressed and hopeless.

Fear of complications that may lead to blindness or possible amputation may create additional anxiety. For some individuals, these feelings are overwhelming. Self-destructive behaviors, such as skipping insulin injections and/or abandoning the diet, both of which can imperil their life, may result.

Many lifestyle changes are necessary for individuals with diabetes mellitus, especially for those with IDDM. Although diet and insulin dosage can be adjusted to account for different types of activities, advance planning is essential. Activities, including exercise and meal times, should generally be consistent from day to day. Eating on the run or skipping meals is not feasible. If the schedule changes, food intake and insulin dosage must be changed accordingly. If activities involve additional walking, comfortable and well-fitting shoes should be worn to avoid formation of blisters that could become infected.

Individuals with diabetes mellitus should check with their physician about insulin and food schedules before traveling, especially across time zones. If traveling by plane, they should request special meals ahead of time, and they should be served at the time required for the regimen. They should carry insulin with them and should protect it against extremes of temperature. With guidance from physicians or dietitians, individuals can learn to accommodate meals served at restaurants or in other people's homes. The quantity and types of foods must be taken into account, however. Individuals with diabetes must learn to judge calories and portions, and fatty, rich foods should be eliminated from the diet. Although concentrated sweets and alcohol should usually be avoided, planning may permit the incorporation of small quantities into the diet for special occasions.

Diabetes mellitus does not usually affect sexual activity unless there are complications. Neuropathy may be the cause of impotence in men and decreased sensation in women. Frequent vaginal infections in women with diabetes may also alter sexual activity because of the physical discomfort involved. Reproductive function is not affected in men who are not impotent. Women with diabetes mellitus who become pregnant generally have more complicated pregnancies and need special medical attention to monitor the progress of the pregnancy and to alter insulin and caloric requirements.

The effects of any chronic disease are not limited to the individuals with the condition. This is especially true of diabetes mellitus, because so many lifestyle factors are involved in the adequate management of the condition. Often, the degree to which individuals follow the prescribed treatment protocol depends on the degree of social support they receive. The eating habits of family members, as well as their understanding of the importance of the diet prescribed for the individual with diabetes, can contribute significantly to the individual's willingness to adapt to and follow the diabetic diet. Acceptance and understanding of diabetes and its restrictions by friends and colleagues also contribute to individuals' self-concept and subsequent acceptance of their condition.

The effect that a diagnosis of diabetes has on the family of individuals with diabetes depends on family composition, the family's usual coping mechanisms, the age of the individual at the onset of diabetes, the regimen prescribed, perceptions of future disability, and how the family functioned before the diagnosis was made. If individuals with diabetes do not control their diet or prepare their own meals, the family member assuming this responsibility has new status and influence. This can create another source of support or, in some instances, a source of sabotage of the regimen itself.

The impact of diabetes on other social relationships varies. In social situations where food and alcohol are the major focus of activity, individuals with diabetes mellitus may need to modify their participation, although they need not totally avoid such situations. Depending on the individual and others in the social setting, modifications may or may not have an impact on the social relationship itself.

Individuals with diabetes mellitus are constantly aware of the need to comply with dietary restrictions, the need to eat at regular times, the need to balance activity with calories, and the need to stick themselves several times a day to inject insulin or to test their blood glucose level. These factors can make them feel alone and different if they do not have social support at work or at home.

Since diabetes mellitus is an invisible disability, couples planning to marry may not discuss diabetes and its effect on the marital relationship or on plans for children. Depending on the maturity, understanding, and expectations of both individuals in the marital relationship, problems related to the presence of diabetes may emerge, especially in the decision to have children or in the management of complications, should they arise.

### Vocational Issues in Diabetes Mellitus

The type of diabetes, the demands of the job, individuals' willingness and ability to carry out treatment recommendations, and the degree to which the prescribed protocol controls their diabetes determine the special needs of individuals in the work environment. Certain modifications in employment may be necessary to accommodate their condition. First, the activity level should be consistent as much as possible, or activity should be planned so that it is balanced with food intake and insulin or the dosage of oral hypoglycemic agents. If at all possible, rotating shifts or irregular schedules should be avoided because of the alterations in insulin and food schedules that would be required for individuals with Type I diabetes.

Work in which there is risk of even minor cuts and scratches, especially to the feet, should be avoided because of the risk of infection. Emotional stress has a direct impact on the blood glucose level. Consequently, individuals with diabetes mellitus should learn coping strategies that enable them to deal effectively with job stress, or they should avoid overly stressful job situations, if possible.

Despite the ability of many individuals to effectively control their diabetes, discrimination in employment still occurs (American Diabetes Association, 2004b). Employers may fear that individuals are a safety risk or that fluctuations in blood glucose levels may cause unexpected incapacity. Many individuals are able to recognize early warning signs of high or low glucose levels and are therefore able to take steps to counteract physical reactions so that risk is minimal. Symptoms of insulin reactions are, however, variable from individual to individual. In some instances, individuals may become desensitized to symptoms and therefore not recognize the need to intervene before the reaction occurs (Martz, 2003).

Employers should generally be informed of an employee's diagnosis of diabetes mellitus so that misunderstandings about the need for regular meal schedules, routine activities, and avoidance of injury do not develop. In addition, employers should be alerted to the symptoms of diabetic coma or insulin shock so that appropriate action may be taken if either of these events occurs.

The potential for complications should be considered in vocational planning. Although following treatment protocol precisely does not guarantee that complications will not develop, maintaining good control of blood glucose levels can decrease the number of days lost from work due to minor complications. When complications do develop, alterations in employment are specific to the type of complication. For example, individuals with peripheral neuropathy or poor circulation to the lower extremities may need to avoid occupations that require excessive walking or standing. Individuals who develop diabetic retinopathy may need special low-vision aids. Development of peripheral neuropathy of the upper extremities may interfere with sensation and manual dexterity. Because of the possibility of diabetic coma or insulin shock, individuals with diabetes mellitus should not work in isolation.

## DIAGNOSTIC PROCEDURES FOR CONDITIONS OF THE ENDOCRINE SYSTEM

### Blood Tests for Thyroid Function

A number of tests are available to assess thyroid function. Examples of blood tests are the *serum thyroxine* (*T4*) and *free thyroxine index* tests. These tests measure either the exact or relative amount of thyroid hormone in the blood. In addition, a blood test that measures the level of TSH in the blood is an accurate assessment of thyroid hormone levels.

### Blood Tests for Diabetes Mellitus

The major blood tests used in the diagnosis of diabetes mellitus are determinations of the *fasting blood glucose* and *postprandial plasma glucose* levels, and the *oral glucose tolerance test*. In the *fasting blood glucose* test, blood is drawn after the individual has not eaten for a number of hours. For a *postprandial plasma glucose test*, blood is drawn several hours after individuals have eaten. Blood is drawn for the *oral glucose tolerance test* while individuals are fasting. Individuals are then given concentrated glucose in liquid form to drink, and blood samples are drawn at 1-, 2-, and 3-hour intervals. All three tests make it possible to compare the level of glucose in individuals' blood with the level expected in persons without diabetes mellitus under similar circumstances.

## GENERAL TREATMENT OF ENDOCRINE CONDITIONS

For many endocrine conditions, treatment involves replacement of hormones if there is insufficient production, or administration of medication to decrease production of hormones if hormones are being overproduced. Although in some instances surgery may be indicated, it is not always curative.

## PSYCHOSOCIAL AND VOCATIONAL ISSUES IN ENDOCRINE CONDITIONS

### Psychological Issues

The changes in hormonal patterns associated with conditions of the endocrine system may cause behavioral changes that result in misdiagnosis, delayed treatment, and subjection of individuals to unnecessary hardships. Individuals with treatable endocrine disorders have been diagnosed as having mental disorders and at times even placed in institutions, while the real cause of their symptoms is left untreated.

Endocrine disorders can cause a broad range of emotional and psychiatric symptoms. For example, individuals with thyroid disease may experience emotional outbursts, irritability, or anxiety symptoms that are not always recognized as manifestations of their disease. Older adults with a thyroid disorder may demonstrate memory impairment, which is misdiagnosed as Alzheimer's disease or another dementia that goes untreated. In most cases, changes in behavior are temporary and steadily improve as the endocrine condition is corrected. In children, unrecognized endocrine disorders can cause permanent disability, such as mental retardation. Recognition of the role of the endocrine system and various hormones in children's cognitive development has resulted in earlier recognition and treatment, in many cases preventing disability from occurring.

Changes in physical appearance, such as the exophthalmos associated with thyroid disease or the physical changes associated with Cushing's syndrome, can disturb individuals' body image, causing subsequent emotional reactions. Treatment of many endocrine conditions involves long-term or lifelong ingestion of medications. For some individuals, taking medication daily creates frustration and resentment, which lead to noncompliance with treatment and the development of subsequent complications or a recurrence of the disease.

### Lifestyle Issues

For most individuals with endocrine disorders, after the condition has been stabilized and barring complications, primary lifestyle changes involve remembering to take medications at the same time every day. The exception is, of course, diabetes mellitus, in which lifestyle changes are a significant part of the treatment of the condition and are necessary for survival.

### Social Issues

Many social issues associated with endocrine disorders depend on the specific condition. For example, individuals with hyperthyroidism may experience social isolation because of associated behavior changes that occur before treatment is instituted. Physical changes caused by endocrine conditions, such as those associated with Cushing's syndrome, may lead to self-consciousness and cause individuals to withdraw from social activities. The demands of diabetes can also cause stress in families, especially to siblings of children with Type I diabetes, causing isolation and resentment (Hollidge, 2001).

## VOCATIONAL ISSUES IN ENDOCRINE CONDITIONS

In most instances, individuals with conditions of the endocrine system that have been identified and are being treated have no special vocational needs. When hormone replacement therapy is part of the treatment, however, the importance of complying with the prescribed medical regimen cannot be overstated. This is, again, especially true of individuals with diabetes mellitus, the vocational implications of which were discussed earlier in the chapter.

## CASE STUDIES

### Case I

Ms. T., a legal secretary with an associate's degree, is 35 years old and has worked for a law firm for the past 15 years. Over the past year her employer expressed increasing concern about her job performance, citing her decreased ability to keep up with work, and she was finally terminated. Ms. T. states that over the past year she had become increasingly fatigued and admits she had difficulty keeping up with work. She is married with two children who are ages 12 and 14. Her family had also noticed a change in her behavior and encouraged her to seek medical attention. Her physician attributed her symptoms to depression and prescribed antidepressant medication. Her symptoms continued to worsen over the next 3 months until during a routine eye examination the ophthalmologist noticed changes suggestive of thyroid disease and recommended that she have a blood test. She was found to have severe hypothyroidism, and when she was placed on thyroid medication, her symptoms improved dramatically.

### Questions

1. Are there limitations resulting from her condition that will affect Ms. T.'s rehabilitation potential?

2. How would you assist Ms. T. in determining her vocational goals?

3. Would you approach Ms. T.'s former employer about reinstating her in her former job?

4. What other factors might you consider in helping Ms. T. develop her rehabilitation plan?

### Case II

Mr. W. is a 49-year-old jewelry distributor and works for a major jewelry company. He lives in Minnesota with his wife and one daughter, who is 12. Mr. W.'s job is to supply jewelry to major department stores in a 300-mile radius of his home, which involves frequent trips away from home. He travels alone by car and must engage in frequent business lunches and dinners with clients. Mr. W. was diagnosed with Type I (insulin-dependent diabetes) when he was 22. He has a bachelor of science degree in business administration. His diabetes has been under moderate control; however, he recently has had increasing visual difficulty from complications of diabetic retinopathy and also has had difficulty with circulation in his lower extremities.

### Questions

1. What factors regarding the demands of his current job would you consider given his diagnosis?

2. What impact might his complications have on his ability to continue in his current line of employment?

3. What other factors should you consider when estimating Mr. W.'s rehabilitation potential?

4. Are there other issues or concerns regarding his diagnosis that should be considered when working with Mr. W. to develop his rehabilitation plan?

## REFERENCES

American Diabetes Association. (2004a). Diabetes statistics. Retrieved May 18, 2004, from http://www.diabetes.org/home.jsp.

American Diabetes Association. (2004b). Hypoglycemia and employment and licensure. *Diabetes Care, 27*(Suppl. 1), S134.

Bode, B. W., Sabbah, H., & Davidson, P. C. (2001). What's ahead in glucose monitoring. *Postgraduate Medicine, 109*(4), 41–49.

Boscaro, M., Barzon, L., Fallo, F., & Sonino, N. (2001). Cushing's syndrome. *Lancet, 357*(9258), 783–791.

Boulton, A. J. M., Kirsner, R. S., & Vileikyte, L. (2004). Neuropathic diabetic foot ulcers. *New England Journal of Medicine, 352*(1), 48–55.

Centers for Disease Control. (2002). Statistics: Diabetes Surveillance System. Retrieved May 18, 2004, from http://www.cdc.gov/diabetes statistics/prev/national/fig1/data.htm.

Chandalia, M., Garg, A., Lutjohann, D., von Bergmann, K., Grundy, S. M., & Brinkley, L. J. (2000). Beneficial effects of high dietary fiber intake in patients with type 2 diabetes mellitus. *New England Journal of Medicine, 342*(19), 1392–1397.

The Diabetes Control and Complications Trial Research Group. (1993). The effect of intensive treatment of diabetes on the development and progression of long-term complications in insulin-dependent diabetes mellitus. *New England Journal of Medicine, 329*(14), 977–986.

Hoffman, R. P. (2001). Eating disorders in adolescents with type I diabetes. *Postgraduate Medicine, 109*(4), 67–74.

Hollidge, C. (2001). Psychological adjustment of siblings to a child with diabetes. *Health and Social Work, 26*(1), 15–25.

Ludwig, D. S., & Ebbeling, C. B. (2001). Type 2 diabetes mellitus in children: Primary care and public health considerations. *Journal of the American Medical Association, 286*(12), 1427–1430.

Martz, E. (2003). Living with insulin-dependent diabetes: Life can still be sweet. *Rehabilitation Counseling Bulletin, 47*(1), 51–57.

Olefsky, J. M. (2001). Diabetes mellitus. *Journal of the American Medical Association, 285*, 628–632.

Plodkowski, R. A., & Edelman, S. V. (2001). Pre-surgical evaluation of diabetic patients. *Clinical Diabetes, 19*(2), 92–94.

Rendell, M. (2000). Dietary treatment of diabetes mellitus. *New England Journal of Medicine, 342*(19), 1440–1441.

Robertson, P. R. (2000). Successful islet transplantation for patients with diabetes: Fact or fantasy? *New England Journal of Medicine, 343*(4), 289–290.

Robertson, P. R. (2004). Islet transplantation as a treatment for diabetes: A work in progress. *New England Journal of Medicine, 350*(7), 694–705.

Shapiro, A. M. J., Lakey, J. R. T., Ryan, E. A., Korbutt, G. S., Toth, E., Warnock, G. L., Kneteman, N. M., & Rajotte, R. V. (2000). Islet transplantation in seven patients with type 1 diabetes mellitus using a glucocorticoid-free immunosuppressive regimen. *New England Journal of Medicine, 343*(4), 230–238.

Sonino, N., Boscaro, M., Fallo, F., & Fava, G. A. (2000). A clinical index for rating severity in Cushing's syndrome. *Psychotherapy Psychosomatics, 69*, 216–220.

Stevens, R. B., Matsumoto, S., & Marsh, C. L. (2001). Is islet transplantation a realistic therapy for the treatment of type 1 diabetes in the near future? *Clinical Diabetes, 19*(2), 51–59.

Strauss, M. B. (2001, November). Diabetic foot problems: Keys to effective, aggressive prevention. *Consultant, 11*, 1693–1705.

Tataranni, P. A., & Bogardus, C. (2001). Changing habits to delay diabetes. *New England Journal of Medicine, 344*(18), 1390–1391.

Taylor, R. (2004). Causation of type 2 diabetes: The Gordian knot unravels. *New England Journal of Medicine, 350*(7), 639–641.

Wilson, J. D. (2001). Prospects for research for disorders of the endocrine system. *Journal of the American Medical Association, 285*(5), 624–631.

Woeber, K. A. (2000). Update on the management of hyperthyroidism and hypothyroidism. *Archives of Internal Medicine, 160*(8), 1067–1071.

Wu, P. (2000). Thyroid disease and diabetes. *Clinical Diabetes, 18*(1), 38–42.

# CHAPTER 10

# Conditions of the Gastrointestinal System

## NORMAL STRUCTURE AND FUNCTION OF THE GASTROINTESTINAL SYSTEM

The gastrointestinal tract (*alimentary canal*) is a hollow, muscular tube approximately 30 feet long (Figure 10–1). Its principal purpose is to provide a mechanism whereby nutrients and liquids can be taken into the body for energy and tissue growth, and through which wastes from the digestive process can be eliminated.

The digestive process begins in the mouth, sometimes called the *oral* or *buccal cavity*, where teeth break food into smaller particles. The teeth at the front of the mouth (*incisors*) provide a cutting action, while the teeth at the back of the mouth (*molars*) provide a grinding action. Chewing is important to the digestive process. Breaking food into smaller particles facilitates the passage of the food into the stomach and also enlarges the surface area available for the gastric juices as the digestive process continues in the stomach. While still in the mouth, smaller particles of food are mixed with *saliva*, a fluid secretion in the mouth that lubricates and softens food and that also facilitates its passage down the throat. Produced by the *parotid glands, submaxillary glands*, and *sublingual glands*, saliva contains an enzyme that begins the breakdown of starches.

Food passes from the throat (**pharynx**) into a muscular tube called the **esophagus**, which leads from the mouth to the stomach. The esophagus and windpipe (**trachea**) have a common opening at the pharynx. Consequently, a flap called the *epiglottis* closes over the opening to the windpipe when food is swallowed, ensuring that food will pass into the esophagus rather than the windpipe. The esophagus is approximately 10 inches long and moves food along through rhythmic, muscular movements called **peristalsis**.

The esophagus passes through a muscular wall called the **diaphragm** that separates the **thoracic** (chest) cavity from the *abdominal cavity*. The abdominal cavity contains the stomach, intestines, and other abdominal organs and is lined with a thin membrane called the **peritoneum**. The esophagus passes through the diaphragm in order to reach the *stomach*. Food enters the stomach from the esophagus through an opening called the lower esophageal sphincter (LES), sometimes called the *cardiac sphincter*. Pressure gradients around this opening prevent the backflow of food and gastric juices into the esophagus from the stomach.

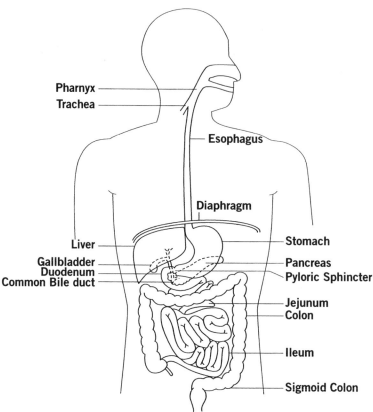

**Figure 10–1** Gastrointestinal System.

The stomach is a muscular organ that stores, mixes, and liquefies food. It contains gastric juices that continue the digestive process. One component of gastric juice, hydrochloric acid, has a sterilizing effect, killing most organisms that enter the stomach. Pepsin, the primary enzyme of gastric juice, digests protein in the presence of hydrochloric acid. Also produced in the stomach is a substance called the intrinsic factor that is necessary for the absorption of vitamin B12. Gastic secretion is stimulated by the *vagus nerve*, as well as by the presence of food in the stomach. The stomach lining is protected from irritation and from the action of the gastric enzymes by a thin layer of mucus secreted by tiny glands within its lining. Although some alcohol, water, sugars, and drugs are absorbed in the stomach, most digestion and absorption take place in the small intestine.

From the stomach, food passes through an opening called the *pyloric sphincter* into the small intestine. The small intestine is approximately 22 feet long and is divided into three parts. The first part of the small intestine, the *duodenum*, is approximately 10 inches long and is connected to the stomach at the *pyloric sphincter*. The middle section, the *jejunum*, is approximately 8 feet long. The last part of the small intestine, the ileum, connects to the *large intestine*, and is approximately 12 feet long. Digested food continues to move through the gastrointestinal tract by *peristaltic movements*. Most nutrients are absorbed in the small intestine. Some fluid is also absorbed in the small intestine; however, most fluid is absorbed in the *large intestine*. Thus the contents of the small intestine tend to be liquid in nature.

The small and large intestines are connected by the *ileocecal valve*, which allows the contents of the small intestine to flow into the large intestine but prevents backflow. The large intestine (**colon**) is only about 5 feet long, but, like the small intestine, it is divided into parts. The part attached to the small intestine at the ileocecal valve is the *cecum*, to which the *appendix* is attached. The major portion of the large intestine, the *colon*, is divided into the *ascending colon*, the *transverse colon*, the *descending colon*, and the *sigmoid colon*. The sigmoid colon leads to the rectum, which leads to the anus, the opening through which solid waste is excreted from the body. The large intestine collects food residue and is the site of most water absorption from intestinal contents. Consequently, waste products (**feces**) contained in the large intestine are more solid. The brown color of feces is due primarily to *bile pigments*.

The *liver*, *gallbladder*, and *pancreas*, sometimes called the *accessory organs of digestion*, are located together in the *upper abdominal cavity*. The *liver* is the largest single organ in the body and is necessary for survival. In addition to aiding in digestion, the liver is important to *carbohydrate*, *protein*, and *fat metabolism*. The liver:

- converts glucose, a product of carbohydrate metabolism, into an energy source, glycogen.
- stores glycogen until the body needs it.
- converts the end products of protein metabolism into urea, which is later excreted by the kidneys.
- manufactures and secretes bile for the digestion and absorption of fat.
- breaks down red blood cells.

- produces substances important for the clotting of blood.
- acts as a detoxification center of the body, detoxifying poisonous chemicals and drugs.

Two major blood vessels enter the liver. The *hepatic artery* carries oxygenated blood for the liver itself. The *portal vein* carries blood to the liver from the *pancreas, spleen, stomach*, and *intestine*. Blood in the portal vein contains nutrients and toxins for *either metabolism* or *detoxification* by the liver. The *gallbladder*, a small sac that stores bile, is located on the underside of the liver. Bile leaves the liver via the *hepatic ducts* and enters the gallbladder through the *cystic duct*. When the gallbladder contracts, bile flows through a structure called the *common bile duct* into the small intestine. Bile, along with bile salts, contains *bilirubin*, an orange pigment formed from the breakdown of red blood cells. Bile salts are important to fat digestion and absorption.

The pancreas, in addition to its *endocrine function* of producing the hormone insulin (see Chapter 9), also plays an important role in digestion. The pancreas lies behind the stomach and produces *pancreatic juice*, which contains enzymes to digest fats, carbohydrates, and proteins. Pancreatic juices enter the common bile duct through the *pancreatic duct* and then continue to the small intestine.

## CONDITIONS OF THE GASTROINTESTINAL SYSTEM

### Conditions of the Mouth

Although not always disabling, disorders of the mouth can contribute to illness and disability by interfering with nutrition. Tooth decay (**dental caries**) and **periodontal disease** (disease of the tissues that surround and support the teeth) can lead to the loss of the teeth. Periodontal disease can also contribute to other systemic diseases, such as cardiovascular disease (Janket et al., 2004). With periodontal disease, gum tissue may separate from the tooth, leading to the destruction of underlying tissues. The early form of the disease is called **gingivitis** (inflammation of the gums). If untreated, **periodontitis** (a more severe form of gum disease) may develop.

Periodontitis can affect the supporting structures of the teeth, causing the teeth to become loose and possibly fall out. Loss of teeth has implications not only for cosmetic appearance but also for nutrition and general health. The inability to chew food adequately may limit the food types taken in as well as interfere with the beginning digestive process. Although dentures may help cosmetically and increase the ability to chew food, they are not as effective as natural teeth for chewing. Dental caries and periodontal disease are best treated through prevention, early detection, and early treatment.

Other disorders of the mouth that interfere with proper nutrition are **stomatitis** (inflammation of the mouth) and **parotitis** (inflammation of the parotid glands). Stomatitis can be the result of infection, injury, toxic agents, or systemic illness. Parotitis can result from inactivity of the glands due to lack of oral intake, can be caused by infection, or can be a side effect of medications or general anesthesia. Treatment of both stomatitis and parotitis is directed toward correcting or alleviating the underlying cause.

## Conditions of the Esophagus

### General Conditions of the Esophagus

**Dysphagia** (difficulty in swallowing) is a major symptom of a variety of disorders. One cause of dysphagia is **stricture** (narrowing) of portions of the esophagus be-
cause of injury or obstruction. When dysphagia is caused by narrowing or constriction of the esophagus, the goal of treatment is to widen the opening of the passageway. The opening may be dilated repeatedly with a dilating instrument, or surgical repair may be necessary.

When narrowing is due to a *tumor*, surgical removal of the tumor or part of the esophagus may be indicated. Dysphagia may also be caused by *neurologic disorders*, such as *stroke* or *multiple sclerosis*; or *cardiovascular conditions*, such as an enlarged heart. **Achalasia** (cardiospasm) is a type of dysphagia believed to be caused by degeneration of the nerves that supply the muscles of the esophagus. As a result, the motility of the lower portion of the esophagus is decreased, and food is unable to pass into the stomach efficiently and accumulates within the lower esophagus, causing *esophageal irritation* (**esophagitis**) and *regurgitation*. Emotional upsets can aggravate the problem. In addition to the discomforts of esophagitis and the embarrassment of regurgitation, aspiration of undigested food particles into the lungs may occur, resulting in *atelectasis* (see Chapter 12).

The aim of the treatment of achalasia is to reduce the amount of pressure at the lower end of the esophagus, thus reducing the extent of the obstruction. The opening between the stomach and esophagus may be dilated mechanically with the use of a dilating instrument, or, in more severe cases, surgery that involves cutting the muscle fibers of the sphincter of the lower esophagus may be indicated.

**Dyspepsia** (indigestion) is also a common symptom of esophageal disease. Dyspepsia may be experienced alone or in combination with dysphagia. Among the causes of dyspepsia is *esophageal reflux*, in which stomach contents flow back into the esophagus, irritating the esophageal lining. Esophageal reflux may be treated by using medications (e.g., *antacids* or *cimetidine*) that decrease acidity, by avoiding smoking, and by avoiding foods or beverages that seem to increase gastric acidity and discomfort. Mechanical measures may include sleeping with the head of the bed raised to minimize the amount of reflux by gravity.

### Hiatal Hernia (Esophageal Hernia; Diaphragmatic Hernia)

The esophagus passes through an opening in the diaphragm to the stomach. When the opening becomes stretched or weakened, the stomach may protrude through the opening in the diaphragm into the thoracic cavity. This condition is called a **hiatal hernia**. It allows gastric juices to come into contact with the esophageal wall, causing **esophagitis** (inflammation of the esophagus), **dyspepsia** (indigestion), and possible ulceration of the esophagus. Individuals with a hiatal hernia may experience mild to severe pain and discomfort with the development of esophagitis.

Although a hiatal hernia may not cause extensive debilitation, the discomfort and potential complications may interfere with individuals' sense of well-being and subsequent productivity. If symptoms are mild, treatment of hiatal hernia may be similar to the treatment of esophageal reflux, as described above. To decrease the frequency of symptoms, individuals with a hiatal hernia may need to refrain from any activity that increases intra-abdominal pressure, such as strenuous exercise and bending. In addition, they may need to modify the timing and size of meals (such as having four to six small meals a day) to decrease the amount of gastric acid the stomach produces. Raising the head of the bed approximately 6 inches while sleeping may also improve symptoms. In other instances, hiatal hernia may be repaired surgically. Surgery returns the stomach to its normal position and makes the opening in the diaphragm smaller so that the stomach cannot again move above the diaphragm.

### Gastroesophageal Reflux Disease (GERD; Reflux Disease)

Gastroesophageal reflux disease (GERD) is a condition of the digestive tract that affects the LES, which connects the esophagus and the stomach. During normal digestion, when food is swallowed, the LES opens to allow food into the stomach. After the food passes the sphincter, the LES normally closes like a door to prevent food and stomach acids from coming in contact with the esophagus. When the sphincter becomes weakened, it may not close adequately, allowing stomach contents to flow backward (**reflux**) into the esophagus (*acid regurgitation*), causing inflammation of the esophagus (**esophagitis**). When this happens, individuals experience symptoms commonly known as *heartburn* or *acid indigestion*. The symptoms are pressure and burning chest pain, often moving upward to the neck and the throat.

A variety of lifestyle and dietary factors have been implicated as playing a role in the cause of GERD; however, there are still conflicting findings regarding the impact of most of these factors, including the role of alcohol and tobacco (Meining & Classen, 2000). Fatty meals, sweets, carbonated beverages, juices and citrus products, large meals, and obesity have all been implicated as potential causes. GERD may also be related to hiatal hernia, as described above.

In addition to causing significant discomfort, GERD symptoms have been found to precede the diagnosis of cancer in about 60 percent of individuals with *esophageal adenocarcinoma* (see Chapter 16) (Lagergren, Bergstro, Lingren, et al., 1999).

Diagnosis is based on symptoms, and in some instances an **endoscopy** (examination of the esophagus through a hollow tube) is performed, usually by a physician specializing in conditions of the gastrointestinal tract (**gastroenterologist**). Short-term treatment of GERD usually consists of using medications such as *H₂ receptor antagonists* (cimetidine) or medications called *proton pump inhibitors* (PPIs) (Cohen & Parkman, 2000). Lifestyle modifications such as avoiding foods, exercises, or positions that seem to aggravate the condition are also incorporated into treatment. In some instances, treatment remains long term and is directed to helping individuals control symptoms when they occur (Dent, 2001).

## Conditions of the Stomach

### Gastritis

**Gastritis** is an inflammation of the lining of the stomach that can be caused by a variety of irritants or infectious agents. *Acute gastritis* is of short duration, with symptoms of nausea, vomiting, and pain. It is generally self-limiting, requiring little except symptomatic treatment. Chronic gastritis, which is of longer duration, may consist of nondescript upper abdominal distress with vague symptoms. Extensive evaluation may be necessary to identify causative factors. It may be due to irritation of the stomach from medications used to treat another condition, or it may be a symptom of a more serious illness. Untreated, chronic gastritis can progress to scarring of the stomach lining, ulceration, or hemorrhage.

### Peptic Ulcer Disease

#### Types of Peptic Ulcers

**Peptic ulcer disease** (PUD) is a chronic inflammatory gastrointestinal disorder characterized by ulcer (sore) formation in the esophagus, stomach, or duodenum. Peptic ulcers in the upper portion of the small intestine are called **duodenal ulcers**; those in the stomach are called **gastric ulcers**. Duodenal ulcers occur more frequently than gastric ulcers.

Until the 1980s, spicy food, acid, stress, and lifestyle were considered major causes of ulcers. In 1982 the bacterium *Helicobacter pylori* (*H. pylori*) was discovered and was found to cause more than 90 percent of duodenal ulcers and up to 80 percent of gastric ulcers (Centers for Disease Control and Prevention, 2004). Other risk factors for PUD include the use of aspirin or nonsteroidal inflammatory drugs, chronic renal failure, chronic obstructive pulmonary disease, hyperparathyroidism, renal transplantation, and alcoholic cirrhosis (Laird, 1999).

Although some foods and beverages (e.g., alcohol and caffeine-containing beverages) increase gastric secretion and can irritate the lining of the gastrointestinal tract, there is no evidence to suggest that the intake of these substances causes ulcer disease.

Another type of peptic ulcer, a *stress ulcer*, may develop after an acute medical crisis, such as a severe injury or a catastrophic illness. Special names are given to stress ulcers that develop with some conditions. For example, stress ulcers associated with burns are called *Curling's ulcers*; those associated with head injury are called *Cushing's ulcers*. The reason that these ulcers develop is unknown; however, they develop rapidly, sometimes within 72 hours of the injury or illness. Symptoms may not appear until the ulcer perforates and massive gastric hemorrhage occurs.

### Symptoms and Complications of Peptic Ulcer Disease

The most common symptom of a peptic ulcer is *epigastric pain*, a gnawing or burning pain located in the lower chest above the heart. Often, pain occurs several hours after eating when the stomach is empty, and it is relieved by the ingestion of food, especially in the case of a duodenal ulcer. Bleeding of the ulcer may also occur, causing symptoms of **hematemesis** (vomiting of blood) or **melena** (black, tarry bowel movements). Individuals may become anemic from blood loss, and in some instances hemorrhage, a severe complication of a peptic ulcer, may occur. Another serious complication of a peptic ulcer is *perforation*, the erosion of the ulcer through the gastric lining. Perforation of the gastric lining allows the contents of the gastrointestinal tract to escape into the *peritoneal cavity*, causing irritation of the peritoneal lining. The resulting inflammation of the peritoneum (**peritonitis**) can be fatal. The complications of hemorrhage and perforation are medical emergencies.

### Diagnosis of Peptic Ulcer Disease

Several types of diagnostic procedures can be used to diagnose peptic ulcer disease and to determine whether individuals have been infected with *H. pylori*. Blood tests may be used to determine whether individuals have the organism. A breath test can also determine if individuals are infected with *H. pylori*. In the breath test individuals are given a drink of a special liquid and an hour later their breath is tested for *H. pylori*. In some instances individuals may have an *endoscopy*, in which a tube with a camera inside is inserted through the mouth and into the stomach to look for evidence of ulcers. During the endoscopy, biopsies or tissue samples of the stomach lining may be obtained and examined for *H. pylori*.

### Treatment of Peptic Ulcer Disease

The overall goals in the treatment of peptic ulcer are to relieve discomfort, to heal the ulcer itself, and to eradicate the organism *H. pylori*. Once the organism is eradicated, reinfection rates are low (Suerbaum & Michetti, 2002). A major treatment is the use of antibiotics and medications to suppress stomach acid secretion, such as $H_2$ *blockers* or *PPIs* (Cutler, 2001). Since the *H. pylori* organism is difficult to eradicate, partly because it is protected by the stomach lining, it is especially important that the individual takes medications as prescribed and completes the entire regimen of medication to prevent the organism from developing resistance. Resistance to antibiotics and noncompliance with the medical treatment are the two most common reasons for treatment failure (Centers for Disease Control and Prevention, 2004).

There is little evidence that dietary intake causes PUD or that dietary therapy is useful in its treatment. Even so, individuals are generally encouraged to avoid foods that produce discomfort and to use alcohol and coffee only in moderation. Other substances that irritate the stomach lining, such as tobacco, aspirin, and nonsteroidal anti-inflammatory medications, are generally discontinued. Individuals who must continue using aspirin, such as for the treatment of arthritis, may be encouraged to use aspirin that is buffered or that has a special enteric coating.

Although surgical treatment of PUD is rare today, if the ulcer does not respond to medical therapy or if there are complications such as uncontrollable bleeding or perforation, surgery is indicated. Several types of surgery may be performed. One procedure, a *vagotomy*, involves cutting the *vagal nerve* to eliminate its ability to stimulate acid secretion in the stomach. Another procedure, *pyloroplasty*, involves widening the opening between the stomach and the small intestine to facilitate stomach drainage. A *gastroenterostomy* is a surgical procedure in which the bottom of the stomach and the small intestine are both opened. The two openings are then connected, creating a passage between the body of the stomach and the small intestine to facilitate stomach drainage. In some instances, the acid-secreting portions of the stomach are removed; this procedure is called an *antrectomy* or *subtotal gastrectomy*.

Surgical resection of the stomach has several possible consequences. One of these is a condition known as *dumping syndrome*, which occurs when food enters the small intestine too rapidly and is not adequately mixed. Individuals with dumping syndrome may experience dizziness, sweating, fainting, rapid heartbeat, and nausea 5 to 30 minutes after eating. The treatment of dumping syndrome involves decreasing the amount of food taken at one time, lying down after meals, and not taking liquids with meals. Dumping syndrome usually subsides 6 months to 1 year after surgery.

Another possible consequence of surgical resection of the stomach includes *pernicious anemia* (vitamin B12 deficiency). Pernicious anemia may occur after the removal of a portion of the stomach because of the absence of the *intrinsic factor*, a substance necessary for the absorption of vitamin B12. In this case, lifelong treatment with injections of supplemental vitamin B12 is necessary. Other nutritional problems, such as reduced absorp-

tion of calcium or vitamin D, may also be experienced because of the rapid emptying of food into the bowel.

### Psychosocial Issues in Peptic Ulcer Disease

In the past, individuals with PUD were advised to avoid certain foods and often were placed on restricted diets. Evidence now shows that special diets have no greater benefit for the treatment of ulcer disease than regular meals. Individuals may need to avoid foods or drinks that appear to be aggravating their symptoms.

Stress had been viewed as a major contributor to PUD prior to the discovery of the organism *H. pylori*. Although treatment now focuses on medical treatment of the condition rather than lifestyle modification, stress as a contributing factor to the development of the peptic ulcers is frequently ignored (Levenstein, 1998), but it cannot be dismissed. An increase in both gastric and duodenal ulcers has been found in survivors of a number of natural disasters and crisis situations (Aoyama, Kinoshita, Fujimoto, et al., 1998; Nice, Garland, Hilton, Baggett, & Mitchell, 1996). Although *H. pylori* may still be present in these individuals, the impact of the organism and stress may be additive, promoting growth of the organism (Levenstein, Ackerman, Kiecolt-Glaser, & Dubois, 1999). Moreover, even if stress may not be a causative factor in PUD, it may worsen symptoms. Consequently, minimizing stress in general or learning stress reduction techniques may still be an important part of overall treatment for many individuals with PUD.

### Vocational Issues in Peptic Ulcer Disease

In most instances, disability from PUD alone is nonexistent. In the past, the disability experienced was mostly related to the side effects of surgery performed for the disease. Now that medications are used predominantly in the treatment of PUD, the incidence of resulting disability has decreased significantly. Most individuals, if undergoing appropriate and timely medical treatment, will be able to continue in their employment. However, those with additional chronic diseases, those who do not have access to appropriate health care, or those who are noncompliant with the treatment and recommendations prescribed have a greater chance of experiencing a reoccurrence and the subsequent disabling effects.

## Conditions of the Intestine

### Hernia (Rupture)

Protrusion of an organ through tissues that normally hold it in place is called a **hernia**. The most common types of *abdominal hernias* are the *inguinal* and *femoral hernias*, in which the intestine protrudes through a weakened part of the lower abdominal wall. *Men* are more likely to develop *inguinal hernias*, and *women* are more likely to develop *femoral hernias*.

Symptoms are often mild, consisting of little more than a lump or swelling on the abdomen underneath the skin. The protrusion may appear when the individuals cough or lift something heavy, but application of manual pressure over the area often pushes it back into place (*reduces it*). The protruding structure can become swollen and constricted by the opening, however, making it impossible to move the protrusion back into place. If this condition, called **incarceration**, is not treated, the blood supply to the herniated portion of the intestine may be cut off, causing tissue death. This condition is called a **strangulated hernia** and is a surgical emergency.

Uncomplicated hernias cause little disability, although it may be necessary to avoid activities such as lifting or pushing heavy objects. Even though there may be little discomfort or disability, because of the danger of hernia strangulation it is important for individuals to seek treatment, even though they have no pain. This is especially true if they engage in strenuous work.

The surgical procedure used to repair hernias is called a **herniorrhaphy**. In this surgery, the protruding organs are replaced and the weakened area in the abdominal wall is repaired.

### Inflammatory Bowel Disease

*Inflammatory bowel disease* refers to a group of disorders that cause inflammation and/or ulceration in the lining of the bowel. Inflammatory bowel disease is chronic and long term, with an unpredictable course. Symptoms usually consist of fever, weight loss, diarrhea, tenderness in the abdomen, and sometimes blood in the stool. Some people experience long periods of **remission** (times when symptoms subside) that alternate with periods of **exacerbation** (times when symptoms become worse). The exact cause of inflammatory bowel disease is unknown, but it appears that susceptibility is inherited in at least some inflammatory bowel diseases (Podolsky, 2002). Two of the most common conditions classified as inflammatory bowel disease are *Crohn's disease* and *ulcerative colitis*.

### Crohn's Disease (Regional Enteritis)

Crohn's disease is a lifelong, relapsing and remitting condition characterized by inflammation of segments of the **ileum** (small intestine). It results in scarring, thickening, and small inflammatory nodules of the intestinal wall that can cause **stenosis** (narrowing) of the intestine. It is characterized by *chronic diarrhea, abdominal pain, fever, loss of appetite*, and *weight loss*. The condition's disabling and unpredictable recurrence pattern causes restrictions in lifestyle and can interfere with work attendance. Three contributing interacting factors—genetic susceptibility, environmental triggers, and altered immune response—appear to be indicated in the development of Crohn's disease (Shanahan, 2003).

Crohn's disease may be complicated by obstruction of the intestine because of stenosis or by the formation of abscesses. In addition, an abnormal tubelike passage (**fistula**) may form between the small intestine and other parts of the abdominal cavity. If there are no complications, complete recovery may follow a single isolated attack; however, Crohn's disease is frequently characterized by lifelong exacerbation.

Treatment of Crohn's disease is aimed at managing symptoms, improving quality of life, and minimizing complications. Treatment varies according to severity and complications. In severe exacerbations of the condition, medications, including antibiotics, steroids, and sulfa preparations to reduce inflammation, are often used in addition to nutrition support through special feedings or *total parenteral nutrition* (discussed later in the chapter) if individuals are unable to tolerate an oral diet for longer than 5 to 7 days (Ireton-Jones, George, Day, & Zeiter, 2000).

### Ulcerative Colitis

In contrast to Crohn's disease, which affects segments of the small bowel, *ulcerative colitis* is an inflammatory condition of the **colon** (large intestine). It starts at the rectum or lower end of the colon and spreads upward, at times involving the entire colon. The colon lining becomes **edematous** (swollen), thickened, and congested with small ulcers that ooze blood. Ulcerative colitis may develop slowly or rapidly. Symptoms usually include crampy abdominal pain and bloody diarrhea. In severe cases, shock may result.

Ulcerative colitis, as a condition with periods of remission and exacerbation, can be a serious, debilitating disease with systemic complications that range from malnutrition to *arthritis* and *ankylosing spondylitis*. Treatment consists of medications, such as steroids, to control inflammation or immunosuppressive drugs to induce remission. There is no evidence that dietary intervention has any specific therapeutic effect. Nearly one-third of individuals with ulcerative colitis eventually require surgical intervention, such as a **colectomy** (removal of the colon), which is curative. Removal of the colon does, however, require permanent *ileostomy* or the creation of a pouch or reservoir for solid waste (*ileoanal pouch*), both of which are discussed below. Because individuals with ulcerative colitis have an increased risk of developing cancer of the colon, regular cancer screening is essential (Ghosh, Shand, & Ferguson, 2000).

### Medical Treatment of Inflammatory Bowel Disease

The treatment of inflammatory bowel disease depends on the location, severity, and chronicity of the disease and on whether it is Crohn's disease or ulcerative colitis. Steroid therapy may be used to reduce inflammation in acute exacerbation of the disease. A sulfonamide known as sulfasalazine is frequently prescribed for individuals with inflammatory bowel disease to prevent or control infections, since the inflamed bowel is susceptible to infection. During acute attacks, individuals with inflammatory bowel disease are directed to keep physical activity to a minimum. They may continue working, but they may need rest at intervals. Some individuals with severe symptoms may be debilitated to the extent that bedrest is indicated.

Specific dietary restrictions vary with different individuals. In general, individuals with inflammatory bowel disease need to avoid foods that cause flareups. Low-fiber diets may be appropriate for those who have a propensity toward bowel obstruction, whereas a high-fiber diet that stimulates the bowel may be advisable for others.

### Surgical Treatment of Inflammatory Bowel Disease

When medical management fails to resolve inflammatory bowel disease or if complications occur, surgery may be indicated. The type of surgery depends on the location and severity of the disease. In Crohn's disease, surgery is not curative but rather is indicated for complications such as obstruction or abscess formation. Surgical treatment of Crohn's disease may involve removing or resecting the diseased portion of the intestine and surgically connecting the two ends of the intestine. This surgical connection is called an *anastomosis*.

The most common surgical procedure for ulcerative colitis is the removal of all or part of the colon, a procedure called a **colectomy**. If removing the entire colon, the surgeon passes a portion of the small intestine (**ileum**) through a surgically created opening to the outside of the abdomen and establishes an **ileostomy**. The part of the intestine that is exposed to the outer surface of the abdomen is called a *stoma*. In this instance, the ileos-

tomy is permanent, and all waste from the small intestine passes through this opening rather than through the rectum. The removal of the entire colon is curative for ulcerative colitis.

If only part of the colon is removed, a surgically created opening between the remaining portion of the colon and the external surface of the abdomen is formed. This opening, called a **colostomy**, is the opening through which solid wastes (**feces**) will be excreted. A colostomy may be temporary or permanent.

Because the stoma of either an ileostomy or a colostomy has no sphincter, individuals have no control over the elimination of waste through the stoma. Individuals with an *ileostomy* have more liquid and more frequent bowel movements than do individuals with a colostomy, because a great deal of liquid is removed from waste products in the large intestine. Thus, although individuals with a colostomy may be able to control the timing of their bowel movements through regular daily colostomy irrigation, individuals with an ileostomy may have more difficulty regulating elimination by this means. Individuals with either a colostomy or ileostomy may wear *ostomy pouches*, which are small plastic bags placed over the stoma to collect fecal waste (see Figure 10–2). The bag is attached by a separate base plate that is individualized to fit snugly around the stoma. A skin barrier paste is usually used to ensure a tight seal and prevent leakage. A variety of products are also available that may be placed in the bag to neutralize odor. For some individuals, especially those with colostomy who are able to control elimination with irrigation, small security pads may be all that are needed over the stoma between irrigations.

Some individuals with an ileostomy have a *continent ileostomy*, in which an

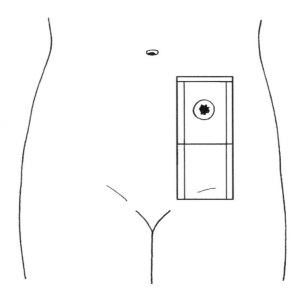

**Figure 10–2**  Colostomy with Bag. Copyright © 1999 Rachel Clarke.

*intra-abdominal pouch*, or *Kock pouch*, is surgically constructed from a portion of the small intestine. Fecal waste collects in the pouch until individuals drain the pouch through the stoma with a catheter. Those who have such a pouch need not wear an external appliance. Individuals insert a catheter three or four times a day, as needed, to remove the waste.

Some individuals are able to have a surgical procedure that creates an *ileoanal pouch*. In this procedure, after the colon is removed, the small intestine is sutured to the anal opening. An internal pouch for storing feces is created from the ileum so that individuals are able to have bowel movements through the anus. A temporary ileostomy may be necessary until the area around the ileoanal pouch heals, but, after 2 to 3 months, the ileostomy may be closed and anal elimination resumed.

Having a colostomy or ileostomy not only alters body function, but also alters body image. *Ostomy support groups* are useful to help individuals learn to live with a stoma and to overcome the self-con-

sciousness that may be associated with having an ostomy. Ileoanal pouches have gained increasing popularity, and for some individuals they have improved the quality of life; however, they have higher complication rates (Seidel, Newman, & Sharp, 2000).

*Psychosocial Issues in Inflammatory Bowel Disease*

The chronic nature of inflammatory bowel disease, with its associated remissions and exacerbations, may cause significant stress, since individuals are unable to predict when there will be a flareup. When surgery is required and a colostomy or ileostomy result, individuals' body image is altered. Since the stomas of a colostomy and ileostomy have no sphincter, and thus no control over elimination, individuals may be concerned about odors or embarrassing sounds when in social situations, and consequently may avoid them. Because of an alteration of body image and the fear of an "accident" during sexual activity, they may also feel self-conscious and have concerns about sexual encounters. The reactions of significant others, family, and friends have a significant impact on individuals' adjustment to their condition. An atmosphere of acceptance and support is important to their self-esteem and ability to live with their condition.

*Vocational Issues in
Inflammatory Bowel Disease*

When in remission, inflammatory bowel disease should have little impact on vocational function. When in exacerbation, depending on the severity of symptoms, individuals may have repeated absences from work. In some instances, if the condition is severe, repeated hospitalizations may be needed.

A colostomy or ileostomy should have no impact on the ability to work; however, individuals' own level of comfort or discomfort with either may be a major determinant of whether they continue to work.

### Diverticulitis

A **diverticulum** is a small balloonlike sac or pouch that develops in the walls of the large intestine. These tiny pouches, or *diverticula*, are formed when pressure causes the inside wall of the large intestine to bulge out through weak spots in the outer wall of the intestine. One of the major causes of diverticula formation is constipation. Once diverticula have formed, there is no way to reverse the process; however, a diet that contains fiber and bulk to promote regular bowel habits may help to control and minimize the condition. **Diverticulosis** is the presence of numerous such outpouchings in the intestinal wall. Individuals with divertic-

ulosis are often symptom-free and even unaware of the condition until it is found accidentally through a radiologic examination for another reason. Individuals with no symptoms usually experience little debilitation and usually require no special treatment; however, they may be advised to avoid activities that increase intra-abdominal pressure, such as bending, lifting, and stooping. They are also instructed to avoid constipation by ingesting a high-fiber diet and drinking plenty of fluids.

Some individuals with diverticulosis develop a condition called **diverticulitis**, in which there is obstruction, infection, and inflammation of a diverticulum. Symptoms of diverticulitis include crampy pain in the lower abdomen and, occasionally, mild fever. Treatment may consist of providing the colon with a period of rest. During this time individuals are permitted to have nothing by mouth and may be given antibiotics. At times diverticula perforate so that bowel contents spill into the abdomen. The resulting complications may consist of hemorrhage and **peritonitis** (inflammation of the peritoneum). Individuals who develop complications may require surgery, which usually involves a *colon resection*, in which a portion of the bowel with the inflamed diverticula is removed and the healthy portions of the bowel are rejoined (**anastomosis**). Individuals who undergo surgery for diverticulitis may be able to resume normal activities within 2 to 4 weeks after surgery, but they are usually advised to continue the therapeutic measures recommended for diverticulosis.

### Irritable Bowel Syndrome (Spastic Colon)

Irritable bowel syndrome is a chronic or intermittent condition of the gastrointestinal tract in which individuals experience chronic, excessive spasms of the large intestine, cramping abdominal pain, and diarrhea, constipation, or both. It is known as a *functional disorder* (with no identifiable organic cause) (Ringel, Sperber, & Drossman, 2001) and, as a biopsychosocial disorder, is thought to result from the interaction of psychosocial factors, altered motility of the bowel, and heightened sensory function of the intestine (Camilleri, 2001; Mach, 2004). Psychosocial factors alone are not the cause of irritable bowel syndrome; however, they can worsen the symptoms and influence the way the condition is experienced. Although the condition does not cause significant functional limitations, it can affect quality of life and have a large economic impact because of the increased health care and the indirect cost due to absenteeism (Camilleri, 2001).

### Symptoms of Irritable Bowel Syndrome

In irritable bowel syndrome, the colon is more sensitive and reacts to mild stimuli more than the colon of most people, resulting in spasm of the bowel. Individuals may experience cramping abdominal pain and a frequent, urgent need to defecate, especially after meals. Symptoms vary in intensity. Although irritable bowel syndrome can cause significant distress, it does not cause permanent harm to the intestines and does not cause ulceration or bleeding.

### Diagnosis of Irritable Bowel Syndrome

Minimal diagnostic tests are advocated in the initial diagnostic approach to irritable bowel syndrome. Diagnosis is usually made through a detailed history of abdominal pain or discomfort associated with chronic altered bowel habits.

### Treatment of Irritable Bowel Syndrome

Since there is no known cause of irritable bowel syndrome, there is also no cure. Treatment is directed toward relieving its symptoms and eliminating stress. Dietary modification may be indicated. Foods and beverages that appear to aggravate the symptoms should be avoided. Individuals who experience constipation may be helped by a diet high in fiber.

Medications such as laxatives for constipation or antidiarrheal medication for individuals who experience diarrhea may also be prescribed. Medications may be prescribed to reduce intestinal activity or to relieve tension and anxiety. Medications such as antispasmodics for pain and tricyclic antidepressants (see Chapter 6) may be used as well.

Psychosocial intervention, such as counseling, psychotherapy, or hypnotherapy, may be necessary in more severe cases (Alaradi & Barkin, 2002; Sach & Chang, 2002). Individuals may be referred to special programs where they can learn techniques to control emotional tension. Behavioral treatments such as relaxation therapy, hypnosis, biofeedback, and cognitive-behavioral treatments directed toward reduction of anxiety and promotion of healthy behaviors may give individuals a sense of control and help them adapt to the condition.

Individuals with irritable bowel syndrome always live with the potential for abnormal function of the colon. If they are able to identify what triggers the symptoms, whether it is a certain food or a stressful situation, they may be able to prevent the occurrence of symptoms. Because the bowel responds to stress, individuals with this syndrome should maintain a healthy lifestyle that includes adequate nutrition, rest, exercise, and recreation.

*Psychosocial Issues in
Irritable Bowel Syndrome*

Irritable bowel syndrome can have a significant impact on individuals' quality of life, and individuals may have a number of concerns related to their social activities, home life, and work. The condition can have debilitating effects, causing frequent absences from work (Camilleri, 2001).

Because of their frequent, intense need to use the bathroom, individuals may be afraid to go to social events or to travel even short distances. They tend to be very concerned about their symptoms and may be quite sensitive to the physical discomfort they experience.

*Vocational Implications of
Irritable Bowel Syndrome*

The prognosis for irritable bowel syndrome is often favorable. It is not linked to other serious diseases, and the mortality rate is zero. Distressing symptoms can be relieved or eradicated, increasing the individual's ability to function.

## Conditions of the Accessory Organs of the Gastrointestinal System

### Pancreatitis

Individuals may develop **pancreatitis** (inflammation of the pancreas) in association with gallbladder disease (*biliary pancreatitis*), certain surgical procedures, some viral infections (e.g., mumps), trauma, chronic alcohol abuse, or *drug-induced pancreatitis* due to hypersensitivity. The most common symptom of pancreatitis is severe abdominal pain, often radiating to the back and often accompanied by nausea and vomiting. Pancreatitis begins

with **edema** (swelling) in the tissues surrounding the pancreas and may progress to hemorrhage and **necrosis** (death) of surrounding tissue. Enzymes produced in the pancreas for digestion of food may begin an autodigestive process of attacking the pancreas itself.

Pancreatitis may be *acute* or *chronic*. *Acute pancreatitis* may be mild or may result in complications such as pancreatic abscess and, in some situations, death. Individuals are usually treated in the hospital with intravenous fluids and pain medications during the initial phase of the disease. If there are no complications and early treatment has been implemented, inflammation and symptoms usually subside with no long-term effects. *Chronic pancreatitis* involves progressive scarring and calcification of the pancreas and is most frequently associated with *chronic alcoholism*. The most frequent symptom is abdominal pain, which can be sudden or chronic. Chronic pancreatitis due to alcohol abuse can progress even if alcohol ingestion is discontinued. With significant damage to the pancreas, individuals with chronic pancreatitis can develop *diabetes mellitus* secondary to the pancreatitis (see Chapter 9). Treatment may involve hospitalization for control of pain, although damage to the pancreatic tissue will be permanent.

### Cholecystitis

Although **cholecystitis** (inflammation of the gallbladder) can occur in individuals with severe trauma or other critical illness even if they do not have *gallstones*, an obstruction of the cystic duct by a gallstone is the most common cause. The presence of gallstones is called **cholelithiasis**. Stones may injure the gallbladder and block passage of the bile that is stored there.

Gallbladder disease can be *acute* or *chronic*. Symptoms of *acute cholecystitis* include severe pain in the upper abdomen, often with nausea and vomiting. When stones block its passage, bile may back up to the liver, interfering with production of more bile. As a result, the level of *bilirubin* circulating in the blood becomes excessive, causing **jaundice** (a yellowish appearance of the skin and whites of the eyes).

Possible complications of cholecystitis include infection and/or perforation of the gallbladder, damage to the liver, and pancreatitis. For individuals with *cholecystitis*, treatment may begin with the elimination from the diet of fatty and highly seasoned foods, which aggravate the condition. The usual treatment for *cholelithiasis* is surgical removal of the gallbladder. The curative treatment is surgical removal of the gallbladder, a procedure called **cholecystectomy**. Cholecystectomy is often now performed through a small tube called a *laparoscope* (in a procedure called *laparoscopic cholecystectomy*). This procedure eliminates the need to make large incisions through the muscles of the abdominal wall. Consequently, cholecystectomy is often now performed in an outpatient surgical setting, with individuals going home 24 to 48 hours after surgery.

### Hepatitis

**Hepatitis** (inflammation of the liver) may be caused by viruses, abuse of alcohol and drugs, or ingestion of other toxic chemicals.

#### Acute Viral Hepatitis

Several different viruses can cause hepatitis. They are transmitted in different ways, but they all produce an inflammatory process in the liver that interferes with its effective functioning. Hepatitis is categorized according to the cause.

Hepatitis A. Hepatitis caused by the type A virus is called *hepatitis A*. It is highly contagious and usually transmitted through the ingestion of food or water that has been contaminated because of poor sanitation or poor personal hygiene. When spread through direct person-to-person contact, it may be called *infectious hepatitis*. Individuals with *hepatitis A* usually experience initial weakness, **malaise** (feeling of general fatigue or discomfort), or body aches.

Hepatitis A is diagnosed through blood tests. There is no specific treatment, and infection is usually self-limited. Although the infection can persist for months, it does not lead to chronic liver disease (Hoofnagle & Lindsay, 2000). Vaccination for Hepatitis A is available for individuals at high risk, such as travelers to areas where the rate of infection is high.

There is no specific medication or treatment that directly affects the viruses that cause hepatitis A. Usually, the hepatitis resolves spontaneously after 1 to 2 months. During that interval, the treatment is directed toward alleviating the symptoms and maintaining the individual's state of health so that he or she can withstand the infection. Rest and adequate nutrition are the cornerstones of therapy. Individuals with hepatitis may generally return to work after jaundice disappears and they feel sufficiently strong to resume their duties.

Hepatitis B. *Hepatitis B*, sometimes called *serum hepatitis*, is caused by the *type B virus* and is a major health problem. Initial symptoms may be flulike. Eventually, jaundice may appear because of **hyperbilirubinemia** (an excess of bilirubin in the blood). Individuals may also complain of **pruritus** (itching of the skin).

The hepatitis B virus can live in all body fluids and is transmitted by blood, semen, and vaginal fluids. Hepatitis B is spread through injection with a contaminated needle when injecting drugs or through tattooing, ear piercing, electrolysis, or acupuncture. It is also transmitted through contact with contaminated body fluids during sexual intercourse or through sharing personal care items such as toothbrushes.

Pregnant women can pass the hepatitis B virus to their baby at birth, causing lifelong, incurable liver problems for the infant. Diagnosis of hepatitis B is made through a blood test.

Although there is no cure, hepatitis B can be prevented. Because of the potential serious consequences of hepatitis B infection, a comprehensive immunization strategy to eliminate transmission of the hepatitis B virus has been adopted in the United States and includes routine vaccination of infants and adolescents and vaccination of high-risk adults. Although most individuals recover from the symptoms of hepatitis B in about 6 months, they continue to be carriers of the virus (Zuckerman & Lavancy, 1999). Not all carriers are infectious; however, they are at risk for developing chronic hepatitis, which can be associated with cirrhosis, liver failure, and liver cancer (Lox, 2002).

Hepatitis C. Hepatitis C (formerly called hepatitis non-A, non-B) is caused by the hepatitis C virus and is contracted primarily through the transfusion of contaminated blood or blood products or from infected needles. Once an individual becomes infected, the disease is lifelong. A major complication of hepatitis C is chronic hepatitis. Hepatitis C is the most common cause of chronic liver disease in the United States, and many individuals with hepatitis C go on to develop end-stage liver disease (Gaster & Larson, 2000). They are also at risk for developing cancer of the liver.

Hepatitis C may be **asymptomatic** (without symptoms) or may begin with flulike symptoms, such as **anorexia** (lack of appetite), distaste for cigarettes, chills and fever, nausea and vomiting, or headache.

Treatment of hepatitis C consists of a course of antiviral therapy that includes a combination of medications such as *interferon* and *ribavirin*, usually three times a week for up to 6 months to a year. Treatment is not curative, but it can have a beneficial effect on survival and development of chronic liver disease (Gaster & Larson, 2000). However, treatment is expensive and may cause side effects so severe that individuals may be prevented from working during treatment periods (Yates & Gleason, 1998). Individuals who develop cirrhosis because of hepatitis C may be candidates for liver transplantation. They are usually required to be free of alcohol or illicit drugs for 6 months prior to being placed on a transplant list.

There is currently no immunization available to prevent hepatitis C infections. Consequently, the best prevention is avoidance of high-risk behaviors.

### Chronic Hepatitis

Chronic hepatitis comprises several diseases that are grouped together because of similar symptoms and because they can all lead to cirrhosis and end-stage liver disease (Lindsay & Hoofnagle, 2000). When liver inflammation continues longer than 3 to 6 months, individuals are said to have chronic hepatitis. This condition may lead to progressive fibrous changes in the liver or cirrhosis. The prognosis is variable, depending on the cause.

*Toxic Hepatitis*

Because the liver metabolizes and detoxifies many drugs as well as other toxic or poisonous substances, overexposure to or the presence of **hepatotoxins** (substances that are harmful to the liver) can cause liver damage and chronic liver disease. The prognosis depends on the extent of the liver damage and the prevention of associated complications.

### *Cirrhosis*

Cirrhosis is a progressive disease of the liver in which liver function is disorganized and altered because of damage that produces fibrous changes in the structure of the liver. Such changes can occur for a wide variety of reasons:

- Infection of the liver, as in viral hepatitis
- Obstruction of bile flow, as in gallbladder disease
- Overexposure to hepatotoxins, such as toxic chemicals
- Alcohol abuse

Some individuals with cirrhosis have no symptoms. As the disease progresses, symptoms may consist of **anorexia** (lack of appetite), nausea, and vomiting. Individuals with advanced cases of cirrhosis may gain weight because of their retention of fluid and the presence of fluid in the abdominal cavity, a condition called **ascites**. Finally there may be vomiting of blood (**hematemesis**) and a general bleeding tendency.

Complications of cirrhosis include hemorrhage, coma, and eventually death. Treatment of cirrhosis is based on its cause and any complications that may be present. Treatment is discussed in further detail in Chapter 7. Prognosis depends on the severity of the condition and the associated complications.

## GENERAL DIAGNOSTIC PROCEDURES FOR CONDITIONS OF THE GASTROINTESTINAL SYSTEM

### Barium Swallow (Upper Gastrointestinal Series)

A radiologic (X-ray) study of the upper gastrointestinal tract, or *barium swallow*, makes it possible to identify abnormalities of the esophagus, stomach, and the upper portion of the small intestine. Immediately before the procedure, individuals drink a white, chalky liquid called *barium* so that the radiologist can visualize the structures of the upper gastrointestinal tract on X-ray film. The test aids in the medical diagnosis of structural abnormalities, ulcers, and tumors of the upper gastrointestinal tract. The test is usually performed by a **radiologist** (a physician specializing in diagnostic or therapeutic use of X-ray film).

### Barium Enema (Lower Gastrointestinal Series)

Like the barium swallow, a *barium enema* is a **radiologic** (X-ray) study. In the case of the barium enema, however, the large intestine is filled by an enema with barium. This procedure enables the radiologist to visualize the large intestine on X-ray film for the diagnosis of structural abnormalities, diverticula, and tumors.

### Esophageal Manoscopy (Manometry)

Although done infrequently, *esophageal manoscopy* is a diagnostic procedure to evaluate the function of the sphincter between the esophagus and the stomach. During the procedure, individuals swallow a catheter that has a small instrument or transducer attached to it. When the transducer reaches the lower end of the esophagus, the pressure around the sphincter is measured.

## Endoscopy (Gastroscopy)

When there are indications of abnormalities in the esophagus, stomach, or small intestine, the walls of these organs may be visualized directly through a specially lighted, flexible tube called a *gastroscope* or *endoscope*. This procedure is called a **gastroscopy** and is usually performed by a **gastroenterologist** (a physician who specializes in the diagnosis and treatment of gastrointestinal conditions). During the procedure, the individual's throat is sprayed with an anesthetic medication to numb the gagging reflex. The gastroscope is then inserted through the mouth, into the esophagus, into the stomach, and, at times, into the small intestine. Through the tube, the physician can visualize ulcerations or other abnormalities, as well as remove stomach contents for analysis, if needed.

## Proctoscopy, Colonoscopy, and Sigmoidoscopy

These procedures are performed by a physician, often a *gastroenterologist*, a *family physician*, or a *general internist*. The procedures are performed to identify problems of the rectum and large intestine, including tumors, obstruction, and bleeding. The procedure used to detect abnormalities of the rectum is called a **proctoscopy**. It involves the direct visualization of the anus and rectum through a special instrument called a *proctoscope* inserted into the rectum. **Colonoscopy** is a procedure that enables physicians to examine the lining of the **colon** (large bowel) for abnormalities by inserting a flexible tube into the anus and advancing it slowly into the rectum and colon.

Similarly, **sigmoidoscopy** permits direct visualization of the sigmoid colon through a special instrument called a *sig-moidoscope* inserted through the anus and rectum up into the colon.

## Cholecystography

If gallbladder disease is suspected, a *cholecystogram* may be performed to detect abnormalities, inflammation, or the presence of stones. Before the procedure, the individual swallows special pills or liquid or receives an intravenous injection of a special substance that allows the gallbladder to be visualized on X-ray film. A **radiologist** (a physician who specializes in the diagnostic or therapeutic use of X-ray) usually performs the procedure.

## Cholangiography

A study called a *cholangiogram* is used to visualize the bile ducts on X-ray film. Dye is injected into a vein or into a drain called a *T tube* that has been inserted into the bile duct (usually after gallbladder surgery). A radiologist performs the procedure to identify any obstruction of the bile ducts.

## Ultrasonography (Abdominal Sonography)

In *ultrasonography*, sound waves are passed into the body and converted to a visual image or photograph of a body structure. *Abdominal sonograms* focus on organs contained within the abdomen and can be used to identify disorders of the pancreas, liver, gallbladder, or any other abdominal organ.

## Computed Tomography (CT Scan, CAT Scan)

A special kind of X-ray procedure, *computed tomography*, produces three-dimensional pictures of a cross-section of a part of the body. The radiologist studies the image produced to identify problems and to determine if further tests are needed. This procedure can be used to diagnose pancreatic disease, tumors, or abscesses in the abdominal area.

### Radionuclide Imaging

For radionuclide imaging, individuals are given a small amount of a radioactive chemical (**radionuclide**) that gives off energy in the form of radiation. Different radionuclides concentrate in different organs. Special types of equipment, such as counters, scanners, and gamma cameras, detect the radiation, producing an image on film or on a special type of screen. A physician who has specialized in nuclear medicine then examines and evaluates the image. In the gastrointestinal system, radionuclide imaging is helpful in detecting tumors, abscesses, or cirrhosis of the liver and in diagnosing gallbladder disease.

### Biopsy

The removal of a specimen of tissue from a specified site for examination is called a **biopsy**. Common sites of biopsy in the gastrointestinal tract are the esophagus, stomach, rectum and colon, and liver. Biopsies are performed by a physician and can be performed on an outpatient basis under local anesthesia.

### Abdominal Paracentesis

A procedure to remove fluid from the abdominal cavity, *abdominal paracentesis*, involves puncturing the abdominal cavity with a hollow needle through which accumulated fluid can be withdrawn. A physician performs the procedure. It may be done for diagnostic purposes to determine the nature of the fluid present, or for

therapeutic purposes to remove accumulated fluid in the abdominal cavity that may be causing respiratory difficulty, pain, or other problems.

### Laparoscopy

Laparoscopy may be conducted for either diagnosis or surgical procedures. The abdominal cavity may be directly examined through a hollow tube called a *laparoscope* or *peritoneoscope*. The instrument is inserted into the abdominal cavity through a small incision. Individuals who have undergone laparoscopy may remain in the hospital overnight for observation after the procedure.

## GENERAL TREATMENT FOR CONDITIONS OF THE GASTROINTESTINAL SYSTEM

### Medications

Various medications are used in treating conditions of the gastrointestinal system; they may act on either muscular or glandular tissues and may be one or more of the following:

- *Antacids* and *acid inhibitors* to counteract excess acidity.
- *Antiemetics* to prevent nausea and vomiting. A side effect of these medications may be drowsiness.
- *Digestants* to replace missing enzyme secretions when there is an enzyme deficiency in the gastrointestinal tract.
- *Antidiarrheals* to prevent diarrhea.
- *Laxatives* and *cathartics* to relieve constipation. Generally, laxatives have mild actions, and cathartics have stronger actions.
- *Anticholinergics* to inhibit the action of the involuntary nervous system. In gastrointestinal conditions, these medications may be given to reduce

activity of the intestine or to decrease secretions.

- *Histamine H₂ receptor antagonists* (e.g., cimetidine) to inhibit cells in the stomach lining from producing acid.
- *Proton pump inhibitors.*
- *Antimicrobials* (e.g., sulfonamides) to inhibit the growth of microorganisms.

## Hyperalimentation
## (Total Parenteral Nutrition)

When individuals are unable to take nourishment by mouth, or when nutritional status is compromised, it is possible to bypass the gastrointestinal tract in order to provide nourishment. **Hyperalimentation** is the infusion of a special nutritional solution into a vein. Because of the nature of the solution, infusion usually takes place in a large vessel such as the *subclavian vein*, located in the upper body. Hyperalimentation may be used in the treatment of any condition that compromises the individual's nutritional status. It may also be used when there is a need to rest the gastrointestinal tract, as in inflammatory bowel disease, or when there is an obstruction or malabsorption problem in the bowel.

## Stress Management

Although stress management may be helpful in the treatment of a variety of chronic illnesses and disabilities, it may be especially useful in the treatment of conditions of the gastrointestinal tract. Stress itself may not be a direct cause of many conditions of the gastrointestinal tract, but it may exacerbate or prolong an acute episode in some patients with existing disease.

The body uses a number of defensive mechanisms in the face of threat or danger. When stress is encountered, a variety of physiologic reactions take place in the body, including in the gastrointestinal tract. The digestive system responds differently to different kinds of emotional stimuli. For example, it may become more or less active, and it may secrete more or less gastric juice. The intensity of the physiologic reaction depends on the individual and on the situation. Stress management helps individuals to control their reactions to stress. Programs in stress management may vary from exercise to techniques that alter the body's response to stress, such as biofeedback.

## PSYCHOSOCIAL ISSUES IN CONDITIONS OF THE GASTROINTESTINAL SYSTEM

### Psychological Issues

Although not a causative factor in all instances, there appears to be at least some association between psychological factors and the gastrointestinal system. Psychological factors that significantly affect gastrointestinal conditions may also include nutritional or lifestyle factors, such as alcohol and tobacco ingestion. In some instances, gastrointestinal conditions may also be directly related to treatment for another condition, such as intake of aspirin for rheumatoid arthritis, which results in gastritis.

Conditions that affect the physical processes of eating and elimination have many psychological implications. Throughout life, eating is often associated with pleasure and social interaction. Treatment of gastrointestinal conditions frequently requires avoiding substances that irritate the gastrointestinal tract or cause the excessive secretion of gastric juices. When certain types of food and beverages are restricted or when special diets are required, individuals may have difficulty in giving up something that they enjoyed.

Elimination is associated with privacy and personal cleanliness. The modification of elimination habits is learned in childhood as part of the socialization process. Individuals with problems of elimination may fear embarrassment and social ridicule as a result of their condition. Those with an *ileostomy* or a *colostomy* may fear the loss of physical and sexual attractiveness because of odor or embarrassing sounds. Individuals who have inflammatory bowel disease accompanied by diarrhea may fear fecal incontinence and concomitant humiliation.

There are other reasons for psychological reactions as well. Individuals with *hepatitis* may fear transmitting the disease, and individuals with *ulcerative colitis* may be preoccupied with their increased risk of cancer. Depression is common in individuals with *irritable bowel syndrome*. The identification and resolution of these reactions may be crucial to rehabilitation.

Emotions affect the involuntary nervous system, which, in turn, affects the gastrointestinal tract. Thus, psychological factors may aggravate conditions of the gastrointestinal tract. For example, anxiety may contribute to flareups of conditions such as inflammatory bowel disease. Although rest and relaxation are of prime importance in the treatment of many gastrointestinal conditions, individuals may find it difficult to modify their schedules, to adjust to new life patterns, or to alter stressful situations at home or work. Often, directions to "rest and relax" are useless unless individuals are assisted with methods and techniques to do so.

Although many conditions of the gastrointestinal tract do not affect body image, individuals with an ileostomy or a colostomy may encounter problems with body image and self-concept. They may perceive themselves as different from others. They may visualize themselves as unattractive and may believe that they must wear shapeless, dowdy clothes to hide the ileostomy or colostomy bag. It is often helpful if they are able to meet other persons who have a similar condition and are leading a normal, active life.

Many conditions of the gastrointestinal tract require permanent alterations in lifestyle and constant control over emotional tension. At times, individuals with such conditions exhibit illness behavior and disability that are out of proportion to the objective findings. These individuals should be helped to make the recommended alterations and encouraged to maintain as normal a lifestyle as possible.

## Lifestyle Issues

Individuals with any chronic disease must have a healthy lifestyle, including adequate nutrition, rest, and exercise, in order to reach their maximal functional capacity. This is especially true of gastrointestinal conditions, because stress, fatigue, and emotions appear to have some direct effect on the digestive system. Individuals who are accustomed to performing in high-pressure, high-stress situations may need to learn ways either to decrease the stressful aspects of their daily life or work or to cope better with the stress that is present.

Many gastrointestinal disorders carry notable nutritional implications, and diet is the cornerstone of therapy. Alterations and restrictions of diet are often based on avoiding foods that appear to cause distress. Depending on the meaning these foods have for individuals, it may be difficult for them to abide by such restrictions. In most instances, eating well-balanced, regular meals is part of the therapeutic regimen. For individuals whose work or daily schedule is somewhat erratic, even this simple task may be difficult.

Alcohol intake should not necessarily be totally restricted, but it may be limited. Tobacco use is restricted for many individuals with gastrointestinal conditions. Depending on the former habits of these individuals, both of these recommendations may be difficult to follow.

In most instances, conditions of the gastrointestinal tract do not directly affect sexual function. However, individuals may be reluctant to engage in sexual activity if their gastrointestinal condition affects their body image or if they fear fecal incontinence. Those with an ileostomy or a colostomy may have fears of defecation during sexual contact or may be self-conscious about the stoma itself. In some cases, men may become impotent as a result of nerve damage caused by the surgical procedure. Open discussion about such issues is important to uncover such fears and concerns, as well as to provide information that can help individuals and their partners deal with such issues.

### Social Issues

Food is a part of celebration and socialization as well as nourishment. When specific conditions of the gastrointestinal system prohibit individuals from eating or from having foods that have typically been part of their social milieu, their social interactions may be affected.

Social situations that are stressful for the individual with gastrointestinal disease may cause a flareup of symptoms. To avoid such stress, some individuals with gastrointestinal symptoms may withdraw from many social activities.

Individuals with ileostomy or colostomy bags may fear fecal incontinence, odors, or spillage and may withdraw from social interactions to avoid potential embarrassment. For individuals with an ileostomy or a colostomy, problems may arise if family members are repelled by the condition or find it impossible to fit the care of a stoma into the household routine. If these individuals have not accepted responsibility for their own personal care, they may become overly demanding or sloppy in the care of the stoma, antagonizing family members. The acceptance of the individual by family members and friends often determines to a great degree the acceptance of the condition by the individual.

## VOCATIONAL ISSUES IN CONDITIONS OF THE GASTROINTESTINAL SYSTEM

In most instances, special work restrictions are not necessary for individuals with gastrointestinal disorders. Those with diverticular disease or hernia may need to avoid activities that increase intra-abdominal pressure, such as lifting or bending.

Modifications in the work environment or work schedule may occasionally be necessary for those with other gastrointestinal conditions. For example, erratic or rotating schedules may make it difficult for individuals with a peptic ulcer to eat regular, well-balanced meals, aggravating the condition. Work situations that cause undue stress may contribute to a flareup of the symptoms of some gastrointestinal conditions. If schedules or workload cannot be changed, individuals may need to learn different ways of expressing tension and coping with stress.

Special accommodations, such as readily available bathrooms with privacy in the workplace, may be necessary for individuals who experience diarrhea as a symptom of a gastrointestinal disorder or for those who have an ileostomy or a colostomy that may need attention during the day.

## CASE STUDIES

### Case I

Mr. A. is a 36-year-old musician who plays with a band at a local club six nights a week. During the day he gives music lessons to a number of private music students. He is unmarried and has a master of arts degree in music. He was diagnosed with Crohn's disease 10 years ago, and since then his symptoms have become considerably worse. He has had to cancel a number of private music lessons each week, and he has been unable to perform with the band several nights a week. This pattern has continued for several months, and several music students have sought out other instructors. The band members have informed him that if the pattern of absences continues, they will need to drop him from the band. He is interested in looking for other career options in the event this should occur.

#### Questions

1. What type of medical information would help Mr. A. evaluate his rehabilitation potential?

2. What factors would you consider in helping Mr. A. to develop a rehabilitation plan or to identify his options?

3. Are there any types of referrals that Mr. A. might find helpful?

### Case II

Mr. Z., a 17-year-old grocery clerk, was shot in the abdomen during an attempted robbery. As a result of his injury, Mr. Z. had a large portion of his colon removed and now has a permanent colostomy. It is now 6 months since his injury, and he is ready to graduate from high school. He has asked you as his high school vocational counselor to help him determine suitable career options.

#### Questions

1. Are there specific limitations associated with Mr. Z. having a colostomy that you would consider when focusing on career goals?

2. In addition to determining Mr. Z.'s vocational interests and abilities, are there other issues you may want to explore?

## REFERENCES

Alaradi, O., & Barkin, J. S. (2002). Irritable bowel syndrome: Update on pathogenesis and management. *Medical Principles and Practices, 11*(1), 2–17.

Aoyama, N., Kinoshita, Y., Fujimoto, S., et al. (1998). Peptic ulcers after the hanshin-Awaji earthquake increased incidence of bleeding gastric ulcers. *American Journal of Gastroenterology, 93*, 311–316.

Camilleri, M. (2001). Management of irritable bowel syndrome. *Gastroenterology, 120*(3), 1527–1528.

Centers for Disease Control and Prevention. (2004). Fact Sheet for Health Professionals. http://www.cdc.gov/nchs/hus.htm.

Cohen, S., & Parkman, H. P. (2000). Diseases of the esophagus. In L. Goldman & J. C. Bennett (Eds.), *Cecil textbook of medicine* (21st ed.). Philadelphia: W. B. Saunders.

Cutler, A. F. (2001, April 15). Eradicating *Helicobacter pylori* infection. *Patient Care*, pp. 91, 92, 94, 97–100.

Dent, J. (2001). The role of the specialist in the diagnosis and short and long term care of patients with gastroesophageal reflux disease. *American Journal of Gastroenterology, 96*(Suppl), S22–S26.

Gaster, B., & Larson, A. (2000). Chronic hepatitis C: Common questions, practical answers. *Journal of the American Board of Family Practice, 13*(5), 359–363.

Ghosh, S., Shand, A., & Ferguson, A. (2000). Ulcerative colitis. *British Medical Journal, 320*(7242), 1119–1123.

Hoofnagle, J. H., & Lindsay, K. L. (2000). Acute viral hepatitis. In L. Goldman & J. C. Bennett (Eds.), *Cecil textbook of medicine* (21st ed., pp. 783–790). Philadelphia: W. B. Saunders.

Ireton-Jones, C., George, M. B., Day, L., & Zeiter, T. (2000). Case problem: Medical nutrition therapy for a patient with Crohn's disease/Response. *Journal of the American Dietetic Association, 100*(4), 472–475.

Janket, S. J., Qvarnstrom, M., Meurman, J. H., Baird, A. E., Nuutinen, P., & Jones, J. A. (2004). Asymptotic dental score and prevalent coronary heart disease. *Circulation, 109*(9), 1095–1100.

Lagergren, J., Bergstro, M. R., Lingren, A., et al. (1999). Symptomatic gastroesophageal reflux as a risk factor for esophageal adenocarcinoma. *New England Journal of Medicine, 340*, 825–831.

Laird, T. W. (1999). Peptic ulcer disease. *Physician Assistant, 23*(2), 14–33.

Levenstein, S. (1998). Stress and peptic ulcer life beyond Helicobacter. *British Medical Journal, 316*, 538–541.

Levenstein, S., Ackerman, S., Kiecolt-Glaser, J. K., & Dubois, A. (1999). Stress and peptic ulcer disease. *Journal of the American Medical Association, 281*(1), 10–11.

Lindsay, K. L., & Hoofnagle, J. H. (2000). Chronic hepatitis. In L. Goldman & J. C. Bennett (Eds.), *Cecil textbook of medicine* (21st ed., pp. 790–796). Philadelphia: W. B. Saunders.

Lox, A. S. F. (2002). Chronic hepatitis B. *New England Journal of Medicine, 346*(22), 1682–1683.

Mach, T. (2004). The brain-gut axis in irritable bowel syndrome: Clinical aspects. *Medical Science Monitor, 10*(6), RA125–RA131.

Meining, A., & Classen, M. (2000). The role of diet and lifestyle measures in the pathogenesis and treatment of gastroesophageal reflux disease. *American Journal of Gastroenterology, 95*(10), 2692–2697.

Nice, D. S., Garland, C. F., Hilton, S. M., Baggett, J. C., & Mitchell, R. E. (1996). Long-term health outcomes and medical effects of torture among U.S. Navy prisoners of war in Vietnam. *Journal of the American Medical Association, 276*, 375–381.

Podolsky, D. K. (2002). Inflammatory bowel disease. *New England Journal of Medicine, 347*(6), 417–429.

Ringel, Y., Sperber, A. D., & Drossman, D. A. (2001). Irritable bowel syndrome. *Annual Review of Medicine, 52*, 319–338.

Sach, J.A., and Chang, L. (2002). Irritable Bowel Syndrome. *Current Treatment Options Gastroenterology, 5*(4), 267-278.

Seidel, S. A., Newman, M., & Sharp, K. W. (2000). Ileoanal pouch versus ileostomy: Is there a difference in quality of life? *American Surgeon, 66*(6), 540–548.

Shanahan, F. (2003). Crohn's disease. *Science and Medicine, 9*(1), 48–58.

Suerbaum, S., & Michetti, P. (2002). *Helicobacter pylori* infection. *New England Journal of Medicine, 347*(15), 1175–1186.

Yates, W. R., & Gleason, O. (1998). Hepatitis C and depression. *Depression and Anxiety, 7*, 188–193.

Zuckerman, A. J., & Lavancy, D. (1999). Treatment options for chronic hepatitis. *British Medical Journal, 319*(7213), 799–800.

# CHAPTER 11

# Cardiovascular Conditions

## NORMAL STRUCTURE AND FUNCTION OF THE CARDIOVASCULAR SYSTEM

The *cardiovascular system* consists of the *heart* and a network of *blood vessels* that carry blood throughout the body. Blood vessels in the circulatory system are composed of:

- **arteries**, which carry *oxygenated* blood *away* from the heart
- **veins**, which carry *unoxygenated* blood *to* the heart
- small branching blood vessels (*arterioles* and *veniuoles*)
- tiny vessels called *capillaries*, which provide a link between arterioles and venules

The heart, acting as a pump, forces blood through two circuits. One circuit carries blood *to* and *from* the lungs (*pulmonary circulation*). The second circuit carries blood *throughout the body* (*systemic circulation*).

The heart is a strong and powerful muscle located somewhat to the left of the center of the chest. The heart muscle itself is called the **myocardium**. It is enclosed in an outer covering (the **pericardium**) consisting of two layers. The space between the two layers of the pericardium contains a small amount of fluid to lessen friction between the two surfaces as the heart beats. The inner surface of the heart is called the **endocardium**. The *myocardium*

is a special type of muscle that has the ability to work continuously with only brief periods of rest between contractions. This resting period, when the heart is relaxed and the chambers are filling, is called *diastole*. The pumping action, or contraction, of the heart muscle is called *systole*. Diastole and systole produce different pressure gradients. The ratio of these two pressures is called *blood pressure*. The amount of pressure produced is dependent on the force with which the heart pumps and the degree to which the blood vessels resist blood flow. Blood pressure is expressed numerically as a fraction, with the systolic reading being the numerator and the diastolic reading being the denominator. For instance, in a blood pressure reading of 120/80, the systolic pressure is 120 and the diastolic pressure is 80.

Like all muscles of the body, the myocardium requires oxygen and nutrients to survive. A separate network of blood vessels called the *coronary vessels* supplies the heart muscle with blood. The coronary vessels consist of **coronary arteries**, which carry oxygen and nutrients *to* the heart muscle, and **coronary veins**, which carry blood used by the heart muscle and containing waste *away from* the heart muscle. Without the blood flow supplied directly to the myocardium, the heart is unable to carry out its function of pumping blood to the rest of the body.

The heart contains four chambers. The two upper chambers are the right and left

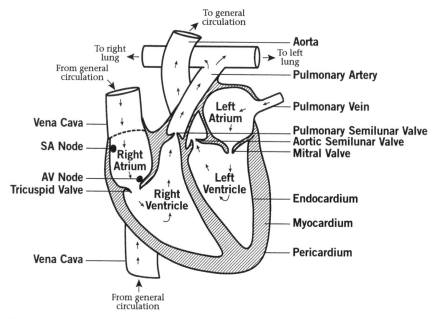

**Figure 11–1**  The Heart. SA, sinoatrial; AV, atrioventricular.

**atria**, and the two lower chambers are the right and left **ventricles**. Four valves help blood move from chamber to chamber in one direction without backflow. Between the right atrium and the right ventricle is the *tricuspid valve*. Between the left atrium and left ventricle is the *mitral (biscuspid)* valve. The *right atrium* receives *deoxygenated blood* from the systemic circulation through a large vein called the *vena cava*. The deoxygenated blood is pumped from the right atrium to the *right ventricle* through the *tricuspid valve*. Blood is then pumped from the right ventricle through the *pulmonary (semilunar) valve* to the pulmonary artery, where it is carried to the lungs (*pulmonary circulation*). The pulmonary artery is the only artery in the body that carries deoxygenated blood. In the lungs, waste in the form of carbon dioxide is released from the blood and excreted from the lungs. Oxygen is taken into the blood from the lungs and the oxygenated blood is then pumped back to the heart through

a vessel called the *pulmonary vein* (the only vein in the body that carries oxygenated blood). Oxygenated blood enters the left atrium of the heart, moves through the *mitral valve* to the left ventricle, and then is pumped out of the heart through the *aortic (semilunar) valve* to a large blood vessel called the *aorta*, which carries it to the *systemic circulation*. (See Figure 11–1.)

Blood carries oxygen and nutrients to all parts of the body through blood vessels in the *peripheral circulation* (outside the heart). Arteries diminish in size as they progress farther away from the heart, eventually leading to tiny vessels called capillaries. Capillary walls are very thin, allowing for the exchange of oxygen and nutrients from the blood with waste products from body tissues. Blood containing waste products is then carried back to the heart through small blood vessels that increase in size until they reach the *vena cava*, which returns to the heart, and the process begins all over again.

A special nerve conduction system in the heart maintains its regular, rhythmic beating. Special cells called the *sinoatrial (SA) node* (also called the pacemaker of the heart), located within the right atrium, initiate the contractions. Impulses from the SA node spread over both atria, causing them to contract simultaneously. The impulse then reaches special cells in the lower right atrium, the *atrioventricular (AV) node.* From the AV node, impulses are transferred to special muscle fibers (*bundle of His*) located on the right and left side of the septum separating the two ventricles. The bundles branch out to small branches (Purkinje fibers), which spread over both ventricles, causing them to contract. At this point, the cycle starts over. Conduction of these nerve impulses throughout the heart occurs involuntarily. Through communication from the central nervous system, the heart adjusts to the changing needs of the body, speeding or slowing the heart rate as needed.

## CARDIOVASCULAR CONDITIONS

### Arteriosclerosis (Atherosclerosis)

The general term *arteriosclerosis* refers to conditions in which walls of the arteries become thickened or less elastic, obstructing circulation and diminishing blood flow to various parts of the body. It is caused by buildup of plaque along the interior vessel wall, which causes **stenosis** (narrowing) of the vessel, impeding blood flow. Symptoms of arteriosclerosis develop slowly and are generally nonexistent until blood flow is diminished to the extent that oxygen supply to a body part is hampered. At this point individuals may experience pain, fatigue, or altered function in the body part affected.

Plaque can also contribute to **thrombus** (blood clot) formation within the nar-

rowed vessel, blocking blood flow even more. Tissue death can occur if all blood flow to a body part is obliterated. A thrombus can be dangerous even when blood flow isn't totally blocked because it can become an **embolus** if it becomes dislodged from the vessel wall and begins traveling in the bloodstream. (The term *embolus* can also refer to other substances traveling in the blood, such as an air bubble, fat globule, or other foreign matter.) The embolus can lodge in a blood vessel too small to allow its passage, thus occluding blood flow. The effects of an **embolism** depend on the body part affected. For example, an embolism of the brain results in stroke, whereas an embolism in a coronary artery causes **myocardial infarction** (heart attack). An embolus lodging in the lungs would be called a *pulmonary embolus.* In all instances, embolism can result in severe tissue damage and can be fatal.

Symptoms experienced by individuals with arteriosclerosis vary depending on the extent of stenosis of the vessels and the location of the impeded blood flow. For example, cognitive changes can result when blood flow to the brain is decreased, such as in *carotid artery stenosis* (narrowing of the vessels carrying blood directly to the brain). A decreased blood flow to the kidneys may contribute to kidney damage, causing chronic renal failure. Decreased blood flow to the heart may cause **angina pectoris** (chest pain) or, if blood flow is severely restricted, heart attack.

Treatment of arteriosclerosis is directed at the complications the condition causes, such as angina pectoris, arrhythmias, myocardial infarction, and stroke (see Chapter 2), kidney failure (see Chapter 13), and peripheral vascular disease (described later in this chapter). Since nicotine further constricts vessels already narrowed in arteriosclerosis, individuals with arteriosclerotic disease should avoid tobacco use.

## Aneurysm

An **aneurysm** is a dilation or ballooning out of a weakened arterial wall.

Although often associated with arteriosclerosis and hypertension, an aneurysm may also result from a congenital abnormality. The weakened wall of the artery, if under increased pressure (e.g., because of hypertension), may burst and lead to hemorrhage. Common sites of aneurysms are in the *brain* and the *aorta* (the major trunk of the arterial system of the body). A *dissecting aneurysm* is a tear in the inner wall of the vessel so that blood leaks between the layers of the wall of the vessel, moving longitudinally to separate the layers along the length of the vessel rather than rupturing into an open body space.

Symptoms experienced as a result of an aneurysm vary according to its location. In some instances, there are no symptoms until the aneurysm becomes large enough to create pressure, causing pain at the site. In other instances, there are no symptoms until the aneurysm ruptures, which could result in sudden death.

Aneurysms may be treated surgically if they are diagnosed early or if surgery is not contraindicated because of associated medical problems. Surgical procedures to correct aneurysms involve removing the weakened area of the artery and then connecting the two remaining ends. A graft to join the two remaining ends is used if a large portion of the vessel has been removed. Controlling hypertension, if present, is an important aspect of continuing treatment after surgery.

## Endocarditis

**Endocarditis** (inflammation of the membrane that covers the heart valves and chambers of the heart) is most often caused by an infection; however, it can also be the result of an immunological reaction. It is characterized by deposits of "vegetation" on the inner lining of the heart (the endocardium) and most frequently on the valves. Damage to the valves can result.

Endocarditis may be associated with systemic infectious diseases or intravenous drug abuse, or it may be a complication of an invasive medical procedure. Sometimes even minor trauma can precipitate the development of endocarditis. Most people have isolated incidents in which bacteria enter the bloodstream (**bacteremia**). Usually the body's own defenses overcome the organism with no untoward results. At times, however, because of the strength of the organism or the reduced effectiveness of the body's defenses, the organism settles on the inner lining of the heart, causing endocarditis.

Individuals with previous cardiac surgery, congenital heart disease, or conditions in which the heart valves have been damaged are more susceptible to development of endocarditis. Individuals with valve replacement (discussed later in the chapter), and especially those with prosthetic valves, are also at higher risk for endocarditis (Levinson, 2000).

Symptoms of endocarditis may be insidious at first, mimicking the flu. As the disease progresses, symptoms such as high fever, weight loss, and extreme fatigue become more pronounced. The condition is diagnosed based on history and symptoms, blood culture, and echocardiogram (discussed later in the chapter). Treatment consists of administering appropriate antibiotics to eradicate the infection before serious complications develop. When severe valvular dysfunction results, surgical replacement of the valve may be necessary.

Complications of endocarditis include **embolism** (obstruction of a blood vessel by a foreign substance), in which some of the vegetation from the affected valve breaks away and occludes a blood vessel in another part of the body. Any organ or part of the body can be affected. Depending on the part of the body affected and the extent of the resulting damage, embolism can result in death.

## Pericarditis

Inflammation of the outer layer of the heart (**pericardium**) is known as **pericarditis**. Most commonly, pericarditis is caused by a virus (Manning, 2000). When inflamed, the pericardial layers can adhere to each other, creating friction as their surfaces rub together during cardiac contraction. The most common symptom is chest pain that is aggravated by moving and breathing because of the rubbing together of the two inflamed surfaces. A low-grade fever may also be present.

Diagnosis is often based on symptoms, physical examination, and at times an *electrocardiogram (ECG)*, which is discussed later in the chapter. Treatment of pericarditis is directed toward alleviating the pain caused by inflammation of the pericardium. Medications such as *nonsteroidal antiinflammatory agents* are commonly used.

Severe inflammation of the pericardium can result in accumulation of excessive fluid within the pericardial sac, a condition known as *pericardial effusion*. Excess fluid in the sac surrounding the heart may constrict the myocardium, causing cardiac dysfunction. If constriction of the heart is severe because of increasing amounts of fluid, a condition called **cardiac tamponade** (severe constriction of the heart that prevents it from filling and emptying properly) may occur. A procedure called **pericardiocentesis** may be performed during which the physician inserts a needle into the pericardial sac to drain the fluid. After severe inflammation, the peri-cardium may become scarred, further constricting cardiac function (*constrictive pericarditis*). This rare condition may need to be treated surgically so that a portion of the pericardium is removed.

## Rheumatic Heart Disease

*Rheumatic heart disease* is a type of heart condition brought about by a condition called *rheumatic fever*. Rheumatic fever is an inflammatory condition that occurs as a type of allergic reaction elicited by an organism called *streptococcus*. Since not everyone develops rheumatic fever after a streptococcal infection, the reason for the allergic type of reaction in some individuals is unknown.

Recovery from rheumatic fever can be complete with no residual effects; however, some individuals experience permanent cardiac damage as a result. Valves of the heart are most frequently affected, resulting in **stenosis** (narrowing), insufficiency, or regurgitation, as described later in the chapter under valvular heart disease.

## Hypertension

Individuals with *hypertension* have a sustained elevation of pressure in the arteries. Both *systolic* and *diastolic* pressure may be elevated. Blood pressure normally fluctuates with physical activity, becoming lower at rest and higher with changes in posture, exercise, or emotion. Individuals whose blood pressure remains high even at rest put increased strain on body organs. This prolonged elevation of pressure can eventually damage other organs, such as the heart, kidneys, or brain. Although this **hypertension** (high blood pressure) in and of itself is not disabling, it is a major health problem because of its associated high risk of myocardial infarction (heart attack), stroke, renal failure, and congestive heart failure, all of which cause significant disability (August, 2003; Oparil, 2000).

The most common type of hypertension is *primary*, or *essential*, *hypertension*, which has a gradual onset and few, if any, symptoms. The exact cause of primary hypertension is unknown. At other times hypertension is a symptom of another medical condition, such as kidney disease, endocrine disorders, neurological disorders, or drug use or abuse. This type of hypertension is called *secondary hypertension*. A less common, but more severe, type of hypertension is *malignant hypertension*, which has an abrupt onset, more severe symptoms, and more associated complications.

Often, primary hypertension is discovered for the first time during a routine physical examination. Because symptoms of hypertension are often vague or even nonexistent, hypertension may go undetected until complications such as heart attack, stroke, or visual problems arise (Glasser, 2001; Setness, 2001). Accurate measurement of blood pressure and verification of elevated blood pressure on several occasions are the chief ways hypertension is diagnosed. Hypertension is most accurately diagnosed when blood pressure is measured under similar conditions over a period of time. Since blood pressure fluctuates throughout the day or may be higher when measured in a health care setting than it would be at home, ambulatory 24-hour blood pressure monitoring is gaining recognition as a more accurate appraisal of blood pressure throughout the day (White, 2003).

The primary goal of treatment of hypertension is to lower blood pressure and reduce the risk of complications such as heart attack, stroke, or kidney failure. In mild cases of hypertension, lifestyle modifications such as maintaining a proper body weight, engaging in exercise, cutting down on alcohol intake, ceasing to use tobacco, and limiting fats, red meat,

sweets, and sodium may be sufficient to lower blood pressure (Appel, Moore, Obarzanek, et al., 1997; Sacks, Svetkey, Vollmer, et al., 2001). Although stress itself may not directly cause primary hypertension, emotional stress does cause physiologic changes that raise the blood pressure. Learning how to reduce stress, or learning to avoid chronic stressful situations, may also be important in the overall treatment of hypertension.

When lifestyle modification is insufficient to control hypertension or when blood pressure is too elevated to control with lifestyle modification alone, an important aspect of treatment is medication. A variety of medications, called *antihypertensives*, are prescribed to control high blood pressure. However, these can also cause a variety of side effects that can interfere with individuals' willingness to take the medication as prescribed.

### Psychosocial Issues in Hypertension

Although there usually are no symptoms associated with primary hypertension, the consequences of untreated hypertension can be severe, including end-stage renal disease, **myocardial infarction** (heart attack), or stroke. Consequently, treatment of hypertension is essential to preventing disability and/or death. Individuals with hypertension frequently experience few symptoms, so there may be less motivation to follow treatment. Treatment also often involves lifestyle changes that individuals may have difficulty accomplishing, such as weight loss, smoking cessation, or exercise. Consequently, they may not comply with treatment and medical recommendations that could help them prevent complications and further disability.

Compliance is defined as the degree to which individuals' behavior corresponds to the medical advice and instructions given. In treatment of hypertension, compliance includes not only taking medications prescribed, but also keeping scheduled medical appointments and making recommended lifestyle changes. Identifying the potential problems that contribute to noncompliance and working toward solutions to overcome them can be beneficial.

### Vocational Issues in Hypertension

There are usually no specific limitations associated with hypertension per se; however, isometric activities such as pushing, lifting, or carrying heavy objects can increase blood pressure during the activity and may need to be avoided. Some degree of emotional stress is inherent in many jobs; however, chronic, sustained stress may also have a detrimental effect on blood pressure. Individuals should either be assisted in learning to manage the stress they experience on the job or should seek ways of modifying the work environment to make it less stressful. The major impact hypertension has on employment is the disability that can occur if it is uncontrolled. Consequently, reinforcing adherence to medical recommendations is of major importance to ongoing employment.

## Coronary Artery Disease: Angina Pectoris and Myocardial Infarction

**Coronary artery disease** is a condition in which the coronary arteries that supply blood and oxygen directly to the heart muscle (**myocardium**) become narrowed. The condition is usually caused by **atherosclerosis**, in which plaque builds up on the inner walls of the blood vessels that supply the heart muscle. Buildup of plaque may narrow the coronary arteries to the extent that insufficient blood passes through the arteries to meet the oxygen demands of the heart muscle (**ischemia**). Lack of oxygen to the heart muscle results in chest pain (**angina pectoris**). Since the heart muscle's need for oxygen is greatest when demands are placed on the heart, angina pain is often triggered by physical activity. Decreasing the activity and thus decreasing the workload of the heart often causes the chest pain to subside. This type of angina is called *stable angina*. When chest pain occurs at rest, with no precipitating activity, or when pain is more severe, more frequent, or more prolonged, individuals are said to have *unstable angina*. Diagnosis of angina is based on symptoms, *laboratory evaluations*, an *electrocardiogram* (ECG) (recording of electrical activity of the heart) or *exercise electrocardiogram* (stress test), or an *echocardiogram* (discussed later in the chapter).

The heart muscle, like all other muscles, cannot live without oxygen. When the myocardium receives *no* oxygen (**anoxia**), **necrosis** (tissue death) of part of the heart muscle occurs. This is called a **myocardial infarction** (heart attack), which means there has been death of part of the heart muscle. Myocardial infarction may occur anytime the blood supply to the heart muscle is insufficient. Not all individuals with angina go on to develop myocardial infarctions, and not all people with myocardial infarctions have first experienced angina, where there is only *diminished* blood supply and oxygen to the heart. Total occlusion of a coronary vessel so that the heart muscle receives no blood supply can occur because of:

- **atherosclerosis**, in which the coronary arteries become totally occluded

- a **thrombus** (blood clot) that has formed in a coronary artery, occluding blood flow

- an **embolus** (blood clot, a particle of vegetation from a diseased valve, or other foreign material that has traveled through the bloodstream) that has lodged in a coronary artery, occluding blood flow

Once a portion of the heart muscle has been destroyed, it cannot regenerate. The ability of the heart to continue functioning as a pump is directly related to the amount of heart muscle damage that has occurred. Myocardial infarction can result in **arrhythmia** (irregular heartbeat), *congestive heart failure* (discussed later in the chapter), or death. Individuals with myocardial infarction often experience pressure in the chest and chest pain that is not relieved by reducing activity. Myocardial infarction is a medical emergency and can be fatal. Consequently, immediate medical attention is required.

Myocardial infarction is diagnosed by the individuals' *symptoms* and by ECG and *laboratory determinations*, which also help physicians determine the most appropriate treatment.

### Treatment of Angina Pectoris and Myocardial Infarction

#### Angina Pectoris

Treatment of angina pectoris includes measures to reduce symptoms and prevent **myocardial infarction** (heart attack), as well as surgical measures to correct the cause. Treatment includes modification of ongoing risk factors, medication, and evaluation of the need for surgical intervention. Cessation of tobacco use, treatment of **hypertension** (high blood pressure), and weight loss, if obesity exists, are important ways to modify risk. Angina pectoris may be helped by *nitroglycerin*, a medication that dilates the coronary arteries and enables the heart muscle to receive more oxygen, thus relieving chest pain.

When angina pain occurs so frequently that limitation of activity becomes severely debilitating, or when occlusion of the coronary arteries becomes so pronounced that myocardial infarction is imminent, surgery may be indicated. One procedure used to enlarge a narrowed coronary artery is *coronary angioplasty* (*percutaneous transluminal coronary angioplasty, PTCA*). In this procedure, a long catheter with a balloon on its tip is guided into the coronary artery. The balloon is then inflated, compressing the occluding material against the vessel wall. The vessel is dilated as the inflated catheter tip is withdrawn, thus increasing the blood flow to the myocardium. Although helpful for some, the procedure may not be appropriate for all individuals. Individuals may also have a *coronary artery bypass graft* (*CABG*) to relieve narrowing or constriction of the coronary arteries. A graft, usually a vein from the individual's leg, is used to bypass an obstructed coronary artery. Often, several coronary arteries are constricted, and more than one graft is needed. The bypass increases the myocardium's blood supply, thus potentially increasing individuals' ability to engage in activity.

#### Myocardial Infarction

Myocardial infarction, a potentially life-threatening condition, requires immediate medical attention. Individuals usually receive initial treatment in the emergency department, where the focus is on assessing the condition, stabilizing the condition, relieving pain, and preventing sudden death. In the initial stages of myocardial infarction, pain may be treated with narcotics, *thrombolytic drugs* may be given to dissolve clots, *anticoagulants* may be given to decrease the likelihood of further clot formation, and oxygen may be given to decrease **hypoxemia** (lowered oxygen in the blood).

After emergency department treatment, individuals are usually hospitalized in a hospital unit called a coronary care unit (CCU), which specializes in critical care of individuals with cardiovascular conditions. The goal of treatment in the CCU is to limit the size of heart damage, promote the electrical stability of the heart, promote comfort, and prevent additional damage to the heart muscle. Here individuals are monitored for life-threatening **arrhythmias** (irregular heartbeat) and also receive continued pharmacologic and medical treatment directed to these treatment goals. Some individuals also undergo surgical revascularization procedures (PTCA or CABG ) as described above.

Cardiac rehabilitation is crucial in the treatment of myocardial infarction so that individuals can improve their exercise capacity, return to work, and reduce the risk of mortality. Most cardiac rehabilitation programs include educational sessions to help individuals achieve necessary lifestyle changes, including dietary restrictions, smoking cessation, and graduated exercise training, to help them reach their maximum activity level and functional capacity. Psychological and vocational counseling are also important components of cardiac rehabilitation programs.

After a cardiac event, the degree of disability and the type of activities in which individuals can engage are based on the energy expended to perform the activity. Energy is expressed in terms of calories per minute and is based on the equivalent of one liter of oxygen equaling five calories. Prior to exercise training, individuals undergo testing to assess their functional capacity so that an appropriate level of activity may be prescribed. Functional capacity is estimated in METs (*metabolic equivalents*). The MET is the unit or level used to estimate the oxygen requirements to perform a task. This measure helps to determine the energy cost (in terms of oxygen consumption) of physical activities and provides a method for describing the functional capacity or exercise tolerance of individuals and the physical activity level in which they can participate safely. The degree of activity individuals may participate in after a cardiac event is determined by an exercise test that focuses on the symptoms and signs shown during exercise. Different types of activity have been classified in terms of how many METs are required. MET requirements range from one (the amount of oxygen an individual consumes at rest while awake) to nine for the heaviest tasks (such as shoveling heavy snow or carrying items over 90 pounds).

### Psychosocial Issues in Angina Pectoris and Myocardial Infarction

The pain associated with angina pectoris, as well as limited activity and the anxiety caused by fear of potential heart attack, can limit the individual's ability to participate in a number of activities. As a result, individuals may experience low self-esteem and depression.

Stresses experienced as a result of myocardial infarction are greatly influenced by individuals' psychological reactions to the heart attack. When individuals have a myocardial infarction, the realization that death could have occurred as well as the realization of the unpredictability and threat of sudden death can precipitate severe depression or anxiety, which can result in emotional disability. In the early stages of recovery from myocardial infarction, denial may be positive because it helps individuals reduce the emotional distress associated with the knowledge that their condition is potentially life-threatening (Livneh, 1999). As individuals progress in recovery, however, denial may become detrimental if they deny the seriousness of the heart attack and fail to alter their lifestyle or to follow other treatment recommendations.

The life-threatening nature of myocardial infarction may cause a variety of reactions in family members, which in turn affect individuals' adjustment to their condition. Because of overwhelming anxiety about the possibility that another myocardial infarction might occur, family members can overprotect the individual, inhibiting his or her return to full functional capacity. The extent to which family members believe individuals contributed to the development of their condition by engaging in activities viewed as precursors of heart disease, such as by smoking, following an improper diet, or eating to the point of obesity, may further influence relationships. Family members may express anger, resentment, or frustration or blame individuals for their behavior. In turn, individuals who have had a myocardial infarction may experience guilt, low self-esteem, and self-blame.

Sexual readjustment after myocardial infarction may also be an issue. Depression and lowered self-esteem may contribute to sexual dysfunction. In addition, some medications commonly prescribed after myocardial infarction may impair sexual function. Individuals and/or their partners may be especially anxious about engaging in sexual activity after a heart attack, fearing that sexual activity is too stressful and may precipitate another heart attack and possibly sudden death. Education and appropriate counseling, as well as reassurance, may be necessary to help individuals and their partners lessen their fears.

### *Vocational Issues in Angina Pectoris and Myocardial Infarction*

Most individuals after appropriate cardiac rehabilitation are able to return to moderate levels of activity; these are determined through a medical evaluation of the energy cost of various activities, as described previously. Work activity should not exceed individuals' limits. For the most part, isometric activities are avoided because of the additional stress they place on the heart. Because of stress that extreme temperatures place on the heart, work environments with controlled temperatures are preferable. The amount of stress experienced on the job as well as the individual's response to it should also be considered.

### Cardiac Arrhythmia

An **arrhythmia** is an abnormality of the heart rate or rhythm. A dysfunction in the heart's electrical conduction system causes irregularities in its rhythm and/or rate. Arrhythmias decrease the heart's ability to work effectively and to supply adequate amounts of blood to all of the body's organs. The heart may beat too fast (**tachycardia**), too slowly (**bradycardia**), or irregularly (**dysrhythmia** or **arrhythmia**).

There are many different causes of arrhythmia and many different types. Types of arrythmias are usually named for the type of disorder or the part of the electrical impulse system that is affected. For example, a *sinus bradycardia* indicates that there is an abnormally slow rhythm arising in the *SA node* of the heart, whereas an *AV block* describes an arrhythmia in which electrical impulses are blocked at the *AV junction*. Some arrhythmias may be the cause of significant disability (such as *atrial fibrillation*, which can cause stroke), some may be life-threatening (such as *ven-*

*tricular fibrillation*), and others may be relatively minor and require little or no treatment.

The symptoms individuals experience with arrhythmia depend on the type and extent of the arrhythmia. Individuals may, for example, experience **palpitations** (in which they feel the heartbeat), **exertional dyspnea** (shortness of breath with activity), fatigue, **vertigo** (dizziness), or **syncope** (fainting). Severe or prolonged arrhythmia can result in sudden death.

### Treatment of Arrhythmia

Treatment depends on the underlying condition. It is directed toward correcting or controlling the factors causing the arrhythmia. Some arrhythmias may be prevented by avoiding stimulants such as caffeine or avoiding alcohol.

#### Medications

Medications called *antiarrhythmics* regulate the heartbeat and are often a central part of treatment. Other medications useful in the control of arrhythmia are *digitalis* preparations, *beta blockers*, and medications called *calcium channel blockers*. Because certain types of arrhythmias (e.g., *atrial flutter*) can contribute to **thrombus** (blood clot) formation and possible **embolus** (traveling blood clot), some individuals may also need to be on *anticoagulant* medications (Hart, 2003).

In more severe arrhythmia, an electrical shock procedure called *cardioversion* may be indicated to return the heart to a normal rhythm. For individuals with a severe, recurrent arrhythmia that could result in a life-threatening arrhythmia (e.g., *ventricular tachycardia*, which can become *ventricular fibrillation*), a device called an *implantable automatic defibrillator* may be surgically implanted. The defibrillator delivers an electric shock automatically to the heart when an arrhythmia occurs (see the following section).

#### Pacemakers and Implantable Defibrillators

When the heart's ability to maintain an effective rate or rhythm is altered, an artificial cardiac pacemaker may be used to stimulate the electrical activity of the heart and to maintain function. Implantable pacemakers and defibrillators are undergoing rapid evolution (Cooper, Katcher, & Orlov, 2002) and can not only decrease the incidence of potentially fatal arrhythmias, but can also enhance quality of life for those with problem arrhythmias (Newman, Dorian, Schwartzman, et al., 2000). The pacemaker consists of a battery-operated pulse generator and a lead wire with an electrode tip. One end of the lead wire is inserted into a vessel and advanced into the individual's heart; the other end is connected to the generator. The generator then sends out an electrical stimulus to the heart muscle. The generator may be external if the need for pacing is only temporary. If the pacemaker is to be permanent, a small battery-operated generator is placed under the skin and fatty tissue of the upper chest or lower thoracic area.

There are various types of pacemakers. They are usually classified according to the chamber of the heart that is being stimulated, the chamber of the heart that is being monitored, and the response that the pacemaker is expected to deliver. The classification system uses a three-letter code to describe pacemaker function. The first letter of the code signifies the chamber being stimulated, the second letter indicates the chamber being monitored, and the third letter indicates the pacemaker response. For example, a code VVI would indicate that a ventricle is being both stimulated and monitored. The *I* stands for "inhibited response," indicating that the pacemaker will not allow impulses from the atria to stimulate the ventricle.

There are several modes of pacing that pacemakers are designed to deliver. The oldest type of pacing, *fixed rate*, is rarely used today. In this type of pacing, the pacemaker is set to fire at a fixed rate, usually about 70 beats per minute, and is unaffected by the heart's own rhythm. Another type of pacing, demand or *standby*, is accomplished with a pacemaker that has a special sensing circuit that is set at a specific rate. When the individual's own conduction system in the heart falls below that specific rate, the artificial pacemaker fires. Other types of pacing, namely, *synchronous* and *bifocal*, use pacemakers that are programmed in similar ways to monitor and deliver specific types of impulses.

The mode of pacing is determined on an individual basis according to the individual's specific arrhythmia. Physicians determine the type of pacemaker to be used and the amplitude of the stimulus based on the individual's condition. For most individuals, even permanent pacemakers may be inserted under local anesthesia with mild sedation.

Complications related to implantation of a pacemaker are rare, but they can include **pneumothorax** (collapse of the lung), dislodgement, inflammation, or infection of the surrounding area (Morady, 2000). The level of activity individuals with a pacemaker can engage in depends on the underlying disease process, age, and the degree of cardiac functional capacity. Normal daily activities can usually be resumed 6 weeks after the implantation of the pacemaker. Activities that could expose the internal pacemaker to a blow, such as contact sports, should be avoided. Although driving may be restricted for a short time after the pacemaker is inserted, most individuals can begin driving in approximately a month if the pacemaker is functioning well.

Individuals who have a pacemaker should at all times wear identification, such as *Medic Alert*, or should carry a card containing information about the type of pacemaker, the date of implant, and the pacemaker's programming. Because the pacemaker's generator is battery-operated, failure of the battery means that the heart returns to beating at its previously abnormal rate or rhythm. Individuals with pacemakers should be aware of the signs of battery depletion, such as a change in the cardiac rate or the appearance of symptoms similar to those experienced before the pacemaker was inserted. The length of time that a battery lasts depends on the model and can vary from one to several years. A physician should evaluate the pacemaker's function regularly. Periodic evaluations may be conducted with special telephone monitoring in which information about the pacemaker's function is transmitted over regular telephone lines to a special device in the physician's office.

Electromagnetic interference with permanent pacemakers and implantable defibrillators may have deleterious effects (Santucci, Haw, Trohman, & Pinski, 1998). Although the shielding around battery-operated generators has been improved significantly, individuals who wear these devices should be aware of possible interference from a variety of external electrical signals in the environment. Since implantable defibrillators are designed to be more sensitive to intracardiac electrical activity, their sensitivity to electromagnetic interference may be increased. Microwave ovens, radar installations, arc welding devices, antitheft devices, cellular phones, and other sources of electrical signals may interfere with pacemaker signals. The pacemaker may also set off metal detection devices installed at airports.

### Psychosocial Issues in Arrhythmia

The psychosocial impact of arrhythmia can be significant. Fearful of triggering a potentially fatal arrhythmia, individuals may curtail many activities related to both work and leisure. In many instances, the fear and anxiety may be more disabling than the arrhythmia itself.

Since arrhythmias can be triggered by caffeine, alcohol, or tobacco use, individuals may also need to modify their life to some extent. Commitment to lifestyle changes varies with the degree to which individuals accept and understand the condition and the necessity for treatment. Individuals who become extremely anxious about their condition may cope by employing denial as a way of decreasing the level of stress. If individuals are in denial, rather than making the necessary lifestyle changes, they may continue activities that could have serious consequences.

### Vocational Issues in Arrhythmia

Any activity that has been identified by the individual as triggering arrhythmia should be avoided. Avoiding excessive emotional stress and learning to manage it may be important components of the individual's ability to continue to perform adequately at work without danger of precipitating an arrhythmia. Individuals being treated with anticoagulants may need to be aware of the potential for excessive bleeding if injury should occur. Excessive anxiety about precipitating an arrhythmia can become disabling, immobilizing individuals and preventing them from carrying out normal tasks and activities. Individuals may develop chronic depression, which can further interfere with their ability to work.

Individuals with pacemakers may need to avoid activities (such as using an air hammer or shooting a rifle) that could potentially cause the pacemaker to dislodge because of vibrations on the side where the pacemaker is located. Individuals should avoid activities such as arc and resistance welding, the use of power tools, or contact with radar transmitters, which could cause the pacemaker to malfunction. A physician should clarify the level of activity allowed, and counseling may be indicated to help individuals deal with their fears and enhance their ability to perform work activities.

## Valvular Heart Conditions

Damage to the valves of the heart is most often the result of rheumatic fever (a condition caused by the body's immune response to a streptococcal infection) or **endocarditis** (inflammation of the inner membrane of the heart), although valvular abnormalities may also be congenital. Two types of problems generally occur. Valves may become weakened or floppy, permitting a backflow (*regurgitation*) of blood from the ventricle to the atria, or valves may become scarred, narrowing the valvular opening (**stenosis**) and causing an obstruction of blood flow from a chamber of the heart. Although some valvular conditions are minimal and may require little intervention, more extensive valvular damage places an increased burden on the heart and can lead to dysfunction of the myocardium, *congestive heart failure* (discussed later in the chapter), and, in some instances, sudden death.

### Types of Valvular Conditions

Valvular conditions are classified according to the nature of the abnormality and the valve affected. One type of valvular condition, **mitral prolapse**, refers to bulging of all or part of the mitral valve into the left atrium during ventricular contraction. *Mitral regurgitation, mitral insufficiency*, or *mitral incompetence* refers to the inadequate closing of the mitral valve, which allows blood to flow backward into the atria. **Mitral stenosis** refers to narrowing of the mitral valve, which obstructs the blood flow from the left atrium to the left ventricle. *Tricuspid regurgitation* and *tricuspid stenosis* are conditions similar to the regurgitation and stenosis conditions described above but occur on the right instead of the left side of the heart. The same process may affect the pulmonary or aortic valves.

Valvular defects of the aortic valve, such as *aortic stenosis* and *aortic regurgitation*, place additional loads on the left ventricle of the heart, possibly resulting in left ventricular heart failure. Symptoms of valvular disease vary in severity but often include fatigue, **dyspnea** (difficulty breathing), and **palpitations** (heartbeat perceptible to the individual).

### Treatment of Valvular Heart Conditions

Specific treatment depends on the severity of the problem. Some conditions may require individuals to avoid strenuous activity. Others require no treatment or may not necessitate taking any precautions. Damaged valves are more susceptible to infection. Consequently, prophylactic antibiotics may be given to prevent *endocarditis* when there is the chance for a generalized bacterial infection, such as after a dental extraction.

Severe damage to the valve may require surgery to open or replace the valve. Surgical interventions for valvular abnormalities are intended either to widen a valve that is narrowed or constricted or, in the case of valvular insufficiency or regurgitation, to replace a diseased valve with an artificial valve. Individuals with stenosis of a valve may undergo a procedure known as **valvuloplasty** in which the **stenosed** (narrowed) valve is dilated with a balloon that is inserted through a peripheral vessel.

When valves are replaced, artificial valves, which are mechanical, or valves made of tissue may be used. Mechanical valves are made entirely from synthetic materials, whereas tissue valves may be made from a combination of synthetic and biologic tissue. Mechanical valves require long-term anticoagulant therapy to prevent thrombus formation. Although tissue valves decrease the risk of clot development, they may not have the long-term durability of mechanical valves. Because prosthetic valves are more vulnerable to infection, individuals may need to take antibiotics before procedures in which infection is a risk (e.g., dental work).

## Congestive Heart Failure

When the heart muscle is weakened or damaged and it cannot pump an adequate amount of blood to the rest of the body, a condition called heart failure occurs. The causes of heart failure include **myocardial infarction** (heart attack); damage from substances toxic to the heart muscle (such as alcohol or other chemicals); *hypertension, arteriosclerosis*, or *valvular dysfunction*; or *lung disease* such as *emphysema*, all of which cause the heart to work harder. When the heart consistently must work harder to pump, over time it becomes enlarged (**hypertrophy**) and ineffective in its pumping action. As a result, fluid accumulates in the lungs, causing congestion, **dyspnea** (difficulty breathing), and difficulty breathing when lying down at night (**nocturnal dyspnea**). The decreased pumping action of the heart and the congestion in the lungs result in an inadequate supply of oxygen to the rest of the body. Individuals with heart failure may consequently also experience fatigue and physical weakness. If the oxygen supply to the brain is inadequate, cognitive changes may also be present. Because of insufficient pumping and circulation of blood, fluid may accumulate in the extremities, causing swelling (**edema**). Blood flow to the gastrointestinal system may be impaired, causing congestion with resulting **anorexia** (loss of appetite) or nausea and vomiting.

### Treatment of Congestive Heart Failure

Treatment of heart failure depends on the type and causes of the condition. It is usually directed toward controlling or correcting the cause of heart failure and toward alleviating the symptoms. Often, medications to lower blood pressure (**antihypertensives**) are prescribed. These medications decrease the vascular resistance, thus decreasing the amount of work that the heart must perform to circulate blood. Medications to help the heart muscle work more efficiently by increasing its pumping action (e.g., *digitalis preparations*) may also be prescribed. **Diuretics** (medications that help rid the body of excess fluid) and a low-salt diet to eliminate some of the excess fluid may also be part of the treatment plan.

### Psychosocial Issues in Congestive Heart Failure

Although some symptoms may be controlled, heart failure usually signifies the end stage of cardiovascular disease. Individuals with heart failure may experience depression and anxiety about their present and future situation. Symptoms of shortness of breath, fatigue, and edema of the extremities can severely limit activities and increase dependency on others, which

may in turn lower self-esteem. Since heart failure is frequently the result of the heart gradually losing its function, individuals also live with the knowledge that their condition can result in increasing disability and death. If individuals are candidates for cardiac transplant (discussed later in the chapter), uncertainty of whether a donor heart will be identified before the condition deteriorates even more may be another source of continuing stress for individuals and their families.

### Vocational Issues in Congestive Heart Failure

The extent to which individuals are able to continue to function in the work environment depends on the severity of the symptoms and the nature of the work. Individuals in sedentary occupations requiring limited activity will be able to function longer than individuals in occupations in which strenuous activity is required.

In general, emotional stress and physical demands on the job should be minimized as much as possible. Extremes in temperatures can put additional strain on the heart, and therefore temperature-controlled environments are better tolerated.

Congestive heart failure is often associated with gradual and progressive deterioration of cardiac function. Consequently, vocational goals may need to be short range to accommodate potential functional decline if it does occur.

## Peripheral Vascular Conditions

Disorders of the peripheral blood vessels (i.e., those in the extremities) can lead to damage of the tissues supplied by those vessels. When oxygen supply is inadequate because of the diminished blood flow, extremities feel cold and appear pale or **cyanotic** (blue). Pain is also characteristic when the oxygen supply is diminished.

### Peripheral Vascular Disease (Arteriosclerosis Obliterans)

When arteriosclerotic changes have narrowed or occluded the larger peripheral vessels, an adequate blood supply cannot reach tissues in the extremities.

Symptoms depend on the extent of the obstruction, the vessels involved, and whether alternate blood supply routes, called *collateral circulation*, have formed. Exercise requires increased demand for oxygen by muscles. Therefore, individuals who have a deficient blood supply to the muscles because of peripheral vascular disease may, with activities such as walking, experience aching, cramping, or fatigue of the muscles in the legs, a condition known as **intermittent claudication**. Stopping to rest decreases the muscles' need for oxygen and consequently relieves the pain. If the condition progresses, however, pain in the extremities may occur even at rest. In severe cases, the feet may become numb and cold, and ulcerations of the foot may appear. Surgical procedures, such as a *bypass graft* of the severely affected vessel, may restore vascularization to the extremity in selected cases. Since smoking constricts blood vessels, use of tobacco products should be avoided.

Because of the diminished blood supply in peripheral atherosclerotic disease, even tiny injuries in the extremities may become infected and not heal properly. If circulation becomes so severely impaired that **necrosis** (tissue death) results, amputation of the extremity may be necessary to prevent complications such as the spread of infection throughout the body.

### Thromboangiitis Obliterans (Burger's Disease)

*Thromboangiitis obliterans* is a rare condition of the small and medium-sized arteries and superficial veins of the extremities that causes diminished blood flow to the affected part. In contrast to peripheral atherosclerotic disease, thromboangiitis obliterans occurs predominantly in individuals between the ages of 20 and 40 who do not have significant atherosclerosis. Symptoms include numbness, tingling, and pain in the upper or lower extremities. Although the exact cause is unknown, thromboangiitis obliterans occurs almost exclusively in individuals who smoke. Consequently, the major treatment of the condition is to stop smoking. If individuals with thromboangiitis obliterans continue to smoke, the disease continues to progress and can ultimately require the amputation of affected extremities.

### Raynaud's Disease

*Raynaud's disease* is a condition in which spasms of the vessels in the fingers or toes impair the blood flow to those areas. Occasionally, the condition also affects the nose and the tongue. In most instances, the cause of the condition is unknown; however, it may be associated with other conditions, such as *rheumatoid arthritis* or *arteriosclerosis obliterans*. Attacks of vasospasm may last from minutes to hours, but they rarely last long enough to cause tissue death. Attacks result in color changes in fingers or toes, either *blanching* (white coloration) or **cyanosis** (blue coloration). Attacks may be precipitated by cold or emotional upsets.

If the Raynaud's phenomenon is secondary to another condition, treatment is directed toward the underlying disorder. In the majority of cases the cause is unknown, and treatment involves taking steps to prevent an attack from occurring, such as protecting oneself from the cold or avoiding emotional upsets. Smoking constricts the blood vessels; consequently, tobacco use should also be avoided. Treatment with biofeedback or the use of relaxation techniques may sometimes be helpful in reducing attacks.

### Venous Thrombosis (Thrombophlebitis; Phlebitis)

A common and potentially lethal complication of bedrest or inactivity is thrombophlebitis. In chronic illness or disability in which activity is limited, thrombophlebitis can be a serious complication causing additional disability or potentially death. **Phlebitis** is the inflammation of a vein. **Thrombophlebitis** is the inflammation of a vein with associated clot formation. Although phlebitis and thrombophlebitis can occur in any vein, they frequently occur in the veins of the lower extremities.

Individuals with thrombophlebitis may experience pain and tenderness in the affected area, especially if the lower extremity is affected. Individuals with loss of sensation as a result of spinal cord injury may be unaware of the condition, and consequently it may not be promptly treated. Other symptoms may include swelling and redness of the affected part, or at times, depending on the location of the inflammation, there may be no symptoms at all. If thrombophlebitis is unrecognized or inadequately treated, clots can break off and travel to the heart, lungs, or other parts of the body and lodge in a vessel, occluding blood supply to the body part. Depending on the location of the occlusion, individuals can experience stroke,

*myocardial infarction* (heart attack), or massive damage to whatever body part is affected. Treatment of phlebitis and thrombophlebitis is directed toward decreasing inflammation and preventing or dissolving clots through use of anticoagulants, antithrombotic agents, or anti-inflammatory agents. Bedrest is usually prescribed during therapy, along with medications that decrease clotting.

### Varicose Veins

When blood cannot be returned efficiently to the heart, backup of blood causes distention and congestion of the veins, or varicose veins. Anything causing stricture or pressure on the veins, such as prolonged standing, obesity, or constriction of the leg by circular garters, can aggravate the condition. Symptoms are a sensation of heaviness in the legs, fatigue, and, at times, pain. In mild cases, treatment may consist of using compression hosiery. Surgery to tie and strip the veins may be indicated when the condition involves severe pain or recurrent phlebitis.

### Vocational Issues in Peripheral Vascular Disease

Individuals with peripheral vascular conditions may be unable to stand for long periods of time or may be unable to walk without pain or muscle fatigue. Their stamina during these activities should be evaluated before they return to work. Environmental conditions, such as cold temperatures, or other factors that reduce blood supply to the extremities should be avoided. The potential for infection in the lower extremities because of inadequate blood supply necessitates avoiding work environments that contain hazards that could cause trauma to the feet or legs.

## DIAGNOSTIC PROCEDURES IN CARDIOVASCULAR CONDITIONS

In addition to a physical examination and medical history, a variety of tests are used to diagnose cardiovascular conditions. These tests may also provide information that is used to make treatment determinations or to evaluate treatment effectiveness.

### Chest Roentgenography (X-ray)

A noninvasive radiographic procedure, *roentgenography* (*X-ray*) makes it possible to visualize organs in the chest cavity on X-ray film. Films may show evidence of congestion or fluid in the lungs, **hypertrophy** (enlargement) of any of the heart's chambers, or other abnormalities in the chest cavity.

### Electrocardiography

An ECG is a graphic representation of electrical currents within the heart muscle. It is helpful in identifying abnormalities of the heart's rhythm, assessing the amount and location of damage to the cardiac muscle, determining whether the cardiac muscle is receiving an adequate supply of oxygen, and obtaining information about the effects of certain medications. An ECG is a painless, noninvasive procedure in which electrodes are placed externally on the skin and then connected to a special machine that transforms electrical impulses from the heart to a graphic printout that records the heart's activity. The ECG is usually performed in the physician's office, hospital, or other medical setting.

### Holter Monitor

The *Holter monitor* is a form of ECG in which several electrodes attached externally to the chest are connected to a small portable device that records the heart's activity. The device is worn on the shoulder or waist so that the individual can go about regular activities at home or work. The advantage of the Holter monitor is that the graphic reading of the heart's electrical impulses is continuous rather than being a one-time reading in a laboratory situation. Readings from the Holter monitor enable physicians to assess the heart's functioning during various normal activities throughout a 24-hour period or longer.

### Cardiac Stress Test

The *cardiac stress test* is a noninvasive exercise test that provides a graphic record of the heart's activity during forced exertion. It may be used diagnostically to determine the extent of cardiac disease. It can also be used as a basis for recommending either medical or surgical treatment, as well as for counseling individuals with cardiac disease about the type and amount of physical activity in which they may safely engage. The stress test is performed in a cardiology unit or clinic by a technician with a physician present.

Electrodes are placed externally on the chest and connected to an ECG monitor. The individual is then asked to step on a motor-driven treadmill or to sit on a stationary bicycle with an *ergometer*. Activity is begun slowly, with a gradual increase of pace. During this time, the physician or technician monitors the individual's ECG reading, pulse, and blood pressure. The test is stopped if the individual is no longer able to keep up the pace or develops chest pain, or if the physician determines that blood pressure, pulse, or ECG readings indicate excessive strain on the heart.

The stress test is performed in a controlled, laboratory environment. Consideration must also be given, however, to additional sources of stress, such as emotional stress, extremes in temperature, and physical terrain (such as steps or ramps), that may be present in the individual's natural or work environment and that may increase the heart's workload beyond that experienced in the laboratory situation.

## Angiography

When it is necessary to study one or more blood vessels, an invasive procedure called *angiography* (a series of X-ray pictures that define the size and shapes of vessels and/or organs) is used. An *angiogram* of the heart enables physicians to identify abnormalities in the size or shape of the vessels, the extent of narrowing or occlusion, and the sequence and time in which the vessels fill with blood.

Angiograms are named for the specific area of the body being studied. If arteries are being studied, the test is called an *arteriogram*. If veins are being studied, the test is called a *venogram*. If vessels of the heart are being studied, the test is called a *cardiac angiogram*. A radiologist (a physician who specializes in X-ray procedures) performs an angiogram. The procedure is usually done in the radiology department. During the procedure, a special catheter is placed into a vein in the arm or leg and dye is injected. At this time, a rapid series of X-rays are taken, enabling the physician to visualize the vessels.

## Echocardiography

Like the ECG, the *echocardiogram* is obtained by means of a noninvasive procedure. Ultrasound is used to record the size, motion, and composition of the heart and large vessels on an echocardiogram. A transducer converts sound waves to electrical signals, which are then recorded as visual images and displayed on a type of television screen called an *oscilloscope*. Images can be photographed for further evaluation by a *radiologist* or *cardiologist*. Echocardiograms are helpful for identifying and evaluating valvular defects or other structural abnormalities of the heart.

## Radionuclide Imaging

The procedure for *radionuclide imaging* begins with the intravenous injection of a radioactive substance that localizes in heart tissue. Multiple views of the heart are taken with a special camera. Additional views are repeated for comparison hours later. The procedure is most useful in evaluating the **myocardium** (heart muscle) or damage to the myocardial tissue. It may also be used to evaluate coronary artery disease or valvular disease. It can be performed with the individual either at rest or during exercise.

## Cardiac Catheterization

An invasive procedure, *cardiac catheterization*, is performed to study the chambers, valves, and blood supply to the heart. A catheter is passed into a vessel in an arm or a leg and then threaded into the heart. A special X-ray machine called a *fluoroscope* enables physicians to visualize the catheter advancing into the heart. When the catheter is in place, internal pressures in the heart are measured. Dye is then injected into the catheter, allowing physicians to visualize the pumping action of the heart and the blood flow through the coronary arteries.

Cardiac catheterization may be performed to determine the extent of coronary artery disease, valvular disease, congenital heart disease, or damage to the heart muscle. Information gained from this procedure may be used to determine whether cardiac surgery is indicated or to assess the function of the heart after cardiac surgery. The procedure may be performed in the radiology department, operating room, or special room within a cardiac clinic.

## GENERAL TREATMENT OF CARDIOVASCULAR CONDITIONS

Individuals with cardiovascular conditions may receive medical and/or surgical treatment. In any case, treatment requires regular medical follow-up to monitor the success of the treatment and the progression of the disease.

### Medical Treatment

Although medical treatment of cardiovascular conditions varies with the type of disorder, treatment generally includes both medication and lifestyle changes. *Hypertension* is frequently associated with other cardiovascular disorders. Consequently, *antihypertensives* (medications that lower blood pressure) and/or medications that rid the body of excess fluid (*diuretics*) are often prescribed. When *arrhythmias* (irregular heartbeat) are present, *antiarrhythmic* medications may also be prescribed. A medication called *nitroglycerin* may be taken to dilate the coronary vessels when there is chest pain from inadequate oxygen supply to heart muscle. Nitroglycerin may also be taken prophylactically before any activity that may increase the heart's workload. *Anticoagulants* may be prescribed to reduce the coagulability of the blood and, thus, the risk of clot formation. *Cardiotonic medications*, such as *digitalis* preparations, may be prescribed to change heart rhythm or rate and generally to strengthen the heart. Regardless of the type of medication prescribed, in all instances, medications are taken under physicians' direction and supervision.

Physicians also prescribe the degree and type of activity permissible for individuals with cardiovascular disease. Because the heart responds to different types of muscular activity in different ways, when prescribing activity, physicians take into account the nature of the condition and the ability of the heart to function under various types of muscle action. Exercise may also be prescribed to increase individuals' tolerance of activity.

Factors that contribute to the development of cardiovascular disease or that place additional burdens on the heart, such as obesity, tobacco use, and stress, are also considered in planning treatment goals. Obesity increases strain on the heart. Consequently, individuals with cardiac disease are often placed on low-calorie diets. Sodium may also be restricted because it contributes to water retention, which increases the heart's workload. Because cholesterol levels have also been associated with cardiovascular disease, individuals may be placed on a low-fat, low-cholesterol diet. Tobacco use is associated with an increased pulse rate, blood pressure changes, and blood vessel constriction. Consequently, individuals with cardiovascular conditions should avoid using tobacco.

### Surgical Treatment

#### Angioplasty and Bypass

Surgical treatment of coronary artery disease consists of PTCA and CABG.

The purpose of PTCA is to reopen a narrowed coronary artery. PTCA, also called *balloon angioplasty*, involves putting a special catheter (thin flexible tube) into the artery in the leg and then threading it under X-ray guidance into the coronary vessel that is blocked. A balloon on the catheter's tip stretches the vessel and flattens the arteriosclerotic plaque against the wall of the artery. The advantage of PTCA is that it is not an open heart procedure, so the recovery time is shorter. The procedure is, however, a temporary solution. Most individuals who have had PTCA need to have the procedure repeated or have a coronary artery bypass at a later date. Other devices, such as a *coronary stent*, a small mesh tube, may be inserted and left in the artery to prop it open.

The CABG procedure, although not a cure, is intended to alleviate symptoms of arteriosclerotic heart disease, prevent myocardial infarction, or, if myocardial has occurred, prevent additional damage from occurring. In addition, it has considerable impact on individual's quality of life as well as ability to return to work (Charlson & Isom, 2003; McMurray, 1998). In the past CABG involved *open heart surgery*, which also required the use of a heart-lung machine. This type of surgery involves a longer recovery time. In recent years less invasive procedures called *port-access coronary artery bypass surgery* and *minimally invasive coronary bypass surgery*, which require much smaller incisions and use tiny cameras and video monitors to guide surgical procedures, have been developed. These minimally invasive procedures do not require a heart-lung machine. Unless complications develop, recovery time is generally shorter than for the regular CABG procedure.

Individuals with valvular disease may have surgical treatment to widen a valve that is narrowed or to replace a valve that is diseased. All of these procedures are described elsewhere in the chapter. When the heart is severely impaired, cardiac transplantation may be performed, as discussed as follows.

### Cardiac Transplantation

Cardiac transplantation is an accepted, established form of therapy when heart disease is so advanced (*end-stage heart disease*) that standard therapy is no longer effective and survival is severely threatened (House-Fancher & Foell, 2004). Individuals who undergo successful transplantation increase their chance for survival and also their chance to return to a normal, productive life. There are approximately 257 transplant centers and 140 programs that perform heart transplants in the United States (United Network of Organ Sharing, 2002).

### Pre-Transplant Procedures

Individuals selected for transplant often have end-stage cardiac disease with a life expectancy of less than 1 year without a transplant (Rourke, Droogan, & Ohler, 1999). Prior to cardiac transplant, individuals undergo a complete physical and diagnostic workup. The individual and family also undergo a comprehensive psychological profile that assesses the coping skills, family support, and motivation in the family to follow the rigorous medical regimen that is required. The evaluation period can be extremely stressful, with individuals becoming fearful they may be found unsuitable for transplant.

Not all individuals with heart disease are candidates for cardiac transplantation. Selection is based on factors such as general physical condition, absence of other systemic disease that would in itself limit survival, the ability to return to normal function after surgery, and the ability to comply with the complex medical regimen that necessarily follows transplantation. Usually a history of drug or alcohol abuse, mental illness, severe obesity, other systemic diseases, or end-stage renal function or altered liver function is a contraindication to cardiac transplant (House-Fancher & Foell, 2004).

To be eligible for transplant, an individual's physical condition must be strong enough to survive the transplant procedure and to be able to comply with the complex medical regimen required after surgery. Individuals accepted for transplant are placed on a waiting list. A 24-hour national computer network links all organ procurement centers. When a donor organ is identified, the computer center searches the list of potential recipients for the best match. Donor and recipient match is based not only on blood type, but also on body and heart size.

The pre-transplant period may be extremely stressful for individuals and their families as they wait for a donor to be identified. Many individuals may put their lives on hold while waiting for a transplant, and the pressure of uncertainty as to whether or when a heart will become available can cause severe stress in family relationships. Individuals and families have no control over when surgery will occur, and in the interim the individual's condition may continue to deteriorate. Feelings of anxiety and depression are common. Individuals may also have feelings of guilt because of receiving a heart donated as a result of someone else's death. Organ preservation time is limited from the time of procurement to the time of implant (about 4 to 6 hours), so that individuals who are to receive the transplant must be readily available for surgery at short notice. This means that if they do not live near a transplant center, they may need to relocate to be closer to the facility. Relocation can be an additional source of stress, not only for individuals but also for their family.

When a donor heart has been identified and matching of donor and recipient blood type has been confirmed, the recipient is taken to surgery. The individual's heart is removed and the donor heart transplanted. Immunosuppressant therapy to block the body's natural response to foreign objects begins immediately.

*Post-Transplant Procedures*

After cardiac transplant, individuals remain in the hospital for approximately 5 to 10 days. After discharge from the hospital, they are required to have checkups by the transplant team biweekly and then every 6 to 8 weeks for 1 to 2 years after transplant. Biopsies of the heart and monitoring of blood are conducted frequently during the first 6 months to assess immune status; then the frequency of biopsy decreases over time. Individuals are also evaluated for possible medicine toxicity or graft rejection as well as other complications of transplant. If there are signs of rejection, additional medications are prescribed to augment immunosuppression.

Individuals undergoing cardiac transplantation must follow a complex medical regimen to prevent rejection of the donor organ and other complications. Because the body never really ceases its efforts to reject the donor heart, immunosuppressants must be taken indefinitely. These medications are a necessary part of treatment, but they have serious side effects that must be monitored on a continuing basis. Too much or too little medication may cause the body to reject the transplant. Potential complications of immunosuppression include an increased susceptibility to infection and an increased rate of malignancy.

Individuals generally take approximately 3 to 6 months after surgery to become fully functional and to adjust to the immunosuppressant medications. Survival rates after cardiac transplant increase as the time after transplant increases. When death after transplant does occur in the first year, the most common cause is tissue rejection or infection (Rourke et al., 1999). After the first year the mortality rate is more frequently related to malignancy.

The cost of heart transplantation can be staggering. Not only are there significant charges for the transplant surgery, hospitalization, and continuing immunosuppressant medication, but there are also costs associated with travel to and from the transplant center for checkups, the cost of food and lodging for the family while the individual is hospitalized, and and the cost of other support services that may be needed when the individual returns home.

Since the demand for cardiac transplantation far exceeds the number of donor hearts available, mechanical support in the form of left ventricular assist devices or artificial hearts has become a temporary therapy that can increase survival while individuals are waiting for a donor heart to become available (Mielniczuk et al., 2004). The mechanical devices have become a reliable bridge until cardiac transplant and also have the psychological and social benefits of enabling individuals to be more self-sufficient, possibly even going home (Morales, Argenziano, & Oz, 2000). These alternative devices do not require immunosuppression. The extent to which they may be used over the long term is, however, still unknown.

*Vocational Issues in Heart Transplant*

Although after transplant many individuals are able to be physically active and return to work, they may experience difficulty and require assistance in making the transition from their pre-transplant state to one in which they return to employment. One barrier to employment is prejudicial attitudes of employers, who may have concerns about individuals' insurability as well as their need for con-

tinuing medical care and follow-up after transplant. The functional limitations experienced by individuals after transplant are individually determined; however, there may be some restriction with heavy lifting or aggressive exercise.

After a transplant, individuals' immune status is compromised because of the continuing use of immunosuppressants to prevent rejection of the transplanted heart. As a result, they may be more prone to infection and should avoid situations in which they may be exposed to contagious infections.

Psychological factors may also be a barrier to individuals' successful return to work. Prior to receiving the transplant, individuals may have been out of work for some time because of their condition. Adjusting to being employed again may be difficult. Individuals may also have difficulty with body image or may be fearful that work-related activity could interfere with their new heart's effective functioning. Fear of contracting an infection or anxiety about potential rejection of the transplant may also be psychologically debilitating, interfering with the individual's ability to work.

## Cardiac Rehabilitation

Cardiac rehabilitation has been described by the U.S. Department of Health and Human Services (1995) as a program consisting of:

- medical evaluation
- prescribed exercise
- education
- counseling

Cardiac rehabilitation is a comprehensive and individualized program, the purpose of which is to reverse the limitations that have developed following the adverse physical and psychological consequences of cardiac events. Specific aims are to:

- curtail physical and psychological consequences
- limit the risk of future cardiac events from occurring
- relieve symptoms
- reintegrate individuals as functional beings in society and at work

Programs in cardiac rehabilitation use a multidisciplinary approach and include exercise training, dietary consultation, smoking cessation (if needed), patient education, and counseling (Balady, Ades, Comoss, et al., 2000). Treatment programs are designed to maximize individuals' physical and psychosocial functioning. Education and increasing awareness of the underlying condition as well as ways to prevent future cardiac events are a cornerstone of cardiac rehabilitation programs. Since some individuals with cardiac conditions become disabled because of excessive fear, anxiety, or depression, interventions directed to helping individuals and their families deal with these feelings are also part of the total rehabilitation program.

## PSYCHOSOCIAL ISSUES IN CARDIOVASCULAR CONDITIONS

### Psychological Issues

The heart has been given symbolic significance for centuries. Consequently, individuals' reactions to conditions involving the heart can be far-reaching. Sudden death is also associated with cardiac malfunction. Therefore, fear and anxiety are common reactions to cardiac conditions. Although many chronic illnesses trigger these reactions, because the heart is considered by many people as the most vital organ, any condition involving the heart can have significant emotional ramifications.

Most individuals come to accept their condition and its associated restrictions or treatment. In other instances, however, individuals' responses seriously affect treatment and rehabilitation. Reactions of anger, anxiety, and depression can be the most debilitating factors in cardiac disease. Such reactions can contribute to inactivity, social isolation, or withdrawal from the activities that were previously enjoyed. Consequently, it is necessary to consider the impact of emotional reactions on the ability to return to a comfortable, productive life.

Individuals with cardiovascular disease may be immobilized by fear and therefore may restrict their activities more than they need to. Excessive concern that additional stress or exertion may lead to cardiac failure may cause individuals to alter job, recreational, and family activities severely. Depression may result from the numerous concerns about work, family activities, sexual activities, and lifestyle changes. When cardiovascular conditions require significant modifications in lifestyle or employment, the changes may be associated with a sense of loss and bereavement.

Denial is part of a normal psychological defense that can be used to cope with severe threat. Although denial can be an effective mechanism for reducing levels of anxiety, it can also have a detrimental effect on treatment. Symptoms may be ignored or trivialized, physical incapacity denied, or recommendations for treatment or lifestyle change ignored. As a result, care and treatment may be inadequate, leading to complications or hastening progression of the condition itself. Although the way in which individuals respond to cardiovascular conditions is dependent to some extent on their personality, the magnitude of the response may be due to their personal situation at the time. Financial, work, and family concerns, in addition to the diagnosis of a cardiac condition and its implications, can intensify the response expressed.

## Lifestyle Issues

Although not all cardiovascular conditions require significant lifestyle changes, some changes are generally recommended. Modifications in diet, a decrease in alcohol intake, or elimination of tobacco use may be required. Because smoking constricts blood vessels, persons with cardiovascular disease, particularly peripheral vascular disease, should not smoke to avoid diminishing blood flow to the heart or extremities further. Changes in exercise may also be recommended. The physician may prescribe exercise such as daily walks as a therapeutic activity. Even when recommended changes are minimal, individuals may perceive the changes as having a negative effect on the quality of life; depression or anger may result.

The degree and the way in which stress contributes to the development of cardiovascular disease are unknown. Even if stress itself does not directly cause pathologic changes in the cardiovascular system, the behaviors used to cope with stress may. Overuse of tobacco and alcohol as a reaction to stress has adverse effects on cardiovascular function. Individuals who used tobacco and alcohol as a means of coping with stress in the past may need to learn different coping strategies.

Stress is not always associated with overcommitment and activity. For some individuals, significantly cutting down on activity and involvement can be more stressful than continuing the activity itself. Therefore, helping individuals learn new ways to cope with stress may be more beneficial than insisting that potentially stress-producing activities be avoided.

Many cardiovascular diseases require long-term treatment with medication. Often individuals' successful rehabilitation and subsequent progress depend on their willingness and ability to take medications accurately. Potential barriers to effective treatment with medication may be financial, attitudinal, or logistical. Appropriate strategies must be developed to maximize an individual's ability to comply with treatment as prescribed.

After diagnosis of a cardiac condition, sexual activity may be a special source of anxiety for individuals, as well as for their partners. In most instances, sexual activity can be resumed; however, associated fear and anxiety can hamper both enjoyment and performance, altering self-esteem and contributing to depression. Often, lack of information contributes to fear and misperceptions. The physician should discuss specific recommendations regarding the resumption of sexual activity, as well as any restrictions or modifications.

## Social Issues

To some degree, the reactions of those in the environment influence the success with which individuals cope with any chronic condition. The quality of individuals' interpersonal relationships at the time of the cardiac event and the presence or absence of social supports can be major determinants of individuals' reaction to their condition.

Cardiovascular conditions can produce profound effects on family dynamics. Depending on the condition and extent of disability, there may be a shifting of family roles and role reversal. Because of the invisible nature of many cardiac conditions, some family members may not understand that individuals may not be able to sustain the activity level they engaged in prior to their diagnosis. Lack of understanding may breed resentment or anger. Family members may be a source of support and consolation. They may also, however, contribute to individuals' fear and anxiety by being overly protective or showing anxiety out of proportion to the medical condition. Qualified professionals should discuss such reactions and their potential impact on individuals' return to function with family members.

Although those with cardiovascular disease may continue most forms of recreation, extremely rigorous activities may need to be curtailed. When recreational activities that were once a major social outlet must be restricted, social isolation and depression may result unless another recreational activity can be substituted.

Cardiac conditions often have few visible signs of disability. Although this may seem advantageous at first glance, the lack of visible cues may contribute to a misunderstanding of the activity restrictions that are part of the treatment protocol. As a result, individuals with such conditions may be pressured into participating in activities that are more strenuous than those at the prescribed level of activity. The absence of outward signs of disability may also foster denial of the condition and subsequent noncompliance with the medical treatment plan.

## VOCATIONAL ISSUES IN CARDIOVASCULAR CONDITIONS

For most individuals, work is a source of pride as well as a financial necessity. The degree to which the cardiovascular condition inhibits the return to regular employment can influence individuals' reactions to the condition. In some instances, attitudes of employers are barriers to the successful return to work. Employers may be reluctant to employ or reemploy individuals with cardiovascular

disease because of fear of liability or of the responsibility for medical costs if the condition should worsen.

Each job must be viewed in relation to the individual's physical and emotional abilities and the effect that the job has on the individual's health status. In some instances, a job change may be necessary, which can be an additional source of stress. In other instances, individuals can return to their former job with little or no modification.

Physicians generally prescribe the degree and type of activity in which individuals with cardiovascular disease may safely engage. Most individuals with heart conditions are able to engage in light to moderate activity.

Because of the effect on the cardiovascular system, environmental conditions such as excessive heat or cold should be avoided. Isometric exercise elevates blood pressure and places an extra burden on the heart; consequently, any exertion that involves muscular activity against a fixed, unmoving resistance is usually to be avoided. Individuals with pacemakers should be aware that certain types of equipment may interfere with pacemaker function.

In most instances, once cardiovascular conditions are stabilized and appropriate treatment is instituted, functional decline is slow or minimal. The greatest barrier to productive vocational activity may be the individual's unwillingness or inability to make recommended lifestyle changes or his or her noncompliance with the medical treatment prescribed.

## CASE STUDIES

### Case I

Mr. C., a 50-year-old high school teacher, has been employed in his current position since graduating from college. He teaches history and physical education. He had a myocardial infarction at the age of 40; however, he went through intensive cardiac rehabilitation and has returned to most of his former functional capacity. Over the past year, however, he has had increasing fatigue and shortness of breath. Upon evaluation by his cardiologist, Mr. C. was found to have beginning stages of heart failure. Although his cardiologist is currently managing his symptoms with medication, he has told Mr. C. that if his cardiac condition continues to deteriorate within the next 5 years, he may need to have a heart transplant. Mr. C. is married and has three stepchildren.

### Questions

1. How would you approach Mr. C. about his rehabilitation potential?
2. Is there additional medical information that would be helpful in establishing Mr. C.'s rehabilitation potential?
3. What other factors should be considered in determining his rehabilitation potential?
4. Is it feasible for Mr. C. to continue in his current job?

5. If Mr. C. would continue in his current job, what modifications might be considered?
6. What would Mr. C.'s rehabilitation potential be if he had a cardiac transplant?

### Case II

Ms. B., age 55, had rheumatic fever as a child and as a result experienced damage to the mitral valve. She is unmarried and lives alone. She has supported herself by cleaning professional offices since she graduated from high school. Over the past year she has noticed increasing fatigue and dyspnea. When evaluated by her physician, she was found to need valve replacement.

### Questions

1. What types of information would you find useful in helping Ms. B. develop a rehabilitation plan?
2. How will Ms. B.'s ability to perform in her current employment be affected by her surgery?
3. What factors should you consider when helping Ms. B. develop a rehabilitation plan?

### REFERENCES

Appel, L. J., Moore, T. J., Obarzanek, E., et al. (1997). A clinical trial of the effects of dietary patterns on blood pressure. *New England Journal of Medicine, 336,* 1117–1124.

August, P. (2003). Initial treatment of hypertension. *New England Journal of Medicine, 348*(7), 610–616.

Balady, G. J., Ades, P. A., Comoss, P., et al. (2000). Core components of cardiac rehabilitation/secondary prevention programs: A statement for health care professionals from the American Heart Association and the American Association of Cardiovascular and Pulmonary Rehabilitation Writing Group. *Circulation, 102,* 1069–1073.

Charlson, M. E., & Isom, O.W. (2003). Care after coronary-artery bypass surgery. *New England Journal of Medicine, 348*(15), 1456–1463.

Cooper, J. M., Katcher, M. S., & Orlov, M. Y. (2002). Implantable devices for the treatment of atrial fibrillation. *New England Journal of Medicine, 346*(26), 2062–2068.

Glasser, S. P. (2001). Hypertension syndrome and cardiovascular events. *Post Graduate Medicine, 110*(5), 29–36.

Hart, R. G. (2003). Atrial fibrillation and stroke prevention. *New England Journal of Medicine, 349*(11), 1015–1016.

House-Fancher, M. A., & Foell, H. Y. (2004). Heart failure and cardiomyopathy. In S. M. Lewis, S. McLean Heitkempei, & S. Ruff Dirksen (Eds.), and P. Graber O'Brien, J. Foret Giddens, & L. Bucher (Section Eds.), *Medical surgical nursing* (6th ed., pp. 838–860). St. Louis: Mosby.

Levinson, M. E. (2000). Infective endocarditis. In L. Goldman & J. C. Bennett (Eds.), *Cecil textbook of medicine* (21st ed., pp. 1631–1640). Philadelphia: W. B. Saunders.

Livneh, H. (1999, July–September). Psychosocial adaptation to heart diseases: The role of coping strategies. *Journal of Rehabilitation, 65*, 24–32.

Manning, W. J. (2000). Pericardial disease. In L. Goldman & J. C. Bennett (Eds.), *Cecil textbook of medicine* (21st ed., pp. 347–353). Philadelphia: W. B. Saunders.

McMurray, D. L. (1998, January–March). Psychological, social, and medical factors affecting rehabilitation following coronary bypass surgery. *Journal of Rehabilitation, 64*, 14–18.

Mielniczuk, L., Mussivand, T., Davies, R., Mesana, T. G., Masters, R. G., Hendry, P. J., Keon, W. J., & Haddad, H. A. (2004). Patient selection for left ventricular assist devices. *Artificial Organs, 28*(2), 152–157.

Morady, F. (2000). Electrophysiologic interventional procedures and surgery. In L. Goldman & J. C. Bennett (Eds.), *Cecil textbook of medicine* (21st ed., pp. 248–252). Philadelphia: W. B. Saunders.

Morales, D. L., Argenziano, M., & Oz, M. C. (2000). Output left ventricular assist device support: A safe and economical therapeutic option for heart failure. *Progress in Cardiovascular Diseases, 43*(1), 55–66.

Newman, D., Dorian, P., Schwartzman, D., et al. (2000). Effect of an implantable atrial defibrilla-

tor on health-related quality of life in patients with atrial tachyarrhythmias. *Circulation, 102* (Suppl. 2), II-715.

Oparil, S. (2000). Arterial hypertension. In L. Goldman & J. C. Bennett (Eds.), *Cecil textbook of medicine* (21st ed., pp. 258–273). Philadelphia: W. B. Saunders.

Rourke, T., Droogan, M. T., & Ohler, L. (1999). Heart transplantation: State of the art (advanced practice in acute and critical care). *Clinical Issues, 10*(2), 1–15.

Sacks, F. M., Svetkey, L. P., Vollmer, W. M., et al. (2001). Effects on blood pressure of reduced dietary sodium and the Dietary Approaches to Stop Hypertension (DASH) diet. *New England Journal of Medicine, 344*, 3–10.

Santucci, P. A., Haw, J., Trohman, R. G., & Pinski, S. L. (1998). Interference with an implantable defibrillator by an electronic antitheft-surveillance device. *New England Journal of Medicine, 339*(19), 1371–1374.

Setness, P. A. (2001). Hypertension. *Postgraduate Medicine, 110*(5), 26.

United Network of Organ Sharing. (2002). Transplant centers. Retrieved from http://www.unos.org/whoWeARE/transplantCenters.asp.

U.S. Department of Health and Human Services. (1995). *Public Health Services, AHCPR: Cardiac Rehabilitation Clinical Practice Guideline*. Rockville, MD.

White, W. B. (2003). Ambulatory blood-pressure monitoring in clinical practice. *New England Journal of Medicine, 348*(24), 2377–2378.

# CHAPTER 12

# Conditions of the Respiratory (Pulmonary) System

## NORMAL STRUCTURE AND FUNCTION OF THE RESPIRATORY SYSTEM

The respiratory system consists of air passages, pulmonary vessels, and the lungs, as well as the muscles involved in breathing. The respiratory system supplies *oxygen* to the blood to be distributed to body tissues, and it also removes *carbon dioxide*, a waste product of tissue metabolism, from the body. Abnormal functioning of the respiratory system affects every system of the body. Diminished oxygen or excess carbon dioxide can also result in loss of consciousness and death.

Breathing is an involuntary activity and under the control of the respiratory center in the brain. Changes in the levels of carbon dioxide and oxygen in the blood bring about automatic changes in the rate and depth of breathing. As the concentration of carbon dioxide in the blood increases, the breathing rate increases to hasten elimination of the waste product.

**Inspiration** refers to the act of breathing in, and **ventilation** refers to the actual movement of gases (oxygen and carbon dioxide) into and out of the lungs. Air first enters the respiratory system through the nose during inspiration. Air entering the nostrils comes in contact with a *mucous membrane* that warms and moistens it. Tiny hairs within the nostrils trap dust particles and organisms before they reach the **pharynx** (throat), which serves as a passageway for both air and food. At the bottom of the pharynx are two openings, one into the *esophagus* for the passage of food and the other into the **larynx** (voice box) for the passage of air. The larynx contains the *vocal cords*, necessary for speech. A flap called the *epiglottis*, located on top of the larynx, closes over the larynx when food is ingested to prevent food from entering the respiratory system. As air is taken in, it passes through the larynx into the main airway to the lungs, the **trachea** (windpipe). The trachea is a cartilaginous tube lined with special hairlike projections called *cilia*. These cilia are part of the body's defense against foreign objects, such as bacteria, or other particles that have not been filtered out by the upper part of the respiratory system. With a rhythmic motion, cilia project mucus or other particles up toward the pharynx where they can be expectorated. After entering the chest cavity, the trachea divides into two branches, called the right and left *bronchi*. Each bronchus, which also contains cilia, enters a lung and con-

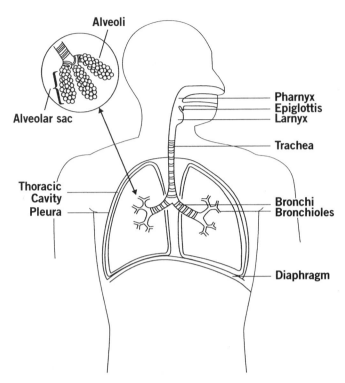

**Figure 12–1** Respiratory System.

tinues to branch into smaller segments called *bronchioles*. The bronchioles terminate in tiny sacs called *alveolar sacs*. Within the alveolar sacs are small pockets of balloonlike structures called *alveoli*, which make up most of the lung's substance. It is within the alveoli that the exchange of oxygen and carbon dioxide takes place through tiny blood vessels called **capillaries**. **External respiration** is the process of exchanging oxygen and carbon dioxide in the lungs. The exchange of oxygen and carbon dioxide at the tissue level is called **internal respiration**. Oxygen diffuses through the alveolar walls into capillaries so it can be distributed by the blood to tissue cells throughout the body. Body cells release carbon dioxide into the blood, where it is then carried to the alveoli. Capillaries in the alveoli release carbon dioxide from the blood; it then diffuses

across the alveolar wall and is expelled from the lungs through **expiration** (the process of expelling air from the lungs).

The lungs are two spongelike structures contained within the *thoracic cavity* (chest cavity) (Figure 12–1). The thoracic cavity is lined by a thin membrane called the *pleura*, which secretes a thin layer of fluid to help minimize friction as the lungs expand and contract against the chest wall during respiration. The thoracic cavity is surrounded by ribs. Muscles around the ribs (*intercostal muscles*) expand when air is inhaled and contract when air is exhaled. The thoracic cavity is separated from the abdominal cavity by the main respiratory muscle called the *diaphragm*.

The left lung contains two lobes, the *upper* and *lower lobes*. The right lung contains three lobes, the *upper*, *middle*, and *lower lobes*. The heart is located between the two lungs. Pulmonary vessels (the pulmonary artery and pulmonary vein) carry blood to and from the lungs from the heart. The *pulmonary artery* carries *deoxygenated blood* from the heart to the lungs, and the *pulmonary vein* carries oxygenated blood to the heart from the lungs.

After delivering oxygen to the body tissues, blood returns to the heart from the general circulation; at this point, it carries an excess of carbon dioxide. The blood is pumped from the right ventricle of the heart into the lungs. Here, the thin walls of the alveoli come in contact with the thin walls of tiny blood vessels called capillaries. Carbon dioxide passes from the capillaries across the alveolar wall to be expelled through expiration of the lungs. In turn, the oxygen that has been taken into the alveoli through inspiration passes across the alveolar wall into the capillaries. The red blood cells take up oxygen, and the blood returns to the heart, where it is pumped into the general circulation to supply body tissues with oxygen.

Air is able to move in and out of the lungs because of pressure changes that occur because of contraction and relaxation of the diaphragm and other breathing muscles. The pressure within the lungs and the thorax must be less than the pressure in the atmosphere for inspiration to occur. As air is taken into the lungs, the diaphragm contracts and moves downward, increasing the size of the thoracic cavity and lowering the pressure within it. The lungs expand and atmospheric air, which is at higher pressure, flows into the lungs, bringing oxygen as inhalation occurs. The diaphragm then moves in the opposite direction, relaxing and moving upward and causing the thoracic cavity to become smaller, thus increasing intrathoracic pressure. As the lungs are squeezed, air is forced out and carbon dioxide is exhaled.

## CONDITIONS OF THE RESPIRATORY SYSTEM

### Infections of the Respiratory System

#### *Upper Airway Infections (Pharyngitis, Laryngitis)*

The upper respiratory tract consists of the nose, the pharynx, and the larynx. **Pharyngitis** (sore throat) is a condition of the upper airway that may be caused from viruses or bacteria. The mucous membrane lining the throat becomes inflamed and may cause symptoms such as sore throat, fever, or difficulty in swallowing. **Laryngitis** (inflammation of the larynx) is usually caused by a virus and can produce hoarseness, loss of voice, cough, and sore throat. Both pharyngitis and laryngitis are relatively minor and self-limiting.

#### *Pneumonia*

Pneumonia is an acute illness caused by inflammation and infection that affect the bronchioles and alveolar tissue in the lung. It is characterized by cough, chest pain, fever, and breathlessness. Although not in and of itself a disability, it can be a major and often life-threatening condition when it is superimposed on other chronic illnesses and disabilities. Individuals with conditions such as heart disease, alcoholism, neuromuscular disease (such as multiple sclerosis), chronic obstructive lung disease, spinal cord injury (especially quadriplegia), dementia, altered immune status, or swallowing abnormalities are at particularly high risk for developing pneumonia.

The term *pneumonia* is usually further qualified to describe the cause or location. For example, *lobar pneumonia* refers to pneumonia that affects one lobe of the lung, and *bronchopneumonia* refers to patchy and diffuse inflammation and infection of one or both lungs. Pneumonia can be caused by a number of organisms, including viruses, bacteria, fungi, yeasts, or others. Pneumonia caused by a virus would be called *viral pneumonia*, whereas pneumonia caused by a bacterium would be called *bacterial pneumonia.*

Usually the defenses of the respiratory system against infection are sufficient to ward off infection. However, when the body is weakened or when the causative agent is overwhelming, defenses in the respiratory system cannot withstand the organism, and pneumonia develops. Individuals with chronic illness or disability, and particularly those who have limited mobility or prolonged inactivity because of bedrest, have an increased susceptibility for developing pneumonia. Pneumonia caused by inactivity or immobility so that the lungs do not expand sufficiently is known as *hypostatic pneumonia.* Another type of pneumonia can result in individuals who have difficulty swallowing or are unconscious. In these situations the epiglottis does not close adequately, so that food, liquid, or other substances can enter the lungs. The consequent accumulation of foreign material in the lung contributes to the development of *aspiration pneumonia.* Those especially vulnerable to aspiration pneumonia are individuals with altered mental status, neuromuscular disorders, or abnormalities of the esophagus. Aspiration of toxic materials such as oils, bile, gastric acid, or alcohol causes additional complications because of direct damage to the alveolar membrane, called *chemical pneumonitis.*

Inflammation and infection of the alveoli interfere with oxygen and carbon dioxide exchange in the lungs. The greater the extent of inflammation and infection, the greater the interference with respiration. Infection triggers changes in the capillary walls in the alveoli that cause fluid to flow into the alveoli and accumulate. The accumulation of fluid serves as an excellent growth medium for organisms, so that the infection becomes worse. Accumulation of fluid in the lungs further interferes with the exchange of carbon dioxide and oxygen. When the infection becomes widespread, there is danger of the organism invading the bloodstream, a potentially life-threatening complication of pneumonia.

### Diagnostic Testing for Pneumonia

Diagnosis of pneumonia is usually determined by symptoms as well as chest X-ray, which help to identify the location and degree of lung involvement. Cultures of sputum specimens may be done to identify the organism responsible for the infection so that appropriate medication can be prescribed. In some instances, if the sputum culture is inconclusive or if the individual's condition deteriorates rapidly, **bronchoscopy** (insertion of a special tube through the mouth extending into the trachea to examine the bronchi) may be indicated.

### Treatment and Prevention of Pneumonia

Once the cause of pneumonia is identified, treatment with medication is directed toward the specific organism. Medications that facilitate removal of secretions from the lungs (**expectorants**) may also be administered. Because individuals with pneumonia may have lowered oxygen content in the blood (**hypoxia**) due to poor gas exchange, oxygen may be administered. Manual chest physiotherapy may also be conducted to facilitate drainage from the lungs.

Individuals at high risk for developing pneumonia should be especially vigilant to prevent an infection that might lead to pneumonia. Good nutrition, adequate hydration, and adequate sleep help to bolster immunity. Individuals should attempt to minimize situations in which they are exposed to infection, especially during cold and flu season. Exposure to others with a cold or flu should be avoided. The position of individuals with limited mobility should be changed frequently to facilitate lung expansion and drainage. Flu and pneumococcal vaccinations may also be important to prevent pneumonia from occurring. Respiratory irritants such as secondhand cigarette smoke or other pollutants can make individuals more susceptible to infection and consequently should be avoided.

### Vocational Issues in Pneumonia

Pneumonia can cause significant morbidity and consequent loss of workdays, not to mention a threat to life itself. Because individuals with chronic illness or disability often have increased susceptibility to pneumonia, the steps mentioned above to minimize the development of pulmonary complications are especially important. The presence in the workplace of conditions that can induce or aggravate lung conditions may require job modification or complete avoidance or exposure to the risk. Although the risk of exposure may be present in a number of work situations, specific exposure to respiratory irritants or to large numbers of people who may have respiratory symptoms should be avoided as much as possible.

### Tuberculosis (TB)

Tuberculosis (TB) is an infectious and potentially fatal disease that is caused by an organism called the *tubercle bacillus*. Although it occurs most frequently in the lungs, TB can occur in almost any part of the body. TB of the lung is called *pul-monary tuberculosis*. Infection occurs primarily through inhalation of infectious droplets that an infected individual has released through coughing. As a result of the infection, nodules form in the lung.

Exposure to the tubercle bacillus may or may not lead to infection or to active disease. Whether infection or active TB develops depends on individuals' general physical condition and the intensity of the exposure. Ordinarily, TB is not contracted from brief exposure to a person with TB. Many factors predispose individuals to develop TB. Lowered body resistance due to inadequate rest and poor nutrition may be one predisposing factor. Persons with other disabling conditions, such as diabetes, alcoholism, HIV infection, and conditions that affect the lungs (e.g., silicosis), are more vulnerable to develop TB if they should come in contact with the infectious agent (Poss, 2000).

Individuals infected with TB for the first time are said to have a primary infection. Primary infections may or may not become active. The infection may be dormant for years until physical resistance is lowered. The most common form of TB is reinfection, or secondary TB. Individuals with active pulmonary TB may have few symptoms until nodules in the lung are large enough to be seen on X-ray. Initial symptoms may be weight loss, anorexia (loss of appetite), and a slight elevation of temperature. Symptoms may then progress to cough, overproduction of sputum, and **hemoptysis** (blood-streaked sputum).

### Diagnosis of Tuberculosis

Infection with the tubercle bacillus is diagnosed through *cultures of sputum, chest X-rays*, and *tuberculin skin tests*. Skin tests can be a valuable screening tool to determine if the individual has been infected with the tubercle bacillus. After being infected by the tubercle bacilli, the body develops an allergic response over time, resulting in tissue sensitivity. This sensitivity can be identified through the tuberculin skin test. A skin test consists of an injection of a small amount of filtrate from dead tubercle bacilli under the skin. If an individual has been exposed to and infected by the tubercle bacillus, there will be a local skin reaction at the injection site. Skin tests are interpreted for reaction at 24 hours and at 48 to 72 hours after injection.

A positive reaction to a skin test indicates that the individual has been exposed to and infected with the tubercle bacillus, but it does not indicate whether the disease is active. Individuals who have a positive skin test but have no symptoms and no evidence of active disease on X-ray or sputum specimens do not have active disease, and they are not contagious to others. It is now recommended that individuals with positive skin tests be treated even though they have no active signs of the disease to prevent the possibility of the disease becoming active at a later date, when their resistance may be diminished from other causes, such as chronic disease or aging (Horsburgh, 2004).

To determine whether the individual with a positive skin test has active TB, physicians obtain *chest X-rays* and *sputum specimens* from the individual. Identification of nodular changes in the lung and/or the finding of the tubercle bacillus in the sputum of other body secretions confirms the diagnosis of active disease. Individuals with active TB are infectious and theoretically would be able to transmit the disease to others.

### Treatment of Tuberculosis

Individuals with active TB should undergo prompt treatment, not only for their own well-being but also for the protection of others. Treatment consists of taking medication for 6 to 24 months. The average length of treatment with medication is from 9 to 12 months. Usually, after 2 to 4 weeks of intensive treatment with medication, individuals are no longer a public health threat and can return to normal activities. It is of the utmost importance that individuals being treated for TB take the prescribed medication accurately and consistently if treatment is to be effective. Because individuals have not always been compliant with the drug regimen prescribed, there are more cases in which the tubercle bacillus has become resistant to the regular medications, which had once been effective. Drug-resistant TB is becoming an increasing problem.

TB that occurs outside the lungs is called *extrapulmonary tuberculosis*. Possible disease sites include the lining of the brain and spinal cord, the kidney, the bones, or the abdomen. TB that is widespread throughout the body is called *miliary tuberculosis*. Treatment of extrapulmonary TB is similar to that of pulmonary TB, but it may continue for a longer period.

### Psychosocial Issues in Tuberculosis

Although anyone of any social class or educational level can be infected by the tubercle bacillus, development of TB is still often associated with crowded conditions and poverty, alcoholism, substance abuse, and homelessness (Campion, 1999). In many cultures, the social stigma of TB may contribute to individuals' denial that they have the condition and abandonment of treatment. Individuals with TB who remember the social stigma once associated with the condition may feel ashamed and embarrassed. They may try to hide their diagnosis from others, ignore the physician's recommendations, or discontinue treatment. Such reactions have serious consequences for both individuals with TB and those in close contact with them.

### Vocational Issues in Tuberculosis

When tubercle bacilli are no longer present in the sputum after beginning treatment, individuals are no longer considered infectious to others and are able to return to work (usually within 2 to 4 weeks). Once individuals are treated, providing there have been no associated complications, the ability to return to work or to perform tasks performed previously should not be affected. Because of the stigma attached to the condition and the misinformation that employers or coworkers may have about it, however, one of the major barriers to employment may be the attitudes of employers and fellow employees.

## Chronic Lung Diseases

### Asthma

**Asthma** is a chronic inflammatory hyperresponsiveness of the airways that leads to reversible airway obstruction (National Asthma Education and Prevention Program, 1997). It is characterized by episodic attacks of wheezing, **dyspnea** (difficulty breathing), chest tightness, and cough triggered by a variety of stimuli. Factors such as exercise, emotional stress, inhalation of cold air, or exposure to respiratory irritants such as fumes from paint or gasoline, cigarette smoke, or perfumes may precipitate an asthma attack. Some people have attacks triggered by food preservatives or to substances found in some medications, such as aspirin. Most triggers initiate an allergic response that causes the immune system to initiate an inflammatory response, causing airways to swell and secrete excess mucus that clogs the passages. At the same time, the muscles that control air passages constrict and go into spasm, causing the airways to narrow. As a result, individuals have difficulty breathing and the lungs work less efficiently.

The severity of symptoms and the frequency of asthma attacks vary with individuals. Some individuals may have a slight cough and shortness of breath during an attack, whereas others may be so restricted by cough and shortness of breath that they are unable to speak more than a few words at a time. *Chronic bronchitis* or *emphysema* may coexist with asthma, especially in older adults.

Asthma may be classified as *mild, moderate,* or *severe.* Individuals with *mild asthma* may have intermittent brief symptoms several times a month but have no symptoms in between attacks, so that medication is required only during an attack. Individuals with *moderate asthma* may have an attack several times a week and require medication almost daily. Individuals are classified as having *severe asthma* when symptoms are almost continuous and physical activities are limited because of the symptoms. Severe asthma requires daily medication and may be accompanied by frequent hospitalizations and potentially life-threatening exacerbations.

**Atelectasis** (collapse of the lung) is a possible complication of asthma. Another is a severe, prolonged attack (**status asthmaticus**). This condition is a severe exacerbation of asthma that is unresponsive to treatment methods, and it can be fatal. The condition requires emergency medical intervention.

### Treatment of Asthma

Treatment of asthma is directed toward the identification and avoidance of precipitating factors, the symptomatic relief of attacks, and the prevention of future attacks. If asthma is due to allergy, individuals should attempt to rid the environment as much as possible of the substance causing the allergic response (**allergen**). Common allergens are dust mites, mold, pollen, and animal dander. When individuals know what triggers a response, whether allergic or not, precipitating factors should be eliminated as much as possible. Common precipitating factors that can aggravate asthma and possibly bring on an attack are irritants such as dust, smoke, exhaust fumes, chemicals, or perfumes. Some food preservatives, such as sulfites, can also bring on an attack. In some instances, attacks may be brought on by stress or fatigue.

Several medications are commonly used to treat asthma. Individuals may take medications daily or may use medications for relief of symptoms during an asthma attack. *Corticosteroids* are substances produced naturally in the body by the adrenal glands that perform a number of vital functions, such as regulating metabolism, maintaining proper water balance, and fighting against inflammation. Corticosteroids prescribed by a physician for treatment of asthma are anti-inflammatory medications that reduce the inflammation and swelling of the lining of the bronchial tubes. They are usually taken on a regular basis to prevent asthma attacks. They may be inhaled or taken orally or by injection. Cromolyn sodium may be prescribed as an alternative to inhaled steroids or to help reduce the amount of steroid needed. It helps to prevent asthma attacks by blocking the release of substances that narrow airways during an asthmatic reaction and may be especially helpful when taken prior to exercises or prior to exposure to triggering factors.

Medications called *bronchodilators*, which dilate the narrow and constricted bronchioles, are commonly used in the treatment of asthma attacks. These medications dilate the bronchioles by relaxing the muscles of their walls, thus creating a larger opening for the passage of air. They may be used to relieve an acute asthma attack. Bronchodilators may be used orally or as *inhalers* or *nebulizers*. A **nebulizer** is a device that converts liquid medication into tiny droplets that individuals then inhale. Nebulizers and inhalers deliver medication directly to the lungs so that the medication begins to act immediately. Individuals with asthma may use special instruments such as *metered-dose* or *aerosol inhalers*. When inhalers are used correctly, medication is delivered directly into the lungs for quick relief of symptoms. Metered-dose inhalers dispense aerosol medication in measured doses, but to receive the full effect, individuals must learn and remember to use the proper technique with the inhalers. *Spacer devices* may also be used. A spacer device is a tube or bag that is attached to the metered-dose inhaler at one end and that has a mouthpiece for the individual to inhale through at the other end. The spacer acts as a holding chamber, slowing down the medication so the individual can inhale it more efficiently. A *peak flow meter* is a device that determines changes in the size of the individual's airways. Individuals are able to measure and record their peak flow rate to help determine the severity of their asthma and how well they are responding to treatment.

Individuals with asthma require periodic medical assessment to ensure that the goals of treatment have been achieved and to monitor their condition. The severity of the condition and the appropriate therapy vary widely among individuals, and their condition can change over time, with new allergies developing or the severity of the asthma increasing or decreasing. One of the most important aspects of the treatment of asthma is patient education and monitoring (Naureckas & Solway, 2001). Individuals should be aware of how to recognize and manage exacerbations of the condition as well as to identify and if possible avoid environmental triggers. Asthma self-management education should be tailored to the needs of each individual with sensitivity to cultural beliefs and practices. In addition, an annual influenza vaccination may be indicated for individuals with persistent asthma.

## Psychosocial Issues in Asthma

Effective management of asthma requires adherence to the medical recommendations to control attacks. However, psychological or behavioral responses may prevent or limit individuals' ability to comply with recommendations. Individuals may experience a variety of obstacles that impede their ability to adhere to medical interventions. Resistance to the treatment plan may be one of the greatest barriers to successful asthma control. Asthma, unlike many other chronic conditions, has associated symptoms that are usually reversible when treated with medications. Consequently, with proper treatment, the condition should only minimally affect daily living. Unfortunately, individuals may feel that adherence to the treatment necessary to control the symptoms draws attention to them. Consequently, they may feel stigmatized and avoid implementing treatment. Individuals with asthma may view daily medications as a negative, constant reminder of their condition. Social opportunities may also be affected by asthma if, depending on the factors that appear to precipitate an attack, there are limitations on certain physical activities or on exposure to certain environmental factors because they trigger attacks. Fear and panic may be experienced during acute asthma attacks.

Individuals who have had asthma since childhood may be especially vulnerable to social adjustment problems because of the stressors experienced from hospitalizations and restrictions, which may have impeded their social development. Obstacles such as lack of medical insurance coverage may encourage episodic care and inadequate follow-up and monitoring. Out-of-pocket expenditures for health care and prescription costs may impose an undue hardship on individuals and their family, making it difficult to obtain necessary medication and medical care. Transportation obstacles that prevent individuals from gaining access to follow-up health care may also cause difficulty.

In other instances, individuals may not understand the importance of certain recommendations, such as taking medication daily even when they are not having an asthma attack, reducing exposure to allergens, or modifying the home or work environment to reduce irritants that can trigger attacks.

Individuals with asthma may experience feelings of anger and low self-esteem, which in turn make it difficult to accept their condition. They may have difficulty coming to terms with the limitation of their condition and may have a sense of loss of control over themselves and their life.

## Vocational Issues in Asthma

Asthma is a common cause of morbidity and mortality in the United States (Marik, Varon, & Fromm (2002) and a major cause of missed school or missed work (Li, 2001). It imposes some limitations on individuals regardless of the level of severity. Since exposure to irritants and allergens can increase asthma exacerbations in individuals who are sensitive to these factors, environmental pollutants or allergens to which the individual is particularly sensitive should be avoided. Environmental factors that can contribute to asthma include chemicals such as cleaning solutions, craft supplies, industrial and vehicle emissions, tobacco smoke or wood stove emissions, pollens, and animal dander. Exertion should be avoided in situations where air pollution is high. Individuals with asthma should also avoid exposure to individuals with respiratory infections.

### Chronic Obstructive Pulmonary Disease (COPD; Chronic Bronchitis and Emphysema)

The term *chronic obstructive pulmonary disease (COPD)* refers to a collection of diseases with the primary characteristic of limited expiratory outflow. It leads to substantial disability and death (Mannino, Homa, Akinbami, Ford, & Redd, 2002). Cigarette smoking is the major risk factor for developing COPD (Barnes, 2004; Petty, 2001); however, not everyone who has COPD has a history of smoking (Rennard, 2004). Environmental pollutants, occupational chemicals, passive smoke, and a genetic predisposition to COPD are also risk factors (Barnes, 2000; Hogg et al., 2004). Although there is no universally accepted definition of COPD (Snider, 2003), all instances of COPD involve airflow limitation that is not fully reversible, that is progressive, and that is associated with exposure to noxious particles or gases (Pauwels, Buist, Calverley, Jenkins, & Hurd, 2001). Included in this definition are *chronic bronchitis* and *emphysema*.

Although chronic bronchitis and emphysema are two distinct conditions, they frequently coexist and share similar symptoms, including **dyspnea** (shortness of breath),

especially on exertion, intermittent cough, and fatigue. This combination of symptoms is a major contributor to disability, with dyspnea in particular significantly altering quality of life (Luce & Luce, 2001). Fatigue is a common symptom in most individuals with COPD. The dyspnea of COPD can affect individuals' ability to exercise or perform tasks of daily living. Those with early COPD may experience dyspnea after walking for short distances, and those in later stages of the condition may experience significant dyspnea with minimal activity such as brushing their teeth.

*Chronic bronchitis* is clinically defined as a chronic productive cough on most days for a minimum of 3 months in the year for not less than 2 consecutive years (Goldman & Bennett, 2000). Symptoms consist of a persistent cough, often in the early morning, accompanied by an excessive volume of mucus and expectoration. The lining of the air passages becomes irritated, swollen, and clogged with mucus. Mucus obstructs airflow in and out of the **alveoli** (the small air sacs in the lung where the air exchange takes place). Sometimes the small muscles around the air passages tighten. This is called *bronchospasm* and makes breathing even more difficult. Chronic bronchitis often leads to *emphysema*. Although bronchitis often predisposes individuals to develop emphysema, emphysema can also result from other conditions of the lung, such as *occupational lung diseases* and *cystic fibrosis*.

*Emphysema* is defined as a permanent enlargement of the alveoli because of the overinflation of and destructive changes in the alveolar walls (Kerstjens, 1999). As a result, the alveoli have less surface available for the exchange of oxygen and carbon dioxide, and the bronchioles close before exhalation is complete. As more and more alveoli are affected, the lungs lose some of their natural ability to stretch and relax, thus diminishing the efficiency of expiration. Airways become obstructed, and stale air, high in carbon dioxide and low in oxygen, is trapped in the alveoli. The lungs become overinflated because all the air cannot be expelled.

The most important risk factor for the development of COPD is cigarette smoking, even though COPD may develop in those who have had chronic asthma for years and do not smoke. Smoking and air pollution in combination may facilitate the development of COPD. The course of COPD varies. In most cases, the condition develops slowly with respiratory function remaining relatively stable for years. In other cases, however, respiratory function deteriorates rapidly. Many people have COPD for years before it is diagnosed. Individuals usually seek medical advice when they note shortness of breath with exercise or at rest. At this point, more than 50 percent of their lung function may already have been lost. Because of airway obstruction, **hypoxemia** (decreased oxygen in the blood) may occur. As COPD becomes more advanced and hypoxemia increases, the oxygen supply to the brain may be inadequate, resulting in impaired judgment, confusion, or motor incoordination. A buildup of carbon dioxide (**hypercapnia**) may also occur because of inadequate gas exchange in the lungs, resulting in drowsiness or apathy. To counteract the low concentration of oxygen, the body's production of red blood cells increases, resulting in a condition called **polycythemia**. The increased number of red cells in the blood increases blood viscosity, which, in turn, can interfere with blood flow. When polycythemia is severe, periodic **phlebotomies** (removal of blood) may be performed to reduce the number of red blood cells, thus decreasing the viscosity of the blood. As COPD advances, individuals may have increased difficulty

expectorating secretions; increased shortness of breath, especially upon exertion; and increased vulnerability to respiratory infections. For individuals with COPD, respiratory infections can be life-threatening, because they further compromise an already diminished gas exchange.

Failure of the right ventricle of the heart (**cor pulmonale**) may develop as a complication of COPD. As a result of the obstruction of airflow in the lungs and the subsequent breakdown of the alveolar walls, many capillaries in the lungs are destroyed. The surrounding capillaries become constricted to compensate for the lower concentrations of oxygen. Constriction of the capillaries channels additional blood flow to areas of the lungs that are better oxygenated; however, it also creates a resistance to the blood being pumped into the lungs by the right ventricle of the heart. Therefore, the right ventricle must pump against resistance and becomes **hypertrophied** (enlarged), losing the ability to pump effectively (see Chapter 11). Because of the inefficient pumping action of the enlarged right ventricle, blood returning to the right side of the heart from the general circulation begins to back up, causing **edema** (swelling) in other parts of the body. Organs of the digestive system may become engorged with fluid, causing nausea and vomiting. There may also be edema of the lower extremities, predisposing individuals to skin ulcerations.

### Diagnosis of COPD

Despite the disabling effects of COPD, it is still grossly underdiagnosed in many individuals (Mannino et al., 2000). Although a history of smoking, smoker's cough, and excess mucus secretion may be indicative of COPD, spirometric measurements are required to diagnosis COPD and document the degree of loss of lung function (Ferguson et al., 2000). In an effort to increase awareness of COPD and to develop consensus for the diagnosis of COPD, the Global Initiative for Chronic Obstructive Lung Disease has introduced a five-stage classification for the severity of COPD based on measurements of airflow limitation during forced expiration as measured through spirometry (Hurd & Pauwels, 2002). Spirometry is discussed later in the chapter.

### Treatment of COPD

COPD is irreversible and incurable. The major goals of treatment include smoking cessation, symptom relief, improvement in functional capacity, and limitation of complications (Sutherland & Cherniack, 2004). Individuals with COPD may be referred to a **pulmonologist** (physician who specializes in evaluation and treatment of lung conditions) for evaluation and treatment. *Pulmonary rehabilitation* is an important nonpharmacologic treatment of COPD and is directed toward increasing the ability to compensate for and live with disease, rather than attempting to cure it (Rochester, 2000). Pulmonary rehabilitation consists of a structured program of education, exercise conditioning, energy conservation, and physiotherapy, as well as psychosocial and vocational counseling. The goals are to provide symptomatic relief, decrease disability, and enhance lifestyle. For individuals who smoke, the most important intervention to alter the clinical course of the condition is smoking cessation (American Thoracic Society, 1995; Petty, 1999).

A variety of medications may be used in the treatment of COPD. Bronchodilators that help to reduce hyperinflation and thus dyspnea are a mainstay of treatment for COPD (Barnes, 2000). Most individuals with COPD have chronic inhaled bronchodilator therapy prescribed. Some individuals with COPD may have features of asthma, and during exacerbation of symptoms, systemic steroids may be prescribed for their anti-inflammatory effect (Irwin & Madison, 2003). Individuals with COPD are susceptible to respiratory infections and pneumonia, which, because of the already reduced lung function, may be fatal. For bacterial lung infections, antibiotics are usually prescribed. In addition, individuals with COPD should have annual vaccines for both flu and pneumonia.

In addition to medication, other forms of therapy may include *postural drainage* or *chest physiotherapy* (to remove secretions from the lungs) or *resistive breathing devices* (to increase breathing capacity). Avoidance of pulmonary irritants, especially smoking, is of primary importance. Many individuals with COPD benefit from learning new breathing techniques that stress *abdominal, diaphragmatic breathing* (to reduce the use of accessory muscles for breathing and to conserve energy) or *pursed lip breathing* (to slow the breathing rate and help remove trapped air from the lungs). Others find it helpful to use a simple resistive breathing device in the home daily in order to "exercise" the muscles of respiration. Physicians may advise individuals with COPD to engage in a daily walking or exercise program to keep in shape, to build strength and endurance, and to maintain their physical condition and improve their work capacity. Physicians may also recommend that individuals with COPD have a series of small meals throughout the day rather than a few large meals because a distended stomach or abdomen can push against the lungs, further interfering with breathing. Foods that cause gas and bloating should also be avoided. Adequate fluid intake is important to facilitate clearance of respiratory secretions.

Supplemental home oxygen therapy may be required, depending on the amount of lung damage and the oxygen level in the blood. Often these individuals have right ventricular failure, **polycythemia** (elevated level of red blood cells), severe dyspnea, and sleep-associated hypoxemia. Oxygen administration during ambulation can reduce the disabling effects of dyspnea and increase endurance and the ability to carry out daily activities. Physicians may prescribe home oxygen therapy for individuals with advanced COPD. The prescription for oxygen therapy usually depends on the degree of hypoxemia experienced at rest or during exercise. The amount of oxygen needed for each person will vary. Some people need oxygen only at night and during exercise, whereas others will require supplemental oxygen 24 hours a day. Supplemental oxygen provides the additional oxygen that the lungs cannot provide.

Oxygen may be supplied from several different sources. Weight, portability, ease of refilling, availability, and cost are taken into account when choosing a system. Compressed gas usually comes in large cylinders, which can weigh up to 200 pounds. These cylinders are stationary and may be mounted near the bed to be used at night during sleep. Small portable devices that contain oxygen and that can be carried and used by the individual throughout the day are also available. Portable systems generally consist of canisters containing liquid oxygen. They weigh 6 to 9 pounds and can be carried by the individual. Larger units are also available, but the difficulty of carrying these devices may make it necessary for them to be wheeled. Therefore, the larger device may limit mobility; in addition, there is the possibility of tripping over the device or becoming entangled in the tubing.

Supplemental oxygen reduces dyspnea and can improve quality of life. However, it is a medicine and should be prescribed and used as such. Although oxygen can improve individuals' functional capacity and quality of life, use of portable oxygen machines can also cause others to perceive the individual as an invalid, hampering social interaction because of false perceptions. Because the body's ability to respond to different concentrations of oxygen diminishes in some respiratory conditions, oxygen should be used only as prescribed, and the use should be carefully monitored. Individuals should never increase or decrease the amount of oxygen prescribed without first checking with their physician. Individuals using oxygen should not smoke or allow smoking around it because of the danger of combustion. Oxygen equipment and tubing should also be kept away from open flames. Combustible material such as aerosol sprays, paint thinners, or petroleum-based products should also be avoided.

### Surgical Intervention for COPD

Surgical interventions for COPD are also available in severe cases. The goal of surgical therapy for individuals with advanced COPD is to prolong life by preventing complications, relieving dyspnea, and enhancing quality of life by improving functional status. Until recently, lung transplantation was the last surgical option available for individuals with limited life expectancy because of emphysema. Lung transplantation may involve one or both lungs. Selection of individuals appropriate for lung transplant is generally based on the individuals' inability to survive without it (O'Brien & Criner, 1998).

More recently, lung volume reduction surgery has been proposed as a palliative treatment for individuals with severe emphysema (Flaherty, Kazerooni, Curtis, et al., 2001; Geddes et al., 2000; Pompeo, Marino, Nofroni, Matteucci, & Mineo, 2000). Since emphysema causes the lungs to become overinflated and lose much of their elastic recoil, the remaining functional part of the lung is essentially compressed within the chest wall. When some of the functionless area of the lung is removed, lung capacity decreases and a more normal physiologic state is restored. A major requirement for lung reduction surgery is severe disease in which individuals without the surgery are not expected to live longer than 18 to 24 months. Individuals must be within normal body weight, abstain from cigarette smoking for at least 6 months, and have no coexisting medical problems or severe psychological problems. Prior to the surgery, individuals are expected to attend pulmonary rehabilitation for at least 6 weeks. This includes exercises with the treadmill, exercise bike, stair climbing, and the like under medical supervision. During exercise the oxygen saturation of the individual's blood is measured. To qualify for surgery, individuals must build an exercise tolerance to 30 minutes while maintaining a predetermined oxygen level in the blood, using supplemental oxygen as necessary. After lung reduction surgery, individuals undergo *pulmonary rehabilitation* for respiratory muscle retraining, in which they learn how to use the diaphragm and accessory muscles of respiration to assist in breathing. Pulmonary rehabilitation is also directed to helping individuals increase their overall fitness and endurance. Although overall lung-volume-reduction surgery has been found to increase the chance of improved exercise capacity and quality of life (Geddes et al., 2000), it has not been found to increase survival rates any more than medical ther-

apy (National Emphysema Treatment Trial Research Group, 2001).

### Psychosocial Issues in COPD

Psychosocial issues can manifest as anxiety, depression, fatigue, and withdrawal from family and social life. Individuals can require extensive psychosocial support to deal with these issues. Many of the psychosocial issues individuals experience are related to dyspnea. Shortness of breath can lead to anxiety and panic, whether a disease process is involved or not. For individuals with COPD, dyspnea may lead to severe anxiety, fear of death, avoidance of all activities that cause dyspnea, and preoccupation with bodily complaints. Because strong emotions naturally raise the respiratory rate, fear of becoming short of breath may in itself increase dyspnea, causing a vicious cycle that can be totally incapacitating. Because shortness of breath is anxiety provoking, individuals may adopt an abnormally and potentially unnecessarily restricted life even though they are physically capable of being more active. Maladaptive avoidant responses may result, severely limiting interpersonal activities and causing individuals to become isolated. Individuals may be unable to work and may feel less interested in participating in social and family events.

Individuals may also experience intense emotions such as anger and depression in reaction to coping with their illness. Suppression of emotions can further compromise individuals' physical condition, causing increased functional decline and restricting individuals' activity and involvement with others even more.

Sexual difficulties may be a particular problem for individuals with COPD. Problems may stem from fear of becoming short of breath rather than from any physical limitation due to the condition. Although it is physically safe for most people with COPD to engage in sexual activity, sexual inhibition may be present if individuals interpret dyspnea that can occur during sexual activity as an exacerbation of their condition or as a life-threatening symptom. These concerns can inhibit further sexual activity and can affect intimate relationships with others. In other instances, sexual function may be negatively affected by depression.

Individuals with COPD confront a number of losses. Employment, physical independence, self-esteem, and social interactions may be lost or limited because of their condition. Some individuals may be reluctant to begin to use portable oxygen in public because of embarrassment, whereas others may become psychologically dependent on it and may be reluctant to venture out without the oxygen source, even when they do not need it. Some insist on using oxygen even though their difficulty in breathing is not the result of lowered oxygen content of the blood. In such instances, the psychological dependency on the oxygen may be more debilitating than the respiratory condition itself.

Individuals may find themselves excluded from activities of their families and friends because of their limited functional capacity. In some instances, coughing and expectoration of foul-smelling mucus may interfere with the ability to interact socially. Counseling and support groups can help to increase self-esteem and help family members cope with the individual's illness. Education of both individuals with emphysema and their family members is important. Both the individual and family members should develop reasonable expectations of what can be accomplished with treatment and should be helped to understand the importance of adhering to medical recommendations.

## Vocational Issues in COPD

The most limiting factor in COPD is dyspnea. Chronic hypoxemia may cause neuropsychological deficits that diminish individuals' ability to perform a number of mental functions, which can further contribute to work difficulties. In later stages of the condition, dyspnea may become so severe that even walking and communicating become difficult.

Until the condition becomes too severe, individuals may need to learn energy conservation so that activities are planned and paced to improve performance within the limitations of their condition. They may need to change their methods of performing more energy-consuming activities to improve energy efficiency. Proper attitude, breathing techniques, body mechanics, pacing, and relaxation can all increase work tolerance. Although stress is a part of every job, when demands are too challenging, muscles tense, the heartbeat increases, breathing becomes more difficult, and more oxygen is required. Working in a relaxed atmosphere can reduce the emotional strain that can contribute to dyspnea. To expend less energy at work, individuals should sit rather than stand. Ensuring the proper height of stools or chairs in relation to tables or desks and placing equipment, tools, or supplies within easy reach can minimize strain on breathing. Unnecessary motions or movements should be eliminated. Therefore, arranging work to make tasks simpler can increase functional ability. Pushing or sliding objects is easier than lifting, placing casters on items can facilitate movement, and pushing a wheelbarrel or cart with a light load of items is less strenuous than carrying the items. Individuals may also need to prioritize tasks. Distributing more difficult tasks throughout the day and breaking activities into constituent parts with periods of rest in between can enable them to accomplish tasks more easily. Individuals with COPD may also be limited in the amount they can use their arms and upper body because of the additional stress placed on accessory muscles of respiration. For this reason, activities that involve lifting or reaching may need to be avoided. Using special long-handled tools to access materials can help individuals avoid stooping, bending, and reaching. These are all ways to make physical work easier. If individuals are in sedentary lines of work, they can work even in the later stages of the condition.

Transportation to and from work should also be considered. Although many people with COPD continue to drive, driving in crowded conditions in which fumes and pollutants are present may be detrimental. Planning to drive alternate routes that are less congested or driving earlier or later in the day can help to conserve energy and decrease exposure to pollutants. The work environment should also be relatively free of allergens as well as free of dust, fumes, or chemicals that are irritating to the airways. Generally, extremes in heat, cold, wind, distance, and duration should be avoided. The work environment should be well ventilated and climate controlled so that the temperature is not too hot or too cold.

## Occupational Lung Diseases (Pneumoconiosis; Asbestosis; Silicosis; Berylliosis; Byssinosis; Occupational Asthma)

Some lung disorders are directly related to matter inhaled from the occupational environment. This group of lung disorders is called *occupational lung disease*. Although disabling, occupational lung diseases are preventable. They are classified by the type of material particles inhaled. The term *pneumoconiosis* refers to a group of lung diseases in which there has been inhalation of dusts. Examples of types of pneumoconiosis are *silicosis*, *coal miner's pneumoconiosis*, *asbestosis*, *berylliosis*, and *byssinosis*.

*Silicosis* is a type of occupational lung disease caused by exposure to silica dust, usually in the form of quartz. It may occur in those with occupations such as quarry workers, metal mining, foundry work, pottery making, sandblasting, or other occupations in which there is exposure to silica. Development of silicosis generally takes 15 to 20 years of exposure. When particles of silica enter the alveoli, special cells within the lungs engulf the foreign material and then die. In response, a special substance is released in the lung, and **fibrosis** (fibrous tissue within the lung) results. There may be no respiratory impairment initially, although damage in the form of nodules may be identified by **roentgenogram** (X-ray).

In the early stages of the disease, individuals may show no symptoms. As damage continues, there is a progressive restriction of lung function with associated **hypoxemia** (decreased oxygen in the blood), shortness of breath on exertion, cough, and expectoration. Symptoms are worse when accompanied by tobacco use. If the condition progresses further, complications such as *right ventricular failure* (see explanation under COPD above) may result.

There is no effective treatment, other than removing the individual from the environment in which silica is present, although the condition can continue to progress without additional exposure. Some individuals are able to continue to work in the environment with the use of an air stream helmet that offers dust protection. Silicosis also predisposes individuals to the development of TB. Diagnosis is based on an occupational history of silica exposure as well as demonstration of nodule filtration on X-ray. Persons with airway obstruction as a result of silicosis are treated similarly to those individuals with COPD, as described previously.

*Coal miner's pneumoconiosis*, or *black lung disease*, is an occupational lung disease in which there has been excessive exposure to coal dust. It is characterized by a wide distribution of coal dust throughout the lungs, leading to a mild dilation of the bronchioles and the development of abnormalities surrounding the bronchioles. Although not all cases of coal miner's pneumoconiosis progress, a small percentage of individuals develop progressive scarring of the lung that, in turn, interferes with air exchange. There is no specific treatment for coal miner's pneumoconiosis. Treatment is similar to that for COPD.

*Asbestosis* is an occupational lung disease resulting from the long-term inhalation of asbestos fibers. Exposure may be through the mining, milling, or manufacturing processes involved in the production of items such as cement, shingles, or siding, or through asbestos products such as insulation. The inhalation of asbestos fibers can cause fibrinous changes within the lung. Individuals usually notice **dyspnea** (difficulty breathing) on exertion. Treatment of asbestosis is symptomatic. Because asbestosis increases the risk of lung cancer, it is recommended that individuals with the condition abstain from smoking.

Inhalation of dust or fumes that contain beryllium compounds may cause another type of occupational lung disease, called *berylliosis*. Exposure to beryllium is common in many chemical plants, in factories (e.g., those that manufacture fluorescent light bulbs), and in the aerospace industry. Symptoms of the condition may not appear for as long as 10 to 20 years after the exposure. Inhaled beryllium creates an inflammatory process in the lungs that alters the lung tissue. Symptoms may include progressive difficulty with breathing on exertion, with progressive loss of respiratory function. The treatment of berylliosis is largely symptomatic.

The occupational lung disease *byssinosis* occurs primarily in textile workers. It is caused by the inhalation of dusts from fibers such as cotton, flax, and hemp. The resulting bronchoconstriction causes chest tightness. Unlike those with other occupational lung diseases, which become worse with increased exposure, individuals with byssinosis experience symptoms after they return to work from days off, but as the week goes on, symptoms gradually lessen. With prolonged exposure over a number of years, chest tightness may extend for longer periods.

*Occupational asthma* is a condition characterized by airway restriction and hyperresponsiveness induced by exposure to sensitizing agents in the work environment (Bernstein, Bernstein, Chan-Yeung, & Malo, 1999). The term *occupational asthma* is not used to describe instances in which environmental factors provoke an attack in someone who already has asthma. Rather, it applies to individuals who become asthmatic because of exposure to environmental agents in the workplace, a process that may take from days to years. The list of agents considered potential causes of occupational asthma is growing daily. If asthma is proven to be occupational, exposure must be reduced or avoided completely, depending upon the severity of the disease. The treatment and management of occupational asthma are individually determined. In some instances, even those who leave the work environment continue to have symptoms for a number of years.

## OTHER CONDITIONS AFFECTING RESPIRATORY FUNCTION

### Restrictive Pulmonary Disease

*Restrictive pulmonary diseases* prevent individuals from receiving an adequate supply of air during inspiration. Conditions that cause restrictive pulmonary disease may include skeletal problems such as **scoliosis** (lateral curvature of the spine) or **kyphosis** (forward curvature of the spine, see Chapter 14) so that chest expansion is decreased. Other conditions that may cause pulmonary restriction are nervous system diseases such as polio, spinal cord injury, or Parkinson's disease (see Chapter 3), in which the muscles that assist in respiration are hampered. Obesity also restricts lung expansion.

### Bronchiectasis

**Bronchiectasis** is a chronic disease in which there is chronic respiratory tract infection and increased inflammatory response of the bronchi and bronchioles so that they become dilated and inflamed and permanently vulnerable to recurrent infection. It is caused by repeated respiratory tract infections associated with conditions such as chronic sinusitis, bacterial infections, cystic fibrosis, or rheumatic conditions or by a genetic or immune deficiency (Barker, 2002). **Purulent** (pus-containing) material collects in the dilated airways. Individuals with bronchiectasis experience cough and chronic sputum production. They may also complain of fatigue, weight loss, or loss of appetite or may experience **hemoptysis** (expectoration of blood).

The condition is usually diagnosed by symptoms, chest X-ray, and in some instances a computed tomography scan to pinpoint the location and extent of damage.

Treatment includes the administration of antibiotics to control the infection, bronchodilators to clear the airways, maintenance of general health through rest and nutrition, and avoidance of further infections. Individuals may also learn special techniques (*bronchopulmonary hygiene*) or receive treatment (*postural drainage* and *chest physiotherapy*) to remove respiratory secretions.

Damaged bronchi do not return to normal. If the inflammatory and destructive process continues, surgical removal of the diseased part of the lung may be necessary, although the role of surgery in treatment of bronchiectasis has declined.

### Cystic Fibrosis

Cystic fibrosis is a multisystem disorder affecting the respiratory, digestive, skin, and reproductive systems (Dickinson-Herbst, 2001). It is a genetic condition in which mucus-secreting organs in the body become obstructed by abnormal, thick mucus (Esmond, 2000). As a result, there is degeneration and scarring of the organs involved.

Individuals with cystic fibrosis once rarely lived beyond childhood; however, with recent improvements in the management of complications, many individuals with cystic fibrosis now survive well into adulthood (Cystic Fibrosis Foundation, 2003).

Lung involvement is one of the most frequent causes of disabling effects of cystic fibrosis, and, when complications occur, it can also result in death. Respiratory involvement occurs because of the formation of thick mucus in the small *bronchi*, which can lead to severe *bronchitis* and *emphysema*. **Atelectasis** (collapse of the lung) is not uncommon. Individuals may have intermittent episodes of acute respiratory infections that persist. Coughing may be pronounced and may produce thick and purulent sputum. As the disease progresses, there is usually a gradual decline in pulmonary function.

Although the lungs are involved, other organs, such as the pancreas, are also affected. The pancreas may also become inflamed so that individuals develop **pancreatitis**. Because ducts of the pancreas are plugged by the thick mucus production, enzymes produced by the pancreas that aid in digestion are unable to function in this capacity, leading to poor digestion of protein and fat. As a result, individuals experience chronic malnutrition and delayed growth.

Individuals with cystic fibrosis also have malfunctioning sweat glands, so that excessive loss of salt occurs, resulting in **hyponatremia** (decreased concentration of salt in the blood).

Fertility problems are also common. Males with cystic fibrosis have high rates of infertility (almost 99 percent; Knowles & Durie, 2002), and women, although they have lower rates of infertility, have higher rates of complications with pregnancy, such as progression of lung disease (Hamlett, Murphy, Hayes, & Doershuk, 1996).

### Diagnosis of Cystic Fibrosis

Because of the increased concentration of sodium and chloride in the sweat of individuals with cystic fibrosis, a *sweat electrolyte* test is an important diagnostic tool in identifying individuals with the condition. The test is noninvasive and involves collecting and analyzing sweat from a small area of the individual's arm. When the test is positive, additional genetic testing may be instituted.

### Treatment and Management of Cystic Fibrosis

Pulmonary symptoms require the administration of antibiotics to prevent or treat infection. Because mucus production is increased, individuals with cystic fibrosis may have difficulty clearing secretions, which is important so that organisms do not have an environment in which they can grow and thrive. To help clear secretions, individuals may be taught specific procedures to facilitate coughing, or they may be encouraged to increase fluid intake in order to liquefy secretions. Other measures include breathing warm humidified air or inhaling steam several times a day. Individuals may also be instructed in various forms of *postural drainage* to be used at home to drain mucus. For example, they may be instructed to lie over the side of the bed with their head lower than the rest of the body several times a day. In some instances, individuals may be referred for *chest physiotherapy*, in which procedures such as *percussion* are used. *Percussion* is a form of massage in which the chest is repeatedly tapped or vibrated to loosen the mucus and allow it to drain. This procedure may be done by a *physical therapist*, or it may be done at home, either with an *electric percussor* or *manually* by a family member. Supplemental oxygen may also be used on an as-needed basis to maintain lifestyle and work activities.

Diet plays a direct role in the treatment of pancreatitis. If pancreatic ducts become blocked, *supplemental enzymes* are taken at mealtimes to aid in digestion and prevent malnutrition. Despite supplemental enzymes, however, individuals with cystic fibrosis still frequently experience delayed growth and malnutrition, and they are often underweight. Because of the increased salt loss characteristic of cystic fibrosis, dietary prescription is necessary to ensure adequate salt intake. Adequate hydration is necessary to liquefy secretions, and other dietary prescriptions may be needed to prevent nutritional deficiencies.

When progression of the lung disease associated with cystic fibrosis reaches a stage in which there is severe disability, double lung transplantation may be performed to halt disease progression and restore function (Dickinson-Herbst, 2001; Lanunza, Lefaiver, & Farcas, 2000).

### Psychosocial Issues in Cystic Fibrosis

Because cystic fibrosis is a genetic condition, with symptoms usually present in childhood, affected individuals grow up with a chronic and potentially fatal disease that can impact their successful passage through normal growth and development. The attitudes of family, teachers, and peers are instrumental in helping children develop their self-concept and their view of their condition, and such attitudes can also affect the individual's future function.

The psychological impact of cystic fibrosis in adulthood varies (Burker, Carels, Thompson, Rodgers, & Egan, 2000; Crews, Jefferson, Broshek, Barth, & Robbins, 2000). Adequate time, energy, and resources are needed to perform many of the home therapy treatments, such as *chest physical therapy, dietary adjustment, monitoring for respiratory infection, enzyme administration* to aid in digestion, and *routine use of other mediations such as bronchodilators and antibiotics*. Special skills are required for monitoring symptoms, interpreting changes, and making decisions about the need for altering treatment. Children who have been encouraged to assume more responsibility for their self-care will be more likely to grow into gradual independence (Esmond, 2000).

During adolescence, the behavioral responses to chronic disease may be made more difficult by the "need to fit in" or by the attitudes of rebellion and defiance that are characteristic of that age. These factors may potentially result in health-compromising behaviors. Without appropriate support, individuals may be less able to adapt and cope with chronic illness; this inability may result in isolation and altered relationships.

Individuals with any chronic condition may find adherence to treatment difficult because of its long-term and complex nature. Adhering to treatment is a daily reminder of the condition. Some individuals may feel that, given the likelihood of increasing deterioration and potential mortality, adherence is not worthwhile.

Fertility problems in individuals with cystic fibrosis may take an emotional toll. In addition to coping with the challenges of daily management of the condition, individuals also must incorporate issues of infertility into their relationship with significant others.

### Vocational Issues in Cystic Fibrosis

Cystic fibrosis is an incurable chronic condition that may produce increasing disability over time. The rate of progression of the condition varies significantly with different individuals. Because of the incurable and progressive nature of cystic fibrosis, employment of adults with the condition has not been considered feasible until recently (Mungle, Burker, & Yankaskas, 2002).

Individuals with cystic fibrosis have heightened susceptibility to respiratory infections and consequently should avoid environments in which exposure to respiratory infections is likely. Flu and pneumonia vaccinations are important to prevent respiratory complications from occurring. Individuals should also avoid exposure to dust or toxic fumes. Individuals may show exercise intolerance if they are placed in an environment where they are exposed to sudden temperature changes or air pollutants. If supplemental oxygen is needed for maintaining work activities, oxygen precautions as discussed elsewhere in this chapter should be instituted.

Because excessive salt is lost through sweat and because adequate hydration is necessary to avoid excessive viscosity of mucus, which can clog airways, hot, humid environmental conditions should be avoided. Although many individuals with cystic fibrosis are able to be employed full-time, the time and energy required to carry out daily treatment routines and the potential disruptions because of periodic hospitalizations must be incorporated into individuals' vocational plans.

## Apnea

The term **apnea** refers to cessation of breathing. Apnea can be caused from a variety of conditions. One of the more common conditions is *sleep apnea*, in which there are repeated episodes of the cessation of breathing during sleep. The condition is more common in middle age. Individuals with sleep apnea may be unaware that they stop breathing during sleep, but they may experience excessive daytime drowsiness, difficulty with attention or concentration, and irritability because of disruption of sleep. Although individuals with sleep apnea may be unaware of periods of apnea during sleep, their sleep partners may complain of being awakened by their loud snoring or sudden body movements during an attack of apnea.

There are several types of sleep apnea. The least common type is *central sleep apnea*, which is caused by a disruption of the signals from the central nervous system that stimulate respiration. This condition may be due to a variety of disease conditions of the central nervous system (see Chapter 2). *Peripheral sleep apnea*, also

called *obstructive sleep apnea*, is the most common type and is caused by an upper airway obstruction. The obstruction can be caused by narrowing of airways due to obesity, **hypertrophy** (enlargement) of tonsils, or structural abnormalities that predispose the airway to narrowing or closure during sleep (Flemons, 2002). *Mixed type sleep apnea* is a combination of central and peripheral sleep apnea. Individuals with sleep apnea, regardless of the type, experience **hypoxia** (decrease of oxygen), resulting in **hypoxemia** (decreased oxygen in the blood) and **hypercapnia** (buildup of carbon dioxide in the blood).

The consequences of sleep apnea go beyond sleep disruption and daytime drowsiness. Individuals with sleep apnea have an increased risk of **hypertension** (high blood pressure), heart failure, **myocardial infarction** (heart attack), and stroke. Because of sleep deprivation, people with sleep apnea are also at increased risk of accidents. The evaluation of sleep apnea often takes place in a sleep laboratory, where breathing during sleep is monitored and recorded. There are also portable monitoring systems that can be used outside the hospital; however, readings may not be as accurate.

### Treatment of Sleep Apnea

Sleep apnea may be treated behaviorally, medically, or surgically. The type of treatment chosen is dependent on individuals' symptoms and the function of the cardiopulmonary system. Treatment goals are directed toward establishing normal breathing and oxygenation of the blood and to eliminating disruption of sleep. Because alcohol consumption reduces muscle tone of the upper airway and increases the frequency of abnormal breathing during sleep, treatment recommendations often include limiting alcohol use. Individuals who are obese are encouraged to lose weight to reduce obstruction. Some individuals have more difficulty with sleep apnea when lying on their back, so in these instances, they are trained to sleep on their side.

The treatment of choice for some individuals with sleep apnea includes *continuous positive airway pressure* delivered through a mask. Machines used for this purpose weigh only about five pounds. They are used at night and fit on a bedside table. Individuals may use a mask that covers only the nose, nasal prongs, or a mask that covers both the nose and the mouth. The amount of continuous positive pressure applied is determined through evaluation in a sleep laboratory. Rather than using the positive airway pressure machine, some individuals choose oral appliances that are worn during sleep to help keep the airway open.

Surgical treatment can range from **tracheostomy** (in which a surgical opening is made through the neck into the trachea to enable the individual to breathe) to surgical correction of the structural abnormalities of the palate or facial structure that contribute to obstruction. Insufficient awareness of sleep apnea among physicians and the public in general may result in sleep apnea that goes undiagnosed and consequently untreated.

### *Vocational Issues in Sleep Apnea*

Sleep apnea can cause significant vocational impairment. Individuals with sleep apnea, in addition to daytime sleepiness, may also experience irritability, impatience, or even depressive manifestations, which can affect their relationship with others at work. Individuals with sleep apnea may also experience cognitive impairments, including difficulty with attention and concentration, visual/motor abilities, and memory. Tasks involving planning, verbal fluency, or general intellectual performance may be impaired. Because of sleep deprivation, individuals with sleep apnea may also be more prone to accidents.

If sleep apnea is diagnosed and treated, symptoms can be reversed. However, unfortunately, in many cases the condition is not diagnosed and a decrease in job performance is attributed to other causes.

### Chest Injuries

Fractured ribs are a common chest injury. Although painful, they are usually treated relatively easily by wrapping a strap or binder around the chest for support. In some instances, however, a fractured rib punctures other organs, such as the lungs or heart, and the consequences are more serious.

An open wound to the chest, such as a puncture wound, may allow air to enter the thoracic cavity. This condition, called **pneumothorax**, may cause the lung on the affected side to collapse. Pneumothorax unrelated to trauma can be secondary to a number of pulmonary conditions, such as COPD, asthma, or cystic fibrosis. This is called *spontaneous pneumothorax* and is caused by a tear or rupture of air sacs in the lung, causing air to escape into the thoracic cavity. Pneumothorax is generally treated by inserting a tube through the chest wall to facilitate expansion of the lung. Individuals who have experienced pneumothorax should avoid smoking, high diving, or flying in unpressurized aircraft, all of which can cause a recurrence.

Escape of blood into the thoracic cavity because of an injury to the chest that damaged vessels in the thoracic cavity is called **hemothorax**, which may also cause collapse of a lung. In both pneumothorax and hemothorax, the lung is compressed and breathing is hampered. A large pneumothorax or hemothorax requires emergency treatment to remove air or blood and repair the injury. The removal of fluid from the thoracic cavity is called **thoracentesis**, a procedure in which a needle is inserted into the thoracic cavity and fluid is aspirated out through the needle.

## DIAGNOSTIC PROCEDURES FOR RESPIRATORY CONDITIONS

### Chest Roentgenography (X-ray)

**Roentgenography** (X-ray) of the chest is a *radiographic* procedure that allows bony structures (e.g., the ribs), the lungs, and other organs in the thoracic cavity to be viewed as a still image on X-ray film. It may be useful in diagnosing tuberculosis, in noting changes in the lungs due to COPD, or in identifying structural abnormalities or tumors.

### Bronchoscopy

Visual examination of the bronchial tubes through a long hollow tube inserted through the mouth and into the bronchus is called **bronchoscopy**. With the *bronchoscope*, the physician can view the walls of the bronchus and note any abnormalities. A **pulmonologist** (physician who specializes in evaluation and treatment of conditions of the lung) usually performs the procedure, although other physicians with special training in the procedure may also do so. Individuals undergoing bronchoscopy are usually given a sedative, but they remain awake during the procedure.

### Laryngoscopy

**Laryngoscopy** is visual examination through a hollow tube called the laryngo-scope. The procedure enables the physician to inspect the structures of the larynx visually and to assess the function of the vocal cords. The procedure is usually performed under a local anesthetic, although the individual may be sedated.

### Pulmonary Angiography

In a procedure called *pulmonary angiography*, a catheter is inserted into a vessel and a *contrast agent* (special dye that enhances visualization of a structure) is injected into the catheter to enable the physician to visualize the pulmonary vessels. X-ray films are then taken and the circulation of the lungs studied. Pulmonary angiography may be used to assess the extent to which emphysema has destroyed lung tissue or may be used prior to surgery for lung cancer to assess the potential benefits of surgery.

### Pulmonary Function Tests

Pulmonary function tests are used to detect abnormalities in respiratory function and to determine the degree of impairment of respiratory function. Physicians use pulmonary function tests to assess the volume of air that an individual can take in and expel from the lungs, as well as individuals' ability to move air in and out of the lungs. Pulmonary function tests may be used to determine the cause of dyspnea, the extent of lung disease, or the effectiveness of treatment for lung disease. Generally done in a *pulmonary laboratory*, the tests involve breathing into a special machine called a *spirometer*, which measures several types of pulmonary function. The results are then printed out in a graphic representation called a *spirogram*. The types of pulmonary functions that are measured are the following:

- Vital capacity: the maximum volume of air that can be inspired and expired.
- Forced expiratory volume (FEV): the volume of air that the individual can forcibly exhale at 1-, 2-, and 3-second intervals. Readings of the FEV are reported as FEV1, FEV2, and FEV3.
- Residual lung volume: the amount of air left in the lungs after maximum expiration.
- Maximum voluntary ventilation: the maximum volume that an individual can breathe in 12 seconds, breathing in and out as rapidly and forcefully as possible.
- Tidal volume: the amount of air breathed in and out at rest.
- Inspiratory capacity: the volume of air taken in by maximal inspiration after normal expiration.
- Functional residual capacity: the volume of air remaining in the lungs after normal expiration.

### Ventilation/Perfusion Scan (Lung Scan)

**Ventilation** is the process by which gases are transported between the atmosphere and the alveoli. **Perfusion** is the process by which blood or other fluid passes to a body part through a vascular bed. The ventilation/perfusion scan is a radiographic procedure that makes it possible to measure the ventilation and/or perfusion of the lung. The test may be performed to determine whether a blood clot has traveled to the lung and lodged there or to diagnose other disease conditions, such as emphysema. For the ventilation scan, the individual inhales radioactive gas; the image taken shows where ventilation is occurring in the lung. For a perfusion scan, a radioactive dye is injected intravenously, enabling the radiologist to visualize blood flow to the lung.

## GENERAL TREATMENT FOR RESPIRATORY CONDITIONS

Because many diseases of the respiratory system are irreversible, treatment may be directed toward controlling symptoms and preventing complications or further deterioration. Pollutants and other irritants, especially cigarette smoke, should be avoided, as they can aggravate respiratory conditions. In areas where pollution is severe or if allergies complicate the condition, special air filters or purifiers may be needed. Even when pulmonary function is compromised, physicians often advise individuals with pulmonary conditions to engage in a daily walking and exercise program to keep in shape and build strength and endurance. A number of medications may be used for respiratory conditions, depending on the nature of the respiratory dysfunction.

- *Bronchodilators* help to open the airways so that more air can move in and out. Bronchodilators come in several forms, including pills, liquids, and sprays.
- *Antibiotics* may be taken for infections. They may be taken by mouth or injected.
- *Diuretics*, sometimes called *water pills*, rid the body of extra fluid, such as the fluid that builds up because of right ventricular failure.
- *Expectorants* are oral medications that make mucus thinner and easier to clear.
- *Steroids* are hormonal preparations that help reduce swelling in the airways, consequently easing breathing. Steroids are usually taken orally but may also be injected. Because of their serious side effects, they are usually prescribed only for temporary relief of severe symptoms rather than for

long-term use. Additional information about steroids can be found in Chapter 14.

A variety of breathing aids may be used in the treatment of respiratory disorders. Many devices are designed to help put medicines, oxygen, or moist air deep into the lungs and to help individuals clear their lungs of mucus. An *intermittent positive pressure breathing* machine is a device used to deliver air under pressure to the lungs. It may have a *nebulizer* attached so that it delivers medication and humidity to the lungs as well. Individuals with cancer or severe chest injuries may require surgery. At times, the removal of the lung (**pneumonectomy**) or a portion of the lung is indicated. Most people are able to function normally even with a portion of the lung removed.

## PSYCHOSOCIAL ISSUES IN RESPIRATORY CONDITIONS

### Psychological Issues

Difficulty breathing can be a frightening and distressing experience. The associated fear and anxiety may lead to inactivity, which, in turn, may result in a variety of additional physical problems. Prolonged breathing difficulty often causes feelings of helplessness and despair. For those individuals who have been active and self-sufficient, the inability to engage in even simple activities without breathing difficulty can be devastating. Depression is common. Individuals may focus on the activities in which they can no longer participate, at least not as vigorously, rather than attempting to attain their highest level of functional capacity.

When a respiratory condition reduces oxygen concentrations in the blood and the oxygen available to the brain is insuf-ficient, associated cognitive changes may result. Clouding of consciousness or changes in cognitive function can be frightening for individuals who experience these changes, as well as for family members who observe them. Close monitoring of the oxygen and carbon dioxide concentrations is important in the care of individuals with respiratory disorders so that low oxygen or high carbon dioxide concentrations can be identified and appropriate measures instituted to reestablish normal concentrations.

Emotional factors can compound the physical symptoms of respiratory conditions. Anxiety or emotional upsets may increase the difficulty in breathing, causing more anxiety and leading to more difficulty in breathing. When it is possible to identify situations that increase anxiety or stress, it is important to institute interventions to decrease anxiety so that the difficulty in breathing does not escalate.

The responses of family and friends to respiratory conditions may affect individuals' ability to cope with their condition. Family members may unintentionally place individuals in an invalid role, reducing expectations of them in the family structure or removing responsibility from them, even though they may be capable of engaging in a number of activities. Individuals may respond by using breathing difficulty to escape from life's demands, to receive emotional rewards, or to manipulate or control the behavior of others. In other instances, family members may overestimate individuals' abilities, not fully understanding the seriousness of the condition and its implications for function. Such reactions may push individuals to go beyond their functional capacity or to ignore physicians' specific recommendations for controlling the condition.

Circumstances that surround the development of a respiratory condition may elicit guilt on the part of the individual with the condition, or anger on the part of family members. Because smoking is linked to a variety of respiratory conditions, individuals who have smoked heavily may feel guilty for their actions. Family members may express anger, blaming the individual for smoking and possibly contributing to the development of the disease. When respiratory conditions are related to occupational factors, individuals and their family members may be angry because of the exposure to unrecognized hazards or, if hazards were identified, the failure of the employer to take proper precautions to protect employees.

Unless individuals have severe respiratory distress or use some type of breathing aid, respiratory conditions are not usually as easily recognizable as conditions in which there are visual cues, such as crutches or a wheelchair. Consequently, employers, coworkers, or casual acquaintances may expect individuals to be able to perform various activities that may not be consistent with their functional capacity. Lack of visual cues may enable individuals to deny their condition and avoid treatment, which can prove hazardous, not only for the individual but also, in the case of infectious disease (e.g., TB), for others with whom the individual has contact.

## Lifestyle Issues

As with other chronic conditions, the lifestyle changes required by respiratory conditions depend on the condition's seriousness and on the individual's previous state of health and functional capacity. In general, it is important for individuals with respiratory conditions to maintain good nutritional status and a normal weight. Because of the increased load that obesity or overeating can place on breath-

ing capacity, individuals with respiratory conditions should be urged to avoid both.

Cessation of smoking is a necessary component of treatment, regardless of the type of respiratory condition. Many individuals consider this task the most difficult part of their treatment. Even when they are aware that smoking exacerbates their respiratory condition, they may find it difficult to alter their behavior. Enrollment in specially designed smoking cessation programs may be necessary to help individuals stop smoking. Some individuals resist participation even in these interventions, however.

Although exertion can cause difficulty breathing, individuals with respiratory conditions are generally able to maintain activity unless they have associated cardiac complications. Exercise programs can improve self-esteem and reduce symptoms somewhat. If individuals experience dyspnea partly because of ineffective breathing patterns and partly from lack of conditioning, it is crucial that they work to increase exercise tolerance through daily breathing or conditioning exercises, in addition to participating in other exercise routines to increase exercise tolerance.

Unless the cause of dyspnea can be corrected, individuals with respiratory conditions need to become accustomed to feeling short of breath and to adapt to the sensation so that they can maintain their maximum level of activity without undue fear or anxiety. They may need extra time to accomplish tasks so that they can take rest periods. They may need to divide some activities into smaller tasks rather than trying to accomplish the complete task at one time.

Although an environment near sea level with a mild climate and minimal air pollution is ideal for individuals with chronic respiratory conditions, it is not always possible to live in this type of environment. Individuals living in less moderate climates should avoid extremes in temperatures. Home and work temperatures should be kept cool. Radiant or baseboard heaters may be better than forced-air heating systems, as the latter have filters that need to be cleaned or changed regularly. If a humidifier is used, it should be cleaned regularly to forestall mold growth. Fireplaces and wood-burning or coal-burning stoves should be avoided as potential sources of air pollution in the home.

Maintaining adequate hydration is important in respiratory conditions in which there is an overproduction of mucus. The environment should be well humidified, and a nebulizer or aerosol may be used periodically throughout the day to deliver humidity directly to the lungs. High levels of humidity may make breathing more difficult, however. Therefore, individuals living in hot, humid environments should have air conditioning to maintain the temperature and the humidity at acceptable levels. Filters on air conditioners should be changed on a regular basis.

If factors in the home contribute to the respiratory disease, environmental modifications, such as removing the cause of the allergic reaction, may be required. This is especially distressing if the offending factor is a pet. The environment should also be kept dust-free. It may be necessary to install special filters to cut down on molds and household dusts.

Individuals with respiratory conditions may become very anxious about participating in any type of physical activity that increases respiratory difficulty. Because both the rate and the depth of respiration are increased during sexual excitement, the fear of suffocation may cause these individuals to be reluctant or restrained when engaging in sexual activity. Although dyspnea may be uncomfortable,

those who have a respiratory condition with no complications can generally maintain sexual activity. They can often increase their tolerance to sexual activity through conditioning, or their partners may assume a more active role.

## Social Issues

Individuals with respiratory conditions may avoid social contacts and social situations that they once enjoyed if dyspnea, especially on exertion, is pronounced. The resulting social isolation can contribute to depression and lowered self-esteem. As much as possible, individuals should continue to participate in social activity, modifying the circumstances as necessary. For example, using a golf cart may reduce the exertion required in golf to the extent that those with respiratory conditions can still enjoy the game as a form of recreation and time to be spent with friends. Outdoor activities should be avoided, of course, when temperatures are very hot or very cold, or if pollution levels are especially high.

Even though crowded, polluted environments aggravate respiratory conditions, individuals with respiratory conditions need not refrain from participating in activities in urban areas. It may be necessary to plan travel time to and from the events so that traveling does not take place during the time of heaviest traffic. Arriving early at events can help cut down on crowding and the potentially anxiety-provoking rush. Establishments that do not prohibit smoking altogether usually provide nonsmoking areas. Individuals should check on smoking rules ahead of time and request seating in no-smoking sections.

Some respiratory conditions cause pronounced coughing, which may be accompanied by excessive, foul-smelling mucus production. Both the cough and excessive mucus can be embarrassing and interfere with communication and social interactions. Individuals with respiratory conditions should be open and honest about their condition with others, not making excuses or excessive apologies. Frequent mouth care can help to alleviate foul-smelling breath.

Because of the potential seriousness of respiratory infections in individuals with lung disease, they should avoid contact with persons who have upper respiratory infections or flu as much as possible. For example, exposure to large groups of people in confined environments at the height of the flu season should be discouraged, although this is not always possible without severely limiting social contacts.

## VOCATIONAL ISSUES IN RESPIRATORY CONDITIONS

The extent to which individuals with respiratory conditions can continue regular employment depends on the type of work, the work environment, and the severity of the respiratory condition. Individuals with severe respiratory incapacity may still be able to function in the workplace if their job requires little physical exertion. On the other hand, individuals with a small degree of respiratory incapacity may be unable to maintain employment in an environment that requires strenuous activity. Work that requires extensive use of upper extremities requires higher levels of ventilation than does work that mostly involves the use of lower extremities.

If factors in the work environment have contributed to or aggravated the respiratory condition, a change may be needed. In some instances, individuals may transfer to another location in the facility where the offending factors are not present.

The extent of activity that individuals with respiratory conditions can tolerate

should be evaluated. If, for example, they can walk the length of the hall but cannot walk up one flight of stairs without severe dyspnea, using an elevator may be indicated, or the individual's workstation may need to be moved to a different floor. The degree to which upper body movements are used in work and the impact of these movements on dyspnea should be considered. If the work demands lifting and carrying that increase dyspnea, alternate strategies may be devised so that the work can be performed with less exertion. Individuals, their employers, and their coworkers should be helped to understand that moderate dyspnea, although uncomfortable, is not in itself life-threatening. Because cough and sputum production can be cosmetically displeasing, they may interfere with individuals' effectiveness in jobs that require close personal contact or continued conversation. The degree to which the workplace demands this type of interaction and the impact of these symptoms on job effectiveness should be assessed.

If any type of breathing device or aid is used, the extent to which the aid will be a hazard in the work environment must be considered. Tubing in some portable devices may be caught in machinery, for example, or cause falls. Oxygen, because of the danger of fire or explosion, should not be used in close proximity to open flame.

In addition to stress in the work setting that could increase anxiety and subsequently add to breathing difficulty, stressors such as those involved in transportation to and from work should also be noted. If commuting necessitates travel in polluted, congested areas, it may be possible to modify the work schedule to allow travel at less busy times. Flexibility of the work schedule may also be important if specific treatments or rest periods are required during the day.

The legal implications of many lung conditions, especially if they are occupationally related, may be barriers to continued employment. For individuals eligible for workers' compensation or other benefits, financial considerations may affect motivation and cooperation with treatment. In other instances, the employer's fear of liability may limit job opportunities for individuals with respiratory conditions. Medical rehabilitation programs for individuals with respiratory conditions can be important to help them increase their activity level to their optimum capacity.

## CASE STUDIES

### Case I

Ms. G. is 48 years old. She has a degree in cosmetology and has worked as a self-employed hairdresser for the past 28 years. She has also been a heavy smoker and was diagnosed as having emphysema 5 years ago. Although she continues to work, she has found that keeping up with the number of customers she had worked with in the past is more difficult. Her physician has recently suggested that she may be helped by having a portable oxygen tank.

### Questions

1. Is it feasible for Ms. G. to continue working as a hairdresser?
2. What factors would you consider when discussing with Ms. G. whether she can remain in her current line of employment?
3. If Ms. G. elects to use a portable oxygen tank, are there specific precautions that should be taken?
4. What is the general prognosis for Ms. G.'s condition?
5. What lifestyle factors need to be considered in working with Ms. G. on her rehabilitation plan?

### Case II

Mr. L., age 29, has been a counselor in a drug treatment facility for the past 3 years. The policy of the facility is to have all employees tested for TB on an annual basis. This year Mr. L. tested positive.

### Questions

1. What vocational implications does a positive TB test have for Mr. L.?
2. What additional steps need to be taken if it is determined that Mr. L. has active TB?
3. What should Mr. L.'s coworkers be told about their exposure?
4. What are the vocational implications for Mr. L.?

## REFERENCES

American Thoracic Society. (1995). Standards for the diagnosis and care of patients with chronic obstructive pulmonary disease. *American Journal of Respiratory Critical Care Medicine, 152* (Suppl. 5), S77–S120.

Barker, A. F. (2002). Bronchiectasis. *New England Journal of Medicine, 346*(18), 1383–1393.

Barnes, P. J. (2000). Chronic obstructive pulmonary disease. *New England Journal of Medicine, 343*(5), 269–280.

Barnes, P. J. (2004). Small airways in COPD. *New England Journal of Medicine, 350*(26), 2635–2640.

Bernstein, I. L., Bernstein, D. I., Chan-Yeung, M., & Malo, J. L. (1999). Definition and classification of asthma. In Bernstein, I. L., Chan-Yeung, M., Malo, J. L., & Bernstein, D. I. (Eds.), *Asthma in the workplace* (pp. 1–3). New York: Marcel Dekker.

Burker, E. J., Carels, R. A., Thompson, L. F., Rodgers, L., & Egan, T. (2000). Quality of life in patients awaiting lung transplant: Cystic fibrosis versus other end-stage lung diseases. *Pediatric Pulmonology, 30*, 453–460.

Campion, E. W. (1999). Liberty and the control of tuberculosis. *New England Journal of Medicine, 340*(5), 385–386.

Crews, W., Jefferson, A., Broshek, D., Barth, J., & Robbins, M. (2000). Neuropsychological sequelae in a series of patients with end-stage cystic fibrosis: Lung transplant evaluation. *Archives of Clinical Neuropsychology, 15*, 59–70.

Cystic Fibrosis Foundation. (2003). *Cystic Fibrosis Foundation, patient registry, 2002 annual data report.* Bethesda, MD: Author.

Dickinson-Herbst, D. (2001). Cystic fibrosis and lung transplantation: Ethical concerns. *Pediatric Nursing, 27*(1), 87–94.

Esmond, G. (2000). Cystic fibrosis: Adolescent care. *Nursing Standard: Harrow-on-the-Hill, 14*(52), 47–59.

Ferguson, G. T., et al. ( 2000). Office spirometry for lung health assessment in adults: A consensus statement from the National Lung Health Education Program. *Chest, 117*, 1146.

Flaherty, K. R., Kazerooni, E. A., Curtis, J. L., et al (2001). Short-term and long-term outcomes after bilateral lung volume reduction surgery: Prediction by quantitative CT. *Chest, 119*, 1337–1346.

Flemons, W. W. (2002). Obstructive sleep apnea. *New England Journal of Medicine, 347*(7), 498–504.

Geddes, D., Davies, M., Koyama, H., Hansell, D., Pastorino, U., Pepper, J., Agent, P., Cullinan, P., MacNeill, S., & Goldstraw, P. (2000). Effect of lung-volume-reduction surgery in patients with severe emphysema. *New England Journal of Medicine, 343*(4), 239–245.

Goldman, L., & Bennett, J. C. (2000). *Cecil textbook of medicine.* Philadelphia: W.B. Saunders.

Hamlett, K. W., Murphy, M., Hayes, R., & Doershuk, C. F. (1996). Health independence and developmental tasks of adulthood in cystic fibrosis. *Rehabilitation Psychology, 41*(2), 149–160.

Hogg, J. C., Chu, F., Utokaparch, S., Woods, R., Elliott, W. M., Buzatu, L., Cherniack, R. M., Rogers, R. M., Sciuba, F. C., Coxson, H. O., & Paré, P. D. (2004). The nature of small-airway obstruction in chronic obstructive pulmonary disease. *New England Journal of Medicine, 350*(26), 2645–2653.

Horsburgh, C. R. (2004). Priorities for the treatment of latent tuberculosis infection in the United States. *New England Journal of Medicine, 350*(20), 2060–2067.

Hurd, S., & Pauwels, R. (2002). Global Initiative for Chronic Obstructive Lung Diseases (GOLD). *Pulmonary Pharmacologic Therapy, 15*(4), 353–355.

Irwin, R. S., & Madison, J. M. (2003). Systemic corticosteroids for acute exacerbations of chronic obstructive pulmonary disease. *New England Journal of Medicine, 348*(26), 2679–2680.

Kerstjens, H. A. M. (1999, August 21). Stable chronic obstructive pulmonary disease. *British Medical Journal, 319*, 495–500.

Knowles, M. R., & Durie, P. R. (2002). What is cystic fibrosis? *New England Journal of Medicine, 347*(6), 439–442.

Lanunza, D. M., Lefaiver, C. A., & Farcas, G. A. (2000). Research on the quality of life of lung transplant candidates and recipients: An integrative review. *Heart and Lung, 27*(3), 180–195.

Li, J. T. (2001). Asthma and allergy. *Postgraduate Medicine, 109*(5), 43.

Luce, J. M., & Luce, J. A. (2001). Management of dyspnea in patients with far-advanced lung disease: "Once I lose it, it's kind of hard to catch it…." *Journal of the American Medical Association, 285*(10), 1331–1337.

Mannino, D. M., et al. (2000). Obstructive lung disease and low lung function in adults in the United States: Data from the National Health and Nutrition Examination survey, 1988–1994. *Archives of Internal Medicine, 160*, 1683.

Mannino, D. M., Homa, D. M., Akinbami, L. J., Ford, E. S., & Redd, S. C. (2002). Chronic obstructive pulmonary disease surveillance—United States, 1971–2000. *MMWR CDC Surveillance Summaries, 51*(SS-6), 1–16.

Marik, P. E., Varon, J., & Fromm, R. (2002). The management of acute severe asthma. *Journal of Emergency Medicine, 23*(3), 257–268.

Mungle, J., Burker, E. J., & Yankaskas, J. R. (2002). Vocational rehabilitation counseling for adolescents and adults with cystic fibrosis. *Journal of Applied Rehabilitation Counseling, 33*(4), 15–21.

National Asthma Education and Prevention Program. (1997). *Expert panel report II: Guidelines for the diagnosis and management of asthma.* U.S. Dept of Health and Human Services publication NIH 97-4051. Bethesda, MD: National Institutes of Health, National Heart, Lung, and Blood Institute.

National Emphysema Treatment Trial Research Group. (2001). Patients at high risk of death after lung-volume-reduction surgery. *New England Journal of Medicine, 345*, 1075–1083.

Naureckas, E. T., & Solway, J. (2001). Mild asthma. *New England Journal of Medicine, 345*(17), 1257–1262.

O'Brien, G. M., & Criner, G. J. (1998). Surgery for severe COPD: Lung volume reduction and lung transplantation. *Post Graduate Medicine, 103*(4), 179–202.

Pauwels, R. A., Buist, A. S., Calverley, P. M., Jenkins, C. R., & Hurd, S. S. (2001). Global strategy for the diagnosis, management, and prevention of chronic obstructive pulmonary disease: NHLBI/WHO Global Initiative for Chronic Obstructive Lung Disease (GOLD) Workshop summary. *American Respiratory Critical Care Medicine, 163*, 1256–1276.

Petty, T. (1999). Rehabilitation options for chronic obstructive pulmonary disease. *Annals of Long-Term Care, 7*(5), 200–205.

Petty, T. (2001, April 15). Early diagnosis of COPD. *Hospital Practice*, pp. 7–8.

Pompeo, E., Marino, M., Nofroni, I., Matteucci, G., & Mineo, T. C. (2000). Reduction pneumoplasty versus respiratory rehabilitation in severe emphysema: A randomized study. *Annals of Thoracic Surgery, 70*, 948–953.

Poss, J. E. (2000). Factors associated with participation by Mexican migrant farm workers in a tuberculosis screening program. *Nursing Research, 49*, 20–28.

Rennard, S. I. (2004). Looking at the patient—approaching the problem of COPD. *New England Journal of Medicine, 350*(10), 965–966.

Rochester, C. L. (2000). Which pulmonary rehabilitation program is best for your patient? *Journal of Respiratory Diseases, 21*(9), 539–550.

Snider, G. L. (2003). Nosology for our day: Its application to chronic obstructive pulmonary disease. *American Respiratory Critical Care Medicine, 167*, 678–683.

Sutherland, E. R., & Cherniack, R. M. (2004). Management of chronic obstructive pulmonary disease. *New England Journal of Medicine, 350*(26), 2689–2697.

# CHAPTER 13

# Urinary Tract and Renal Conditions

## NORMAL STRUCTURE AND FUNCTION OF THE URINARY TRACT

The urinary system enables the body to rid itself of the byproducts of metabolism and to regulate body fluids and their electrolyte content. It consists of two *kidneys*, bean-shaped organs lying on the **posterior** (back portion) of the abdominal cavity on either side of the vertebral column; the *urinary tract*, consisting of two *ureters* or tubes (one from each kidney, leading from the kidneys to the bladder); the *bladder* (the storage place for urine until it is eliminated); and the *urethra*, a single tube leading from the bladder to the outside opening (urinary meatus) through which urine is eliminated (see Figure 13–1). The term **renal** refers to the kidney, and the term *urinary tract* refers to the collecting system for urine (i.e., the ureters, bladder, and urethra).

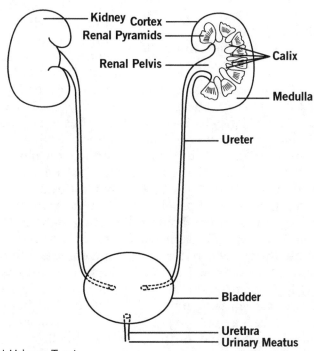

**Figure 13–1**  Kidneys and Urinary Tract.

The kidneys have multiple functions:

- They maintain the body's internal chemical balance (**homeostasis**) by regulating its water content and the concentrations of *electrolytes* (electrically charged particles of substances that are important to many of the body's internal functions).
- They rid the body of metabolic waste products (i.e., *urea, uric acid, creatinine*).
- They remove foreign chemicals from the body (i.e., drugs, pesticides; etc.).
- They secrete hormones:
  - *Renin* influences blood pressure and the sodium and potassium balance in the body. Renin stimulates a hormone (angiotensin) that stimulates an endocrine gland, the adrenal cortex (see Chapter 9), to secrete a hormone called aldosterone, which influences how the kidney regulates potassium and sodium levels in the body.
  - *Erythropoietin* controls the production of red blood cells.
  - *Vitamin D* regulates calcium absorption from the intestine and influences calcium balance in the body.

A thin layer of white fibrous tissue called the renal capsule surrounds the kidney. The outer layer of the kidney is called the *cortex*; the inner portion, the *medulla*. Urine passes into the ureters through a funnel-shaped structure called the *renal pelvis*. The medulla contains 10 to 15 triangular structures called *renal pyramids*, which serve as a portion of the drainage system. Within the cortex and medulla lie units called **nephrons**, which are the functional units of the kidney. There are approximately 1 million nephrons in each kidney. Each nephron contains an initial filtering system called a *renal corpuscle* (located within the cortex) and tiny tube-like structures extending from the renal corpuscle called *renal tubules* (located within the medulla). The renal corpuscle consists of a **glomerulus** (a bunch of capillary loops, or *glomerular capillaries*) and the *Bowman's capsule*, which surrounds the glomerulus. Extending from the glomerulus are the renal tubules, which end in a collecting duct called the *calyx*. Calyces from each nephron merge to empty into the renal pelvis.

The kidney filters a large volume of blood each day. Approximately 20 percent of the body's blood flow passes to the kidney through the renal arteries at a rate averaging about one liter of arterial blood per minute. The remaining 80 percent of blood remains in the general body circulation. Blood enters the kidney through the *renal artery* and leaves from the kidney to enter the general body circulation through the *renal vein*.

Blood entering the kidney flows first to the glomerular capillaries, where it is filtered, and then to a second capillary bed surrounding the tubules (peritubular capillaries), which form the veins through which blood leaves the kidney. The process by which the kidney removes waste products from the blood is called *glomerular filtration*. Initial filtration, which occurs as the blood enters the glomerulus, removes some waste products. As the *glomerular filtrate* continues to move through the tubules of the nephrons, substances are either reabsorbed into the bloodstream or continue through the tubules. As the filtrate moves into the collecting system, it eventually drains into the *calyx* at the mouth of each pyramid and empties into the *renal pelvis* as urine. From the renal pelvis, urine drains into the *ureters* to the *bladder*, where it is stored until ready to be excreted through the *urethra* and *urinary meatus*.

Metabolic end products and toxic substances are removed from the blood through the filtration process so they can be eliminated from the body as urine. Other substances, such as sugar and *amino acids* (the building blocks of protein), are reabsorbed into the bloodstream. Electrolytes (e.g., sodium and potassium) are also returned to the bloodstream, along with 99 percent of the water in the filtrate. *Potassium* is important to muscle contraction and nerve and heart function, and *sodium* is important to heart and nerve function as well as to water balance. The amounts of water and electrolytes reabsorbed vary and are regulated according to the body's specific needs; this internal chemical balance is crucial for the general function of most other organs.

Because of the kidneys' many functions, disorders of the kidney affect many body systems.

## URINARY TRACT AND RENAL CONDITIONS

### Cystitis (Lower Urinary Tract Infection)

The bladder and the urine contained within it are usually sterile. **Cystitis** is a condition in which bacteria have entered the bladder, causing it to become infected and inflamed. Bacteria can invade the bladder through the external *urinary meatus*, or infection of the bladder can be secondary to an infection in another location of the urinary tract. Although cystitis itself is generally not a disabling condition, it can be a serious complication for individuals with chronic illness or disability.

Symptoms of cystitis may include frequent urination even though the bladder may not be full; **dysuria** (painful urination); pain in the lower abdomen or lower back; and, at times, **hematuria** (blood in the urine). Recurrent or inadequately treated cystitis can produce more serious consequences if infection travels up the urinary tract to the kidney, causing kidney infection (**pyelonephritis**). If the infection continues and bacteria enter the blood (**septicemia**), a systemic infection that is potentially life-threatening can result.

Cystitis is diagnosed by the symptoms reported and by examination of the urine for evidence of bacteria, white blood cells, or other indication of infection or inflammation. Treatment of uncomplicated infections includes the administration of medications, such as *antibiotics*. If cystitis is recurrent, treatment may include identifying and removing or correcting factors that contribute to the development of urinary tract infections. Examples are structural conditions, such as a stricture or narrowing of part of the lower urinary tract that prevents adequate emptying of the bladder, thus predisposing individuals to infection.

Immobility, use of an external catheter, or a generally weakened physical condition can also predispose individuals to develop cystitis. Because of the potentially serious nature of this complication in individuals with chronic illness or disability, symptoms that suggest the presence of lower urinary tract infection should be treated promptly. Prevention of cystitis is important to reduce the risk of serious complications. Proper bladder care, adequate fluid intake, maintenance of urine acidity, or periodic urine analyses and cultures for early detection of unsuspected infection can help individuals prone to cystitis prevent or lessen the chance of its occurrence.

### Pyelonephritis

**Pyelonephritis** (infection of the kidney) can be a complication of cystitis in which bacteria have progressed to the kidneys from an infection of the lower urinary tract, or it can be caused from the spread of infection elsewhere in the body to the kidney. It can also be caused by obstruction or stricture of a portion of the urinary tract that leads to **stasis** (stagnation) of urine, which enhances the growth of bacteria. Pyelonephritis may be acute or chronic. No long-term debilitation is usually associated with *acute pyelonephritis*, although individuals may be acutely ill with fever and chills, flank or abdominal pain, nausea, and vomiting. Prompt treatment with appropriate *antibiotics* can eradicate the infection. If an obstruction or stricture is causing the infection, surgical intervention to remove it can prevent acute pyelonephritis from recurring. If acute pyelonephritis is not adequately treated, or if treatment is not permanently successful because of urinary tract obstruction or stricture, *chronic pyelonephritis* can develop. Chronic pyelonephritis can cause irreversible degenerative changes to kidney structure and function, leading to *renal failure*, described later in the chapter.

The diagnosis of pyelonephritis is based on symptoms and on examination of urine for the presence of bacteria and white blood cells.

## Urinary or Renal Calculi (Kidney Stones; Nephrolithiasis; Urolithiasis)

Ranging in size from a stone as tiny as a grain of sand to a stone large enough to fill the inner portion of the kidney, kidney stones (**renal calculi**) may occur anywhere in the urinary tract. They cause severe pain and can be a source of obstruction and secondary infection. Some individuals appear to be more prone to develop kidney stones than others. Structural or metabolic abnormalities, prolonged immobility or bedrest, and a variety of chronic illnesses and disabilities can predispose individuals to develop kidney stones.

Kidney stones may produce no symptoms, or they may cause excruciating pain in the flank or kidney area, along with

nausea and vomiting, **hematuria** (blood in the urine), or frequency of urination. Diagnosis is based on the symptoms, together with an examination of the urine for hematuria or bacteria. A radiologic examination called an *intravenous pyelogram* or *retrograde pyelogram* (described later in the chapter) may also be performed to detect the presence of stones and, if they are present, to evaluate the extent of the obstruction. If a stone severely obstructs urine flow, urine may back up to the kidney (**hydronephrosis**), causing kidney damage. Most calculi are passed through the *urinary meatus* spontaneously. If a stone does not pass spontaneously, it may have to be removed surgically. The type of surgery depends on the size and the location of the stone. Where available, a procedure called *lithotripsy* (described below) may be used to break up the stone through the use of ultrasound.

### Treatment of Renal Calculi (Kidney Stones)

*Lithotomy*

When kidney stones do not pass out of the body with the urine flow, it may be necessary to remove them surgically. This procedure is called **lithotomy**. Several surgical techniques may be used. The surgeon may make an incision in the lower part of the abdomen (a *suprapubic incision*) and remove the stone through the incision. At times, surgeons can remove stones from the bladder by inserting a *cystoscope* into the bladder through the *urethra*, passing a special instrument through the cystoscope, and then grasping and crushing the stone with the instrument; this procedure is called **litholapaxy**. The crushed fragments of stone are then passed in the urine.

Depending on the location of the stone, other surgical procedures may also be used. A special instrument called a *nephro-*

*scope* may be inserted through the skin directly into the kidney to remove the stone. If the kidney pelvis is entered, the procedure is called **pyelolithotomy**. If the renal calyx is entered, the procedure is called a **nephrolithotomy**. Surgical removal of stones from the *ureter* is called **ureterolithotomy**. In this procedure, an incision is made through the lower abdomen or flank, the affected ureter is surgically opened, and the stone is removed.

### Lithotripsy

*Lithotripsy* refers to a procedure used for crushing kidney stones. This may be accomplished in several ways. A noninvasive procedure, *extracorporeal shock wave lithotripsy*, disintegrates kidney stones with shock waves. Because it is not a surgical procedure, it may be performed on an outpatient basis or, if done in the hospital, with only a minimal hospital stay. Individuals undergoing the procedure may be positioned in a padded chair that is lifted into a stainless steel tub of warm water, or a fluid bag may be placed between the individual and the source of the shock waves to serve as a buffer. Once the individual is positioned to receive maximum effect, shock waves from a machine called a *lithotriptor* are directed to the stones, which are visualized radiographically. The stones are broken apart by the sound waves, and the fragments can then be passed in the urine.

Another lithotripsy technique uses a **laser** instead of shock waves. The laser is directed to the location of stone and disintegrates the stone to small particles so it may be excreted.

### Hydronephrosis

An obstruction can occur anywhere in the urinary tract and may be caused by a stone or a stricture that is related to an infection, an injury, a congenital abnormality, or a tumor. Obstructions prevent urine from flowing through the urinary tract so that urine backflows into the kidneys. Because the kidneys continue to produce urine even though there is backup of urine from the urinary tract, the kidney pelvis eventually becomes swollen and distended. This distension is called **hydronephrosis**. Obstruction of the urinary tract and backflow of urine also predispose individuals to infection of the kidney (**pyelonephritis**).

Individuals with hydronephrosis may experience pain or may feel little discomfort. Diagnosis of hydronephrosis is usually made through X-rays. The kidney must be drained and the obstruction removed to prevent further damage to the kidney. The degree of disability experienced because of hydronephrosis depends on the degree of permanent damage to the kidney. In severe cases hydronephrosis can result in renal failure.

### Glomerulonephritis

**Nephritis** is an inflammation of the kidney. **Glomerulonephritis** is a type of nephritis characterized by inflammation of the *glomeruli* of the kidney. Glomerulonephritis does not result from an invasion of the glomeruli themselves by an infectious organism, but rather occurs as an immunologic response to bacteria or viruses. The immunologic response often follows an infection elsewhere in the body, such as *streptococcal pharyngitis* ("strep throat") or *bacterial endocarditis* (see Chapter 11).

Glomerulonephritis may be *acute* or *chronic*. With the acute form, symptoms may be mild, going undetected. When symptoms are present, they often include **hematuria** (blood in the urine); **proteinuria** (protein in the urine); some impairment in kidney function with the retention of salt and water, possibly leading to elevated blood pressure (**hypertension**); and **edema** (swelling), especially in the face and hands. Generalized edema (**anasarca**) may also occur and may be accompanied by other symptoms, such as **dyspnea** (difficulty breathing) on exertion, visual disturbances, and headache.

Although many individuals recover completely, glomerulonephritis that is not adequately treated or that goes undetected can result in irreversible, permanent structural changes in the kidney leading to *end-stage renal disease* (ESRD). The extent of kidney damage depends on the speed and the effectiveness with which the process can be stopped through appropriate treatment. Treatment of glomerulonephritis focuses on the symptoms and the underlying cause.

### Nephrosis (Nephrotic Syndrome)

*Nephrosis* is general term used to describe conditions in which a kidney has been damaged by something other than direct infection of the kidney itself (such as *glomerulonephritis*). It is a collection of signs and symptoms that can be caused by a variety of kidney conditions. It may be the result of *hypertension* (see Chapter 11), *diabetes*, *glomerulonephritis* (described above), or the **hyperproliferation** (overgrowth) of renal cells because of a tumor. It may also be mediated by the immune system and appear secondary to a systemic disease, such as *rheumatoid arthritis* (see Chapter 14).

The collection of symptoms experienced in nephrosis is termed the *nephrotic syndrome*. This syndrome may include a variety of symptoms, but **proteinuria** (protein in the urine) or **albuminuria** (albumin in the urine) is its hallmark. When the kidneys are damaged, certain substances that normally would be reabsorbed into the bloodstream during the filtering process are passed through the membranes of the *glomerular capillaries* and excreted in the urine. Protein is one of these substances. Thus, an important complication of nephritic syndrome is severe protein malnutrition, which may require nutritional supplementation. Although the kidneys may sometimes repair themselves, nephrosis may also result in renal failure.

### Polycystic Kidney Disease

Polycystic kidney disease is a hereditary disease characterized by the presence of many cysts in the kidneys. The cysts enlarge, compressing and exerting pressure on functioning kidney tissue. The disease progresses slowly over many years. Consequently, individuals may be unaware that they have the disease. Physicians may discover the condition by accident during a routine examination, or, as cysts enlarge, individuals may begin to experience symptoms such as low back pain, **hematuria** (blood in the urine), or frequent urinary tract infections.

The condition eventually progresses to ESRD, but progression sometimes takes as long as 20 years. Treatment of ESRD may include dialysis and/or kidney transplantation (both discussed later in the chapter). Although transplantation is feasible for those with polycystic kidney disease, close family members may not be appropriate donors because of the hereditary nature of the condition.

### Nephrectomy

If trauma has severely injured the kidney, if stones have caused severe damage or are too large to remove, or if the kidney is chronically infected or nonfunctional, the entire kidney may be removed. This surgical procedure is called **nephrectomy**. Individuals can live normal lives with one functioning kidney, but they should guard against infection or injury that could compromise the function of the one remaining kidney.

## Renal Failure

When the kidneys become so damaged, or the functional capacity of the kidneys has declined to the extent that it is insufficient to meet the body's demands, individuals are said to be in *renal failure*. Renal failure can be *acute* or *chronic*, *temporary* or *permanent*. Signs and symptoms of renal failure, whether acute or chronic, depend on the:

- cause of renal failure
- degree of dysfunction of the kidney
- rate of renal failure

The symptoms experienced by individuals whose kidneys have failed depend on the stage of the condition. Individuals may lose a significant amount of kidney function before any symptoms are noted. Both acute and chronic renal failure diminish the kidneys' ability to filter blood adequately and remove water and wastes. As a result, wastes that once would have been excreted by the kidney through the urine continue to circulate in the body. This decreased function affects the body's delicate internal chemical balance. Because the kidneys have multiple functions, kidney dysfunction has an impact on all other organ systems. Kidney damage can eventually progress to **end-stage renal disease**, in which the kidneys essentially cease to function at all.

### Acute Renal Failure

Acute renal failure is sudden and can occur as a complication of other medical conditions, surgery, or trauma. Diminished blood volume (**hypovolemia**) due to hemorrhage or severe dehydration, extreme low blood pressure (**hypotension**), **septicemia** (bacteria in the blood), urinary tract obstruction, and **nephrotoxins** (substances harmful to the kidney, such as certain drugs, solvents, or metals) are all potential causes of acute renal failure.

Treatment of acute renal failure is directed toward removing the cause of the kidney failure when possible, preventing permanent damage to the kidney and complications, and restoring the body chemistry to its normal state. Depending on the cause of acute renal failure, it can often be reversed with no permanent damage to the kidney. If the causative factor can be corrected before irreversible structural changes occur in the kidney, acute renal failure may be temporary. To prevent permanent kidney damage, treatment must begin immediately. Dialysis may be instituted temporarily to take over kidney function until the cause of the kidney failure can be corrected. Dialysis may also be used to remove toxic substances from the body, such as in drug overdose.

### Chronic Renal Failure (End-Stage Renal Disease)

*Chronic renal failure* (ESRD) can result from acute renal failure in which irreversible damage occurs before the cause of the acute failure can be corrected, or it can result from complications of a number of other conditions related to the kidney, such as *glomerulonephritis*, *pyelonephritis*, or *polycystic kidney disease*, all discussed earlier in the chapter. ESRD can also result from the complications of a number of systemic conditions, such as *hypertension* (see Chapter 11, *diabetes* (see Chapter 9), autoimmune diseases such as lupus erythematosus (see Chapter 14), or *vascular disease* resulting in **nephrosclerosis** (condition in which the arteries of the kidney become thickened). It can also result from exposure to *nephrotoxins, drug toxicity,* or *drug overdose.*

### Symptoms of End-Stage Renal Disease

Whereas acute renal failure occurs rapidly, chronic renal failure may progress gradually over time. ESRD is usually broken into stages:

- Early-stage renal disease, with 40 to 75 percent loss of nephron function (*renal impairment*)
- Second-stage renal disease, with 75 to 80 percent of nephron function (*renal insufficiency*)
- ESRD, with less than 15 percent nephron function (*renal failure*) (Sosa-Guerrero & Gomez, 1997)

In early-stage renal disease, symptoms may be barely perceptible. Difficulty concentrating or development of shortened attention span may be the first symptom of renal failure. In the early stages there may also be increased urine production (**polyuria**). Examination of the urine (**urinalysis**) may reveal protein in the urine as an early sign. Since protein is usually reabsorbed into the regular body circulation after being filtered through the kidney, the presence of protein in the urine is an indication of failure of this mechanism.

As kidney function declines, waste products of metabolism (*urea* and *creatinine*) build up in the blood, a condition called **uremia**. As waste products continue to increase and circulate in the general circulation, individuals may experience overall itching (**pruritus**).

The final stage of renal disease is *end-stage renal disease*. At this stage individuals must be treated through dialysis or receive a kidney transplant if they are to survive. Individuals with ESRD are unable

to regulate water balance in their body. Urine production is severely diminished (**oliguria**) or nonexistent (**anuria**). Consequently, water that would have been excreted as urine remains in the body, creating fluid overload. Although some water is excreted through the gastrointestinal and respiratory systems, as well as through perspiration, the kidneys are the main source of fluid excretion. Overload of fluid in the body causes stress on the circulatory system, contributing to **hypertension** (high blood pressure) and especially stressing the heart, potentially causing cardiac dysfunction and failure. Outward symptoms of fluid overload consist of *weight gain, edema,* and *difficulty breathing* (**dyspnea**). The problem of fluid overload is compounded if there is also increased sodium in the blood, as discussed in the following paragraph.

*Sodium,* an electrolyte, helps regulate the fluid content of the body's tissues and, along with *potassium* and another electrolyte (*chloride*), regulates the body's internal chemistry. In ESRD, the kidneys are unable to excrete sodium. Too much sodium in the body causes retention of fluid and swelling (**edema**). As a result, individuals may experience sudden weight gain and puffiness or swelling of the face, feet, ankles, legs, and at times the arms and abdomen. Individuals may have high blood pressure and complain of feeling uncomfortable and bloated. They may also experience difficulty breathing because of the fluid overload on the heart and lungs.

Another electrolyte, *potassium,* is important for the stimulation and relaxation that allows muscles, including the heart muscles and the muscles used for respiration, to contract. When there is too much or too little potassium, *muscle weakness* can occur as well as dangerous disturbances in *heart* and *respiratory function.*

Normally most potassium taken in through the diet is excreted by the kidney; however, in ESRD the kidney is unable to secrete potassium, so it is retained and builds up in the blood (**hyperkalemia**). Excessive amounts of potassium in the blood can adversely affect organs such as the heart, potentially causing cardiac arrest.

*Calcium* in the blood is decreased below normal levels in ESRD, partially because the kidney is unable to produce sufficient amounts of *vitamin D*, necessary for calcium absorption, and also because calcium absorption in the intestine is decreased. ESRD also causes overactivity of the *parathyroid glands* (see Chapter 9), causing calcium loss from the bone (**osteoporosis**), further contributing to bone pain and fractures.

Individuals with ESRD may become *malnourished* because of **anorexia** (loss of appetite), nausea and vomiting, or lack of appetite due to depression. **Anemia** (reduction of circulating red blood cells) accompanied by iron deficiency is characteristic in renal failure, not only because of diet, but also because the kidneys are no longer able to produce *erythropoietin*, a hormone responsible for initiating red blood cell production, and because individuals with ESRD have decreased ability to absorb iron from the intestine. As a result, they experience weakness and low exercise tolerance. It may be difficult for many individuals with ESRD to walk very far without resting.

Walking may be further impeded by a condition called *peripheral neuropathy*, which is common in individuals with ESRD. Uremia has toxic effects on nerves, and especially the peripheral nerves of the hands and feet, resulting in **peripheral neuropathy**, which causes weakness and loss of sensation in the arms and legs. The central nervous system may also be affected in ESRD. Intellectual impairment may coincide with worsening *uremia*, so that individuals have increased difficulty concentrating or demonstrate a shortened attention span.

Because of both the physical and emotional changes present in ESRD, individuals with ESRD may also experience impaired sexual function (Ifudu, 1998). Not only may there be diminished interest in engaging in sexual activity, but there may also be diminished physical response to sexual stimulation in both males and females.

### Treatment and Management of End-Stage Renal Disease

Because there is no cure for chronic renal failure, treatment is directed at control. In very early stages of chronic renal failure, treatment may include restricting water to an amount equal to urine output, carefully monitoring body weight, and managing the diet to provide adequate nutrition without overtaxing the kidney with metabolic waste products. The kidney can normally continue to function with as little as 10 percent of its function; however, loss of function beyond this point requires either dialysis or renal transplant in order for individuals to survive (Teichman, 2001).

Diet. When kidney function is significantly reduced, individuals' diet and fluid intake must be regulated to conform to the limited or absent function of the kidneys. The intake of protein, sodium, potassium, fluid, and calories must be carefully regulated and monitored to:

- minimize waste products in the body
- maintain electrolyte levels in the body within normal limits
- avoid either too much or too little fluid in the body

Diets are prescribed individually. There is no one diet that is appropriate for all individuals with ESRD. Individuals with ESRD work closely with *dietitians* (individuals who specialize in the science of applying nutritional information to the regulation of diet) to develop a diet plan right for them. The type of dietary prescription is based on individual needs and the type of kidney disease the individual has.

Since, in ESRD, the kidney is no longer able to filter out the waste products of protein metabolism, the dietary intake of protein must be controlled. Consequently, dietary intake of foods especially high in protein, such as meat, fish, eggs, poultry, and dairy products, is restricted.

Because in ESRD the kidneys are unable to excrete potassium and because of the adverse, and potentially fatal, effects of high levels of potassium on heart muscle as well as on other muscles in the body, potassium buildup in the blood (**hyperkalemia**) must be avoided. Dietary intake of foods rich in potassium must, therefore, be restricted. Examples of foods high in potassium content are listed in Table 13–1. The more severe the loss of kidney function, the more carefully potassium levels must be regulated.

Because sodium is important in the regulation of fluid in the body, as well as in maintaining the body's internal chemical balance, and because the kidneys in ESRD cannot excrete sodium effectively, individuals with ESRD must also regulate their dietary intake of sodium. Sodium restrictions affect the intake of not only salt but also a number of other foods high in sodium. Foods containing high levels of sodium must be restricted. (See Table 13–2.)

Since individuals with ESRD are unable to regulate fluid balance, the amount of fluid taken orally must be restricted. Included in fluid intake are ice cubes, gelatin desserts, sherbet, or any other food that liquefies at room temperature. Physicians calculate the amount of fluid individuals may have based on the amount of fluid lost through perspiration and respiration. Adequate fluid intake is based on the patient's weight gain at specific intervals. In some instances fluid intake may be restricted to no more than one cup of fluid per day.

**Table 13–1**  Foods High in Potassium

| | |
|---|---|
| oranges, orange juice | strawberries |
| grapefruit, grapefruit juice | raisins |
| bananas | beets |
| apricots | cabbage |
| cantaloupe | carrots |
| kidney beans | celery |
| pears | many breakfast cereals |
| potatoes | many breads |
| spinach | many nuts |
| tomatoes | salt subtitutes |
| peaches | |

**Table 13–2**  Foods High in Sodium

corned and chipped beef
bacon
ham
cold cuts such as bologna
pork sausage
canned tuna, salmon, sardines
pork sausage
hot dogs
cheddar and Swiss cheese
snack foods such as pretzels, popcorn, potato chips, some crackers
most canned vegetables
olives
soft drinks

Because of food restrictions, individuals may have difficulty maintaining sufficient caloric intake. Foods low in sodium, potassium, and protein may be needed throughout the day as supplements to add additional calories. For in-between snacking, the dietitian may recommend specialized products that are high-calorie, low-protein, and low-electrolyte foods.

Medications. Because of dietary restrictions in the intake of dairy products and other foods high in calcium, individuals with ESRD may experience calcium depletion. Consequently, calcium supplements as well as supplements of vitamin D derivatives normally produced in the kidney are also given by mouth. The physician may also prescribe supplementary vitamins and certain minerals.

Oral iron supplements are frequently given as part of the medical treatment of ESRD, as well as **erythropoietin** (a substance normally produced in the kidney that stimulates production of red blood cells). The medication is given **subcutaneously** (into the fatty tissue under the skin) three times a week after each dialysis treatment (discussed later in the chapter).

Individuals with ESRD are often placed on *antihypertensive medications* to help control blood pressure. Excess fluid is removed through the process of dialysis, discussed below.

Dialysis. Individuals with renal failure, whether acute or chronic, cannot survive unless there is a method for compensating for kidney function. Dialysis performs the function of the kidney, that of removing waste and fluid from the body. It may be used *temporarily*, as in the case of *acute renal failure*, or it may be used to sustain life when kidney damage is irreversible and permanent, as in ESRD. For individuals with acute renal failure, dialysis is a life-saving necessity. When individuals reach ESRD, either dialysis or a transplant is necessary for survival.

If individuals with chronic renal failure or ESRD are suitable candidates for renal transplantation, dialysis may be used until an appropriate donor kidney is available. Not all individuals with ESRD are suitable candidates for kidney transplant. If a transplant is not feasible, individuals with ESRD must remain on dialysis the rest of their lives.

There are two types of dialysis, *peritoneal dialysis* and *hemodialysis*. Both types simulate kidney function in that:

- waste products of metabolism are removed from the blood
- an appropriate balance in the body chemistry is maintained
- excess fluid is removed from the blood

Both types of dialysis involve the use of a *semipermeable membrane*, a porous material that allows some substances to pass through but keeps other substances in the blood. The blood of individuals undergoing dialysis is on one side of the membrane, and a specially prepared solution called a **dialysate** is on the other side of the membrane. Difference in concentrations of the blood and dialysate allow certain particles, but not others, to pass from the blood, through the membrane, and into the dialysate, where they can then be removed through dialysis.

The development of hemodialysis for ESRD has enabled many people who normally might have died from their condition to live useful and productive lives (Himmelfarb, 2002). However, dialysis is not without risk. The mortality rate for individuals with acute renal failure is high (Bonventre, 2002). Individuals with ESRD receiving dialysis have a first-year mortality rate of approximately 25 percent (US Renal Data System, 2001). Since most peo-

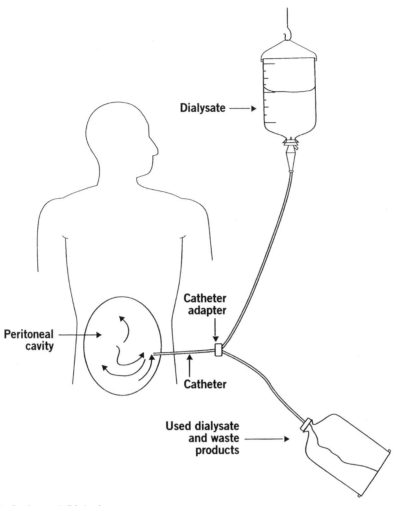

**Figure 13–2**  Peritoneal Dialysis.

ple with ESRD have other systemic conditions that have caused or contributed to
their renal failure, improved outcomes in
dialysis may depend on improved medical
care in the early stages of chronic renal
disease (Kinchen, Sadler, Fink, et al., 2002).

*Peritoneal Dialysis.* In *peritoneal dialysis*
the semipermeable membrane needed for
dialysis consists of the **peritoneum** (the thin
membrane that lines the abdominal cavity). A tube or catheter is surgically placed
within the abdominal cavity. During peri-

toneal dialysis, **dialysate** from a bag is
drained through the catheter into the
abdominal cavity (see Figure 13–2). The
catheter is clamped, and the dialysate is
left in the abdominal cavity for a specified
amount of time. During this time, waste
products and excess fluid pass from the
blood, through the peritoneal membrane,
and into the dialysate. At the end of the
specified period, the catheter is unclamped,
and the dialysate, which now contains the
waste products and excess fluid, is drained
from the body through the catheter. The

tube is again clamped and remains in place for the next dialysis treatment.

Peritoneal dialysis is performed at home, manually or with a machine. There are several methods of peritoneal dialysis:

- *Continuous ambulatory peritoneal dialysis (CAPD)*
- *Intermittent peritoneal dialysis (IPD)*
- *Continuous cycling peritoneal dialysis (CCPD)*

Regardless of the method used for peritoneal dialysis, the principles remain the same. With CAPD, dialysate is instilled into the abdominal cavity manually, using gravity. A bag of dialysate solution is connected to the catheter. The individual then elevates the bag, causing the dialysate to flow into the abdominal cavity. The catheter is clamped and the dialysate left in place for 4 to 8 hours. The catheter is then unclamped and the bag lowered so that the dialysate drains from the abdominal cavity by gravity. When the bag is full, the individual detaches the bag from the catheter, attaches a new bag of dialysate, and begins the process again. Individuals change the dialysate manually three to five times a day. Individuals using this type of peritoneal dialysis are able to continue their regular daily activities, stopping only for periodic intervals to drain the dialysate and attach a fresh bag.

IPD and CCPD both use a machine. *Intermittent peritoneal dialysis* is performed *three or more times a week*, with each exchange lasting for 10 or more hours. With IPD, the catheter is connected to the cycling machine at night. The exchange takes place while individuals sleep; consequently, they are free to engage in their regular activities during the day. CCPD also uses a cycling machine but is performed daily. In CCPD the catheter is connected to the cycling machine, which performs multiple solution exchanges while the individual sleeps. In the morning, individuals disconnect the catheter from the machine, leaving the last solution in the abdomen all day while they engage in their regular activities.

Peritoneal dialysis may be chosen as the dialysis method for individuals who have, in addition to kidney disease, other medical conditions that increase the risk of complications associated with hemodialysis. In other instances, peritoneal dialysis may be chosen because of the relative ease of the procedure and the limited use of sophisticated equipment, factors that enable individuals to use peritoneal dialysis in the home. Depending on the type of procedure used, individuals may enjoy more mobility with peritoneal dialysis than with hemodialysis. If severe vascular disease interferes with the blood supply to the peritoneum or there is an increased vulnerability to infection, however, peritoneal dialysis may be contraindicated.

Although generally a safe procedure, peritoneal dialysis can have a number of associated complications. The most common is **peritonitis** (inflammation of the peritoneum) caused when the peritoneum is contaminated with bacteria. If peritonitis develops, antibiotics may be used to treat the infection, or peritoneal dialysis may be discontinued and hemodialysis begun. Other complications that may occur as a result of peritoneal dialysis are *plugging or displacement of the catheter, development of hernias,* or *pain* during dialysis. Over time, infection or the dialysate concentration itself may damage the peritoneum. Peritoneal dialysis is usually a limited procedure because of the loss of membrane function.

*Hemodialysis.* The most common type of dialysis used for individuals with ESRD is **hemodialysis**, in which an artificial kidney machine (**dialyzer**) circulates and filters the blood outside the body to remove waste products and excess fluid. Hemodialysis requires that there is access to individuals' circulation. Access routes through which blood is removed from the individual to be circulated through the dialysis machine and then returned to the individual's circulation may be surgically created through a *graft*, an *external arteriovenous shunt* (less commonly used today), an *internal arteriovenous fistula* (Figure 13–3), or a *subclavian cannula* (see Figure 13–4).

Access routes are created surgically, most often in the forearm. *Grafts* that connect an artery and a vein may be made by surgical placement of synthetic material or of a vein that has been removed from another part of the individual's body. The *external arteriovenous shunt* consists of surgical placement of a tube (**cannula**) under the skin to connect an artery to a vein. The *internal arteriovenous fistula* is also created surgically. In this procedure, an artery is joined to a vein underneath the skin, establishing an opening called a *fistula* between the two. Shunting arterial blood into the vein causes the vein to become thickened and enlarged so it can be repeatedly used as an access to the circulation for dialysis. It may take from 2 to 6 weeks for the fistula to become thickened and enlarged enough so that it can be used for dialysis. In the meantime, temporary access may be maintained through the subclavian artery.

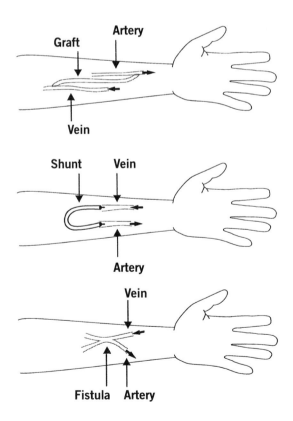

**Figure 13–3** Access for Hemodialysis Through a Graft, a Shunt, or a Fistula.

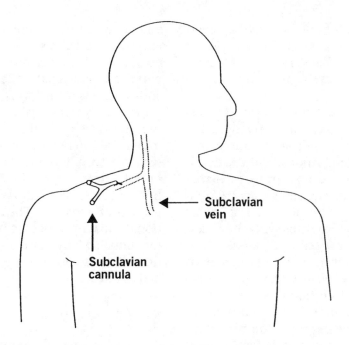

**Figure 13–4** Access for Hemodialysis Through a Subclavian Cannula.

For hemodialysis, a large needle is placed into the artery side of the access route. Another large needle is placed in the vein side of the access. Tubes are attached to the needles and connected to the dialysis machine. Blood moves from the first tube to the dialysis machine, where it is cleansed and filtered. The cleansed blood is then returned to the individual through the second needle in the vein.

The artificial kidney has two compartments, one for the individual's blood and one for the dialysate solution. A synthetic semipermeable membrane separates these compartments within the artificial kidney. Blood cells and other important substances are too large to pass through the pores of the membrane, so they remain in their compartment. Most waste products, however, are small enough to pass through the membrane into the dialysate, and they are washed away. The

cleansed blood then returns through the tube to the individual.

Hemodialysis is usually performed for 3 to 6 hours a day three times a week (Owen, Pereira, & Savegh, 2000). It has also been performed successfully on a daily basis for 2 hours a day (Schiffle, Lang, & Fischer, 2002). Hemodialysis can be performed at a kidney dialysis center or, in some instances, at home. Because home hemodialysis requires a high degree of individual control, self-destructive tendencies in individuals or unwillingness of family members or caregivers to participate in the procedure is a contraindication for home hemodialysis. Home dialysis requires someone (a family member, or someone who has been hired) who has been trained to assist with the procedure. The level of responsibility as well as the need to be always present at specified times of dialysis can cause considerable stress for the helper, especially if he or she is a family member. Stress levels associated with home hemodialysis are usually evaluated and monitored before such a home dialysis program is implemented.

The success of hemodialysis depends on individuals' level of motivation, the presence of other medical conditions that may cause complications, and the development of complications from the hemodialysis itself. The numerous potential complications related to hemodialysis range from technical problems with the access route to more generalized complications that could result in death. Arteriovenous grafts and subclavian catheters are especially prone to infection that can result in **septicemia** (toxins in the blood), a potentially life-threatening complication. Cardiac-related complications, such as **pericarditis** (inflammation of the outer layer of membrane surrounding the heart), **myocardial infarction** (heart attack), **arrhythmias** (irregular heartbeat), or **hypertension** (high blood pressure), may also occur (Ifudu, 1998). Another possible complication of hemodialysis is stroke or some other thrombolytic event. Because of the risk of clot formation in the access route, individuals on hemodialysis may receive *anticoagulant medication* during the procedure. Administration of this medication, however, may also increase the risk of bleeding. Hemodialysis itself is painless, although some light discomfort may occur when needles are inserted for dialysis. Although during dialysis individuals are confined to the dialysis unit, they can read, watch television, or sleep.

Rapid changes that occur in fluid and chemical balances in the body during dialysis cause some individuals to experience nausea, vomiting, headaches, or muscle cramps in association with hemodialysis. Some individuals may become anemic, and some experience sleep disturbances or mental cloudiness. Individuals on prolonged hemodialysis may have changes in nerves of the extremities resulting in **peripheral neuropathy** (loss of sensation and weakness in the arms and legs).

Hemodialysis can relieve many of the symptoms of renal disease, but not all. Individuals on hemodialysis may develop secondary conditions that increase the risk of bone fractures, or the procedure may not adequately clear all wastes, leading to feelings of weakness. The degree of functional capacity varies from individual to individual. Many continue to lead near-normal lives, however, except for their dialysis treatments.

### Renal Transplantation

Renal transplantation involves surgically placing a kidney from another individual inside the body of an individual with renal disease. The diseased kidney is not removed from the individual receiving the renal transplant. Transplants may be received from a family member (*living-related donor*), an individual who is not related to the individual (*living-unrelated donor*), or an individual who has recently died (*cadaver donor*). Regardless of the status of the donor, the donor's blood and tissues must closely match those of the recipient to decrease the chances of the body's rejection of the transplant (El Nahas, Harris, & Anderson, 2000).

Although renal transplant is commonly performed because of ESRD, it may also be performed if one kidney has been removed and the second kidney is injured or ceases to function. Renal transplant frees individuals from the restrictions associated with dialysis, diminishes many symptoms of chronic renal failure, and improves overall quality of life.

Before being considered for renal transplant, recipients undergo careful and thorough medical evaluation to see if they are suitable candidates. General health, including the presence of other diseases that may potentially affect the success of the transplant or make it impossible, are evaluated. Pre-transplant evaluation also includes a thorough psychological evaluation. Discussion of the risk of rejection and infection and the lifelong need to use immunosuppressants with their corresponding risk (discussed below) is a part of the pre-transplant protocol.

Expectations for the transplant are discussed with both the recipient and the living donor. Also evaluated is the recipient's ability to adjust to the transplant as well as his or her ability to adjust should the transplant fail. The degree of family and social support is also assessed. The cost of the kidney transplant itself, as well as the cost associated with travel to the transplant center, lodging for family, and the lifelong medication needed after the transplant, can be staggering. Consequently, the *social service* evaluation also includes the financial status of candidates for transplant and the identification of resources that can help to cover costs.

Scarcity of donors is the major factor that inhibits renal transplantation. Whether the donor is a living donor or cadaver donor, compatibility of tissue type and blood type and a variety of other factors determine the degree of success of the transplantation. Tissue typing is most important in decreasing the possibility of rejection. The most desirable sources of kidneys for transplantation are closely related, living donors, but surgeons in new protocols are attempting to use living, unrelated, and blood type-incompatible donors (Delmonico, 2004).

At the time of transplant, both donor and recipient are hospitalized. The individual with ESRD has dialysis the day before the transplant. The donor has renal angiography (discussed elsewhere in the chapter) to determine which kidney will be used for the transplant. The surgical procedure for the kidney transplant consists of removing the kidney from the donor and placing it in a surgically constructed pocket in the lower abdomen of the recipient.

Once the donor kidney has been transplanted, it may begin to function immediately. Early functioning of the transplanted kidney is a good prognostic sign for success of the transplant. When the recipient is discharged from the hospital, he or she must be careful to avoid infection due to the immunosuppressant drugs used to prevent rejection of the new kidney. Risk of infection is greatest the first 6 months after surgery (Soulillou, 2001). During this time, the individual needs to be particularly careful to avoid contact with persons with communicable disease. After transplant, prophylactic antibiotics are to be administered prior to any dental work. After transplant, the individual receiving the kidney may return to work within 3 weeks to 1 month. Because of the extensive surgical procedure necessary for removing the kidney from the donor, recovery time for the donor is considerably longer.

The major complication of kidney transplantation is rejection, which can destroy the transplanted kidney (Pascual, Theruvath, Kawai, Tolkoff-Rubin, & Cosimi, 2002). Although the rejection rate in the first year after renal transplant has dramatically decreased over the last decade (Hariharan et al., 2000), long-term success is less dependable, with about half of individuals receiving a cadaver kidney losing it after 10 years (Marsden, 2003). The body's defense system, or immune system, naturally attacks foreign substances in the body. Unfortunately, the immune system does not distinguish between a life-saving transplanted kidney and harmful substances. To prevent rejection, medications called *immunosuppressants* are prescribed after transplant. These medications block the body's normal immune response. Unfortunately, immunosuppressants can cause a number of complications, including an increased rate of **malignancy** (cancer), *susceptibility to infection, formation of cataracts*, and *degeneration of bone*. If rejection takes place immediately, it may be necessary to remove the transplanted kidney to avoid a generalized body reaction that could be fatal. Rejection most commonly occurs within the first 6 weeks after the transplantation; however, chronic rejection may occur months or years later.

### Psychological Issues in End-Stage Renal Disease

The initial shock and realization of kidney failure and its ramifications may be immobilizing. Reactions vary in degree from severe depression to total denial. Denial can be helpful in reducing stress levels, but it can be life-threatening if it leads to noncompliance with the recommended treatment.

Individuals who begin dialysis may also have a period of adjustment. When first beginning dialysis, individuals may be hopeful and confident because of the immediate physical improvements they experience after dialysis. In the early sessions of dialysis, individuals may experience apprehension or uneasiness about the possibility that the machine may malfunction. As they become more comfortable with dialysis, these fears generally subside.

As the individuals continue in dialysis, they may become discouraged and disenchanted when they come to the realization that there is no hope that the kidneys will miraculously begin to function again. They may experience loss of self-esteem and feelings of helplessness and inadequacy as they come to recognize that they are dependent on the dialysis machine for their existence. Fears of death may then conflict with fears of continuing to live a life sustained by dialysis with its subsequent restrictions. Many individuals reach a stage of acceptance in which the limitations and complications of dialysis are incorporated into their lives. Even when individuals reach this stage of adjustment, however, there may be alternating periods of depression.

Anger and hostility are frequent manifestations of conflicts between dependency and independence—even conflicts between living and dying. Feelings of hostility may be expressed openly, but they may also be internalized as individuals on dialysis realize their degree of dependence not only on a machine, but also on those who provide their care. These internalized feelings can be self-destructive if individuals rebel against the necessary care and treatment. Feelings of sadness, hopelessness, and despair may become so severe that individuals with ESRD consider suicide as a way to resolve the problems surrounding the condition. Suicide attempts may be subtle and covert, such as not adhering to the diet, taking in too much fluid, or in other ways failing to cooperate with treatment.

Transplantation involves a number of psychological issues as well. Individuals identified as eligible recipients of a transplanted kidney are often elated about the anticipated improvement in their quality of life after the transplantation. Consequently, rejection of the transplanted kidney can be devastating. Even if rejection does not occur and quality of life is significantly improved, individuals with a transplanted kidney may express disappointment that long-term care and evaluation are still necessary. In addition, they may be disappointed if transplantation has not restored the state of health that was theirs before the onset of ESRD. Even after the initial postoperative period, the chance of later rejection or the risk that infection will damage the transplanted kidney may be sources of anxiety.

Individuals may also go through several stages of adjustment after transplantation. Despite significant psychological preparation usually prior to transplantation, postsurgical psychological reactions may still occur. If the donor is a family member or friend of the recipient, the relationship may be altered. At times the relationship is strengthened, but it may also become weakened. Recipients may experience guilt, anxiety, or depression because of the donation of the kidney they received. If the donor felt pressure, either real or imagined, to donate a kidney, he or she may experience stress, conflict, or guilt, especially if he or she decided to decline, or resentment if he or she donated the kidney under duress. If the kidney was received from a cadaver donor, recipients may have fantasies about embodying the spirit of someone who is dead. Whether the transplant was from a living or cadaver donor, recipients may still feel that the kidney is not a part of them.

### Lifestyle Issues in End-Stage Renal Disease

Individuals with renal failure face profound changes in the activities of daily living. When kidney function is impaired or nonexistent, intake of foods and fluids must be carefully monitored. Such restrictions are necessary to minimize the amount of waste products and to avoid the presence of too much or too little fluid in the body. Because in chronic renal failure or ESRD the kidney is no longer able to ex-

crete adequately, total fluid intake between dialysis sessions must also be monitored. Fluid intake includes not only beverages, but also water contained in foods. Individuals are weighed before and after each dialysis treatment to monitor fluid gain so that the dialysis procedure may be adjusted accordingly.

Although there are no limitations or restrictions regarding sexual activity, sexual function is impaired in many individuals on dialysis. Some men with ESRD experience impotence or have a diminished interest in sexual activities. Women with ESRD often report general disinterest or a diminished interest in sexual activities, or a decreased response to sexual stimulation. Sexual dysfunction among individuals on dialysis probably results from a combination of generally poor health and emotional reactions to a life-threatening illness. The reproductive capacity of both men and women on dialysis is severely diminished. Sexual function may improve after renal transplant, and conception is possible. If the transplant is rejected or the individual is heavily medicated, sexual function may be impaired.

### Social Issues in End-Stage Renal Disease

Renal conditions may not affect individuals' social activities until the kidneys become dysfunctional, causing restrictions or alterations in regular activities. Although family, friends, and associates play an important supportive role in individuals' adjustment to kidney failure, an overindulgent attitude can impede individuals' return to the earlier level of independence. Individuals on dialysis may have to alter activities, both because of their physical condition and because of the dialysis schedule. Those with shunts should avoid any activity that could expose the shunt area to potential injury. Because heat intolerance is often associated with ESRD, activities requiring exposure to heat should be avoided.

Previously existing relationship problems may be amplified after a diagnosis of ESRD. Additional stress brought on by dialysis or the wait for transplantation may intensify discord if it exists. If dialysis is conducted at home, the family member assisting with dialysis may feel burdened and strained by the added responsibility and regimen of the dialysis program, since activities must be programmed around the dialysis schedule. Individuals' physical complaints, fatigue, and loss of interest in sexual activities may compound the problem. Although financial assistance for dialysis is usually available through government or private agencies, the overall financial burden of medical bills, dialysis, and lost income if the individual with kidney disease is not able to continue working exerts additional stress on relationships. Even if these individuals feel well enough to participate in social activities, many activities may be altered because of dietary and fluid restrictions. Individuals may be reluctant to accept the dinner invitations of friends because of dietary restrictions, or they may themselves give up entertaining because of the limitations of their condition. Increasing social isolation can increase loss of self-esteem, feelings of depression, and hopelessness.

Vacations are still possible but require careful planning for individuals who are on hemodialysis. Dialysis units near the vacation spot must be located, and arrangements must be made for dialysis at the center prior to departure. Peritoneal dialysis, although offering more flexibility, also requires that individuals plan for travel. Depending on the amount of time away and the method of travel, they may need to prearrange shipment of dialysate or the cycling machine to their destination.

Although transplantation can free individuals from some limitations, other issues may arise. If the donor is a family member or friend, a strong bond may develop between the donor and the recipient; in some cases, however, problems occur in the relationship. The donor may resent the attention paid to the recipient after the transplant or may feel abandoned. The recipient, on the other hand, may have feelings of guilt because of the potential jeopardy to the donor, who is left with only one kidney.

### Vocational Issues in End-Stage Renal Disease

As ESRD progresses and symptoms become more pronounced, the impact on vocational function increases. Fatigue may necessitate a shortened workday or rest periods during the day. Problems of impaired judgment, difficulty with memory, or irritability may interfere with adequate job performance. Peripheral neuropathy may make it difficult or impossible to perform tasks such as lifting or to complete tasks that require manual dexterity.

Individuals on dialysis may need a flexible work schedule to accommodate the dialysis schedule. Many dialysis centers are operational 24 hours each day, enabling individuals to arrange dialysis in off-hours. Blood access routes, such as shunts, require protection; occupations that pose a potential threat of damage to the shunt should be avoided. Fatigue or the decreased ability to walk caused by peripheral neuropathy may necessitate a change to a more sedentary line of work. Environmental issues should also be considered. Work that requires exposure to high temperatures should be avoided because of the heat intolerance associated with kidney diseases.

## DIAGNOSTIC PROCEDURES FOR RENAL AND URINARY TRACT CONDITIONS

### Urinalysis

Urine may be examined by direct visualization, under a microscope, or through other laboratory tests. The urinalysis report contains information about the concentration, acidity, and appearance of the urine, as well as the presence of any other components such as protein, sugar, blood, bacteria, or various types of cells in the urine. A urinalysis not only provides a gross estimate of kidney function, but it also permits identification of other potential problems (e.g., infection) or systemic conditions (e.g., diabetes) that may exist.

A urinalysis is often a screening test to help determine what, if any, other tests are needed. Collection of urine can be external or, if a sterile specimen (one that is uncontaminated by organisms outside the urinary tract) is needed, through a tube or catheter passed through the external opening (urinary meatus) into the bladder.

### Urine Culture

Laboratory examination of a sterile urine specimen, a *urine culture*, helps to determine whether there is an infection within the urinary tract and, if so, which organisms are causing the infection. Specimens for a urine culture are usually obtained through catheterization.

### Blood Urea Nitrogen

A blood test in which the level of *urea nitrogen* (a waste product of protein metabolism) in the blood is measured can be helpful in evaluation of kidney function.

The kidneys normally excrete urea nitrogen. The presence of urea nitrogen in the blood indicates potential kidney impairment. The urea level may also be elevated in conditions other than renal disease. Conditions such as starvation, dehydration, or conditions in which the blood supply to the kidneys is poor may also cause elevated urea nitrogen levels.

### Serum Creatinine

*Creatinine* is a waste product of a high-energy compound (creatine phosphate) found in skeletal muscle tissue, and it is usually filtered out of the blood through the kidney. Elevation in creatinine levels in the blood indicates damage to a large number of *nephrons*. Determination of the creatinine level is a more sensitive test than that of the blood urea nitrogen level and is a better reflection of kidney function.

### Creatinine Clearance Test

The *creatinine clearance test* is used to determine the kidneys' *glomerular filtration rate*. It involves a comparison of the amount of creatinine in the blood serum (*serum creatinine*) with the amount of creatinine excreted in the urine over a specified period of time. For the test, individuals collect and save all their urine during a specified period of time. Blood tests are performed at various points during that time period, and the amounts of creatinine in the blood serum and in the urine are compared. A decreased creatinine clearance rate indicates decreased glomerular function and, thus, kidney dysfunction. The creatinine clearance rate is a better indicator of renal dysfunction than is the measurement of serum creatinine alone. Creatinine clearance tests may be used to diagnose kidney dysfunction or to evaluate the progress of renal disease.

### Kidney, Ureter, and Bladder Roentgenography (KUB)

A simple X-ray of the kidney, ureters, and bladder is called a *KUB*. The X-ray film outlines the size, shape, and location of these structures, but it does not indicate kidney function.

### Intravenous Pyelogram

Radiologic examination of the kidneys, ureters, and bladder through an *intravenous pyelogram* may be done on an outpatient basis. During the test, a special dye is injected into a vein in the individual's arm. The dye is filtered by the kidney and excreted through the urinary tract, during which time X-ray films are taken at intervals for approximately 1 hour. The intravenous pyelogram helps to identify not only any structural abnormalities of the kidney, but also any problems with passage of the dye through the urinary system. Because some individuals are hypersensitive to components of the dye and may have severe allergic reactions, questions about known allergies and skin tests are usually routine prior to testing.

### Cystoscopy

A **urologist** (a physician who specializes in the diagnosis and treatment of conditions of the urinary tract) may visualize the *urethra* and *bladder* directly through a special tube, called a *cystoscope*, inserted through the *urinary meatus* and *urethra* into the *bladder*. This procedure is called *cystoscopy* and can be used either as a diagnostic procedure or as a part of treatment. It may be performed on an outpatient or inpatient basis and may be performed under local or general anesthesia. The cystoscopic examination makes it possible to identify any abnormalities in the internal structure of the bladder, as well as to remove foreign objects or calculi from the bladder, to remove tumors or other abnormal tissue from the bladder, or to perform a *retrograde pyelogram*, described below.

### Retrograde Pyelography

*Retrograde pyelograms* are performed to assess the function of the *kidneys* and *ureters* and to detect possible abnormalities or obstructions in the collecting system. During a retrograde pyelogram, a small catheter is inserted through a tube (*cystoscope*), which is then directed into the *ureters* to the *pelvis* of the kidney. A special dye is injected through the catheter and X-ray films are taken to visualize the collecting system. The procedure may be done on an outpatient or inpatient basis.

### Renal Biopsy

In some cases, it is necessary to remove a small piece of kidney tissue for the diagnosis of kidney disease. This procedure is called a *renal biopsy* and may be done in several ways. One method involves a surgical incision over the kidney so that the physician can directly view the kidney and remove the specimen. Because this procedure is done under a general anesthetic in a hospital setting, it has a prolonged recuperation period. The second, more commonly used method involves the insertion of a specially designed needle through the skin over the kidney. The needle is then inserted into the kidney, and a small amount of kidney tissue is removed. This technique is called a *percutaneous renal biopsy*. It is generally performed under a local anesthetic in a hospital setting. Because it requires no incision or general anesthesia, only limited recuperation time is needed.

## Renal Angiography

In order to examine the vascular function of the kidney, a diagnostic procedure called *renal angiography* may be done. The procedure is performed by inserting a needle into the *femoral artery* (located in the groin). A small catheter is passed through the needle into the artery and advanced until it reaches the renal arteries. Dye is then injected through the catheter, and X-ray films are taken at 2- to 3-second intervals to examine the functioning of the renal artery.

## PSYCHOSOCIAL ISSUES IN RENAL AND URINARY TRACT CONDITIONS

### Psychological Issues

Not all kidney conditions are life-threatening, and they do not all impose major changes in functional capacity. Although they may cause some pain and discomfort, conditions such as *cystitis* frequently leave no functional or psychological sequelae. ESRD, however, has a profound impact on all areas of individuals' lives, causing significant psychological stress.

Psychological changes are associated both with emotional reactions to a life-threatening disease and with the physiological changes that occur with ESRD. Emotional reactions to end-stage kidney failure vary. Mourning over the loss of body function or loss of control, feelings of disconnectedness, and anger are all emotional reactions commonly reported (Moua, 2000). Elevated levels of toxic waste in the blood can produce cognitive changes, such as impaired judgment, drowsiness, and difficulty with concentration. Other possible cognitive changes include memory loss, speech impairments, and irritability. The physical

discomfort associated with dialysis, such as interrupted sleep patterns, nausea, lethargy, and shortness of breath, may increase the individuals' psychological distress. Individuals eligible for kidney transplant may also experience the stress of waiting for a transplant as well as fear of rejection if the transplant takes place.

Uncertainty is also an issue in ESRD. Treatment choices are not always final. Individuals who choose peritoneal dialysis rather than hemodialysis may need to switch if complications from peritoneal dialysis occur. Individuals using hemodialysis may later consider a kidney transplant should one become available. Even after individuals receive a kidney transplant, uncertainty remains because there is always the chance that rejection of the transplant may occur.

### Lifestyle Issues

Many renal and urinary tract disorders require lifestyle changes during the acute phase of the condition; however, after treatment, few limitations may exist. The exception is those individuals with ESRD, for whom lifestyle implications are profound. Not only are there stringent dietary restrictions, but the requirement of regular dialysis treatments restricts individuals' freedom of time. Even when individuals receive a successful transplant, the medical regimen is demanding both before and after the transplant.

Exercise can increase strength and endurance and reduce stress. Individuals with ESRD may be unable to tolerate as much physical activity as before; however, exercise programs individually tailored to and prescribed for individuals' specific needs and abilities may be possible. Although many of their daily activities can be continued, individuals should approach activities with flexibility, since their physical tolerance of various activities from day to day may be unpredictable.

The desire for sexual activity may change for individuals with ESRD, both because of side effects of medications and because of the physical manifestations of ESRD itself. Sexual desire may also change for emotional reasons. If individuals experience depression or anxiety, or if relationship problems exist, sexual desire and/or function may also be altered.

Traveling is possible whether individuals are using hemodialysis or peritoneal dialysis if arrangements are made well in advance. Individuals on hemodialysis must locate a dialysis unit in the area to be visited so that dialysis sessions can be scheduled well in advance. Individuals with peritoneal dialysis need to make plans for backup medical care as well as for the availability of dialysate and a cycling machine if used.

### Social Issues

Many conditions of the kidney and urinary tract have little impact on social functioning. There may be significant impact, however, on individuals with ESRD, a serious chronic condition that fluctuates and requires lifelong management and treatment for survival. Dialysis regimes, dietary restrictions, and medications may limit activities and socialization to some degree.

Preexisting social or relationship problems are frequently made worse by problems associated with ESRD.

Physiologic changes, treatment demands, and the chronic nature of ESRD affect not only the individuals with the condition but also the whole family unit. Family members' reaction and stability can help or hinder individuals' acceptance of their condition. Family members can be over-solicitous or rejecting, making it more dif-

ficult for individuals to reestablish their own emotional balance and their role within the family. Individuals and their families may focus on ESRD as the center of family functioning. They may require assistance in developing a life that incorporates ESRD into family structure, rather than overwhelming it.

Individuals with ESRD may become withdrawn from family and friends because of feelings of inadequacy. They may struggle to resolve their need for dependence on dialysis and on others for assistance with their treatment. Individuals with unresolved dependency conflicts may become uncooperative and ill-tempered. Rather than confronting the individual, family and friends may excuse their behavior, reinforcing the sick role.

### VOCATIONAL ISSUES IN RENAL AND URINARY TRACT CONDITIONS

Many renal and urinary tract disorders have no long-term impact on individuals' ability to work. Renal failure, however, has an impact on psychological, social, and vocational function, and a variety of alterations in individuals' daily life may be necessary. The degree to which kidney disease affects employment depends on individuals' occupation, previous work history, medical condition and treatment, and status of any secondary disabilities. Individuals with beginning renal failure can generally continue their previous job, especially if it is sedentary and does not require strenuous activity. Individuals with ESRD may experience reduced work tolerance due to impaired concentration and/or fatigue. If they are no longer capable of the physical activity that the work requires, a job modification or change may be necessary.

Work schedule flexibility may be necessary to accommodate recurring medical problems, periods of hospitalizations, dialysis treatment, and time away due to normal medical checkups. Other possible barriers to employment are financial disincentives or employer concern about lost work time.

Individuals with ESRD who experience decreased attention span or inability to concentrate may require jobs that accommodate these limitations. Excess heat in the work environment should be avoided since individuals with ESRD are unable to adequately regulate body heat. Individuals with peripheral neuropathy as a result of renal failure may have difficult with manual dexterity or walking. In addition, individuals with a shunt or graft for hemodialysis may have limited use of the arm containing the access route.

## CASE STUDIES

### Case I

Mr. H. is 42 years old and has worked as a metalworking machine operator for the past 22 years. As part of his job he operates powerful, high-speed machines that require strict adherence to safety rules to avoid accidents. He normally works 40 hours a week, but at times of increased production he is asked to work overtime. The metalworking shop in which he works operates two shifts daily that workers are required to alternate every other month. Mr. H. has polycystic kidney disease. He is now in ESRD and requires dialysis. He is now on hemodialysis but hopes to obtain a kidney transplant.

### Questions

1. Given Mr. H.'s type of work, what specific factors related to his medical condition would you consider when establishing a rehabilitation plan?
2. What factors regarding hemodialysis would you consider?
3. Are there special accommodations that will need to be made if he is to continue in his current line of employment while still on dialysis?
4. What issues related to a kidney transplant might be a factor in Mr. H.'s rehabilitation plan?

### Case II

Ms. L. is 36 years old and experienced severe kidney damage several years ago as a result of a drug overdose that was part of a suicide attempt. She is now on CAPD. She has a high school education and had experience as a cab driver in a large city in the past. Ms. L. has expressed interest in returning to cab driving. She now lives in a moderately sized midwestern city.

### Questions

1. What specific factors might you consider in evaluating Ms. L.'s rehabilitation potential?
2. Is her goal of returning to cab driving in her current situation realistic? Why or why not?
3. What specific issues related to her peritoneal dialysis would you consider when helping Ms. L. establish a rehabilitation plan?

## REFERENCES

Bonventre, J. V. (2002). Daily hemodialysis: Will treatment each day improve the outcome in patients with acute renal failure? *New England Journal of Medicine, 346*(5), 362–364.

Delmonico, F. L. (2004). Exchanging kidneys: Advances in living-donor transplantation. *New England Journal of Medicine, 350*(18), 1812–1814.

El Nahas, A. M., Harris, K., & Anderson, S. (Eds.). (2000). *Mechanisms and clinical management of chronic renal failure* (2nd ed.). New York: Oxford University Press.

Hariharan, S., Johnson, C. P., Bresnahan, B. A., Taranto, S. E., McIntosh, M. J., & Stablein, D. (2000). Improved graft survival after renal transplantation in the United States, 1988–1996. *New England Journal of Medicine, 342*, 605–612.

Himmelfarb, J. (2002). Success and challenge in dialysis therapy. *New England Journal of Medicine, 347*(25), 2068–2070.

Ifudu, O. (1998). Care of patients undergoing hemodialysis. *New England Journal of Medicine, 339*(15), 1054–1062.

Kinchen, K. S., Sadler, J., Fink, N., et al. (2002). The timing of specialist evaluation in chronic kidney disease and mortality. *Annals of Internal Medicine, 137*, 479–486.

Marsden, P. A. (2003). Predicting outcomes after renal transplantation: New tools and old tools. *New England Journal of Medicine, 349*(2), 182–184.

Moua, M. N. (2000). End-stage. *Rehabilitation Counseling Bulletin, 45*(1), 53–55.

Owen, W. F., Pereira, B. J. G., & Savegh, M. H. (Eds). (2000). *Dialysis and transplantation: A companion to Brenner and Rector's The kidney.* Philadelphia: W.B. Saunders.

Pascual, M., Theruvath, T., Kawai, T., Tolkoff-Rubin, N., & Cosimi, A. B. (2002). Strategies to improve long-term outcomes after renal transplantation. *New England Journal of Medicine, 346*(8), 580–588.

Schiffle, H., Lang, S. M., & Fischer, R. (2002). Daily hemodialysis and the outcome of acute renal failure. *New England Journal of Medicine, 346*(5), 305–310.

Sosa-Guerrero, S., & Gomez, N. J. (1997). Dealing with end-stage renal disease. *American Journal of Nursing, 97*(10), 44–51.

Soulillou, J. P. (2001). Immune monitoring for rejection of kidney transplants. *New England Journal of Medicine, 344*(13), 1006–1007.

Teichman, J. M. H. (Ed). (2001). *Twenty common problems in urology.* New York: McGraw-Hill, Health Professions Division.

U.S. Renal Data System. (2001). Excerpts from the United States Renal Data system 2001 annual data report: Atlas of end-stage renal disease in the United States. *American Journal of Kidney Disease, 38*(Suppl. 3), S1–S247.

# CHAPTER **14**

# Conditions of the Musculoskeletal System

## NORMAL STRUCTURE AND FUNCTION OF THE MUSCULOSKELETAL SYSTEM

### The Skeletal System

Bones make up the general framework of the body. The skeletal system, which is made up of 206 bones, supports the surrounding tissues and assists in movement by providing leverage and attachment for muscles (see Figure 14–1). It also protects vital organs, such as the heart and brain. The tough outer covering of bone is called the *periosteum*. Bones also have a network of sensory nerves and a network of tiny vessels to supply blood. They have many functions other than support, movement, and protection. Red blood cells are manufactured in the red bone marrow by means of a process called *hematopoiesis*. Bone also stores calcium and other mineral salts. New bone is constantly being produced and old bone replaced, creating a dynamic relationship between calcium in the bone and calcium in the blood.

### *Types of Bone*

Bones are classified according to shape. *Long bones* are found in the arms and legs (e.g., the *humerus* and the *femur*). *Short*

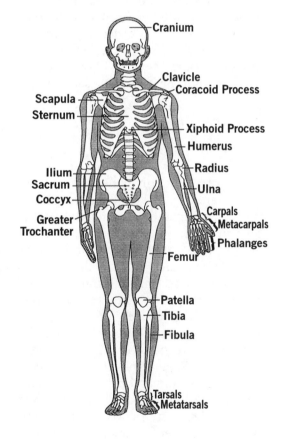

**Figure 14–1** Anterior View of the Skeleton. *Source*: Reprinted with permission from S. M. Jacob and W. J. Lossow, *Structure and Function in Man*, 4th ed., p. 93, © 1978, W. B. Sanders Company.

*bones* are found in the hands and feet (e.g., the *carpals* and the *tarsals*). *Flat bones* are those like the skull (**cranium**) and *ribs*, and *irregular bones* have differing shapes, such as the *vertebrae* and **mandible** (jaw bone).

The **vertebrae** (irregular bones that surround the spinal cord) support the head and trunk of the body, protect the spinal cord, and enable bending and flexing. The seven vertebrae at the neck and upper back are called **cervical vertebrae**. The 12 that extend from the upper to lower back are called **thoracic vertebrae**. In the lower back there are five **lumbar vertebrae**; a bony prominence called the **sacrum**, which consists of fused bone; and the **coccyx** or small residual "tail bone," which extends from the end of the sacrum.

### Connective Tissue

*Connective tissue* supports and, as its name implies, connects other tissues and tissue parts. Not only bones but also *ligaments*, tendons, and cartilage are connective tissue. **Ligaments** are tough bands of fiber that connect bones at the joint site and provide stability during movement. **Tendons** are bands of tissue that connect muscle to bone, enabling muscle movement. **Cartilage** is a dense type of connective tissue that creates form, maintains structure, and can withstand considerable tension. There are several different types of cartilage. For example, there is cartilage between the vertebral disks of the spine and in the joint of the knee to absorb shock and prevent friction, while the cartilage in the external ear and nose provide form.

Between each two vertebrae that surround the spinal cord are disks of cartilage called **intervertebral disks**. They act as cushions against shock. The tough, fibrous outer portion of the disk is called the *annulus*, and the spongy inner portion is called the *nucleus pulposus*. Vertebrae are connected by ligaments and are surrounded in part by a joint capsule containing *synovial fluid* like other *synovial joints*.

### Joints

A joint is the place where two or more bones are bound together. The coming together of two bones at a joint is called *articulation*. Some joints, such as those in the skull, are fibrous, or fixed, meaning that they provide no movement. Other joints, such as the *pubis symphysis* (pubic bone) in the pelvis, are **cartilaginous** (contain cartilage) and provide slight movement. **Synovial joints** are freely movable, enabling both motion and change of position (Figure 14–2). They are enclosed in a sac called the *bursa*, which is lined with a

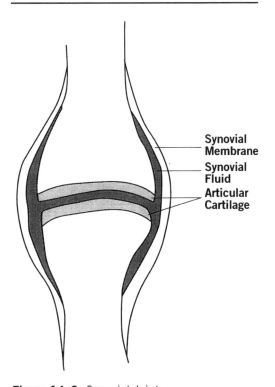

Synovial
Membrane

Synovial
Fluid

Articular
Cartilage

**Figure 14–2** Synovial Joint.

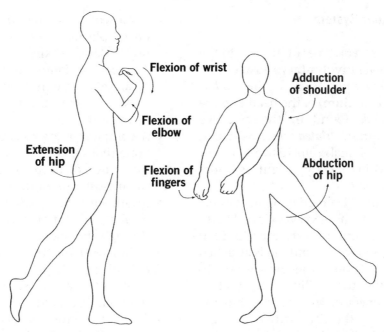

**Figure 14–3** Movement of Synovial Joints. *Source*: Copyright © 1999 Rachel Clarke.

*synovial membrane.* This membrane secretes *synovial fluid*, which aids joint movement by acting as a lubricant. Synovial fluid also helps cushion the joint against the shock produced by joint movement. *Articular cartilage* lines the end of each bone, helping to absorb shock. It receives its nourishment from the synovial fluid.

Synovial joints are capable of various different types of movements (see Figure 14–3):

- **Circumduction:** circular movement
- **Eversion:** movement in which a body part is turned outward
- **Inversion:** movement in which a body part is turned inward
- **Flexion:** bending movement
- **Extension:** straightening movement
- **Abduction:** movement of a body part away from the midline of the body
- **Adduction:** movement of a body part toward the midline of the body

- **Ulnar deviation:** lateral movement of the hand away from the body
- **Radial deviation:** lateral movement of the hand inward, toward the body
- **Pronation:** turning movement of a body part downward
- **Supination:** turning movement of a body part upward
- **Dorsiflexion:** backward movement of a body part

The type of motion of a particular synovial joint depends on the type of joint:

- *Circular motion* is provided by ball-and-socket joints, such as those found in the hip and shoulder.
- *Back-and-forth motion* is provided by hinge joints, such as those in the elbow and knee.
- *Gliding motion* is provided by joints of the vertebrae.
- *Pivotal motion* is provided by vertebrae that connect the head and the spine.

## The Muscular System

There are several types of muscles in the body. Some are **involuntary muscles** that work *automatically*, such as the *cardiac muscle* (**myocardium**) of the heart and the *smooth muscle* found in the digestive tract. In contrast, *striated muscle* (**skeletal muscle**), which makes up 40 to 50 percent of an individual's body weight, is under *voluntary control.*

A *muscle sheath* (a hard band of connective tissue) contains blood vessels and nerve fibers and surrounds every muscle. Each of the two ends of the muscle is attached to a different bone. The muscle attachment closer to the midline of the body is called the *origin* of the muscle, and the attachment of the end farther from the midline of the body is called the *insertion.*

Muscles produce movement by the contraction of opposite muscle groups. They are classified by their function. Muscles that *bend* a limb are called **flexors**; those that *straighten* a limb are **extensors**. Muscles that move a limb *laterally*, away from the body, are called **abductors**, whereas muscles that move a limb *closer* to the body are called **adductors**. Muscles that bend a body part *backward* are called **dorsiflexors**. Because of continuous nerve stimulation to muscle, muscles maintain a partial state of contraction (tone) even when they are at rest and aren't being used.

## CONDITIONS OF THE MUSCULOSKELETAL SYSTEM

### Trauma

#### Fractures

Any break or disruption in the continuity of bone is a fracture. There are several types of fractures with different levels of severity (see Figure 14–4):

- A closed or simple fracture is an uncomplicated break in a bone with no breaking of skin.
- An open or compound fracture is a break in a bone in which the skin is broken so that the bone protrudes through it.
- A complete fracture is a break in a bone that extends through the bone from one side to the other, including the periosteum, or outer cover.
- An incomplete or partial fracture is a break that does not extend all the way through the bone.
- A transverse fracture is a fracture that extends straight across the bone.
- An oblique fracture is a fracture across the bone at a slant.
- A spiral fracture occurs in a spiral around the bone and is usually caused by a twisting injury.
- An impacted fracture is a break in which one portion of the bone is impacted, or forcibly driven, into another portion of the bone.
- A comminuted fracture is a break in which the bone has been shattered, leaving fragments of bone at the site of the break.
- A displaced fracture is a break in a bone in which the two ends of the bone are separated.
- A complicated fracture is a break in a bone in which the tissue surrounding the bone, such as blood vessels and nerves, has also been injured.
- A compression fracture is a break in which the ends of the bones are pressed against each other. Compression fractures often occur in the vertebrae.
- A pathologic fracture is a break in a bone due to disease of the bone itself, rather than to an injury.
- A Colles' fracture is a break in a bone near the wrist.

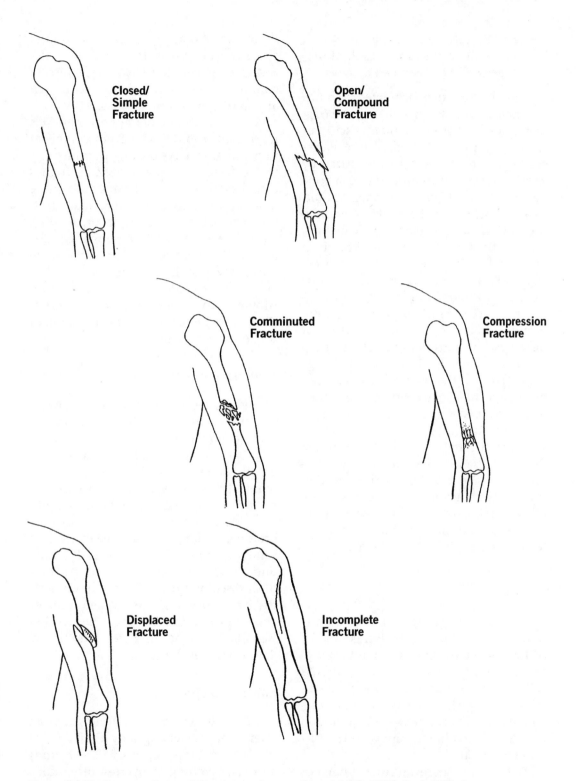

**Figure 14–4** Common Types of Fractures. *Source:* Copyright © 1999 Rachel Clarke.

• A stress fracture is a small break in a bone that occurs as the result of prolonged or unaccustomed activity.

Some fractures may be treated by *closed reduction*, a procedure in which bone fragments are realigned manually, without surgery, and immobilized with a plaster cast. Other fractures must be treated by *open reduction*, a procedure in which bone fragments are realigned and stabilized surgically. *Traction* may be used in combination with either closed or open reduction.

Many fractures heal well and result in no disability. In other instances, however, complications can occur that can cause significant disability. Bone edges or fragments of compound, displaced, or comminuted fractures may injury tissue or nerves in the surrounding area, causing permanent damage. In fractures of large bones, such as the femur, blood loss can be significant. Open or compound fractures can become infected, leading to osteomyelitis (infection of the bone). When individuals with another chronic illness or disability fracture a bone, complications related to the fracture, in addition to complications related to immobility can develop and can pose a significant threat not only to function but also to general health and well-being.

### Dislocations

Displacement or separation of a bone from its normal joint position is called a **dislocation**. If the bone is not totally separated from the joint, the condition is called a **subluxation**. In addition to causing extreme pain, a dislocation causes a partial loss of movement at the joint and can impede the blood supply to the surrounding tissue.

Dislocations can result from trauma or from a congenital weakness or abnormality of a joint that predisposes individuals to dislocation when the joint is moved a certain way. The shoulder and the hip are common sites of dislocation, although any joint can become dislocated.

Prompt treatment of joint dislocation is important in order to prevent complications, such as nerve damage or injury due to the decreased blood supply. The bones can usually be slipped back into place manually. If there has been no damage to the nerves, blood vessels, or surrounding tissue, there is usually no permanent disability. If dislocations recur in the same joint, however, individuals may need to avoid movements that appear to contribute to the dislocation. When dislocation recurs frequently, surgical fixation of the joint may be necessary.

### Contusions

Musculoskeletal injuries may not always involve bone; sometimes the injury involves underlying structures, such as the soft tissue under the skin. A **contusion** is a soft tissue injury that results from a blunt, diffuse blow. Although the skin is not usually broken and no bones are broken, local hemorrhage with associated bruising, swelling, and damage to the deep soft tissue under the skin occurs. Bleeding under the skin is responsible for the purplish discoloration at the site of injury— the bruise (**ecchymosis**). When a major vessel or a muscle is injured, a **hematoma** (sac filled with accumulated blood) may develop under the skin.

### Strains and Sprains

Although the terms *strain* and *sprain* are often used interchangeably, they refer to two different types of injuries. A **strain** is an overstretching or overuse of tendons and muscles, whereas a **sprain** is an injury or overstress of a ligament and its attachment site.

Strains may be acute, resulting from a sudden twisting or wrenching movement, or they may occur with unaccustomed vigorous exercise. Chronic strain may be the result of repetitive muscle overuse. Individuals with strains may be treated with analgesics, muscle relaxants, or anti-inflammatory drugs. One goal of therapy is to increase muscle strengthening. Consequently, immobilization is usually not recommended.

Sprains are categorized as mild, moderate, or severe (first-, second-, or third-degree sprains). First- and second-degree sprains are usually treated with analgesics, anti-inflammatory agents, or muscle relaxants. Treatment of second-degree sprains may also include immobilization of the injured joint and therapeutic exercises and physical therapy to promote early return to motion. A severe sprain tears a ligament completely from its attachment and may require surgical repair.

### Lacerations

An injury that has torn or cut the skin and underlying tissues is referred to as a **laceration**. Puncture and penetration injuries generally have a small entrance wound but cause extensive damage to tissues under the skin. Stabbing wounds and gunshot wounds are puncture and penetration wounds, respectively.

The degree of disability experienced with lacerations, puncture wounds, or penetration wounds depends on the location; the amount of damage to the underlying tissues, such as nerves, blood vessels, and internal organs; and associated complications, such as infection. The risk of infection is dependent on the source and circumstances of the injury.

## Overuse and Repetitive Motion Injuries

### Bursitis

Inflammation of the *bursa* (the sac that contains the synovial fluid in the synovial joints) is called **bursitis** and may be acute or chronic. It may result from chronic overuse of a joint, trauma to the joint, or the invasion of the bursa by infectious organisms. Although it may affect any synovial joint, bursitis commonly occurs in the shoulder, elbow, or knee.

Bursitis is characterized by pain and tenderness over the joint and by limitation of joint motion. Acute attacks may last for days to weeks, and they may recur. Splinting and rest of the joint are generally recommended. Bursitis may become chronic, causing varying degrees of disability.

### Tendonitis and Tendosynovitis

The term **tendonitis** describes a condition in which there is an inflammation of a *tendon*. The term **tendosynovitis** describes a condition in which there is an inflammation of the sheath of tissue that surrounds the tendon. The two conditions usually occur simultaneously. Although the exact cause is unknown, tendonitis may be associated with trauma, strain, or unaccustomed exercise. The primary symptom is pain on motion at the site of inflammation. The condition usually subsides with appropriate treatment, although surgery may be indicated on rare occasions.

### Carpal Tunnel Syndrome

**Carpal tunnel syndrome** is a condition in which there is compression of the median nerve in the wrist, causing pain and **paresthesia** (tingling, pricking sensation) in the hand. This condition is classified as a compression or entrapment neuropathy. It can be associated with rheumatoid arthritis (discussed later in this chapter) or diabetes (see Chapter 9), or it can result from strenuous or repetitive use of the hand (sometimes called a repetitive motion injury) (Sequeira, 1999). Muscle strength in the hand may be weakened to the extent that individuals have difficulty opening jars or twisting lids. They may experience pain that can be dull and aching or that can radiate into the forearm. Individuals may complain of waking at night because the affected hand is numb, or they may complain of numbness in the hands in the morning, feeling they have to shake their hands to get the circulation back. Symptoms may be mild and of short duration, or they may become chronic.

### Treatment of Carpal Tunnel Syndrome

Irreparable nerve damage may occur if carpal tunnel syndrome is left untreated. In mild cases, a wrist splint at night may be sufficient to help the symptoms, along with medications such as nonsteroidal anti-inflammatory drugs. If the splint does not interfere with activity, the individual may also wear the splint or wrist support during the day. Corticosteroids are sometimes injected into the area if the splint is unsuccessful at relieving symptoms; however, improvement may be temporary. When the hand becomes weakened, or when the symptoms become intolerable, surgery to relieve pressure on the nerve may be indicated.

### Vocational Issues in Carpal Tunnel Syndrome

Individuals whose work places biomechanical stresses on the hands and wrists,

especially those whose work involves repetitive motion of the hands, are especially vulnerable to carpal tunnel syndrome. In some instances the condition becomes severe enough to limit individuals' ability to work. It can be of particular concern to individuals who rely on sign language as a major form of communication (Smith, Kress, & William, 2000). With continued exposure to risk factors without adequate care or rest, permanent damage to the soft tissue and nerves can result.

When carpal tunnel syndrome is related to activity, both the nature of the work and the amount of time spent on a task contribute to the potential for injury. If carpal tunnel syndrome is related to a specific activity, ergonomic modifications such as providing forearm support when typing, adjusting the height of the keyboard or work area, or positioning the hands differently may be indicated. For individuals with carpal tunnel syndrome that is aggravated by work-related activity, the factors in the work environment may need to be modified. Office workers and those using computer keyboards may need to take periodic rest breaks throughout the day. When using a desk and chair, different body positions may help reduce muscle fatigue and prevent exacerbation of carpal tunnel syndrome symptoms. Individuals should avoid bent, extended, or twisted hand positions for long periods. When possible, they should alternate hands for work tasks and avoid awkward hand positions.

## Degenerative Conditions

### Osteoporosis

Osteoporosis is a condition in which the bone mass (the amount of bone) is reduced, causing bones to become weakened, fragile, and easily broken (Prestwood & Raisz, 2002). In some instances, although there has been no bone fracture, individuals may experience aching in various bones and often have chronic backache. Vertebral fractures, a serious consequence of osteoporosis, can lead to acute and chronic back pain as well as spinal deformity (Meunier et al., 2004).

Individuals with osteoporosis commonly have no symptoms until a bone is broken as a result of little or no trauma. Frequent sites of bone fractures are the hips, especially in older or frail individuals, and the wrist (**Colles' fracture**). *Crush* or *compression* fractures may occur in the vertebrae.

### Risks for Osteoporosis

Although osteoporosis commonly occurs in individuals after middle age, secondary osteoporosis may occur as a result of other medical conditions or as a side effect of the overuse or long-term use of steroid medication. Individuals with a disability may be at higher risk of osteoporosis. Individuals with physical disability may be nonambulatory and have bone loss due to immobility. Individuals on medications, such as anticonvulsants, may also have increased risk. Women with physical and cognitive disabilities are at especially high risk for osteoporosis and osteoporosis-related fractures (Schrager, 2004).

### Treatment of Osteoporosis

Osteoporosis is progressive, but appropriate treatment may slow the disease process. Fractures related to osteoporosis can result in substantial morbidity and mortality (Solomon, Finkelstein, Katz, Mogun, & Avorn, 2003). Consequently, prevention is a key component of treatment. The best treatment for osteoporosis is prevention through the daily intake of adequate amounts of dietary calcium; engagement in weight-bearing exercise throughout life; avoidance of the long-term use of steroid medications, which promote bone loss; and prevention of falls (Boskey, 2001; Marcus, 2000).

When osteoporosis does occur, analgesics, heat, or rest may relieve the pain. In some instances, braces or splints may be indicated. Exercise that strengthens muscles, thus providing additional support, may be beneficial. Although general activity is encouraged, heavy lifting or any activity that increases the risk of falls should be avoided.

Calcium supplements are usually prescribed for both men and women with osteoporosis. Women with osteoporosis may be given hormones to decrease bone loss and to increase absorption of calcium. When calcium absorption is impaired, supplemental vitamin D may also be given.

### Osteoarthritis (Degenerative Joint Disease)

Associated with "wear and tear" of the joints, **osteoarthritis** is a local joint disease, *not* a systemic disease. Although any joint may be affected, joints in the knees are frequently affected. Risk factors for osteoarthritis of the knee are previous surgery or injury of the knee, occupational kneeling and squatting, and obesity (Rajan & Kerr, 2000).

Since osteoarthritis is not systemic, symptoms are located around the affected joint. Bone spurs (*osteophytes*) develop on the surface of the joints, eroding the cartilage so that it can no longer serve as a cushion or shock absorber. Consequently, the ends of the bones at the joint rub on each other, causing pain and inflammation. Weight-bearing joints, such as the knees, hips, and spine, are frequently affected. Finger joints may also be affected. When osteoarthritis affects the knees or hip, it may be considerably disabling, interfering with mobility.

Joints affected by osteoarthritis may have been previously injured or exposed to long-term strain. Obesity places extra strain on joints and is thought to be one predisposing factor for osteoarthritis. The reason that some individuals who have no known predisposing factor develop osteoarthritis is unknown, although the condition may be associated with aging.

Osteoarthritis is generally unremitting. Overuse of the affected joints, cold and damp weather, or other factors may intensify symptoms. The amount of disability experienced depends on the type and magnitude of joint damage, the number of joints involved, the particular joints involved, and the daily activity of the individual.

### Treatment of Osteoarthritis

Treatment of osteoarthritis is directed toward increasing function and preventing further dysfunction. Specific exercises, including range-of-motion and strengthening exercises, are often part of the treatment prescribed to meet this goal. It may be necessary to balance rest of the joint with its use.

The use of assistive devices, such as canes or crutches, may prevent undue weight bearing on joints. If individuals with osteoarthritis are obese, weight reduction may be advisable to remove undue pressure on the joints. Oral administration of *aspirin* or *nonsteroidal anti-inflammatory agents*, as well as injection of *steroids* into the joint, may also be helpful. In cases of severe joint damage, total joint arthroplasty (surgery to replace damaged joints with artificial joints) can restore individuals to pain-free functional independence in many cases (Ritz & Mann, 2000).

### Vocational Issues in Osteoarthritis

Osteoarthritis can be a cause of long-term disability (Hawker et al., 2000). The limitations experienced depend on the specific joints affected. Individuals with osteoarthritis of the knees, for instance, may be unable to walk long distances or stand for long periods of time. They also may have difficulty with bending or stooping. Individuals with osteoarthritis of the upper extremities or vertebrae of the spine may have difficulty lifting, turning, and reaching. When fingers are affected, individuals may be unable to perform tasks that require significant finger motion.

## Back Pain

Back pain can be caused by a variety of conditions and can produce a number of symptoms in addition to pain, depending on its location. Some back pain may be *psychogenic* in origin, meaning that no organic cause of the pain can be found. Because of the subjective nature of pain and the different meaning of pain to different individuals, diagnosis and treatment of back pain in these individuals may be different. Even if back pain is psychogenic in nature, however, the pain that individuals experience is real and no less debilitating. It is important that the cause of back pain be established so that appropriate treatment can be implemented.

Back pain is classified as *mild, moderate,* or *severe.* Since pain is a subjective measure, the extent of impaired function associated with back pain is often an indicator of the severity.

### Types of Back Pain

#### Low Back Pain

Low back pain is one of the most common conditions experienced. It is defined

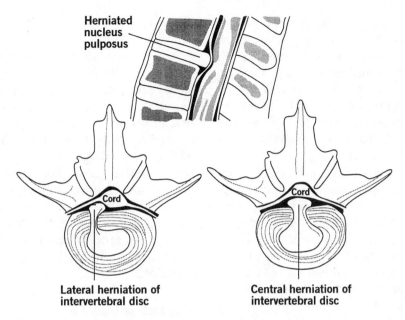

Herniated
nucleus
pulposus

Cord

Cord

**Lateral herniation of
intervertebral disc**

**Central herniation of
intervertebral disc**

**Figure 14–5** Forms of Vertebral Herniation. *Source*: Reprinted with permission from J. Luckman and K. C. Sorenson. *Medical Surgical Nursing: A Psychological Approach*, 1st ed., p. 407, © 1974, W. B. Saunders Company.

as pain in the lumbar or sacral region of the lower back. It may be experienced in the erect, nonmoving spine (*static pain*) or during movement (*kinetic pain*). Low back pain may be caused by:

- mechanical problems due to poor posture, such as **lordosis** (swayback posture)
- poor body mechanics at work, causing sprain or strain
- injury due to falls, motor vehicle accidents, or sports
- **spondylolisthesis** (forward slippage of a vertebra)
- **spondylolysis** (breakdown or degeneration of a vertebra)
- arthritis or osteoporosis
- infection of the bones of the spine or tissue between vertebrae
- tumors in the spine, or metastasis of cancer from another part of the body

- herniation of an intervertebral disk
- *referred pain* from other organs of the body, such as kidneys or uterus

Back pain may be accompanied by *sciatica* or may occur alone. **Sciatica** is a syndrome of pain that radiates from the lower back into the hip and down the leg. It may be accompanied by numbness, tingling, and muscle weakness. Sciatica can accompany a number of disorders of the lower back, herniated disk being the most common.

*Herniated or Ruptured Disk (Herniated Nucleus Pulposus)*

Rupture of the soft, inner portion of the intervertebral disk (*nucleus pulposus*) through a tear in the tougher outer portion of the disk (*annulus*) is called a *herniation* (see Figure 14–5). A sprain or strain of the back or a disease that weakens the annulus may cause herniation of a disk.

It results in back pain, often accompanied by spasms of the back muscles. Protrusion of the herniated disk exerts pressure on the nerves that surround the area. Pressure on the nerves can cause a partial loss of sensation and/or weakness in lower extremities. In severe cases, pressure on the nerves can also cause problems with bowel or bladder function.

The pain experienced with a herniated disk is frequently exacerbated by straining, coughing, or lifting. Symptoms may be intermittent at first but later may progress to continuous pain or loss of sensation. Treatment, consisting of *physical therapy* and the use of *anti-inflammatory medication*, usually eliminates pain; however, a herniated disk is the most common reason for back surgery (Deyo, 1998). When surgical treatment of herniated disk is necessary, **diskectomy** (removal of the disk) may be performed (Deyo, Nachemson, & Mirza, 2004).

### Degenerative Disk Disease

*Degenerative spondylolisthesis* is characterized by slippage of the vertebral body into the one below. It is associated with degeneration and narrowing of the involved disk. The major symptom is back pain, especially with bending, lifting, or twisting. Individuals may also complain of leg pain or may have neurologic signs.

Flexion exercises are often prescribed as one form of treatment. Some individuals find corset support to be helpful. Individuals may also be treated with *nonsteroidal anti-inflammatory drugs* (NSAIDs). Most important are lifestyle changes such as avoidance of repetitive bending, heavy lifting, or twisting of the trunk of the body. *Spinal fusion surgery* (spinal arthrodesis), in which two disks are fused, may also be necessary for treatment of instability and deformity of the disk.

### Scoliosis

Scoliosis is a lateral, S-shaped curvature of the spine that can be **congenital** (present at birth) or can be a complication of amputation or other medical condition that alters posture, such as poliomyelitis or cerebral palsy. Scoliosis can be corrected with early recognition and proper treatment. If the spinal deformity becomes fixed, however, the condition is difficult to reverse. In severe cases, scoliosis can interfere with respiratory capacity and can cause pressure on organs in the thoracic or abdominal cavity, interfering with organ function.

### Diagnosis of Back Pain

Back pain can sometimes be diagnosed by a history of symptoms and observation of individuals in various body postures and activities, as well as by physical examination. X-rays can be helpful in identifying bony abnormalities of the spine; however, conditions such as ruptured disk cannot be seen on a regular X-ray. Other diagnostic tests may involve electromyography, which provides information about nerve function and nerve damage. *Computerized tomography* (CT scan) or *magnetic resonance imaging* may also be used to identify disk degeneration or a ruptured disk.

### Treatment of Back Pain

Exercise is an important part of prevention as well as treatment of either acute or chronic back pain. Although in the past bedrest was thought to be the treatment of choice, little evidence has shown that individuals who maintain bedrest have any different outcome than those who maintain regular activities during the acute period of back pain (Deyo, 1998;

Deyo & Weinstein, 2001). Maintaining activity is, of course, dependent on the demands of individuals' regular activities, such as the need for heavy lifting.

Back pain may be treated with muscle relaxants, or antidepressants may be used for some individuals if they show symptoms of depression (Deyo & Weinstein, 2001). Physical therapy or acupuncture may provide symptomatic relief.

Preventive measures, such as conditioning of the muscles of the back or the use of proper body mechanics, are helpful in avoiding recurrences; however, adhering to specific exercise routines after symptoms have subsided may be difficult. Although most back pain symptoms subside spontaneously, a complication of back pain can be a overreaction to the condition that leads to drug-seeking behavior, which can precipitate a more serious disability of substance dependency.

Low back pain persisting for 6 months or more is considered chronic back pain. *Chronic back pain* may be an extension of symptoms due to injury or may be due to osteoporosis, degenerative spondylolisthesis, or a narrowing (**stenosis**) of the spinal canal. It may be more difficult to resolve chronic back pain, depending on the cause, and extensive, long-term therapy may be necessary. Chronic back pain may be treated medically or surgically. Medical treatment may consist of exercise, biofeedback, stress management, and medication such as muscle relaxants or steroids to reduce inflammation and nonnarcotic analgesics to reduce pain. Spinal surgery has a limited role in alleviating chronic back pain and is usually reserved for those individuals who also have neurologic symptoms, such as loss of urinary or bowel control or footdrop. Surgical interventions are varied, depending on the cause of the pain. Some surgical interventions include simple diskectomy.

### Vocational Issues in Back Pain

*Acute back pain* caused by strain or sprain may significantly impair function from days to weeks. Pain is precipitated by repeated twisting or lifting, prolonged sitting, or operation of vibrating equipment. Individuals may have difficulty standing erect and may need to change position frequently. Most individuals with acute back pain return to work within 6 weeks; however, recurrences are common, and disability caused by back pain has steadily risen (Deyo, 1998). Although low back pain is rarely permanently disabling, return to work after an episode of low back pain is influenced by clinical, social, and economic factors (Deyo & Weinstein, 2001).

Prevention is the best way to reduce back injury. Education about good body mechanics and conditioning can help to reduce further injury. Individuals who are not physically active are more likely to have acute lower back injury; consequently, exercises that increase strength and muscle tone can help prevent injury. Modification of the workplace to reduce mechanical stresses may also be important to decrease both the frequency and cost of lower back injuries.

Individuals whose job requires lifting or heavy physical work may need mechanical assistance devices or tables to allow lifting from the waist. Regular rest breaks may be needed as well as instruction regarding good lifting techniques. An ergonomics review of the workstation and equipment can help to ensure that individuals are sitting and moving in ways that reduce the risk of strain. As much as possible, equipment that causes whole-body vibration should be modified to reduce vibration as much as possible. Individuals using equipment with significant vibration should schedule frequent rest periods or should rotate workstations to a less strenuous task.

## Chronic Pain

Pain is a complex human experience that can dramatically affect the quality of life. It is a multidimensional concept that includes physical, psychological, spiritual, and social functioning (Glajchen, 2001). The purpose of pain is mainly protective; pain is a signal or warning that an area of the body needs attention. Pain and pain-related problems may be associated with a number of body systems and disease conditions. Chronic pain can be experienced because of a number of conditions, ranging from cancer to pain experienced with chronic headaches. It may also be associated with a number of conditions of the musculoskeletal system, from trauma to rheumatoid arthritis.

Pain is subjective, is difficult to quantify, and has different meanings to different individuals. *Pain perception* may be influenced by anxiety, fear, and depression as well as by cultural, ethnic, and other life influences. Individuals also have different *pain thresholds* (points at which sensation is perceived as pain) as well as different levels of *pain tolerance* (points at which the individual finds the pain unbearable). Individuals with heightened pain tolerance may minimize the importance of symptoms and delay seeking medical attention until the pain is severe. Individuals with low pain tolerance may tend to have an exaggerated reaction to pain. Therefore, *pain intensity* is difficult to determine if it is based on the reactions of the individual, and it is not always a reliable index of the seriousness of the condition. Individuals' response to pain (*pain expression*) is influenced by a number of cognitive, emotional, behavioral, and cultural factors. Some cultures encourage a stoic response to pain, whereas other cultures permit a free expression of feelings in response to pain. Different individuals may not respond to the same pain stimuli in the same way. Similarly, the same person may react differently to pain in different circumstances. Anxiety and fear tend to enhance the perception of pain and the intensity of the pain response, whereas distractions tend to lessen the perception of and response to pain.

### Acute Versus Chronic Pain

Pain can be classified as acute or chronic. Acute pain is defined as pain that occurs with the onset of illness or injury and is generally of short duration. It usually has an identifiable cause. As healing occurs or the cause of pain is corrected or removed, the pain usually decreases within an established course of time. The control of most acute pain is based on treatment of the underlying cause.

When pain becomes chronic, however, it is often treated as a condition in itself.

Chronic pain is defined as pain that continues more than 3 months. As it persists over time, chronic pain loses its biologic function of signaling injury or disease and imposes psychological and physical stress on individuals who experience it. Individuals experiencing chronic pain may develop *chronic pain syndrome*, a condition characterized by physical, social, and behavioral dysfunction. These individuals often have marked alteration of behavior, including depression or anxiety, restriction in daily activities, excessive use of medications, and frequent use of medical services. Pain becomes a central issue in their lives.

### Types of Chronic Pain

Chronic pain may be of three types:

- Pain that persists beyond the normal healing time (e.g., pain at the site of a fractured bone after the bone has

healed; phantom pain in an amputated limb)
- Pain related to a chronic, degenerative, or malignant disease (e.g., rheumatoid arthritis, osteoporosis, cancer)
- Pain that persists for months or years but has no readily identifiable organic cause (psychogenic pain), such as back pain or headache with no identifiable physical reason for the pain

For some people, pain is unrelenting and persists at intolerable levels despite analgesic medication and futile attempts for other medical cures. Some individuals with chronic pain engage in cycles of false hope, frustration, and guilt. They may be unable to work and begin to withdraw from family and social activities. Personal relationships may deteriorate. They may believe no one else has ever endured the type of pain they are enduring and may become demoralized, depressed, and angry.

### Treatment of Chronic Pain

Treatment of pain that cannot be controlled or eradicated is directed toward helping individuals learn to cope with the pain. Physicians may find treatment of chronic pain difficult because various treatments for chronic pain are ineffective and because individuals may become addicted to medications used in treatment (Foley, 2003). Consequently, they may refer individuals with chronic pain to a clinic that uses multiple, simultaneous therapeutic approaches to chronic pain. Alternate forms of pain control may be used alone or in combination with analgesic medication.

### Medications

Generally, medications are used more often in the treatment of acute pain than in the treatment of chronic pain. When medications are used as part of pain man-

agement, the type chosen depends on the cause and the type of pain. *Muscle relaxants* may be prescribed to relax tight muscles or muscle spasms. *Analgesics*, which range from medication such as aspirin to *narcotics* such as Demerol or morphine, may also be used, but professionals often limit their use of narcotic analgesics for the long-term treatment of chronic pain (unless pain is part of a terminal illness) because of their fear of physical and/or psychological dependence or addiction, even though studies have shown that there is little risk of addiction in individuals who have had no history of substance abuse (Portenoy, 1994). Because individuals with chronic pain frequently experience depression as well, *antidepressant medications* may occasionally be prescribed.

### Noninvasive Procedures

Physical Therapy. *Physical therapy* may be prescribed to help individuals with chronic pain gradually increase their exercise tolerance and activity level. It is directed toward stretching and strengthening specific muscles and joints. It may also be used to improve functional activity and reduce muscle spasm. Splints or braces may be used to support painful body parts or may be prescribed to help individuals increase their activity.

Transcutaneous Electrical Nerve Stimulation (TENS). *Transcutaneous electrical nerve stimulation* may help to relieve pain. In this technique, electrodes of a small, battery-operated device are placed over the painful area. When the unit is on, it stimulates nerve fibers electrically, providing a counterirritation that, in turn, blocks pain impulses. The treatment itself is painless. The length of time individuals wear the unit varies, ranging from all day to only 1 or 2 hours a day.

The success of TENS depends to some degree on individuals' understanding of the technique and motivation to use it. The degree and duration of pain relief with TENS units are variable. For some individuals, the effects wear off after a few months. Others may use the TENS unit successfully for a longer period of time. Because of the expense of TENS units, long-term or permanent use is usually not feasible.

Stress Management.   Other specific techniques may be used to help individuals reduce the stress response. When individuals are tense, the heart beats faster, blood pressure rises, and muscles tighten. These responses can make pain more intense. *Stress management* includes specific procedures designed to reduce stress and promote relaxation.

Stress management may be useful in the treatment of a variety of disorders, but it may be particularly useful in the treatment of chronic pain. Because tension and anxiety tend to accentuate pain perception, removing tension and anxiety can also serve to reduce the perception of pain. There are many types of stress management. Some individuals may be helped to identify the sources of stress and learn ways to control their reaction to it. Other individuals may learn specific relaxation techniques.

Guided Imagery. Another technique, *guided imagery*, uses audiotaped instruction or descriptive narrative provided by a trained therapist. This technique is directed toward helping the individual relax and visualize positive outcomes. The technique is based on the assumption that images can directly or indirectly influence physiologic processes in the body (Rakel & Shapiro, 2002).

Relaxation Therapy. *Relaxation therapy* is a technique aimed at helping individuals learn the relaxation response, which decreases blood pressure, heart rate, oxygen consumption, and alpha wave (type of brain wave) activity on electroencephalogram. The technique can be learned through practice and may include breathing techniques as well as progressive relaxation.

Individuals who undergo progressive relaxation training are taught to tighten and relax different muscle groups gradually. The procedure promotes relaxation, decreases anxiety, and lessens muscle tension. When used daily, these techniques can help the individual cope with stress.

Meditation. *Meditation* is a technique that helps individuals obtain a relaxed state by focusing attention on a repetitive event, usually a word or phrase recited repeatedly. This new focus removes individuals' focus on the painful sensation. Individuals concentrate on a variety of other focuses, such as breathing, chanting, or forming a visual image.

Hypnosis. *Hypnosis* is a procedure by which individuals are induced into a trance state, during which suggestion is used to alter attitudes, perceptions, or behavior. The hypnotic state is obtained by focusing on a soothing image or situation, purposefully relaxing voluntary muscles, and controlling one's breathing. For individuals with chronic pain, hypnosis may be used to alter the reaction to painful stimuli or the perception of pain. Skilled hypnotherapists may help individuals distract their thinking of pain through posthypnotic suggestion. Hypnosis should be conducted only by trained, certified individuals. It has varying degrees of success in the management of chronic pain.

Biofeedback. Some individuals find biofeedback helpful in controlling pain, especially if pain is due in part to muscle tension. *Biofeedback* is a technique based on operant conditioning and feedback learning of a physiologic response. In principle, biofeedback is a technique of measuring a naturally occurring body function and amplifying it so that individuals can acquire the ability to control that function. Through biofeedback, individuals learn to elicit the relaxation response and control the physiologic mechanisms that produce the stress-related symptoms.

Individuals receive feedback from a specific physiologic measurement such as heart rate, muscle tension, or skin temperature. Electrical equipment is used to provide this feedback. Electrodes are placed on the skin over localized muscles. Wires from the electrodes are attached to an electromyogram machine, which measures the electrical activity of the muscles. Individuals receive information through a tone or lights. After learning different methods to reduce the amount of muscle tension, individuals can monitor the effectiveness of these methods in controlling muscular activity through the feedback system. With practice, individuals can learn to reduce the stress response at will without the benefit of physiologic monitoring.

Operant Conditioning. A behavioral technique designed to decrease the functional impairment associated with chronic pain, *operant conditioning*, does not cure or reduce the pain itself but rather alters the individual's behavioral response to the pain. The technique is based on theories of learning and conditioning. The pain experience often results in a series of behaviors that communicate discomfort (e.g., grimacing, guarding, or limping) and usually elicit responses from others in the form of sympathy, decreased expectations for performance or success, or even monetary compensation. Behavioral responses to pain may also be reinforced by the fact that they may help individuals avoid activities that they find unpleasant. Such reinforcement of these pain behaviors may condition individuals to display them and, as a result, may increase the functional impairment associated with the pain behaviors. Operant conditioning involves withdrawing reinforcement for "pain" behaviors and reinforcing "well" behaviors.

Pain Groups. Joining a *Chronic Pain Anonymous (CPA)* group is another way individuals can learn to live with their pain when no other technique or medical intervention has helped. The CPA model borrows from Alcoholics Anonymous (AA) and is based on the concept that similar psychological and emotional disturbances are seen in alcoholism and intractable benign pain in that both disrupt personal and work relationships; both cause loss of control, obsession, and isolation; and both are chronic conditions. CPA uses the same 12 steps as AA, substituting the word *pain* for the word *alcohol*.

*Invasive Procedures*

Acupuncture. *Acupuncture* has gained increased acceptance in the treatment of chronic pain. It is an ancient Chinese form of analgesia in which long, fine needles are inserted into selected points (*trigger points*) of an individual's body to eliminate the pain sensation.

There is no simple explanation for the mechanisms that underlie the analgesic effects of acupuncture. Although it is considered an invasive technique, it has few, if any, complications when it is done under sterile conditions by those who have been trained and certified in acupuncture techniques.

Nerve Blocks. *Nerve blocks* eliminate pain locally. They are commonly used for surgical procedures, as well as in the treatment of chronic pain. Local anesthetics are injected close to nerves, thus blocking their ability to conduct the painful stimuli. Generally, nerve blocks are given for the temporary relief of pain; however, in cases of severe pain, such as in terminal cancer, nerve blocks may be performed so that the effects are irreversible.

Neurosurgical Procedures. *Neurosurgical procedures* in which surgeons sever the sensory nerves supplying the painful area may be used when severe pain cannot be ameliorated or controlled by other means. Cutting the nerves removes not only the sensation of pain, but also the sensations of pressure, heat, and cold. Consequently, individuals who have undergone these procedures must be aware of the necessity of protecting the area from injury. The type of neurosurgical procedure used depends on the type and location of the pain. For example, *sympathectomy* involves the autonomic nervous system; *neurectomy*, either the cranial or the peripheral nerves; and *rhizotomy* and *chordotomy*, the nerves close to the spinal cord (see Chapter 3).

## Amputation

The general term for loss of all or a portion of a body part is called **amputation**. Amputation can result from injury (*traumatic amputation*), such as loss of an extremity in an explosion or in a motor vehicle accident (Blank-Reid, 2003; Proehl, 2004). Amputation may be performed surgically to treat disease, such as amputation of a breast (**mastectomy**) because of cancer or amputation of a leg because of gangrene. Amputation may also be *congenital*, such as when individuals are born without a limb.

Upper-extremity amputations are often associated with accidents, burns, explosions, or other types of traumatic injury, whereas lower-extremity amputations are more frequently associated with disease, such as peripheral vascular disease (see Chapter 11).

### *Levels of Extremity Amputation*

Amputation of an extremity may be performed at different levels. In order to provide for maximal length of the stump of the extremity and, thus, maximal function with a prosthesis, surgeons usually perform an amputation as **distal** (farthest from the center of the body) as possible. The levels of upper-extremity amputation are as follows:

- Forequarter or interscapular-thoracic amputation: the most severe upper-extremity amputation, in which the entire arm, clavicle, and scapula are removed
- Shoulder disarticulation: removal of the arm at the shoulder joint
- Above the elbow: removal of the arm anywhere between the shoulder and the elbow joints
- Elbow disarticulation: removal of the arm at the elbow joint
- Below elbow: removal of the arm anywhere between the elbow and the wrist
- Wrist disarticulation: removal of the hand at the wrist
- Partial hand: amputation of one or more fingers or the loss of a portion of the hand

The levels of lower-extremity amputation are as follows:

- Hemipelvectomy, or hindquarter amputation: the most severe lower-extremity amputation, in which the entire lower limb and half of the pelvis are removed

- Hip disarticulation: removal of the leg at the hip joint
- Above the knee: removal of the leg anywhere between the hip and the knee joints
- Knee disarticulation: removal of the lower leg at the knee
- Below the knee: removal of the lower leg anywhere between the knee and the ankle
- Syme's amputation: removal of the foot at the ankle
- Transmetatarsal or partial foot: removal of a portion of the foot

It is especially important to retain the maximal length of the stump in lower-extremity amputations, because the amount of energy required to use an artificial limb increases with the height of the amputation. Individuals with a below-the-knee amputation, for example, require approximately 10 to 37 percent more energy for movement than do individuals without an amputation (Wilson, 1998).

### Treatment of Amputation

#### Surgery

When an underlying disease such as cancer or arteriosclerosis necessitates amputation, the type of surgical amputation performed, the postoperative course, and the type of rehabilitation depend to a great extent on the circumstances surrounding the amputation and the individual's general condition. Individuals with an amputation due to an underlying disease may be at risk for additional amputations because of the disease process itself or because of complications that result from the disease.

#### Reimplantation

An extremity, or portion of an extremity, that has been totally severed by an injury can sometimes be surgically reattached to the body with partial restoration of function. This process is called *reimplantation*. Reimplantation may be especially important after amputation of an upper extremity, since upper-limb prostheses provide limited function (Daigeler, Fansa, & Schneider, 2003).

With the evolution of surgical techniques and scientific technology, reimplantation has become more successful. The degree of success depends on the general condition of the individual, the availability of rapid transportation to a reimplantation center, and appropriate care of the severed body part prior to reimplantation. The goal of reimplantation is to preserve quality of life by improving function and appearance (Brown & Wu, 2003). Studies have demonstrated that reimplantation can, in many cases, achieve 50 percent function and 50 percent sensation in the replanted part (Wilhelmi, Lee, Pagensteert, & May, 2003), although in some cases return of motor function is greater than return of sensory function (Wiberg et al., 2003). The success of this surgery in increasing quality of life and function is partly determined, however, on individuals' appropriate and realistic expectations of the appearance and function of the body part after reimplantation (Wilhelmi et al., 2003).

#### Prostheses

A **prosthesis** is a fabricated substitute for a missing body part, such as an artificial limb that replaces an amputated limb. Prosthetic devices may either enable individuals to regain independent function or may be prescribed only for cosmetic purposes. The type of prosthesis, its purpose, and its maximal use are dependent on the reason for the amputation, the type and level of the amputation, the presence of any underlying disease, the development of any complications, and, most important, needs of the individuals and their motivation to use the prosthesis (Bussell, 2000). The physician who performed the surgery, usually the *orthopedic surgeon* (physician who specializes in surgical treatment of bones), also prescribes the prosthesis on the basis of the individual's daily activities, occupation, and cosmetic needs. A *certified prosthetist*, an individual who specializes in making prosthetic devices, then fabricates the prosthesis.

In some instances, the surgeon may place a *temporary prosthesis* on the stump of a lower extremity immediately after surgery. In this case, a rigid total contact dressing is applied to the stump in the operating room, and a pylon or adjustable rigid support structure is attached. An *ankle-foot assembly* is then attached to the lower end of the pylon. The immediate placement of a temporary prosthesis may have a psychological benefit for individuals, fostering a sense of independence and optimism as soon as they wake from surgery. It also promotes ambulation, thus reducing the risk of complications associated with immobility. Immediate placement of a temporary prosthesis is contraindicated, however, when there is severe underlying disease, such as diabetes or infection, or if there has been extensive damage as a result of injury. It is also contraindicated for individuals with limited mental capabilities, who may be unable to understand instructions or to regulate the weight placed on the stump in the early postoperative period.

When immediate prosthetic fitting is not advisable, individuals receive a temporary prosthesis 2 to 3 weeks after surgery. Placement of a temporary prosthesis is necessary, whether the fitting is immediate or delayed, so that **edema** (swelling) can subside and the stump can shrink before the permanent prosthesis is fitted. A *permanent prosthesis* can usually be placed within 3 months.

As much as possible, lower-extremity prostheses are designed to enable ambulation. Generally, the lower the level of amputation, the easier the use of the prosthesis. The *ankle-foot attachment* may be immovable or movable. A commonly used ankle-foot mechanism is the solid ankle-cushion heel foot. In above-the-knee amputations, the prosthesis must also replace knee function, providing a joint that is stable for both standing and walking. The socket of the prosthetic device must be aligned well and fit well for optimal balance and support. Because proper alignment varies with the heel heights of shoes, individuals who wish to wear shoes with different heel heights on occasion may need several removable prosthetic feet designed to accommodate the varying heel heights.

Prosthetic devices for use after *hemipelvectomy* are more difficult to use. The increased energy needed for ambulation often makes the use of a prosthesis after hemipelvectomy unrealistic for other than cosmetic use, although such a prosthesis can be functional. For example, a prosthesis may be worn after hemipelvectomy to help individuals maintain proper posture while sitting in a wheelchair. When using the prosthesis for ambulation, individuals with hemipelvectomy can usually only walk at a slow pace and only on level ground. Most individuals who have undergone hemipelvectomy choose to use crutches or a wheelchair for their daily activities, reserving the prosthesis for special events when cosmetic appearance is more important than ambulation (Amputee Coalition of America, 2000).

Upper-extremity prostheses vary in type and purpose and are custom-made according to individual need. The complex function of the hand cannot be replaced, but functions such as lifting, grasping, and pinching can often be restored with a prosthesis. A *terminal device* is a prosthesis that substitutes for a hand. The level of amputation and individuals' needs determine the type of terminal device used. In general, the greater the cosmetic appearance of the device, the less its functional capacity. Individuals who need grasping, holding, or lifting actions may find a hook more beneficial as a prosthesis. For others, prosthetic hands that have grasp or pinch function for light objects may be most useful. The cosmetic appearance of the prosthetic hand may be more important to some individuals than its functional capacity.

A prosthesis is activated by using the muscles in the remaining portion of the limb. For this reason, a prosthesis for a high-upper-extremity amputation may have limited function. A prosthesis placed after a *shoulder disarticulation* or an *interscapular-thoracic amputation*, for example, may be mostly cosmetic with little, if any, functional capacity. *Myoelectrical prostheses*, which are activated by electrical potentials produced by muscles, may be considered in some instances. In this type of prosthetic device, electrodes are placed over the skin of the muscles to be used. The electrodes pick up electrical impulses from the muscles, transferring them to a motor in the prosthesis that then activates the hand to open and close. The function of the myoelectric prosthesis does not, however, approximate the function of normal hand movement and dexterity. Myoelectrical prostheses are best suited for individuals with below-the-elbow prostheses. They are heavier because of the battery and motor that they contain, and they are more expensive than regular prosthetic devices.

### Complications of Amputation

Complications may develop after either upper- or lower-extremity amputation. It is extremely important that the prosthesis fits well and that there is no undue pressure or rubbing that could lead to ulceration. All individuals, but especially those whose amputation was necessary because of underlying peripheral vascular disease, must be careful to avoid skin ulceration that could become infected and necessitate a higher-level amputation.

Swelling (**edema**) of the stump after the permanent prosthesis has been placed not only can interfere with the proper fit of the prosthesis, but it can also increase pressure and restrict the blood flow to the stump, contributing to the likelihood of ulceration. An improper fit of the prosthesis, rubbing, or swelling of the stump should be immediately brought to the attention of the physician and prosthetist so that appropriate adjustments of the prosthesis can be made.

Individuals undergoing amputation must also concentrate on preserving the range of motion in the remaining joints of the amputated limb. **Contractures** (deformities in which permanent contraction of a muscle makes a joint immobile) may occur because of the improper positioning or limited activity of the remaining joints. Contractures impede or prevent effective use of the prosthetic device. They are easier to prevent through regular range-of-motion exercises of joints than they are to cure. When contractures develop, they may be corrected with extensive *physical therapy* and, occasionally, surgery.

Other complications of amputation include bone spurs, scoliosis, and phantom pain. Bone spurs or bone overgrowth may develop at the end of the stump, changing its shape and causing pain. **Scoliosis** (S-shaped lateral curvature of the spine) may occur after a lower-extremity amputation because of the improper alignment or because of improper use of the prosthesis. After a higher-upper-extremity amputation, scoliosis may develop if the prosthetic device unbalances the trunk. In both instances, scoliosis can be prevented by making sure that the prosthesis is in good alignment. Individuals who have had an upper-extremity amputation may also perform exercises to strengthen the muscles that support the prosthesis.

Although all individuals who have had an amputation experience some degree of **phantom sensation** (sensation that the amputated extremity is still present), the sensation usually diminishes over time. Some individuals, however, experience chronic, severe pain sensation in the amputated extremity, called **phantom limb pain** (Kooijman, Dijkstra, Geertzen, Elzinga, & van der Schans, 2000). Phantom limb pain may gradually diminish over time, but it sometimes becomes disabling. In some instances, treatment to block the nerves that serve the amputated extremity may alleviate the pain. At times, **neuromas** (bundles of nerve fibers) imbedded in the scar tissue of the stump may cause pain and can be removed; however, this may not totally alleviate phantom limb pain. Individuals with chronic disabling phantom pain may need chronic pain management.

### Psychosocial Issues in Amputation

Individuals with amputation have to make permanent behavioral, social, and emotional adjustments to cope with the multiple problems that can exist with amputation (Gallagher & MacLachlan, 1999). Amputation forces individuals to make a major adjustment not only to a change in body image, but also to a change in functional capacity. When individuals are fitted with a prosthetic limb, they are confronted with the irrevocable fact that not only have they lost a limb, but they must now learn how to incorporate the false limb into daily function.

Traumatic amputation produces psychological and social impacts that can be overwhelming if not openly and candidly addressed. The earlier psychosocial intervention can be implemented, the more likely it is that psychological factors will not impede functional outcome (Meyer, 2003). Individuals whose amputation was due to chronic disease may find it less difficult to adjust, especially if the body part amputated was a source of pain or immobility prior to the amputation. Individuals who have lost a body part suddenly, such as with amputation of the breast because of breast cancer or loss of a limb due to traumatic injury, may have more difficulty with adjustment because they have had inadequate time to prepare for the loss.

Regardless of the reason for the amputation, it is important to understand individuals' interpretation of the loss. Individuals' ability to adapt to amputation depends on the circumstances surrounding the amputation, the usefulness of the prosthetic device, and individuals' perception of the disability. Some individuals who have lost a limb no longer consider themselves whole. They may fear that they will never again be able to function as they did prior to the amputation. For these individuals, a prosthesis is a reminder of perceived inadequacy rather than a restoration of function. In some instances, loss of a limb is comparable to the loss of a loved one. Individuals may need sufficient time to grieve and adjust to their loss.

Individuals who have undergone amputation, especially loss of a lower extremity because of disease, must guard against injury and infection to the stump. Consequently, skin care is a vital part of rehabilitation. Bathing in the evening rather than in the morning is advisable, since damp skin may swell and stick to a prosthesis, causing irritation and rubbing.

Many limitations of activity depend on the level of the amputation. Most individuals who have had a lower extremity amputated can bicycle, swim, dance, and participate in many athletic activities with adaptive equipment. Driving a car is usually not a problem, although automatic transmissions may allow individuals to drive more easily. Activities such as climbing, squatting, and kneeling may be more difficult; however, even these tasks are mastered by some individuals. Individuals with upper-extremity amputation may require a number of assistive devices, in addition to the prosthesis, in order to perform some activities of daily living.

Although the amputation of an extremity has no direct effect on sexual activity, psychological factors and/or the reaction of sexual partners to the amputation may alter sexual function. Partners can be supportive or unsupportive. The stability of the relationship prior to amputation, as well as communication and understanding, are important components to adjustment and subsequently to the quality of the relationship.

### Vocational Issues in Amputation

Individuals with amputation who wear a prosthesis may need to avoid hot, humid environments, which can cause skin breakdown or contribute to the deterioration of the prosthesis. Dust or grit can be abrasive to the skin, exacerbating skin problems, and can also interfere with the functioning of the movable parts of the prosthesis.

In the case of lower-extremity amputation, the physical demands of the job, such as walking, climbing, or pushing, should be evaluated and altered, if necessary. The increased energy expenditure required in the use of a prosthesis should also be considered part of the physical demands of the job. Individuals in professional or managerial careers may have fewer limitations following the amputation of either an upper or lower extremity. Those with upper-extremity amputation may have a greater cosmetic need for a prosthesis, however, than do those workers whose jobs require the prosthesis for tasks such as lifting.

### Rheumatoid and Autoimmune Conditions

There are over 105 disorders classified as rheumatic conditions, many of which are also considered *autoimmune conditions*. Autoimmune conditions are thought to be mediated by an autoimmune response in which the body's immune system fails to recognize body tissue and attacks the tissues as if they were foreign objects. The reason for this autoimmune response is unknown.

The term *rheumatic disease* describes conditions that produce symptoms that affect the *joints*, *connective tissues*, and *muscle*. Rheumatoid conditions are characterized by *pain, inflammation, fatigue*, and *loss of motion in joints*. The term **arthritis** is a general term used to describe inflammation of the joints. The term **myositis** refers to inflammation of the muscle.

The effects of rheumatoid conditions are diverse, with symptoms ranging from mild to severe. Most commonly, however, symptoms are unpredictable, so that individuals with rheumatoid conditions can never predict when pain, stiffness, or deformity may occur.

### Rheumatoid Arthritis

**Rheumatoid arthritis** is a chronic, progressive, systemic disorder that causes significant pain, joint destruction, and disability (Kvien, 2004). It is characterized by inflammation and swelling of the *synovial joints*, resulting in pain, stiffness, and deformity. It is one of the most common of the rheumatoid conditions. The course of the disease is unpredictable and fluctuating.

Rheumatoid arthritis is thought to result, in part, from an autoimmune response in which the body's normal mechanisms of defense produce an inflammatory type of reaction against itself, leading to cell destruction. Although much of the focus of rheumatoid arthritis is on the joints, rheumatoid arthritis is a *systemic disease* affecting other body systems as well. Individuals experience symptoms such as fatigue, weight loss, or fever as well as joint pain and deformity. The inflammatory process may also affect other body organs (e.g., the eyes, heart, lungs, or spleen), causing changes that alter organ function.

Rheumatoid arthritis is a progressive condition, but not all individuals are affected to the same degree. The condition may be severe in some individuals, causing moderate joint deformity in a relatively short amount of time. In others, it may progress more slowly or may never become severely debilitating.

Rheumatoid arthritis may be characterized by a series of remissions, in which symptoms subside for a period of weeks to years, and exacerbation, in which symptoms become worse. During exacerbation, joints may sustain increased damage so that they never return to their normal state, even during remissions.

During the exacerbations of rheumatoid arthritis, the synovial membrane becomes inflamed; the joints become warm, swollen, and painful; and the synovial membrane thickens. As the condition progresses, a layer of scar tissue forms over the synovial membrane. This tissue, called *pannus*, interferes with provision of nutrients to the cartilage of the joint, thereby leading to erosion and joint destruction. Scar tissue becomes so tough and fibrous that **ankylosis** (stiffness and fixation of the joint) occurs, impeding movement.

Rheumatoid arthritis may not affect all joints, or it may affect different joints at different times. The most common joints to be involved are:

- wrists
- ankles
- knees
- elbows
- joints of the fingers and toes

Occasionally, shoulder, hip, and neck joints are also involved. Joints are usually affected symmetrically. For example, both knees, rather than one knee, are affected. Joint pain and stiffness are generally worse in the morning, subside somewhat during the day, and again become painful at night.

The prognosis for individuals with rheumatoid arthritis is variable. Some individuals may experience rapid progression of debilitating symptoms, whereas others remain in a state of remission for years, continuing their normal employment and full activity.

### Medical Treatment of Rheumatoid Arthritis

Physicians who specialize in the treatment of rheumatoid conditions, including rheumatoid arthritis, are called **rheumatologists**. Since there is no cure for rheumatoid arthritis, the goals of treatment are to induce and maintain remission, which include decreasing joint destruction, maintaining joint function, and preventing deformity (O'Dell, 2004). The cornerstones of therapy are *rest* and *exercise*.

Exercise. Exercise is almost always directed toward strengthening and increasing the flexibility of muscles without placing additional wear and tear on the joints. Although activity alone is not necessarily therapeutic, prescribed exercise is important in the treatment of rheumatoid arthritis to restore muscle strength, to maintain joint mobility, and to prevent contractures. Individuals should follow the specific exercise plan recommended by their physician.

Exercises usually consist of specific range-of-motion exercises for joints. They are performed regularly and daily to prevent deformity. Other exercises are used to help strengthen muscles to prevent flexion deformity.

Rest. Complete bedrest may be recommended for short periods during the acute phases of the condition. In other instances, rest periods throughout the day may be prescribed.

Splinting of specific joints may occasionally be prescribed to reduce local inflammation. When there is acute inflammation, active exercises may not be possible and splints may be prescribed for various joints. Splints, if used, are usually used only at night and at rest and are designed to maintain the joints in extension. When used, they are prescribed only as a temporary measure and are always prescribed under the direction of a physician. Long-term use of splints can cause deformity because of the lack of mobility in the affected joints.

Thermal Treatment. Thermal treatment (applications of either hot or cold) may be used to relieve pain. Treatments may include *hydrotherapy*, such as a whirlpool bath, or treatments using *paraffin baths*, in which the affected body part is placed in a bath of hot paraffin. The body part is then removed from the paraffin bath. As the paraffin cools externally, warmth to the body part is held in, reducing both pain and inflammation.

Occupational and Physical Therapy. *Occupational therapists* and *physical therapists* may be consulted to help individuals increase their functional capacity. Occupational therapists generally focus on tasks of daily living, whereas physical therapists focus on mobility issues.

Medications. Medications are also a mainstay of treatment in rheumatoid arthritis (Olsen & Stein, 2004). Medications are used to reduce inflammation, thereby also reducing pain. They are divided into three main classes: NSAIDs, corticosteroids, and *disease-modifying antirheumatic drugs* (DMARDs) (O'Dell, 2004). Often these medications are used in combination.

NSAIDs provide partial relief of pain and stiffness. However, they have not been shown to slow the progression of rheumatoid arthritis, and consequently are usually used in combination with DMARDs (American College of Rheumatology Subcommittee on Rheumatoid Arthritis, 2002). Long-term administration of these medications can also result in stomach irritation, gastrointestinal ulcer, and in some instances perforation and hemorrhage (O'Dell, 2004).

In some instances *salicylates* (e.g., aspirin) may still be prescribed in large doses, to nearly the toxic level, to obtain the desired therapeutic effect. This high concentration of salicylates in the blood may exceed the liver's ability to metabolize it, causing toxic effects, such as ringing in the ears (**tinnitus**). Because of the large doses required, individuals may experience other side effects as well, such as stomach discomfort and/or bleeding due to irritation of the stomach lining.

*Corticosteroids* are added to the treatment regimen to suppress the inflammatory response. When and how they are used in the treatment of rheumatoid arthritis remains controversial (Moreland & O'Dell, 2002). Corticosteroids have serious side effects, such as thinning of skin, cataracts, osteoporosis, and hypertension. For this reason, these drugs are not usually used on a long-term basis and are more commonly used when individuals are having a major exacerbation of the disease. To prevent serious complications, individuals taking steroids must not stop medication suddenly but must gradually withdraw from the medication under a physician's supervision.

DMARDs are used to retard or halt the progression of rheumatoid arthritis by suppressing inflammation. One example of a DMARD is methotrexate, which is often selected for initial therapy (Mikuls & O'Dell, 2000).

Complementary and Alternative Therapies. Complementary and alternative medicine therapies are usually diverse products or practices outside the mainstream of Western medical practice for promoting health and preventing or treating disease (Harpham, 2001). Several studies have demonstrated that over 40 percent of individuals with rheumatoid conditions use some form of complementary or alternative therapy (Boisset & Fitzcharles, 1994; Resch, Hill, & Ernst, 1997; Vecchio, 1994).

The types of alternative therapies used in the United States vary. Some individuals use topical ointments ranging from silicon lubricant to alcohol extract from marijuana leaves; others use copper bracelets or other special jewelry to relieve

symptoms; others use dietary supplements such as glucosamine, vitamins, or herb preparations, as well as acupuncture (Kolasinski, 2001).

Many complementary and alternative therapies have few side effects; however, since individuals with rheumatoid arthritis also often continue to receive traditional medical treatment, interactions between traditional therapies and alternative therapies may be of concern. Consequently, individuals should make both traditional health care providers and alternative health care providers aware of all methods of treatment they are currently using.

### Surgical Treatment of Rheumatoid Arthritis

Most individuals with rheumatoid arthritis are treated with a combination of medication, exercise, and rest. At times, however, because of severe joint inflammation or joint deformity, surgical procedures are necessary. Common surgical procedures for rheumatoid arthritis are *synovectomy* and *arthroplasty* with joint replacement. **Synovectomy** is surgical removal of the synovial membrane surrounding a joint. Synovectomy prevents recurrent inflammation, thus reducing joint pain and further joint destruction.

**Arthroplasty** (surgical replacement, formation, or reformation of a joint) may be necessary when the joint has become nonfunctional because of destruction or when movement of the joint becomes so painful that activity is severely hampered.

### Psychosocial Issues in Rheumatoid Arthritis

The debilitating nature of rheumatoid arthritis, with its associated pain, can affect individuals' ability to work or fulfill responsibilities at home and can also curtail their social life and ability to engage in recreational activities (Walsh, Blanchard, Kremer, & Blanchard, 1999). Living with pain is a factor to which individuals with rheumatoid arthritis must adjust. Awareness of the fact that there is no cure for the condition and that it is progressive may lead to feelings of hopelessness. Individuals with rheumatoid arthritis may also experience sleep disturbances, which increase fatigue and contribute to depression and irritability.

In the early stages, before there is deformity, rheumatoid arthritis may be essentially an invisible disease. This invisibility may lead to misunderstanding by family and friends, who perceive individuals as merely seeking attention with their complaints of pain or attempting to avoid work or other activities. The unpredictable nature of rheumatoid arthritis not only contributes to this misunderstanding but can also cause stress for affected individuals, who are unsure on a day-to-day basis whether they will be able to participate in various activities.

Individuals may develop learned helplessness from the unpredictable, chronic, and incurable nature of the condition. Helping individuals gain a feeling of control by increasing their self-management of arthritic pain and ability to cope with the vagueness of the disease can improve their social functioning and overall quality of life.

Independence is a critical issue for individuals with rheumatoid arthritis. Loss of the ability to perform certain tasks or associated role changes may require significant adjustment. Homemakers with rheumatoid arthritis may have to ask their partner to assume some of the housekeeping duties, and adjustment may be difficult for both. Individuals with rheumatoid arthritis who once prided themselves as being self-sufficient and strong may view having someone else perform what they consider simple tasks a sign of weakness.

If individuals have had to leave their job because of rheumatoid arthritis, their social identity may be threatened. Family roles may also be changed, with other family members taking over tasks once performed by the individual. As rheumatoid arthritis progresses and individuals become more dependent on others or on assistive devices, they may feel a loss of control, which can lead to poor self-esteem.

Also contributing to poor self-esteem is altered body image resulting from the joint deformity or assistive devices that accompany joint changes. However, the use of devices can help individuals gain independence and overcome feelings of helplessness. For grooming needs, individuals may use devices such as adaptive handles for combs and brushes or toothbrushes. They may use a long-handled sponge that has a compartment to hold a bar of soap. Devices such as a zipper pull or a button aid may be of help with dressing. Some individuals may be resistant to using an assistive device, viewing it as "giving up" or fearing that if they use the device rather than their joint, they will lose their ability to perform the task. Others may be concerned about appearances or fear that using the assistive device calls attention to their condition. Thus the use of assistive devices can be an emotionally charged issue. The degree of support from family and friends can make a difference in the individual's willingness to use the device.

### Vocational Issues in Rheumatoid Arthritis

Individuals with rheumatoid arthritis experience a number of work barriers, ranging from physical barriers, such as handling, writing, and energy-related barriers to psychosocial barriers, such as hostility of others in the workplace (Allaire, Li, & LaValley, 2003). Because not all individuals with rheumatoid arthritis are affected in the same way, vocational implications will vary with the severity of the disease and its progression. Not all individuals with rheumatoid arthritis will become totally disabled; however, most individuals will experience reductions across a broad spectrum of activities.

A major limitation of the condition is its unpredictability and not knowing when the condition will change and additional disability will occur. Occupations that have significant physical demands may be more difficult for individuals to maintain than those that are sedentary or require light activity. Even when individuals are still able to perform moderate physical work, the progressive nature of the condition and its potential for affecting mobility should be considered. Pain on motion, limited motion, and muscle weakness may also affect individuals' ability to perform tasks. Tasks requiring manual dexterity or pinch grip may also be difficult, if not impossible, if deformity of the hands has occurred. Work that places stress or strain on joints may exacerbate the disease and should be avoided.

If joints in the lower extremities are involved, standing for long periods of time or walking long distances may be affected. Individuals may have difficulty with climbing, stooping, bending, reaching, and kneeling. They may find it uncomfortable or difficult to remain in one position for long periods of time and may need to change position frequently, since arthritic joints should not stay immobile for long periods. If they spend long periods of time traveling, they should take frequent stops, and if on trains or planes, walk around frequently.

Individuals should attempt to organize and plan tasks as much as possible to conserve energy, protect joints, and minimize fatigue. They may attempt to do as much as they can while seated. If cervical joints are affected, individuals should avoid working with their neck bent over. They may use a slanted or elevated table or desk to avoid neck flexion. Individuals should set priorities, giving up activities of least importance. They may consider alternating more difficult tasks with those requiring less energy. In all cases, they should learn to pace themselves, stopping to rest occasionally rather than persisting with the task until they are exhausted.

If individual symptoms are increased by temperature and humidity, an indoor, climate-controlled environment may be preferable. In most instances, sudden, frequent changes in environmental conditions are more bothersome than the exact level of temperature or humidity itself. Consequently, going in and out of excessively cold or warm environments should be avoided.

Rheumatoid arthritis affects all activities of daily living, not just work. Consequently, individuals may require extra time to get ready for work or to perform tasks at home, and this can, in turn, affect their work schedule. The need for prescribed periods of rest and exercise must also be considered, both at home and in the work environment. A variety of environmental alterations may assist individuals with rheumatoid arthritis to maximize their functional capacity, whether at work or at home. The need for reaching and bending can be reduced with modifications such as storing heavy objects on lower shelves and using pullout shelving or baskets to retrieve them. Pullout shelves can also be used to minimize bending and stretching for hard-to-reach items. Counters can be raised or lowered, permanently or with adjustable components.

Assistive devices can help individuals manage their work environment and their essential daily activities more easily and should be used as appropriate. Devices may be of use for impairments in muscle strength, endurance, range of motion, manual dexterity, and mobility. Assistive devices such as long-handled reachers may be used to open cabinets. Knobs can be replaced by levers so that the whole hand can be used. This may be helpful if manual dexterity or hand strength is affected. Individuals with moderate to severe rheumatoid arthritis may use a motorized wheelchair to increase mobility and to conserve energy.

Although there is no impairment in intellectual functioning or cognitive ability with rheumatoid arthritis, the effect of pain on individuals' ability to concentrate should be considered. The combination of pain and the disabling consequences of rheumatoid arthritis may be associated with depression, which in turn can affect functional capacity. Treatment of depression when identified, as well as interventions to enable individuals to decrease their pain and cope more effectively, may be beneficial in maintaining their vocational status.

### Systemic Lupus Erythematosus

The potential variety and severity of its manifestations and the unpredictable course of systemic lupus erythematosus present significant challenges to individuals living with the condition (Sohng, 2003). An autoimmune disease of unknown cause, **systemic lupus erythematosus** can affect the skin, joints, kidney, heart, lungs, nervous system, blood, and other organs of the body (Giffords, 2003). It is most common in young women and does not usually develop in individuals past middle age (Trethewey, 2004). The condition produces inflammation and structural changes in many body organs and has many neurological and psychiatric manifestations, including cerebrovascular disease, movement disorders, seizure disorders, cognitive dysfunction, and anxiety disorder (ACR Ad Hoc Committee on Neuropsychiatric Lupus Nomenclature, 1999). It may progress rapidly or slowly, or it can become chronic with associated remissions and exacerbations.

Symptoms vary from individual to individual, but they may include a characteristic "butterfly rash" on the face, increased sensitivity to sunlight, loss of appetite, and weight loss. As the condition progresses, it may have more serious effects, such as kidney damage; accumulation of fluid around the heart or lungs; and mental changes, including forgetfulness, confusion, and, in some instances, seizures.

The prognosis for individuals with systemic lupus erythematosus depends on which organs are involved and the degree of autoimmune reaction experienced. The condition is not curable and requires long-term management. For many individuals, appropriate treatment controls or suppresses the symptoms; however, it may also result in death (Ruiz-Irastorza, Khamashta, Castellino, & Hughes, 1999). Some individuals experience years of remission in which they are almost symptom-free, whereas others rapidly develop kidney damage. Women may experience flareups of disease activity at certain periods of the menstrual cycle and during or after pregnancy. Complications such as cardiac symptoms or renal damage are treated as appropriate. Persons with severe kidney involvement may require dialysis (see Chapter 13).

### Treatment of Systemic Lupus Erythematosus

Mild cases of systemic lupus erythematosus may require little or no therapy. When therapy is necessary, the type and location of the condition determine the therapy prescribed. If major organs such as the heart or kidney are involved, treatment is directed toward preserving function and preventing organ failure that could result in disability or death. In mild cases, *salicylates* or NSAIDs may be used. In more severe cases, *steroids* may be indicated.

Individuals with systemic lupus erythematosus may need more than the normal amount of rest. The more active the disease, the more rest they need. Exercise to the point of exhaustion and stressful situations should be avoided, because both can cause exacerbation of the disease.

### Psychosocial Issues in Systemic Lupus Erythematosus

Although the diagnosis of systemic lupus erythematosus may cause emotional reactions and psychological issues, some psychological symptoms may be manifestations of the condition itself. Individuals with systemic lupus erythematosus may need considerable emotional support. Not only is lupus a potentially fatal disease, but most individuals are affected in young adulthood, when the psychosocial and vocational impact of the condition can have a profound effect.

Individuals with systemic lupus erythematosus may need considerable rest, which may be difficult because of other responsibilities. Since the stress of pregnancy and childbirth may exacerbate symptoms, the decision of whether or not to have children may be a difficult one for women with the condition. The degree of psychosocial distress resulting from the condition depends, to some degree, on the severity of the symptoms.

### Vocational Issues in Systemic Lupus Erythematosus

Individuals with systemic lupus erythematosus are often sensitive to sunlight, which may trigger symptoms. They may need to give up outdoor activities or at least activities that entail exposure to the sun. When they cannot avoid sunlight, they may need to wear extra clothing or hats or use umbrellas to protect themselves from the sun. Other musculoskeletal conditions may become worse in cold, damp environments. As stated previously, individuals with systemic lupus erythematosus may need more than the normal amount of rest. The more active the disease, the more rest they need. Exercise to the point of exhaustion and stressful situations should be avoided, because both can cause exacerbation of the disease. While in remission, and if there is no associated, permanent organ damage, individuals may have few physical or emotional disabilities.

### Gout

Gout is an arthritic disease that is characterized by **hyperuricemia** (buildup in the body of a substance called *uric acid*). Uric acid is a waste product of the metabolism of substances called *purines*, which are found in a variety of foods. It is normally carried in the blood until it is excreted by the kidneys. With gout, uric acid levels in the blood increase, either because the kidneys are not excreting uric acid fast enough or because the body is making too much uric acid. Excess uric acid changes into crystals, called *urate crystals*, which settle in the joints, causing swelling and excruciating pain. Individuals with gout are more likely than others to develop kidney stones (**urolithiasis**) (see Chapter 13), which occasionally cause obstruction and severe kidney damage (Terkeltaub, 2003).

### Symptoms of Gout

Gout can be inherited, or it can be a complication of another condition. Symptoms, which appear suddenly, may be precipitated by the intake of foods and beverages rich in purines, such as organ meats (e.g., liver, sweetbreads), gravies, and alcohol. Symptoms may also be precipitated by minor injury, stress, or fatigue. Attacks may last only a few days at first, but if the condition is not adequately controlled, later attacks may last weeks.

If untreated, gout may result in chronic joint symptoms with permanent joint deformity and limitation of motion. Although gout cannot be cured, prophylactic treatment can control its symptoms.

### Treatment of Gout

The objectives in the treatment of gout are to terminate the acute attack and to prevent recurrent attacks. Treatment involves not only treating acute arthritic inflammation and urinary tract stones (urolithiasis), but also lowering urate levels in an attempt to prevent recurrent attacks and progression of the disease (Schlesinger & Schumacher, 2001; Wortmann, 2002).

During acute attacks, the affected joint is placed at rest and *anti-inflammatory agents* are prescribed. Prevention of further attacks may require daily use of medications for lowering the level of uric acid in the blood or for increasing its excretion by the kidneys. Occasionally, surgery is nec-

essary to remove *tophi* (deposits of crystals in the joints).

Individuals with gout should increase fluid intake to decrease the risk of kidney stones; follow a diet that excludes foods high in purines and fats, such as sardines, anchovies, organ meats, veal, or bacon; and avoid excessive alcohol intake.

### Vocational Issues in Gout

Since gout can cause significant pain in affected joints, individuals may be unable to work during a gout attack. The extent of absences from work is dependent on the frequency and severity of the attacks. Not all joints are affected. Consequently, the degree of functional impairment that occurs if there is resulting joint deformity or loss of motion is dependent on the joint involved and the degree to which the joint is crucial to job performance. Because stress can precipitate gout attacks, individuals should avoid stressful situations or should be helped with stress management.

### Ankylosing Spondylitis

**Ankylosing spondylitis** is a rheumatic condition that affects the joints and ligaments of the spine. At times, it may also affect the hips, ankles, or elbows. It is a progressive condition that frequently leads to deterioration in spinal posture (Swinkels & Dolan, 2004). The inflammatory process around these joints causes pain and can result in a fusing of the joints, with subsequent loss and/or restriction of motion. Back pain of varying intensity is the most common initial complaint. It is often worse at night. Other complaints may include morning stiffness that is relieved by activity and systemic symptoms, such as fatigue, weight loss, loss of appetite, and anemia. Postural abnormalities may develop with resulting spinal deformities. If the condition is untreated, a permanent postural deformity called **kyphosis** (hump back) may occur.

The course of ankylosing spondylitis and its severity are highly variable (Cush & Lipsky, 2000). With proper treatment, many individuals with ankylosing spondylitis have little permanent disability. There may be occasional flareups when the symptoms become worse, but there may also be long periods with no symptoms (Cornell, 2004).

### Treatment of Ankylosing Spondylitis

Management of ankylosing spondylitis involves relieving pain and inflammation and maximizing function through physical therapy and exercise. NSAIDs may be administered to decrease inflammation and pain, thereby facilitating exercise.

Exercises are designed to strengthen supporting muscles and to maintain good posture and function. Good posture is essential to prevent spinal deformity. Physical therapy should begin early to keep the spine as straight as possible and thus to preserve the chest's ability to expand. In the case of severe deformity, surgical intervention may be indicated.

### Vocational Issues in Ankylosing Spondylitis

Individuals with ankylosing spondylitis experience no limitation with regard to cognitive skills, vision, or motor coordination. Because of the stiffness and potential fusing of joints of the spine, however, twisting and turning motions as well as lifting may be limited. If individuals develops kyphosis, altered self-image may be accompanied by embarrassment and a reluctance to work in situations in which the public is encountered.

## Other Conditions of the Musculoskeletal System

### Osteomyelitis

**Osteomyelitis** (infection of the bone) can be a debilitating condition with a long course of treatment (Calhoun, Laughlin, Mader, & Maher, 1998).

### Causes of Osteomyelitis

There are several ways in which **osteomyelitis** can occur. Pathologic organisms can enter the bone directly through an injury, such as an open or compound fracture in which the broken bone fragment has penetrated through the skin. Osteomyelitis may also result from infection of surrounding tissue that then extends to the bone. For example, ulceration of tissue in a lower extremity that occurs because of *vascular insufficiency* (inadequate blood and oxygen to a body part) in conditions such as arteriosclerosis or diabetes may become infected, and infection may then extend to the bone. In other instances, pathologic organisms that are present in the blood may settle and localize in the bone.

### Treatment of Osteomyelitis

Osteomyelitis is often difficult to cure. If initial treatment is ineffective, osteomyelitis can lead to chronic infection or amputation. Treatment may be medical or surgical. Medical treatment consists of the administration of antibiotics to treat the infection and bedrest until the infection has been eradicated. Surgical intervention may be indicated to remove infected tissue, replace a portion of bone with a graft, or replace an infected prosthetic joint. In some instances, amputation may be required.

### Fibromyalgia

**Fibromyalgia** is a rheumatologic condition characterized by widespread pain, aching, and stiffness in muscles and/or joints, with associated sleep disturbance, fatigue, and extensively distributed areas of tenderness known as tender points (Millea & Holloway, 2000). Symptoms may range from mild to moderate to severe.

The pain and discomfort associated with fibromyalgia are diffuse, involving the neck, shoulders, lower back, and hips, as well as other sites. Fibromyalgia is not a progressively degenerative disease and does not cause damage to bones or joints; consequently, there are no objective findings or a definitive diagnostic test that can legitimize the condition. As a result, the condition is often perplexing for individuals with the symptoms, as well as for their physicians, who are unable to establish a clear-cut diagnosis (Clauw, 2000).

Since there are no definitive laboratory or radiographic tests used in the diagnosis of fibromyalgia, diagnosis is based on individuals' self-report of symptoms and history, with the identifiable tender points being a prime diagnostic marker. Individuals with fibromyalgia can also experience symptoms other than musculoskeletal pain, including headache or manifestations of irritable bowel syndrome (see Chapter 10). Complaints of sleep disturbances and fatigue are common. Any significant life stress can exacerbate symptoms.

Fibromyalgia can occur concomitantly with other serious rheumatic disorders such as lupus and rheumatoid arthritis. Psychological symptoms of anxiety and depression frequently accompany the condition. Fibromyalgia can interfere with individuals' quality of life and may cause interpersonal difficulties because of the symptoms. Individuals often find it helpful to be reassured that the condition is "real." Legitimizing individuals' complaints of symptoms can help reestablish self-control and self-esteem, enabling them to cope with their symptoms.

### Treatment of Fibromyalgia

Fibromyalgia is a chronic condition in which only relative improvement can be expected. Individuals may find neck support during sleep or abdominal exercises to relieve stress on the lower back helpful. Some individuals may find aerobic exercise such as walking or swimming effective in reducing pain and tenderness as well as in helping with sleep disturbances. Recent studies have suggested that hyperbaric oxygen therapy (discussed later in the chapter) may also be useful in treatment of fibromyalgia (Yildiz et al., 2004).

Although simple *analgesics* such as acetaminophen or NSAIDs may be recommended by physicians, medications such as systemic *corticosteroids* or stronger pain relievers are not recommended. Low-dose *tricyclic antidepressants* (see Chapter 6) may also be beneficial to assist individuals with sleep. If individuals are experiencing stress or have other underlying psychological factors that exacerbate sleep disturbances or pain perception, stress management, relaxation, or counseling may be needed to help them cope with the condition. Some individuals also find support groups useful. It is important that individuals remain physically and socially active and that they identify and eliminate the stresses or environmental disturbances that may exacerbate the symptoms.

### Vocational Issues in Fibromyalgia

Individuals with fibromyalgia may have repeated absenteeism at work because of pain, fatigue, or both. The direct effect on individuals' ability to work depends on a number of factors, including the nature of the job, the motivation to follow suggested lifestyle changes, and the presence of any underlying psychological factors.

Many individuals with fibromyalgia may need to learn how to pace themselves, since certain physical activities may take longer than before. Very active individuals may have to cut back on activities. Individuals should be encouraged to remain active but not to push themselves beyond their limit.

Flexibility in scheduling may be beneficial. Some job modification and restructuring may be necessary to prevent overuse or overexertion of muscle groups. Physical stressors that are identified should also be avoided. Because sleep disturbance is an accompanying symptom, individuals may have difficulty concentrating while at work. Because of the vague nature of the symptoms and the fact that there presently is no definitive test to diagnose fibromyalgia, individuals may be subject to the scrutiny of coworkers or their employer, who may question the legitimacy of their diagnosis and their symptoms. Individuals may be labeled as malingerers, and resentment from coworkers may result. Education of employers and coworkers can help to dispel myths and misinformation.

## DIAGNOSTIC PROCEDURES FOR CONDITIONS OF THE MUSCULOSKELETAL SYSTEM

### Roentgenography (Radiography, X-rays)

The most widely used diagnostic tool for musculoskeletal disorders is roentgenography (X-ray). The painless procedure involves positioning the body part to be studied against photographic film and exposing the film by irradiation. A radiographic technician generally takes the X-ray films, and a **radiologist** (physician who specializes in radiation and the use of radioactive materials for the diagnosis and treatment of disease) interprets them. For musculoskeletal conditions, X-ray is useful for identifying deformity or injury of bones.

### Arthrography

To perform an **arthrogram** (radiographic study of a joint), the radiologist first injects the joint to be examined with a local anesthetic and then injects a special material or contrast medium and/or air into the joint cavity. The joint is then moved through its range of motion and a series of X-ray films are taken. This diagnostic procedure is done to identify injury to the joint or supporting ligaments.

### Diskography and Myelography

Although diskography and myelography are similar to arthrography, they involve the study of different areas of the body. **Diskography** is a radiographic study of the *cervical* or *lumbar disks*, and **myelography** is a radiographic study of the *spinal cord*.

### Arthroscopy

**Arthroscopy** is the visualization of a joint through a small instrument called an *arthroscope* that is inserted into the joint to be studied. Videotaped pictures may be taken of the internal joint structures.

### Arthrocentesis

**Arthrocentesis** is a procedure in which the physician aspirates *synovial fluid* with a needle that has been inserted into the joint cavity. The synovial fluid is then examined for abnormalities, such as blood, crystals, or infection. In some instances, arthrocentesis may be used to remove fluid from the joint to relieve pain. If the joint has been injured or is infected, examination of blood or pus in the synovial fluid can help in determining the type or degree of injury or infection.

## Bone Scan

A bone scan is a procedure in which radioactive substances, called *radioisotopes*, are injected intravenously. The radioisotopes concentrate in the bone, and the amount of concentration is measured by a special machine, called a *scanner*. The scanner produces a picture of the bone (*scan*), enabling physicians to identify any abnormalities.

## Magnetic Resonance Imaging (MRI)

A painless, noninvasive procedure, *magnetic resonance imaging* produces rapid detailed pictures of body tissue. It is widely used to assist in the diagnosis of a number of musculoskeletal disorders, as well as disorders of other body systems. The procedure requires no radiation. It may be performed without *contrast* (substance that is injected and enables visualization) or with contrast, meaning that individuals are injected with a contrast substance intravenously.

For magnetic resonance imaging, individuals are placed in a horizontal cylinder, where they are exposed to a magnetic field much greater than the earth's. As a result, hydrogen atoms within the body line up parallel to the magnetic field. Low-energy radio waves are then directed into the individual's body, causing protons in the body to move out of alignment. This process is called *resonance*. When the radio

waves are discontinued, the protons realign. The machine picks up the amount of energy released by the protons as they swing back into alignment and converts it into an image of the body part being studied.

Because of the strength of the magnetic field used for the procedure, individuals with metal in their body should not undergo magnetic resonance imaging. Thus, the procedure is contraindicated for individuals with a cardiac pacemaker, metal clips that have been placed in the body as part of a prior surgical procedure, or small pieces of metal embedded by injury (e.g., shrapnel).

Magnetic resonance imaging is used for diagnosing diseases of many body systems. In the musculoskeletal system, magnetic resonance imaging is helpful in diagnosing diseases of the joints, confirming infection of the bone (**osteomyelitis**), discovering small fractures of the bone that may not be detectable by other means, and identifying soft tissue and bone tumors.

## Computed Tomography (Computed Axial Tomography, CAT Scan, CT Scan)

*Computed tomography* (*CT scan*) is a noninvasive radiographic procedure that may be performed with or without contrast (as described above). It may be used to diagnose a number of types of conditions in many different body systems. In the musculoskeletal system, it may be helpful in identifying fractures, tumors, bone deformities, or soft tissue damage. During the procedure, individuals are placed within a hollow tube where X-rays are passed through the body part at many different angles, resulting in the CT image. Because each tissue contains a different density, each density is given a numerical value, which is computed and displayed on a screen. The image is then recorded on film. The CT scan is performed by the radiologist.

## Blood Tests

In and of themselves, blood tests are not diagnostic of specific disorders of the musculoskeletal system; however, some blood tests indicate inflammation or tissue injury and, thus, may be used as part of the diagnostic process. For example, a determination of the *erythrocyte sedimentation rate* may be part of the diagnostic workup for conditions such as rheumatoid arthritis. Another test, *C-reactive protein*, may also be used to identify inflammatory processes or tissue destruction.

A blood test commonly used in the diagnosis of rheumatoid arthritis is the *rheumatoid factor (RF)*. These *latex fixation* or *agglutination tests* for RF are not definitive tests for rheumatoid arthritis but merely provide supportive evidence when individuals have corresponding symptoms. The blood test determines whether there is abnormal protein in the serum. Many individuals with rheumatoid arthritis have such protein, although those with many other conditions (e.g., tuberculosis and bacterial endocarditis) may also have it.

Another blood test that may be used, especially in the diagnosis of systemic lupus erythematosus, is the *antinuclear antibodies test*. Antinuclear antibodies are proteins found in the blood of some individuals with autoimmune diseases. The antinuclear antibody test is a blood test that identifies the presence of these proteins. However, since the test may be positive in many different autoimmune diseases or may be positive as a result of some medications, the test is not definitive.

## GENERAL TREATMENTS FOR CONDITIONS OF THE MUSCULOSKELETAL SYSTEM

### Medications

Pain and inflammation are common manifestations of many musculoskeletal and connective tissue disorders. *Salicylates* (e.g., aspirin) are commonly the first choice of medication to reduce pain and inflammation. For some conditions, such as rheumatoid arthritis, it may be necessary to prescribe as many as 15 or more tablets of salicylate a day to reach a therapeutic dosage. This high concentration of aspirin in the blood may exceed the liver's ability to metabolize it. The side effects of a high salicylate dosage include gastric irritation and ringing or noise in the ears (**tinnitus**).

NSAIDs may also be used to reduce the pain and inflammation associated with musculoskeletal conditions. Like salicylates, these drugs can irritate the stomach lining, causing pain and, in some instances, bleeding. *Corticosteroids* can produce dramatic short-term anti-inflammatory effects, but they do not prevent progression of joint destruction and, because of their potency and subsequent side effects, can be used only on a short-term basis. Some side effects of prolonged use include cataracts, demineralization of bone, delayed wound healing, poor resistance to infection, and symptoms similar to those of Cushing's syndrome (see Chapter 9). More serious systemic effects may involve severe *adrenal insufficiency* following withdrawal (see Chapter 9). Steroid use should always be carefully monitored by a physician, and steroids should never be discontinued suddenly. Although steroids for musculoskeletal conditions are generally taken orally, they are sometimes injected directly into an inflamed joint for the temporary suppression of the inflammation.

## Hyperbaric Oxygen Therapy

Hyperbaric oxygen therapy is a treatment in which 100 percent oxygen is given at two to three times the atmospheric pressure at sea level. It is used for a number of conditions in addition to musculoskeletal conditions, including carbon monoxide poisoning, decompression sickness, radiation-induced tissue injury, and severe skin injury. Specific conditions of the musculoskeletal system for which hyperbaric oxygen therapy is used include chronic osteomyelitis (Sugihara et al., 2004); crush injuries or other severe traumas to the extremities that cause insufficient blood flow to the extremity resulting in **necrosis** (tissue death) (Chen, Ko, Fu, & Wang, 2004); thermal burns and skin grafts or flaps (see Chapter 15) that have inadequate blood flow or oxygen and are thus not healing properly; and foot and leg ulcers associated with diabetes (see Chapter 9) (Kranke, Bennett, Roeckl-Wiedmann, & Debus, 2004).

Hyperbaric oxygen therapy works by restoring the body's defense against infection and increasing the rate at which the body is able to kill common bacteria. Individuals inhale hyperbaric oxygen in the atmosphere of a special cylindrical single-occupant chamber in which they have been placed or through masks, hoods, or special tubes that are inserted into their **trachea** (windpipe).

The length and amount of treatment depend on the reason for the treatment. Single treatments can range from 45 minutes for carbon monoxide poisoning to almost 5 hours for severe decompression disorders. For musculoskeletal disorders, treatments may average 90 minutes for 20 to 30 treatments. Although hyperbaric treatment can be costly, when comparing the cost with hospitalization and disability for conditions that are not successfully treated, the savings can be extensive.

## Physical Therapy

Many types of musculoskeletal disorders can be improved through physical therapy. These techniques are usually performed by a *physical therapist* or a *physical therapy assistant*. A *physical therapist* is an individual with a bachelor's degree in physical therapy who provides services that help develop, restore, or preserve physical function. A *physical therapy assistant* is generally an individual with an associate's degree who works under the direction of a physical therapist.

The type of physical therapy administered depends on the particular musculoskeletal condition. Physical therapy may be directed toward increasing or maintaining a joint's range of motion, increasing muscle strength, relieving pain or muscle spasms, or teaching techniques for ambulation.

Some techniques used in physical therapy involve therapeutic exercise, which may be passive or active. In *passive exercise*, the therapist or a mechanical device exercises the body part. In *active exercise*, individuals independently perform a specified exercise regimen under the direction or supervision of the physical therapist or physical therapy assistant. Exercise may be designed to increase or maintain range of motion, prevent **atrophy** (shrinking of the muscles), prevent deformity due to contractures, or increase muscle strength.

Other physical therapy techniques may involve applying heat or cold or massaging the muscles for relaxation or relief of pain. Heat may be applied through hot packs, hot soaks, infrared radiation, or whirlpool baths. Another procedure for applying heat is diathermy, a process in which the temperature of the body part is raised through high-frequency ultrasonic waves. Because cold has a numbing effect, it may also be used to relieve pain. Cold packs or chemical packs may be applied to the painful area. Massage, the manipulation of muscles through rubbing or kneading, may be used to relax muscles, improve muscle tone, relieve muscle spasm, or increase blood flow to the area.

## Casts

A variety of musculoskeletal conditions are treated with casts. Although casts may be synthetic, they are more commonly made of plaster of Paris. Casts provide immobilization and support for a body part while it is healing. They may also be used to prevent or correct various musculoskeletal deformities. The type and size of cast depend on the condition and the purpose of the casting. In addition to casts used on extremities, there are spica casts, which extend the entire length of the lower extremity from the middle of the trunk of the body. In some instances, a *full body cast* is necessary.

## Assistive Devices

Individuals with musculoskeletal disorders may use assistive devices to aid in ambulation, to prevent undue strain on a body part, or to restore or enhance functional capacity. Assistive devices may be used therapeutically in the healing period after musculoskeletal injury or on a continuing basis. Some examples of assistive devices that aid in ambulation or prevent excessive weight bearing on a lower extremity are *canes, crutches,* and *walkers*. Other examples are those special devices used for individuals with upper-extremity deformity who need help in performing activities of daily living, such as *long-handled grippers, zipper pulls,* or *jar-opening devices* (see Chapter 17 for a fuller discussion of assistive devices).

## Orthoses

Orthoses are devices used to straighten or correct a deformity; they are mechanical devices applied to the body to control the motion of joints and the force or weight distribution to a body part. A brace, for example, is an orthotic device used to provide support or to prevent or correct a deformity. The type of device used depends on the purpose of the bracing and the condition itself. An **orthotist** is an individual who constructs orthotic devices to meet individual needs.

Orthoses may be prescribed for any musculoskeletal area, depending on the nature of the problem. For example, *lower limb orthoses* are orthopedic shoes or orthoses for the foot, ankle, knee, or hip. *Spinal orthoses* may be used to relieve compression forces on the spine, to restrict movement of the spine, or to modify the alignment of the spine. There are at least 50 types of spinal orthoses, classified according to the level of application. *Cervical orthoses* may be prescribed for a wide variety of problems, ranging from whiplash to fracture of the cervical spine. The *Taylor,* the *Jewett Hyperextension TLSO,* and the *CASH* are spinal orthoses prescribed to restrict trunk flexion and rotation or to provide hyperextension and reduce flexion in the thoracic-lumbar spine. *Lumbar-sacral spinal* orthoses, such as the *Knight Chairback* and the *Williams,* are prescribed primarily for low back pain and may consist of flexible or semirigid corsets that provide support and protection. The *Milwaukee brace* is an orthotic device designed for treatment of **scoliosis** (lateral S-shaped curvature of the spine).

Orthotic devices may also be used for the upper extremities. In these instances, they are most frequently prescribed because of injury. Upper-extremity orthoses may be applied to the shoulder, elbow, or wrist/

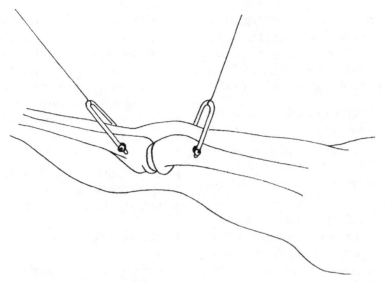

**Figure 14–6** Skeletal Traction. *Source:* Copyright © 1999 Rachel Clarke.

hand. Newer orthotic devices, called *fracture orthoses*, are designed to allow early ambulation on fractures of the lower extremity. These devices permit functional use of the extremity much earlier than does conventional casting. Recently, some upper-extremity fractures have also been treated with fracture orthoses.

### Traction

Individuals with a variety of musculoskeletal conditions may benefit from traction, a therapeutic method in which a mechanical or manual pull is used to restore or maintain the alignment of bones or to relieve pain and muscle spasm (see Figure 14–6). It may be applied in several ways. When traction exerts a constant pull, it is said to be *continuous*. If the pull is relieved periodically, the traction is said to be *intermittent*. Traction may be applied *externally* or *internally*.

*Skin traction* is applied by fastening straps, belts, or other external devices around the body and then to a source of countertraction. In contrast, *skeletal traction* is applied internally; *metal wires* (Kirschner wires), *pins* (Steinmann pins), or *tongs* (Crutchfield tongs) are inserted through the bone surgically and attached to a source of countertraction outside the body. Kirschner wires and Steinmann pins are typically used to *reduce* (align) fractures of the long bones of the extremities in order to promote bone healing or to stabilize the fracture until surgical treatment can be undertaken to correct it. Crutchfield tongs are inserted into the skull for injuries of the cervical spine.

The use of traction may prevent surgical intervention in some cases, and it offers more freedom of movement than does a cast. However, it usually requires prolonged hospitalization. Furthermore, in the case of skeletal traction, there is a risk of complications, such as osteomyelitis, that can contribute to permanent disability.

### Surgical Treatment

Individuals with musculoskeletal conditions may require surgical treatment to correct, remove, or replace injured or diseased structures. Surgery may be performed on an emergency basis in the case of traumatic injury or on an elective basis in the case of disease, deformity, or an old injury. There are several types of surgical interventions:

- **Open reduction:** surgical alignment of the fractured bone.
- **Internal fixation:** placement of screws, pins, wires, rods, or other devices through the bone to hold the bone fragments together.
- **Arthroplasty:** replacement of all or part of a joint with a prosthetic device to relieve pain or to restore function. Common sites of arthroplasty are the hip, shoulder, knee, and elbow. Reasons for arthroplasty include a broken hip (*total hip replacement*) or arthritis.
- **Arthrodesis:** surgical *fusing* (joining) of two joint surfaces, making them permanently immobile. The procedure was once commonly performed to relieve joint pain. With improved arthroplasty procedures, however, arthrodesis is now less common.
- **Synovectomy:** surgical removal of the *synovial membrane* surrounding a joint. Synovectomy prevents recurrent inflammation, thus reducing joint pain and further joint destruction.
- **Laminectomy:** surgical removal of a portion of a vertebra, exposing the spinal cord. It is usually performed to facilitate the removal of any source of pressure on the spinal cord (e.g., to remove bone fragments from spinal cord injury; to remove tumor from the spinal cord).
- **Spinal fusion:** grafting of bone from another area of the body into the disk interspace after a surgical procedure on the spine (e.g., laminectomy). After spinal fusion, mobility at the point of the fusion is lost.

- **Carpal tunnel repair:** a surgical procedure in which the median nerve is decompressed by the transection of surrounding ligaments. It is performed when the symptoms of carpal tunnel syndrome are severe and include progressive sensory loss in the fingers and hand.

## PSYCHOSOCIAL ISSUES IN CONDITIONS OF THE MUSCULOSKELETAL SYSTEM

### Psychological Issues

The emotional needs of individuals with musculoskeletal conditions often relate to prolonged dependence on others, the long-term nature of the condition, and uncertainty about the ability to resume normal responsibilities and activities. Restrictions on mobility and natural movements because of casts, braces, or traction or because of pain, deformity, or absence of a limb are, for many individuals, unbearable. Depending on the extent of immobility, they may have a sense of powerlessness leading to anger, hostility, and, later, depression. If the musculoskeletal condition necessitates giving up some valued activity permanently, depression may deepen. Some individuals who have a strong athletic identity may fail to disclose their condition, continuing the activity even though it may cause additional damage.

The prolonged pain associated with many musculoskeletal system conditions consumes energy and may contribute to increased self-centeredness and dependence as pain becomes the central issue in individuals' lives. The discomfort, as well as the limitations on mobility, can contribute to irritability, discouragement, and depression. Pain perception is related not only to various personality factors, but also to factors such as workers' compensation, litigation, or other benefits that may decrease individuals' motivation to reduce pain or restore function.

Individuals planning to undergo musculoskeletal surgery may experience a mixture of fear and anticipation regarding the extent to which the surgery will restore lost function. Those having repeated surgery, such as a second joint replacement for arthritis or continuing treatment for osteomyelitis, may lose patience and hope.

Individuals with chronic conditions of the musculoskeletal system may force themselves to do more than they comfortably can because of fear of being a burden to others. Inability to maintain previous activity levels may cause continued frustration. The unpredictability of conditions that have remissions and exacerbation (e.g., rheumatoid arthritis) may also be a source of tension.

The deformity associated with many musculoskeletal conditions, such as rheumatoid arthritis, ankylosing spondylitis, osteoporosis, or amputation, alters body image. Most individuals react to any body image change with anxiety and fear of rejection. Concern about appearance can lead to continual worry about acceptance by family, friends, and acquaintances.

## Lifestyle Issues

Although many conditions of the musculoskeletal system require only short-term treatment and impose only temporary disability, some conditions require lifelong adaptation and significant lifestyle changes. Restrictions of body movement resulting from a loss of muscle strength, deformity of joints, or pain alter the activities of daily living, as well as social and recreational activities. Individuals may need to learn new ambulation and transfer techniques and find alternatives to

activities that place undue stress on joints. It may be necessary to install grab bars and safety rails in the home to provide stability and prevent falls.

Conditions affecting the ankles or the feet may require that individuals wear special shoes for comfort and protection of the joints. Sitting while performing many tasks, such as meal preparation, may save wear and tear on weight-bearing joints. Conditions affecting joints of the hands, such as rheumatoid arthritis, may require the use of assistive devices, such as hooks, zipper pulls, special openers, or other self-help aids, if individuals are to perform activities of daily living independently. Adaptive handles for combs and brushes may be of help for grooming. Soft lead pencils and felt-tipped pens may be useful for decreasing pressure on finger joints when writing.

At home, work centers may be established where all the items needed for a specific task are kept within easy reach. It may be necessary to lower tables and cabinets so that individuals with a musculoskeletal disorder may be seated while they work and to raise beds, toilet seats, and chairs so that sitting and arising are easier. Organizing and planning daily tasks can help to reduce strain and fatigue.

Dietary modifications may also be necessary in some conditions of the musculoskeletal system. Obesity places extra strain on joints; consequently, if obesity is an issue, a weight reduction diet may be prescribed. Specific conditions, such as gout, also require dietary modifications. Individuals with pain or deformity in the hands or those who have undergone upper-extremity amputation may need special adaptive eating utensils for activities such as cutting meat.

Many conditions of the musculoskeletal system require some form of therapeutic exercise to maintain joint function, restore strength and/or joint motion, or prevent deformity. Such exercise programs must be incorporated into the daily routine. Conditions such as rheumatoid arthritis may require specified rest periods during the day.

Most conditions of the musculoskeletal system do not hamper sexual activity; however, pain, deformity, decreased range of joint motion, or alteration in body image may affect sexual function. Positioning may be difficult or painful, as in the case of rheumatoid arthritis or low back pain. In some instances, the medications used for the treatment of musculoskeletal disorders can affect sexual function. Steroids prescribed for a number of musculoskeletal conditions may decrease libido, and pain may inhibit sexual desire.

## Social Issues

Because conditions of the musculoskeletal system can impair mobility and because in some cases individuals must depend on others for assistance, the support and understanding of family and friends are paramount. Reassurance that physical changes or deformities are unimportant can be valuable to individuals' self-esteem and confidence; however, such reassurance by family and friends is not always forthcoming.

Depending on the extent of discomfort, limitation of motion, and deformity, individuals may be unable to perform all of their previous tasks, making it necessary for other family members to share household chores and duties. Their willingness or lack of willingness to accept necessary alterations in home life can affect how individuals adjust to their condition. When work or social activities are significantly altered by the individual's musculoskeletal condition, his or her social identity may be altered. These role changes may be

a source of stress. If friendships have developed around specific activities that now must be altered because of the condition, individuals may feel a sense of social isolation and of no longer fitting in.

When mobility is altered because of a musculoskeletal condition, it may be necessary to plan vacations around the condition. Other manifestations of the musculoskeletal condition may also need to be considered when planning vacations. Individuals with systemic lupus erythematosus may have to avoid hot, sunny beaches, whereas individuals with other musculoskeletal conditions may need to avoid colder climates. Individuals who are experiencing severe pain may be reluctant to venture on vacation at all.

Family and friends may have difficulty in coping with the feelings of hostility, frustration, or irritability expressed by individuals because of pain or increased dependency. Others may view these individuals as demanding, manipulative, and difficult. Depending on the premorbid functioning of the family and the degree and quality of communication between family members, family dynamics can be an increased source of tension.

Individuals with musculoskeletal disorders, especially those with ongoing pain, are especially vulnerable to unorthodox, unproven "miracle cures." Although alternative and complementary practices have a place in the treatment of musculoskeletal conditions (Pelletier, Astin, & Haskell, 1999), some unscrupulous individuals can take advantage of individuals' vulnerability by marketing and selling methods that are dubious. In addition to the expense, many fraudulent measures have dangerous side effects that, in some instances, can be fatal. Even if there are no side effects, individuals may use these methods in place of recommended treatment, thus losing the therapeutic effects of legitimate treatment. When complementary and alternative methods are used by individuals to treat musculoskeletal conditions, the safety of the method and the legitimacy of the individuals providing it should always be determined before use.

## VOCATIONAL ISSUES IN CONDITIONS OF THE MUSCULOSKELETAL SYSTEM

The disability associated with work-related musculoskeletal disorders is an increasing problem. Although many individuals with work-related injury return to their job, a substantial number of individuals do not (Turner et al., 2004). The impact of musculoskeletal disorders on vocational function depends on the type of job previously held and on individual factors related to job history and motivation, as well as on the type of musculoskeletal disorder (Rahman, Ambler, Underwood, & Shipley, 2004). The amount of sitting, bending, stooping, or lifting that the job requires must be considered. Modification of the work environment, such as by raising or lowering worktables or chairs, may be necessary. Generally, it is important that individuals return to work and daily activities as soon as possible to maintain good work habits.

Injured worker programs and work-hardening programs have gained popularity for helping individuals return to work. These programs use a systemic approach of case management, evaluation, and treatment that prepares workers for successful and safe reentry into the workforce after injury (Schonstein, Kenny, Keating, & Koes, 2003; Weir & Nielson, 2001).

In injured worker programs, individuals' physical capacity or level of function is evaluated as they are progressed through graded levels of job simulation tasks. Evaluation provides objective data regarding their physical and functional capacity so that goals and a treatment plan can be established. Services are provided on an outpatient basis. Work tolerance screening focuses on individuals' musculoskeletal strength, endurance, speed, and flexibility. Functional capacity evaluation documents individuals' ability to return to work from a physical, behavioral, and ergonomic perspective. Work conditioning (work hardening) prepares individuals to return to competitive employment (Johnson, Archer-Heese, Caron-Powles, & Dowson, 2001). The goal is to increase work tolerance, increase work rate, help individuals learn to control symptoms, increase confidence and proficiency, and help individuals learn to use work adaptations and assistive devices. The program is highly structured. Along with simulated or real-work tasks, this structure instills expectations for the real-world environment, such as promptness, attendance, and appropriate dress.

Assistive devices such as crutches, walkers, or canes may make ambulation slower and more difficult. In addition, the use of such devices makes it difficult, if not impossible, to carry objects from one point to another.

Rheumatoid arthritis, ankylosing spondylitis, systemic lupus erythematosus, and a number of other connective tissue disorders are progressive in nature and often unpredictable. Although not all individuals with these conditions become severely disabled, ongoing medical care and evaluation are necessary. When the condition has remissions and exacerbations, individuals may have unexpected periods of exacerbation in which work is missed. Individuals may need to avoid overexertion, stress, and fatigue, which may in turn necessitate altered or shortened work schedules to accommodate periods of rest.

Overuse of damaged joints should be avoided. For example, individuals with osteoarthritis of the knees should avoid excessive walking; those with carpal tunnel syndrome should avoid repetitive activities with the hands. Deformity of joints not only may interfere with occupational function, but also may be potentially embarrassing to the individual in personal interactions at work. Occasionally, barriers such as financial disincentives, the status of legal claims, and other disability and compensation protocols can interfere with effective rehabilitation of individuals with musculoskeletal disorders. Individuals may be hesitant to learn new skills or use devices that help them to maintain independence if, in so doing, they imperil possible financial benefits or are expected to return to a work environment they did not or will not enjoy.

## CASE STUDIES

### Case I

Mr. P., a 52-year-old self-employed farmer, was mowing his pasture when his tractor hit a hole, throwing him from the tractor and subsequently running over his right leg, crushing it. He was rushed to the hospital; however, the injury was so severe that his leg was amputated above the knee. Mr. P. received a lower-extremity prosthesis but experienced considerable depression after his injury, and he was unmotivated to learn to walk with his prosthesis. His wife, a homemaker, has continued to be supportive, although she has expressed concern about his lack of responsiveness to the support she and friends have attempted to provide to him. Mr. P. grew up on a farm and has had no other type of employment. He has a high school education.

### Questions

1. What factors in addition to his injury will contribute to Mr. P.'s effective rehabilitation?
2. What other sources of referral might be helpful to Mr. P. in his rehabilitation?
3. How would you approach Mr. P. about his rehabilitation?
4. What special equipment or adaptive devices might be helpful to Mr. P. if he chooses to go back to farming?
5. What special equipment or adaptive devices might be helpful to Mr. P. in terms of his functional capacity on a day-to-day basis unrelated to farming?
6. What environmental factors might you consider when helping Mr. P. with a rehabilitation plan?

### Case II

Mrs. R., a 45-year-old medical transcriptionist, has worked in her current occupation for the past 20 years. Her job involves using a transcribing machine with a headset and foot pedal to transcribe dictated reports. She began noting morning stiffness in her hands several years ago. The stiffness has become worse and now also involves her elbows and shoulders. She has been diagnosed as having rheumatoid arthritis. Currently her rheumatoid arthritis is in remission with the help of large quantities of aspirin each day, which are causing her to experience tinnitus.

### Questions

1. What medical factors about Mrs. R.'s condition should be considered when assessing her rehabilitation potential?

2. Is Mrs. R.'s current job a good choice for employment given her current medical condition? Why or why not?
3. Are there assistive devices or job modifications that could help Mrs. R.

maintain her current employment as a medical transcriptionist?
4. Is there additional medical information that could be helpful in establishing Mrs. R.'s rehabilitation plan?

## REFERENCES

ACR Ad Hoc Committee on Neuropsychiatric Lupus Nomenclature. (1999). The American College of Rheumatology nomenclature and case definitions for neuropsychiatric lupus syndromes. *Arthritis Rheumatology, 42*, 599–608.

Allaire, S. H., Li, W., & LaValley, M. P. (2003). Work barriers experienced and job accommodations used by persons with arthritis and other rheumatic diseases. *Rehabilitation Counseling Bulletin, 46*(3), 147–156.

American College of Rheumatology Subcommittee on Rheumatoid Arthritis. (2002). Guidelines for the management of rheumatoid arthritis: 2002 update. *Arthritis and Rheumatism, 46*, 328–346.

Amputee Coalition of America. (2000). *First step: A guide for adapting to limb loss.* Knoxville, TN: National Limb Loss Information Center.

Blank-Reid, C. (2003). Traumatic amputations: Unkind cuts. *Nursing, 33*(7), 48–51.

Boisset, M., & Fitzcharles, M. A. (1994). Alternative medicine use by rheumatology patients in a universal health care setting. *Rheumatology, 21*, 148.

Boskey, A. L. (2001). Musculoskeletal disorders and orthopedic conditions. *Journal of the American Medical Association, 285*(5), 619–623.

Brown, R. E., & Wu, T. Y. (2003). Use of "spare parts" in mutilated upper extremity injuries. *Hand Clinics, 19*(1), 73–87.

Bussell, M. H. (Ed.). (2000). *New developments in prosthetics and orthotics.* Philadelphia: W.B. Saunders.

Calhoun, J. H., Laughlin, R. T., Mader, J. T., & Maher, L. (1998). Osteomyelitis: Diagnosis, staging, management. *Patient Care, 32*(2), 93–94, 99–102, 105–106, 109.

Chen, C. E., Ko, J. Y., Fu, T. H., & Wang, C. J. (2004). Results of chronic osteomyelitis of the femur treated with hyperbaric oxygen: A preliminary report. *Chang Gung Medical Journal, 27*(2), 91–97.

Clauw, D. J. (2000). Treating fibromyalgia: Science vs. art. *American Family Physician, 62*(7), 1492–1495.

Cornell, T. (2004). Ankylosing spondylitis: An overview. *Professional Nurse, 19*(8), 431–432.

Cush, J. J., & Lipsky, P. E. (2000). The spondyloarthropathies. In L. Goldman & J. C. Bennett (Eds.), *Cecil textbook of medicine* (pp. 1499–1507). Philadelphia: W.B. Saunders.

Daigeler, A., Fansa, H., & Schneider, W. (2003). Orthotopic and heterotopic lower leg reimplantation: Evaluation of seven patients. *Journal of Bone and Joint Surgery (Br), 85*(4), 554–558.

Deyo, R. A. (1998, August). Low-back pain. *Scientific American, 279*(2), 49–53.

Deyo, R. A., Nachemson, A., & Mirza, S. K. (2004). Spinal-fusion surgery: The case for restraint. *New England Journal of Medicine, 350*(7), 722–726.

Deyo, R. A., & Weinstein, J. N. (2001). Low back pain. *New England Journal of Medicine, 344*(5), 363–370.

Foley, K. M. (2003). Opioids and chronic neuropathic pain. *New England Journal of Medicine, 348*(13), 1279–1281.

Gallagher, P., & MacLachlan, M. (1999). Psychological adjustment and coping in adults with prosthetic limbs. *Behavioral Medicine, 25*(3), 117–124.

Giffords, E. D. (2003). Understanding and managing systemic lupus erythematosus (SLE). *Social Work and Health Care, 37*(4), 57–72.

Glajchen, M. (2001). Chronic pain: Treatment barriers and strategies for clinical practice. *Journal of the American Board of Family Practice, 14*(3), 211–218.

Harpham, W. S. (2001). Alternative therapies for curing cancer: What do patients want? What do patients need? *A Cancer Journal for Clinicians, 51*, 131–136.

Hawker, G. A., Wright, J. G., Coyte, P. C., Williams, J. I., Harvey, B., Glazier, R., & Badley, E. M. (2000). Differences between men and women in the rate of use of hip and knee arthroplasty. *New England Journal of Medicine, 342*(14), 1016–1022.

Johnson, L. S., Archer-Heese, G., Caron-Powles, D. L., & Dowson, T. M. (2001). Work hardening: Outdated fad or effective intervention? *Work, 16*(3), 235–243.

Kolasinski, S. L. (2001, April 15). Complementary and alternative therapies for rheumatic disease. *Hospital Practice*, pp. 31–39.

Kooijman, C. M., Dijkstra, P. U., Geertzen, A. E., Elzinga, A., & van der Schans, C. P. (2000). Phantom pain and phantom sensations in upper limb amputees: An epidemiological study. *Pain, 87*, 33–41.

Kranke, P., Bennett, M., Roeckl-Wiedmann, I., & Debus, S. (2004). Hyperbaric oxygen therapy for chronic wounds. Cochrane Database System Review, 2004(2): CD004123.

Kvien, T. K. (2004). Epidemiology and burden of illness of rheumatoid arthritis. *Pharmacoeconomics, 22*(Suppl. 2), 1–12.

Marcus, R. (2000). Musculoskeletal health and the older adult. *Journal of Rehabilitation Research and Development, 37*(2), 245–254.

Meunier, P. J., Roux, C., Seeman, E., Ortolani, S., Badurski, J. E., Spector, T. D., Cannata, J., Balogh, A., Lemmel, E. M., Pors-Nielsen, S., Rizzoli, R., Genant, H. K., & Reginster, J. Y. (2004). The effects of strontium ranelate on the risk of vertebral fracture in women with postmenopausal osteoporosis. *New England Journal of Medicine, 350*(5), 459–468.

Meyer, T. M. (2003). Psychological aspects of mutilating hand injuries. *Hand Clinics, 19*(1), 41–49.

Mikuls, T. R., & O'Dell, J. (2000). The changing face of rheumatoid arthritis therapy: Results of serial surveys. *Arthritis and Rheumatism, 43*, 464–465.

Millea, P. J., & Holloway, R. L. (2000). Treating fibromyalgia. *American Family Physician, 62*(7), 1575–1582.

Moreland, L. W., & O'Dell, J. R. (2002). Glucocorticoids and rheumatoid arthritis: Back to the future. *Arthritis and Rheumatism, 46*, 2553–2563.

O'Dell, J. R. (2004). Therapeutic strategies for rheumatoid arthritis. *New England Journal of Medicine, 350*(25), 2591–2599.

Olsen, N. J., & Stein, C. M. (2004). New drugs for rheumatoid arthritis. *New England Journal of Medicine, 350*(21), 2167–2179.

Pelletier, K. R., Astin, J. A., & Haskell, W. L. (1999). Current trends in the integration and reimbursement of complementary and alternative medicine by managed care organizations (MCOs) and insurance providers: 1998 update and cohort analysis. *American Journal of Health Promotion, 14*(2), 125–133.

Portenoy, R. K. (1994). Opioid therapy for nonmalignant pain: Current status. In Fields, H. L., & Liebeskind, J. C. (Eds.), *Progress in pain research and management: Vol. 1. Pharmacological approaches to the treatment of chronic pain; new concepts and critical issues: The Bristol-Meyers Squibb Symposium on Pain Research* (pp. 247–287). Seattle: IASP Press.

Prestwood, K. M., & Raisz, L. G. (2002). Prevention and treatment of osteoporosis. *Clinical Cornerstone, 4*(6), 31–41.

Proehl, J. A. (2004). Accidental amputation. *American Journal of Nursing, 104*(2), 50–53.

Rahman, A., Ambler, G., Underwood, M. R., & Shipley, M. E. (2004). Important determinants of self-efficacy in patients with chronic musculoskeletal pain. *Journal of Rheumatology, 31*(6), 1187–1192.

Rajan, M., & Kerr, H. (2000). Rheumatology. *British Medical Journal, 321*(7265), 882–886.

Rakel, D., & Shapiro, D. (2002). Mind-body medicine. In Rakel, R. (Ed.) *Textbook of Family Practice* (6th ed.) (pp. 52–64). Philadelphia: W. B. Saunders Company.

Resch, K. L., Hill, S., & Ernst, E. (1997). Use of complementary therapies by individuals with "arthritis." *Clinical Rheumatology, 16*, 391.

Ritz, E., & Mann, J. F. E. (2000). Disparities in the use of total joint arthroplasty. *New England Journal of Medicine, 342*(14), 1043–1045.

Ruiz-Irastorza, G., Khamashta, M. A., Castellino, G., & Hughes, G. R. (1999). Systemic lupus erythematosus. *Lancet, 357*, 1027–1032.

Schlesinger, N., & Schumacher, H. R., Jr. (2001). Gout: Can management be improved? *Current Opinions in Rheumatology, 13*, 240–244.

Schonstein, E., Kenny, D. T, Keating, J., & Koes, B. W. (2003). Work conditioning, work hardening and functional restoration for workers with back and neck pain. *Cochrane Database System Review*, CD001822.

Schrager, S. (2004). Osteoporosis in women with disabilities. *Journal of Women's Health, 13*(4), 431–437.

Sequeira, W. (1999). Yoga in treatment of carpal-tunnel syndrome. *Lancet, 353*(9154), 689.

Smith, S. M., Kress, T. A. H., & William, M. (2000). Hand/wrist disorders among sign language communicators. *American Annals of the Deaf, 145*(1), 22–25.

Sohng, K. Y. (2003). Effects of self-management course for patients with systemic lupus erythematosus. *Journal of Advanced Nursing, 42*(5), 479–486.

Solomon, D. H., Finkelstein, J. S., Katz, J. N., Mogun, H., & Avorn, J. (2003). Underuse of osteoporosis medications in elderly patients with fractures. *American Journal of Medicine, 11*(5), 398–400.

Sugihara, A., Watanabe, H., Oohashi, M., Kato, N., Murakami, H., Tsukazaki, S., & Fujikawa, K. (2004). The effect of hyperbaric oxygen therapy on the bout of treatment for soft tissue infections. *Journal of Infection, 48*(4), 330–333.

Swinkels, A., & Dolan, P. (2004). Spinal position sense and disease progression in ankylosing spondylitis: A longitudinal study. *Spine, 29*(11), 1240–1245.

Terkeltaub, R. A. (2003). Gout. *New England Journal of Medicine, 349*(17), 1647–1655.

Trethewey, P. (2004). Systemic lupus erythematosus. *Dimensions of Critical Care Nursing, 23*(3), 111–115.

Turner, J. A., Franklin, G., Fulton-Kehoe, D., Egan, K., Wickizer, T. M., Lymp, J. F., Sheppard, L., & Kaufman, J. D. (2004). Prediction of chronic disability in work-related musculoskeletal disorders: A prospective, population-based study. *BMC Musculoskeletal Disorders, 5*(1), 14.

Vecchio, P. C. (1994). Attitudes to alternative medicine by rheumatology outpatient attenders. *Journal of Rheumatology, 21*, 145.

Walsh, J. D., Blanchard, E. B., Kremer, J. M., & Blanchard, C. G. (1999). The psychosocial effects of rheumatoid arthritis on the patient and the well partner. *Behaviour Research and Therapy, 37*, 259–271.

Weir, R., & Nielson, W. R. (2001). Interventions for disability management. *Clinical Journal of Pain, 17*(Suppl. 4), S128–S132.

Wiberg, M., Hazari, A., Ljungberg, C., Pettrsson, K., Backman, C., Nordh, E., Kwast-Rabben, O., & Terenghi, G. (2003). Sensory recovery after hand reimplantation: A clinical, morphological, and neurophysiological study in humans. *Scandinavian Journal of Plastic and Reconstructive Surgery and Hand Surgery, 37*(3), 163–173.

Wilhelmi, B. J., Lee, W. P., Pagensteert, G. I., & May, J. W., Jr. (2003). Replantation in the mutilated hand. *Hand Clinics, 19*(1), 89–120.

Wilson, B. A., Jr. (1998). *A primer on limb prosthetics.* Springfield, IL: C.C. Thomas.

Wortmann, R. I. (2002). Gout and hyperuricemia. *Current Opinions in Rheumatology, 14*, 281–286.

Yildiz, S., Kiralp, M. Z., Akin, A., Keskin, I., Ay, H., Dursun, H., & Cimsit, M. (2004). A new treatment modality for fibromyalgia syndrome: Hyperbaric oxygen therapy. *Journal of Internal Medicine Residents, 32*(3), 263–267.

# CHAPTER 15

# Skin Conditions and Burns

## NORMAL STRUCTURE AND FUNCTION OF THE SKIN

The skin is the largest organ of the body. It has a number of functions:

- Protection of the body's inner structures from microorganisms, drying, and trauma
- Regulation of body temperature through evaporation of perspiration for cooling and constriction of superficial blood vessels to conserve heat
- Excretion of water and electrolytes through perspiration
- Sensory perception of touch, pressure, and pain

The skin consists of two layers, the *epidermis* and the *dermis* (see Figure 15–1). The outer layer of the skin (**epidermis**) protects the deeper tissues from drying, from invasion by organisms, and from trauma. The epidermis has several layers. The deepest layer of the epidermis constantly produces new cells, which are pushed to the surface of the skin; there they die, are shed, and are replaced by new cells. Cells called *melanocytes* contain the skin pigment **melanin**, which is responsible for skin color. Dark-skinned people have more melanin than do light-skinned people.

The inner layer of skin (**dermis**) lies beneath the epidermis. It contains blood vessels, nerves, lymphatics, hair follicles, and sebaceous and sweat glands, as well as various types of cells that promote wound healing. The dermis also contains major sensory fibers responsible for distinguishing pain, touch, heat, and cold.

With the exception of the palms of the hands and the soles of the feet, hair follicles are located in the dermis throughout the body, although they are more numerous is some areas, such as the scalp, axillae, and pubic area. Hairs are continually falling out and being replaced by new ones. When this process is excessive, thinning or baldness results.

*Sebaceous glands*, contained within the dermis and surrounding hair follicles, produce an oily substance called *sebum* that protects the skin from excessive dryness. *Sweat glands*, also located in the dermis, are present all over the body but are concentrated in the axillae, forehead, palms of the hands, and soles of the feet. They produce perspiration, which aids in temperature regulation of the body as well as excretion of water and electrolytes. When the environment is warm, evaporation of perspiration cools the body. When the environment is cool, constriction of superficial blood vessels conserves body warmth.

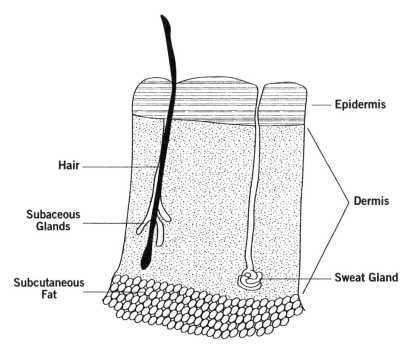

**Figure 15–1** Section of Normal Skin.

Interfacing with the dermis at its lower level is a **subcutaneous** (under the skin) layer of fat, or *adipose tissue*. This subcutaneous fat not only provides insulation for the body, but it also gives shape and contour over bone.

## PSYCHOLOGICAL, SOCIAL, AND VOCATIONAL IMPACT OF SKIN CONDITIONS

The skin is readily visible, and its condition determines to a great extent how individuals appear to the world. Therefore, skin conditions, although not generally life-threatening, can have an impact on quality of life, restricting work, social, family, leisure, and sexual activities (Lamberg, 1997; Morgan, McCreedy, Simpson, & Hay, 1997). Healthy skin is correlated with self-esteem and self-image. A skin disorder that may seem trivial to others can have a major psychological impact on the individual who experiences it. Society places great emphasis on appearance, and appearance often helps to determine how individuals interact with society. Not only does society place great value on clear, healthy skin, but skin disorders are sometimes perceived as being associated with uncleanliness or contagion.

Even though few skin conditions are actually contagious, people may avoid contact with individuals with skin conditions because of fear that they are contagious. Disfiguring skin conditions have a negative effect not only on individuals' self-image but also on interpersonal relationships, often leading to stigmatization by society. Individuals with obvious skin disease or scarring due to burns or trauma may experience stares, expressions of revulsion, or avoidance by others so that they become social outcasts. As a result, they may experience significant secondary psychological symptoms, including depression, social phobia, or paranoia. The psychological implications of skin conditions may extend to all domains of individuals' lives, including the workplace.

## SKIN CONDITIONS

Because the skin is in constant contact with the environment, it is vulnerable to injury and irritation. It is also vulnerable to changes in the internal body environment, and it may reflect systemic conditions, such as *lupus erythematosus* (see Chapter 14). Emotional factors can also precipitate or contribute to disorders of the skin. Skin disorders may be localized or may involve the entire body. They may cause mild discomfort or severe pain and disfigurement.

### Dermatitis

The general term **dermatitis** describes a superficial inflammation of the skin. *Atopic dermatitis*, also called *eczema*, is a type of dermatitis characterized by redness (**erythema**), swelling (**edema**), and itching (**pruritus**). It is more common in childhood, but it can be a lifelong condition. Depending on its location, it can affect appearance, especially if on the face. Constant scratching of the skin can cause tenderness and bleeding. If the skin's protective outer layers crack, individuals are also at risk for infection.

Treatment of atopic dermatitis includes avoiding prolonged contact with hot water (i.e., taking lukewarm showers rather than long, hot baths), avoiding drying soaps, and using moisturizers on the skin. Medications such as antihistamines or steroid creams and ointments may be used to control itching; however, lengthy use of steroid medications is contraindicated because of their potential side effects. New medications called topical im-

munomodulators are also now used. In severe cases, phototherapy (light therapy) or photochemotherapy (combination of ultraviolet light and special medication) may be used.

*Contact dermatitis* is a localized skin inflammation that results from contact with a specific substance. The symptoms occur at the site of contact. The substance may produce a localized allergic response (*allergic contact dermatitis*) as a result of a previous exposure, or the substance may be a primary irritant that causes a nonallergic skin reaction (*irritant contact dermatitis*) following exposure. Common causes of localized allergic contact dermatitis are chemicals, dyes, cosmetics, and industrial agents. Alkalis, acids, metals, salts, solvents, and various dusts can cause irritant dermatitis. Usually, only the skin that comes into contact with the substance is involved, so the area of skin affected is rather clearly demarcated. Symptoms generally disappear when contact with the offending agent is avoided. In addition to localized allergic reactions, individuals can experience generalized allergic reactions, as described below.

### Allergic Reactions

An allergy is a hypersensitivity to a specific substance or substances. Some individuals experience allergic reactions after exposure to certain substances that cause an immune response within the body. Their sensitization to the substance may take days or weeks, but, once the response has been established, the next contact with the substance produces allergic symptoms.

Allergic responses may be external or systemic. External allergic reactions consist of symptoms such as hives (**urticaria**), redness, swelling, itching, or rash. Systemic allergic responses, usually caused by allergic reactions to medication or certain foods, may include skin manifestations in addition to generalized body symptoms, some of which can seriously compromise respiratory function. The treatment of allergy is usually directed toward avoiding contact with the offending agent, reducing sensitivity to the substance if contact cannot be avoided, or reducing or eliminating the symptoms associated with the allergic response.

## Psoriasis

Psoriasis is a chronic, inflammatory disease in which there is greatly accelerated epidermal cell turnover. As a result of the rapid formation of these cells, individuals develop noticeable skin lesions. There are different variations of psoriasis. It is categorized as localized or generalized depending on the severity of the condition and its overall impact on the individual's quality of life and well-being (Pardasani, Feldman, & Clark, 2000). *Plaque psoriasis* is characterized by plaques of **erythema** (redness), covered with silvery scales, which tend to shed. Patches or plaques may occur on localized areas, such as the elbows and knees, lower back, and the scalp, or they can cover the entire body. In some instances, individuals develop *pustular psoriasis*, in which small pustules are spread over the body; these can sometimes lead to systemic infection. Some individuals with psoriasis develop *psoriatic arthritis*, which causes aching and disfigurement of joints.

Although the primary cause of psoriasis remains unknown, it is considered an immune-mediated disorder (Pardasani et al., 2000). Psoriasis may be triggered by a combination of genetic, systemic, or environmental factors. There are periods of **remission** (when symptoms become better) and periods of **exacerbation** (when symptoms become worse) of varying frequency and duration. The course of the psoriasis is often unpredictable and can improve or get worse for no obvious reason. Emotional stress and anxiety may aggravate the condition. Climate change or warm temperatures also tend to make the condition worse.

### Psychosocial Impact of Psoriasis

Psoriasis ranges from being cosmetically annoying to being physically disabling and disfiguring. It does not affect the individual's general health, but the psychological and social stigma associated with an obviously unsightly skin disease may cause frustration and despair. It can cause difficulty with work performance, problems with social rejection, sexual dysfunction, and depression. Itching may be mild or severe and can cause loss of sleep and general fatigue, which can contribute to irritability. The condition can be a burden on financial and time resources, interfere with work, and disrupt the individual's lifestyle. Although psoriasis is not infectious, it may be a source of stares, embarrassing questions or comments, or outright avoidance of the individual by others. The prognosis depends on the extent and the severity of the disease. In general, the earlier the disease begins, the more severe are the manifestations.

### Treatment of Psoriasis

There is no known cure for psoriasis, so treatment is directed toward controlling the condition. The goal of treatment is to suppress the immune-mediated response, which causes the symptoms. Any aggravating factors should be identified and removed if possible. Since injury to the skin can trigger flareups, trauma to the skin should be avoided as much as possible.

Treatment depends on the severity of the condition. Psoriasis can be treated with topical agents, or, if symptoms do not respond to topical treatment, it may be treated with a systemic agent. If the condition is limited, most **dermatologists** (physicians who specialize in diagnosis and treatment of conditions of the skin) initially treat psoriasis with a *topical steroid*. There are seven potency levels of topical steroids. The strength prescribed depends on the area to be treated and the thickness of the plaques. For example, a weaker strength of steroid would be applied to the face. Topical steroids are applied one to three times a day with an aim to decrease immune activity locally. Emollients are often used in combination with topical steroids to increase their efficacy. Although they are relatively safe and have few, rare systemic side effects, topical steroids cannot be used indefinitely. If applications are applied too frequently or if too strong an agent is used, **atrophy** (shrinkage) or thinning of the skin can occur. Long-term use of steroids can lead to a phenomenon called **tachyphylaxis**, a condition in which the body becomes immune to the effects of the medication because of repeated use.

Topical steroids can also be used in combination with other agents, such as vitamin D analogs or topical retinoids. Combination therapy allows lower doses of individual agents to be used, helping to minimize side effects and maximize efficacy.

Older, but still effective topical treatments include the use of coal tar preparations or *anthralin*, a cream most often used to treat scalp psoriasis. Coal tar can be formulated into shampoos, gels, or solutions for soaking. Although the mechanism of action is not clear, coal tar seems to reduce inflammation. Coal tar preparations are inexpensive but can be messy to use, staining both skin and clothing. Anthralin can also stain skin, clothing, and bedding. Because of some reports that link coal tar to cancer, some countries and states prohibit its sale.

Individuals with moderate to severe psoriasis may have any of the above treatments used in conjunction with *phototherapy*, which can lead to remission. Both ultraviolet B and ultraviolet A are used. In phototherapy, individuals come to the physicians' office and spend several minutes in a light booth, where they receive a regulated dose of ultraviolet light. The light decreases the activity of the immune system. Ultraviolet B therapy can be either broadband or, more recently, narrow band. The dose of light is based on individuals' skin type and the minimal dose that produces redness (**erythema**). When combined with other topical or systemic medications, care must be taken not to increase individuals' **photosensitivity** (sensitivity to light), which could result in burns.

Some individuals do not respond to phototherapy, or they may be unable to receive it because of the traveling distance between the treatment facility and their home, or because of their work schedule. In these instances, systemic medications may be used instead. Medications such as methotrexate, aceitretin, or cyclosporine may be used to treat moderate to severe psoriasis. Although all three are effective, they have side effects that require frequent blood monitoring (Lebwohl, 2000), including liver damage, renal damage, increased blood lipids, and bone marrow suppression. Other side effects include hypertension and dryness of the skin and mucous membranes. In addition, the medications can be **teratogenic** (causing fetal abnormalities) and so should not be used when there is a chance of pregnancy.

The newest treatment options for psoriasis are *biological drugs*. This class of medication consists of substances derived from living material that are injected or given intravenously. They act at the cellular level and affect various targets in the immune system that are involved in the pathophysiology of psoriasis. These medications have been shown to have equal or better efficacy than older systemic treatments of psoriasis, and they appear to have few side effects. A major limitation to their use is, however, expense, since they cost up to $1,000 per month.

### Infections of the Skin

A number of organisms, including bacteria, fungi, parasites, and viruses, may infect the skin. Infection may be the primary cause of a skin disorder, or it may be a secondary condition associated with another skin disorder. The degree and length of disability associated with infections of the skin depend on the type and severity of the infection. Effective treatment requires that one accurately identify the causative organisms and institute treatment that is appropriate to those particular organisms.

### Acne

Acne is the most commonly encountered skin condition. It results from interaction between bacteria in the skin, excess oil production, and hormones. The face, neck, and trunk of body are most frequently affected. Although acne is most common in adolescence, some individuals, especially women, have acne that continues into young adulthood. Acne in itself is not frequently thought of as a disabling condition; however, it can have a devastating effect on the individual's self-image and self-esteem. The goal of treatment is to prevent the clogging of hair follicles, reduce inflammation, cut down

on infection, and minimize scarring. Treatment usually consists of topical application of medication and, occasionally, systemic medication in severe or prolonged cases. In some instances individuals with severe scarring from acne may choose to have cosmetic procedures such as resurfacing or **dermabrasion** (a procedure in which scars, wrinkles, or other skin blemishes are worn away) to diminish the scarring once their acne is no longer active.

### Herpes Zoster (Shingles)

*Herpes zoster*, or *shingles*, is a reactivation of the virus that caused chickenpox in individuals at a younger age. After the individual has had chickenpox, the virus lies dormant in the nervous system. When an individual's immune system becomes weakened because of aging or because of medical conditions such as organ transplantation, cancer, or HIV infections, the virus can become reactivated. **Vesicles** (fluid-filled blisters) erupt along a peripheral sensory nerve route. The blisters, which form a band along the nerve, are usually located on the trunk of the body, causing pain, itching, burning, and tenderness along the nerve route. Although vesicles usually appear on the trunk of the body, they may also affect the face and eye. Pain in the affected area may be severe. The condition may last up to a month. Since the reactivated virus is contagious, individuals who have never had chickenpox or who have never been immunized against chickenpox should avoid contact with individuals with herpes zoster.

#### Treatment of Herpes Zoster

The goal of treatment is to relieve pain, reduce potential complications, and shorten the duration of the outbreak. Antiviral medication, administered either orally or intravenously, is often required. Steroids or anti-inflammatory medication may also be used. The pain accompanying herpes zoster is often treated with analgesics.

Herpes zoster usually has no residual effects; however, complications of the condition can include prolonged pain at the site of the skin lesion even after lesions have subsided. Complications can also include scarring, which may be quite disfiguring if the scars involve the facial area. If the eye is affected, another complication may consist of ulceration, which could result in blindness.

### Skin Cancers

Cancer of the skin occurs more frequently than does cancer of any other organ. Because *basal cell carcinoma* is directly visible, it can be diagnosed earlier and, therefore, has a high cure rate. *Malignant melanoma*, a cancer originating in the **melanocytes** (cells containing skin pigment), is a more dangerous and potentially fatal type of skin cancer because it spreads rapidly into deeper skin layers and metastasizes to other body organs (see Chapter 16). Because of the seriousness of the condition, surgical removal of the melanoma itself, as well as large portions of surrounding tissue, may be necessary to eradicate the cancer; this can cause significant deformity, depending on the location.

### GENERAL DIAGNOSTIC PROCEDURES FOR CONDITIONS OF THE SKIN

#### Biopsy

**Biopsy** consists of removing a specific tissue specimen for microscopic examination. Biopsies are performed to diagnose a variety of conditions, including skin cancer and many other types of skin lesions. It is a relatively simple procedure that can be performed on an outpatient basis.

### Scrapings, Cultures, and Smears

Scales of a skin lesion may be gently *scraped* from the surface of the skin and examined under a microscope. If there is an **exudate** (fluid or matter from tissue), a sample is removed with a swab and implanted in a *culture medium*, where it is later examined for growth of organisms. In other instances, the exudate is placed on a slide and examined immediately under the microscope; this procedure is known as a *smear*.

### Patch Tests

In order to identify the substances that are responsible for allergic reactions, *patch tests* may be performed. Small amounts of various substances that are suspected of causing the reaction are applied to the skin, and the area is later examined for possible reactions.

### GENERAL TREATMENT OF CONDITIONS OF THE SKIN

#### Medications

Many skin disorders are treated with topical medications that are applied directly to the skin surface (*topical application*) in the form of lotions, creams, ointments, or powders. The type of medication chosen is dependent on the cause of the skin disorder. For example, *antifungals* are used for fungal infections, *antibiotics* or *antibacterials* for bacterial infections, and *antivirals* for viral infections. Topical *antipruritics* may be applied to reduce the discomfort due to itching. Topical *corticosteroids* are sometimes prescribed to reduce local inflammatory responses.

Because topical medications can have side effects, prolonged use or overuse of medications such as corticosteroids should be avoided. Some skin conditions may be treated with *systemic medication* (medications that are injected or taken orally to be carried throughout the body), such as antibiotics and corticosteroids. Although corticosteroids can produce dramatic improvement, they also have serious potential side effects. Consequently, the use of corticosteroids requires careful monitoring by a physician.

### Dressings and Therapeutic Baths or Soaks

Treatment of skin conditions in which there is excessive skin scaling or in which crusts have formed over lesions may include wet soaks or therapeutic baths to reduce the drying effects of air, relieve discomfort, or enhance the removal of scales and crusts so that healing may take place. In some instances, dressings are applied to skin lesions to protect the skin from injury and infection from the environment.

### Light Treatment (Phototherapy)

Artificial light sources may be used for localized or generalized treatments of various skin conditions. Light therapies are frequently accompanied by therapeutic baths or soaks, or they may be used in combination with topical medication.

### Dermabrasion

Dermabrasion consists of buffing, or abrading, the top surface of the skin in order to reduce scarring.

### Chemical Face Peeling

This procedure produces a controlled chemical burn and destruction of the upper layer of the skin. It is generally done for cosmetic purposes to remove fine lines or blemishes, but it can also be helpful in the treatment of acne and precancerous growths. Individuals with chemical face peeling should avoid the sun and be aware that the skin will not tan evenly.

### Plastic and Reconstructive Surgery

*Plastic* and *reconstructive surgery* is a branch of surgery involving the correction of deformity, the restoration of function of parts of the body, or the enhancement of physical appearance. It plays an important part in rehabilitation, not only to enhance healing and establish or reestablish function, but also to enhance individuals' self-image and minimize limitations.

Although plastic surgery is important to conditions of the skin, plastic surgeons do not limit surgery to only one body part, but rather use concepts and techniques of plastic surgery on many parts of the body. For example, it may be used to minimize or correct congenital anomalies such as cleft lip or cleft palate. It may be used to restore function lost due to **contractures** (tightening or shortening of tissue around a joint that limits range of motion). It may be used to correct deformity and restore function after hand injury or to promote healing and correct deformity caused from complications such as **decubitus ulcers** (also known as pressure sores, caused by immobility and lack of blood supply to tissue so that tissue death occurs). Plastic and reconstructive surgery may also be used to correct deformities secondary to a variety of medical conditions or their treatment, such as cancer, in which a large portion of tissue has been removed.

Plastic and reconstructive surgery can help to restore function and minimize disfigurement, thus helping individuals adjust to their condition and reenter the workplace and the community. The extent to which reentry is possible varies from individual to individual and depends on the part of the body affected and the extent of the remaining limitations, as well as on individuals' own psychological characteristics.

## BURNS

The most traumatic of all skin injuries is that caused by burns (Balasubramani, Kumar, & Babu, 2001). Any tissue injury resulting from direct heat, chemicals, radiation, or electrical current is a burn. The treatment and prognosis of individuals with burns are dependent on the cause or type of burn, the depth of burn, and the amount of body surface that has been burned.

### Types of Burn Injury

#### Thermal

The most common burns, **thermal burns**, are caused by fire, hot liquids, or direct contact with a hot surface. In addition to causing direct injury to the skin, thermal burns can cause severe damage to underlying structures if the heat has been intensive or if the exposure has been prolonged.

#### Chemical

Chemical burns result from direct contact with strong acids (e.g., sulfuric acid) or alkaline agents (e.g., lye), gases (e.g., mustard gas), or other chemicals, such as sulfuric acid, that cause tissue death. The extent of injury from chemical burns depends on the duration of the contact, the concentration or strength of the chemical, and the amount of tissue exposed to the chemical source. Some chemicals cause burns directly through the production of physiologic changes in the tissue with which they come into contact, whereas other chemicals cause burns indirectly through the heat produced by their chemical reaction with the skin.

#### Radiation

The degree of damage caused by a radiation burn depends on the dose of radiation received. Sources of radiation burns may include *ultraviolet radiation*, such as the sun, as well as *ionizing radiation*, such as nuclear materials and X-rays. Localized skin reactions to low doses of radiation may cause discomfort but usually heal spontaneously. Larger doses of local radiation may damage underlying tissues and organs, however, requiring more extensive treatment.

#### Electrical

Electrical burns result from direct contact with *electrical current* or *lightning*.

Injuries from electrical burns range from local tissue damage to sudden death because of cardiac arrest. The effects of electricity on tissue depend on the current, the voltage, the type of current (e.g., direct or alternating), and the duration of contact. Because the entry point of the electric current may be relatively small, electrical burns may appear to have caused little external damage. However, usually extensive internal damage results because as the current travels through the body tissues it damages nerves, blood vessels, and other major organs. The electrical current may also interfere with the electrical activity of the heart, causing the heart to stop (*cardiac arrest*). Electrical burns are generally *full-thickness* burns and are associated with severe postburn disabilities that may include multiple amputations because of damage to blood vessels, nerves, bones, or muscles. If clothing of the individual caught on fire as a result of exposure to the electricity source, thermal burns may also be present. Individuals may also experience secondary injuries such as *fractures*, *dislocations*, or *spinal cord injury* because of falls associated with the injury. They may also have some sensorineural hearing loss, which generally improves over time.

*Lightning injuries* may be classified as mild, moderate, or severe. Being struck by lightning can, of course, be fatal; however, a number of people survive. In mild cases, individuals may appear dazed and confused, having only mild physical injury. In more severe cases, individuals may experience sensory organ damage, such as rupture of the *tympanic membrane* in the ear or *cataract formation* in the eye, which may not show up for weeks or months after the incident. If cardiac arrest occurred and the individual experienced **hypoxia** (decreased oxygen) before resuscitation could occur, he or she may have brain damage or develop a seizure disorder. People who survive lightning injury may also have residual effects of insomnia or other sleep disturbances, anxiety, or reduced fine intellectual function.

### Inhalation

Inhalation injury to the respiratory tract is caused by inhalation of steam, toxic gases, or vapors. Individuals with inhalation injury experience cough, increasing hoarseness, shortness of breath, anxiety, and wheezing. Inhalation of noxious gases alone may lead to brain injury or death. Direct injury to the respiratory tract may also cause swelling, compromising the patency of the airways. Treatment usually involves administrating 100 percent oxygen and maintaining open airways (Nelson & Thompson, 1998).

### Burn Depth

The degree of tissue damage caused by a burn varies with the source of the burn, but several other factors also affect burn severity. One such factor is the burn depth. Burn depth depends on the temperature of the burning agent and the length of exposure. Burn injuries may consist of only one burn depth, or there may be a combination of different burn depths. Burn depth is typically divided into four categories.

- *Superficial* (first-degree) burn: a burn that affects only the *epidermis* (outer layer of the skin). The skin becomes reddened and painful, but no underlying structures are damaged.
- *Partial-thickness* (second-degree) burn: a burn that affects both the *epidermis* and the *dermis*. The skin is reddened and blisters erupt, providing a portal of entry for organisms that can cause infection at the burn site. In addition, second-degree burns are very painful because of the stimulation of sensitive nerve endings in this layer of the skin.
- *Full-thickness* (third-degree) burn: a burn that destroys the dermis and epidermis, as well as skin appendages, such as hair follicles, sebaceous glands, and sweat glands. There is little pain, because nerve endings have been destroyed. Full-thickness burns cannot heal spontaneously and are more susceptible to infection.
- *Fourth-degree burn:* a burn that extends to the underlying subcutaneous fat, muscle, or bone.

In addition to the source of the burn and the burn depth, the percentage of body surface affected determines the severity of the burn. A common method of calculating the amount of body surface injured is the *Rule of Nines*, by which the body is graphically divided into areas that represent different percentages of the total body surface (see Figure 15–2). A more accurate method of estimating the total body surface burn is the *Lund and Browder method*. Since body proportions are different in children and adults, this method calculates the surface area of different body parts according to age. The chart lists various body sections and the percentage of body surface each section represents from 1 year of age to adult. Each burned area is thus given percentage points based on the age of the individual. Points are then added to estimate the total area of the body surface burned.

## Burn Severity

The location of the burn also affects burn severity. For example, those with burns to the upper body, especially the head and neck, may be prone to respiratory complications because of possible smoke inhalation, heat damage to the respiratory structures, exposure to the toxic byproducts of combustion of material such as the synthetic material used in home furnishings, or restriction of air passages due to swelling caused by the injury. For electrical burns, the points of contact and the pathway that the current followed through the body are important considerations in determining the severity of tissue damage. Individuals' age and medical history are also important considerations. Individuals who are very young or very old are most vulnerable to the effects and complications of burns. Pre-

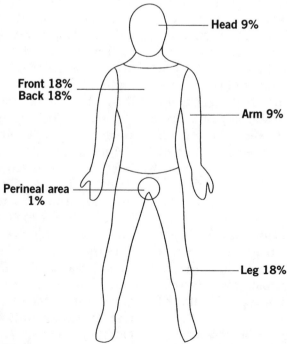

**Figure 15–2** Rule of Nines.

existing debilitating systemic conditions, such as heart disease, diabetes, lung disease, or chronic abuse of drugs or alcohol, can further complicate recovery and severely affect recovery and prognosis.

Individuals experience a systemic response after major burns. Severe burns disrupt the body's internal balance. Because of tissue injury, plasma seeps from blood vessels into surrounding tissues, causing swelling and decreasing the amount of fluid in the general circulation. As a result, the body's general **homeostasis** (equilibrium) is lost, which can affect all body systems. A second danger affecting the prognosis for individuals with burns is infection, especially for those with *partial-thickness* or *full-thickness burns*. After burns have healed, individuals with burns may experience severe **pruritus** (itching) for a year or longer after the injury because of tissue regeneration.

Depending on the extent and location of the burn, individuals may experience a variety of disabilities. For example, burns involving the hand may result in contracture of the fingers, limiting joint motion. Severe burns of a leg may necessitate amputation. Burns around the head and face may involve loss of vision or loss of nose, ears, or hair. Other causes of disfigurement may be *hypertrophic scars*, large ropelike configurations of scar tissue that form on the skin surface. Scar development often becomes worse over time.

### Burn Treatment

The type of treatment used for burns depends on the severity of the injury and the treatment philosophy of the burn center treating the individual. Not all institutions engage in the same type of treatment protocols.

Burns may also be combined with other injuries if they were associated with a vehicle accident or explosion. Although individuals with minor burns and no complications may be treated at home, those with moderate or severe burns require hospitalization. Most individuals who have been moderately or severely burned are transferred to a hospital that has a specialized burn center. Burn centers are specially equipped to provide multifaceted care for individuals with moderate to severe burn injury. The staff are specialists in burn care and are trained to use a multidisciplinary approach. Professionals working in the burn unit may include *physicians, nurses, psychologists, psychiatrists, physical therapists, occupational therapists, dietitians,* and *rehabilitation counselors*. Although the amount of time individuals with burns spend in the hospital varies with the amount, degree, and location of the burn and their general condition prior to the burn injury, a general rule of thumb is one day of hospitalization for every percentage of body burned. During the acute phase, treatment of moderate or severe burns is directed toward stabilizing individuals' general condition, restoring fluid balance, and preventing complications. The major task for the individual during this phase is survival. The greater the surface area of the body burned and the greater the degree of the burn, the greater the risk of complications.

A major complication of burn injury is infection, which, unless controlled, can result in widespread infection throughout the body (**sepsis**). Therefore, during the acute phase, the **eschar** (charred, dead tissue) must be removed (**debrided**) to reduce the risk of infection and to promote wound healing. *Debridement* involves clipping away dead, charred tissue to prevent growth of bacteria under the burn's surface. Debridement is a very stressful and painful procedure that is often performed on a daily basis until all **necrotic** (dead) tissue has been removed. Individuals may be taken to surgery for surgical debridement of dead tissue; in the past, debridement was often performed while the individual was in a whirlpool bath.

Since individuals who have been severely burned are vulnerable to infection, precautions must be taken to prevent them from being exposed to harmful organisms. Most danger comes from organisms within the individual's own body; however, in some burn units individuals with severe burns are placed in a room with a special *air filtration system* that screens out harmful organisms.

In some burn units persons who provide care may also wear caps, gowns, gloves, and masks to protect individuals with burns from infection. Visitors may be restricted, or when allowed to visit, may also be asked to wear masks and gowns. As a result, individuals with burns may also experience an increased sense of social isolation. Because of the stress these restrictions impose and the growing evidence that the risk of infection from outside sources is minimal, some burn units now restrict the environment much less, so that caps and gowns are not worn by personnel or visitors and the time frame for visiting is more liberal.

The nutritional needs of individuals with severe burns are great. In the early postburn period, individuals may lose up to one pound or more per day. Thus, a high caloric intake is essential to meet the increased energy requirements during the postburn period. To supply extra calories, it may be necessary to administer special fluids intravenously, as well as to provide a high-calorie diet. In many instances individuals are given feedings through a tube that has been placed down the esophagus rather than through intravenous feedings, to diminish the chances of infection through the injection site.

Burn wounds are treated in different ways. At times, burns are treated with an exposure method in which no dressing or covering is applied to the wound. In these instances, more sterile conditions are essential to prevent infection. In other instances, the wound may not be covered, but topical medication, such as *silver sulfadiazine* to inhibit bacterial growth, may be applied. In some cases, burn wounds are covered with dressings that are changed daily. The method of treatment depends on the type and extent of the burn wound, as well as on the general philosophy of the burn unit in which individuals are being treated. Individuals with severe burns require daily hygiene to deter infection. Some burn centers use *"tubbing,"* which involves placing the individual in a whirlpool bath filled with a solution of water and a chemical that helps to fight infection. Other centers have the individual bathe daily with antimicrobial soap, just as they might at home. During bathing the burn area may also be scrubbed to remove dead cells. Both of these treatments are extremely painful.

Certain parts of the body require special care when burned. When hands, arms, legs, or the neck have been burned, special care is necessary to prevent the loss of function due to scarring or **contracture** (fixation of a joint in a position of nonfunction). In some cases, affected joints may be splinted in a position of function to prevent the formation of contractures. Facial burns not only can cause disfigurement, but also can damage the ears or eyes. Every effort must be made to prevent complications that could further interfere with function.

After the acute phase of treatment, *grafting procedures* usually begin. A **graft** is tissue that is transplanted to a part of the body to repair an injury or defect. At times, *biologic dressings* (also known as grafts as listed below) are used to cover a burn wound temporarily and prepare it for grafting. The types of biologic dressings include the following:

- **Xenograft** (heterograft): a graft taken from another species. Porcine (pig skin) grafts are often used for burn wounds.
- **Homograft** (allograft): a graft taken from the same species, but not the same person. Homografts may be taken from a living donor or from a cadaver skin bank. Another type of homograft is *amnion*, which consists of placental membrane.
- **Biosynthetic graft**: a graft that has been chemically manufactured. Synthetic skin substitutes are alternatives as temporary wound covering. The material is semitransparent and sterile. It adheres to the wound and prevents infection, and it can help in debridement. It is left in place for 3 to 4 weeks and gradually separates from the wound as new skin is formed.

It is often necessary to change biologic dressings every several days. Biologic dressings can decrease the amount of pain individuals experience by covering nerve endings. They also help to prevent infection until permanent grafting occurs, or until the wound heals. Most biologic dressings are changed every 2 to 5 days to prevent the body from rejecting the graft.

When the burn wound appears healthy, a skin graft is applied. An **autograft** is a section of the individual's own skin that has been removed from an uninvolved site. Depending on the size of the graft needed, the same donor site may be used repeatedly. A **split-thickness graft** is the epidermis and part of the dermis and consists of two types. The first type, a sheet graft, is a single layer. A **mesh graft** is a graft in which many little slits have been made to allow it to expand and cover a larger area. A **full-thickness graft**, which includes the epidermis and the dermis from the donor site, may be used for reconstruction. The graft area may be bandaged or not, depending again on the area involved as well as the philosophy of the burn unit. The grafted part of the body should be kept immobilized. If the graft is on an extremity, a splint may be applied to prevent movement, which could disrupt the graft. When lower extremities are involved, the legs may be kept elevated to reduce swelling and subsequent rupture of small blood vessels. Elastic hose may also be worn when the individual is up. If the individual's face has received a graft, strenuous exercise, which could disrupt the graft, should be avoided.

When larger quantities of tissue are needed, a *flap* may be used. A flap is a tissue in which one area remains attached to the donor site and consequently has its own blood supply. The free end of the flap is then placed over the injury, sutured into place, and allowed to heal. Because flaps maintain their own blood supply, they may produce better cosmetic results than grafts, which may not maintain natural skin color.

The healing burn area may be compressed with elastic dressings to prevent or decrease the formation of hypertrophic scars. Special elasticized garments, such as gloves, vests, face masks, or neck garments, are available to be worn continually over the body part for a year or more to prevent this type of scar formation (see Figure 15–3). The garments are customized to fit the specific body part involved.

Individuals may be required to wear compression garments for 1 to 2 years after the initial injury. The garments must be worn 23 hours per day. Because they are unattractive and are hot and uncomfortable, individuals may have a difficult time emotionally adjusting to this phase of treatment. If contractures have occurred as a result of the burn, physical therapy may be necessary to return mobility to a joint. When the measures are unsuccessful or if the contracture is severe, surgical intervention may be necessary.

Many individuals with severe burns require reconstructive or plastic surgery after the wound has healed, especially if there has been severe deformity or disfigurement. Such surgical interventions may be performed to reconstruct a body part, such as the nose or the ear, or to remove hypertrophic scar tissue. Surgery may be performed for cosmetic purposes, to restore or improve function, or both. Many of these procedures take place over a number of years after the initial burn injury. Corrective cosmetics (camouflage therapy) can also be used for skin discoloration or to minimize scars or suture lines. Correc-

tive cosmetics differ from standard make-up in that they provide heavier coverage and adhere better to the skin (LeRoy, 2000). If individuals with severe burns experience major hair loss, wigs or toupees may also be worn.

## Psychosocial Issues in Burn Injury

Burn injury is often devastating, with long-term physical and psychosocial effects. It threatens the integrity of both the physical and psychological identity of the affected individual (McQuaid, Barton, & Campbell, 2000). Burn scars are cosmetically disfiguring and force individuals to deal with alterations in body appearance. In addition to the traumatic nature of the burn accident, individuals also undergo painful treatment, which may induce additional emotional and psychological responses. Responses to burn injury vary;

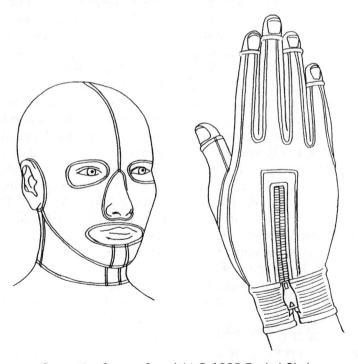

**Figure 15–3**  Pressure Garments. *Source:* Copyright © 1999 Rachel Clarke.

the individual's premorbid personality traits, the characteristics of the burn injury, and the psychological meaning of the injury to the individual all play a part (Gilboa, 2001).

Individuals who have been scarred or disfigured by burns must make psychological and physiologic adjustments, not only to their disfigurement but also to the immediate injury and to the long-term course of hospitalization and treatment. The suddenness of the injury itself produces a primary emotional stress. The impact of the injury is heightened by a variety of other situational factors, such as the separation from family, friends, and other sources of gratification; the experience of pain; the disruption of future life plans; and the threat to the sense of desirability and attractiveness to others. Recovery for individuals with severe burns is long and sometimes dehumanizing. In the initial stage of burn recovery, individuals frequently experience anxiety, partly because of the traumatic nature of the injury and the loss of independence, but also because of the painful treatments and the fear of death. Looking at the injury for the first time can be a traumatic event for which individuals need reassurance and optimism as well as a realistic view of their injury and their potential for recovery (Birdsall & Weinberg, 2001). During this stage of recovery, individuals may become agitated and hostile. They may experience sleep disruption and deprivation, which increase their irritability. As recovery progresses and individuals become more aware of their circumstances, they may regress, becoming overly dependent. Loss of independence, fear of disfigurement, and exposure to continuing painful treatments and procedures are a constant source of stress.

Treatment of burns often involves isolation, pain, multiple operations, and procedures over an extended period of time.

Depression is prevalent in individuals who have been burned (Van Loey & Van Son, 2003). Depression frequently results from feelings of helplessness and grief over loss of function or appearance. Individuals in a burn unit are subjected to numerous painful treatments and procedures, and they may also feel isolated. They may feel they have little power over what is done to them and for them, which can be frightening and frustrating. They may feel a loss of both personal and social satisfaction, as well as an alteration in their relationships with others. As already mentioned, anxiety is also a common psychological response to burns. Individuals with burns may be apprehensive, and realistically so, because of the painful procedures that they must endure. For some, the pain associated with the treatment procedures is a reminder of the initial injury, thus increasing the anxiety and intensifying the pain. Reactions may become generalized so that, even after the treatment period, individuals may continue to experience anxiety about unknown or unrecognized dangers.

Individuals with burns are at high risk for the development of posttraumatic stress, not only because of the trauma of the initial injury, but also because of the ongoing pain associated with treatment, which serves as an additional source of anxiety and as a continuing reminder of the incident (Yu & Dimsdale, 1999). Because burns are frequently associated with accidents, individuals may experience anger, guilt, regret, or resentment, depending on the circumstances. If the accident was caused by the negligence or actions of others, individuals may experience hostility and anger. If the accident was caused by their own actions or if others were also injured as a result, self-blame and guilt may intensify individuals' reaction to their injury.

As individuals begin to think about the future after the immediate burn treatment period, psychological responses may be characterized by false hopes and magical optimism, particularly when skin grafting and reconstruction begin. They may have unrealistic expectations about the results of surgery or deny that there will be a permanent deformity. When continuing disfigurement and/or limitations become apparent, they may again sink into a state of depression and withdrawal before gradually adjusting to their condition.

Discharge from the hospital does not mark the end of stress for individuals with burns. Discharge often marks a new set of stresses when individuals integrate into the larger social setting after having been sheltered in the burn unit. It is difficult psychologically for individuals who have been disfigured by burns to reenter the community, where they may be subjected to the pity and curiosity of strangers as well as to stares and rude remarks. Individuals may test family and friends with unusual requests or with behaviors designed to get attention. Adjusting to the reactions of others, dealing with social stigma, and realistically accepting limitations are important psychological issues with which the individual with burns must deal.

The lifestyle issues that arise in relation to burns depend on the extent, nature, and location of the burn. For example, severe burns of the hands can result in contracture of the hands and fingers, necessitating the use of assistive devices for the activities of daily living. Burns to the face that result in loss of vision may also make it necessary to use adaptive devices.

The sexuality of individuals with burns is often a neglected part of treatment and rehabilitation. Sexual concerns are important during acute treatment in the burn unit and also during discharge and ongoing rehabilitation. Sexuality encompasses much more than sexual activity or sexual function; it encompasses the whole person and is an important part of identity, self-image, and self-concept. The disfiguring nature of burn injury can challenge individuals' view of themselves as sexual beings and can affect their adjustment and adaptation.

Individuals who have been burned severely often require a series of reconstructive operations over several years. Thus, frequent hospitalizations and/or clinic visits interrupt work and home activities. Relationships may be altered because of the absences from the social environment necessitated by these repeated hospitalizations. Increased dependence and length of hospitalization due to burns can disrupt relationships within the family, as well as other social relationships. Friends and family may be shocked at the sudden change in an individual's appearance after a burn injury. Depending on the circumstances of the accident, family members and friends may feel anger, guilt, or resentment, which can be manifested in a variety of ways. In an attempt to make sense of the tragedy and its aftermath, family members, friends, and coworkers may focus on the question of responsibility for the accident. Those who were present at the time of the injury may feel they should have done more or that they were to blame. Others may wonder why they escaped the same type of injury. These feelings may affect their reactions to the individual and their further social interactions with him or her. Families may grieve for the image they once had of the individual, or they may grieve for the potential they feel the individual had that now will not be realized. Family reactions can range from oversolicitude to emotional withdrawal. Concerns about financial considerations and altered social roles may cause additional family stress. Support groups can help individuals and their families share common concerns. Groups such as the *National Phoenix Society* help individuals and their families cope with the ongoing difficulties of returning to society.

## Vocational Issues in Burn Injury

The ability of individuals who have been burned to return to their former occupation is dependent not only on the occupation itself, but also on the extent and location of the burn. At times, the main factor in determining how successful individuals can be in returning to their former position is the attitudes of others in the workplace. Acceptance of the burn survivor in the workplace by fellow employees may be difficult for a variety of reasons. If the injury was work related, depending on the circumstances, coworkers may feel guilty and treat the individual differently. Others may feel uncomfortable because of the individual's appearance and avoid contact with him or her. In some instances, even though individuals who have been severely burned may not consider themselves disabled, they may be perceived as such by others because of their appearance.

The emotional stress on the part of coworkers can prevent the individual from effectively reentering the workplace. Employers may not have confidence in individuals' ability to return to the former job or may be concerned about others' reaction if there has been disfigurement. Considerable work with coworkers and employers is sometimes necessary to provide a smoother transition for individuals returning to work after burn injury. Those with severe burns that necessitate extensive reconstructive surgery may require intermittent hospitalizations over a 1- to 2-year period after the initial injury. The disruption to work activity associated with these hospitalizations should be considered before individuals return to regular employment. Those who have other disabilities resulting from burns, such as the loss of a limb or the loss of vision, have other vocational limitations as well (see related chapters). Contracture as a result of burns may also limit mobility and, if the hands are involved, manual dexterity.

Individuals who must wear compression garments to prevent hypertrophic scarring may need to avoid extremely warm work environments because of the excessive warmth of the garment. Those who wear compression gloves also have decreased manual dexterity. A facial mask may be a cosmetic disability if dealing with the public is a requirement of the occupation. The degree to which cosmetic appearance due to the burn is a factor in employment depends on the individual, the occupation, and the employer.

Skin that has been grafted may be more sensitive than normal skin is. Consequently, grafts should not be exposed to extremes of temperature. Because of this skin sensitivity, individuals should take sun precautions and avoid mechanical trauma that could injure the skin. In addition, there may not be as much fat insulation in burned areas as there is in healthy normal tissue, which affects the individual's ability to tolerate extremes of temperature. Extremely dry climates may exacerbate the itching that may be associated with the new skin growth of skin grafts; thus a more humid environment may be desirable. Other residual problems from burns may also affect the appropriateness of the work environment. For example, individuals who have experienced altered lung function as a result of inhalation injury should avoid work settings in which there is air pollution or exposure to smoke and dust. Individuals with burns to the lower extremities may have difficulty standing for prolonged periods and may need more sedentary employment.

## PSYCHOSOCIAL AND VOCATIONAL ISSUES IN CONDITIONS OF THE SKIN

### Psychological Issues

The skin, exposed and readily observable, determines to a great extent individuals' appearance to others, and it is through personal appearance that others build an image about someone. Individuals, in turn, observe the reaction of others and incorporate it into their own self-image. Consequently, conditions affecting the skin can have considerable impact on individuals' perception and attitudes. Disease or injury affecting the face may be particularly devastating. More than any other body part, the face is tied to personal identity. Although clothing can cover other body parts, the face is left exposed so that disfigurement is readily observable. Our society places considerable emphasis on a clear, radiant appearance. When disease or injury mars this image, it is not surprising that the psychological impact on the affected individuals is considerable.

Disease of and injury to the skin may isolate individuals perhaps more than any other condition. Some people, because they associate skin diseases with uncleanliness and contagiousness, may avoid individuals with skin disorders even though these associations are unfounded. Because of the reactions of others, individuals with skin disease or injury may become very sensitive. Having experienced stares or other negative reactions, they may develop an accentuated state of awareness and assume that others are focusing totally on their appearance. They may become extremely self-conscious and withdraw from social contact.

Although conditions of the skin may not affect sexual function directly, society places considerable importance on physical attractiveness, especially when related to issues of sexuality. Consequently, skin disease or disfigurement, particularly of the face, as well as the reactions of others, may alter individuals' feelings of desirability. The anxiety or depression that accompanies skin conditions may further disrupt sexual function.

### Lifestyle Issues

Changes in lifestyle resulting from skin conditions are dependent on the severity of the condition and on the extent and circumstances of the disability. Skin conditions resulting from exposure to or contact with certain substances within the environment make it necessary to avoid those substances. The discomfort associated with some skin conditions, such as itching, may affect daily activities to some degree. If special baths or dressings are required, these treatments must be provided for within the daily routine. Acute skin conditions may be treated and prevented. Chronic skin conditions require ongoing treatment or intervention. Stress affects some skin conditions, and individuals with these conditions may need to learn ways to reduce stress in their environment or ways to alter their reaction to stress.

### Social Issues

Visible disabilities provoke greater discrimination and social stigma than do invisible disabilities. Physical attractiveness is highly valued in society, where attractiveness is viewed as a salable commodity. Skin conditions, especially if they involve the face, evoke even more profound responses from others. People may feel uneasy in the presence of individuals with disfigurement or deformity and uncertain as to what to do or say. In social settings, individuals with deformity or disfigurement due to a skin condition or injury may encounter staring, feelings of pity, or repulsion. These reactions may cause individuals to limit or avoid social activities or to restrict their social interactions with others.

## Vocational Issues

Most individuals with skin conditions continue in their regular line of employment, although individuals whose skin condition is precipitated or exacerbated by exposure to substances in the work environment may require special considerations. In these instances, alterations in the work site or precautions in the performance of certain work-related activities may be necessary. If stress precipitates or exacerbates the skin condition, measures to decrease stress at the work site or to improve the individual's reaction to stress should also be taken. In some instances, it may be necessary to alter the work site.

Because skin cancer appears to be related to exposure to the sun, those who work outside should take precautions to avoid excessive exposure, such as by wearing protective clothing or sun shields. Those who have had skin cancer or who have a propensity toward it should take additional precautions to avoid direct exposure to the sun as much as possible. Likewise, individuals who are being treated with medications that cause photosensitivity, or individuals who have new skin grafts, may also need to avoid the sun.

The attitudes of employers and coworkers may create barriers to employment for individuals with skin conditions, especially when the condition alters their appearance considerably. Coworkers may fear contagion or may be uncomfortable because of the individual's appearance. Consequently, education and strategies to alleviate misperceptions may be important factors in facilitating the individual's successful reentry or continuation in the work setting.

## CASE STUDIES

### Case I

Ms. N. was a passenger in a small commuter plane when it crashed during a severe storm 2 years ago. Although all other passengers were killed, Ms. N. survived; however, she experienced second- and third-degree burns over 60 percent of her body. As a result of her injury she received severe facial scars and the amputation of her left hand. She has had a number of reconstructive surgeries since her injury. She uses a terminal device for her left hand that is cosmetic. Other than her facial scarring and amputation of her hand, she has no other physical limitations. Ms. N. has a bachelor of science degree in finance. Before her injury she was a teller at a bank. She is 29 years old. She asks you to help her explore her rehabilitation potential.

#### Questions

1. What specific issues regarding the scarring would you consider?
2. What other issues might be important to consider in Ms. N.'s case?
3. What vocational options might be feasible for Ms. N. given her situation?
4. What additional medical information would you like to obtain in working with Ms. N. to develop her rehabilitation plan?

## Case II

Mr. A. and four other men were burned at a construction job because of a gas explosion from a gas leak that was ignited when he lit a cigarette. The accident occurred 2 years ago. Mr. A. is now 30 years old. Mr. A.'s burns were localized over his chest and upper extremities and were second- and third-degree burns. As a result of the burns he also lost one ear and both of his thumbs. He has undergone a number of surgeries since his injury. The construction company is willing to have him return to work, but he does not believe he is psychologically able to return. He has a high school education and no other skills other than those he learned on the job. He had worked for the construction company for 5 years. Previously he had been a gas station attendant. He has been divorced for 5 years but has no children. He had been dating a woman before his injury, but since his injury she has told him she no longer wants to see him.

### Questions

1. What issues related to the accident might be important to address?
2. How will the specific injuries Mr. A. received in the accident affect his rehabilitation potential?
3. What additional issues might be important to address?
4. What types of information would you want to obtain in working with Mr. A. to develop a rehabilitation plan?

### REFERENCES

Balasubramani, M., Kumar, T. R., & Babu, M. (2001). Skin substitutes: A review. *Burns, 27*(5), 534–544.

Birdsall, C., & Weinberg, K. (2001). Adult patients looking at their burn injuries for the first time. *Journal of Burn Care Rehabilitation, 22*(5), 360–364.

Gilboa, D. (2001). Long-term psychosocial adjustment after burn injury. *Burns, 27*(4), 335–341.

Lamberg, L. (1997). Dermatologic disorders diminish quality of life. *Journal of the American Medical Association, 277*(21), 1663.

Lebwohl, M. (2000). Psoriasis treatment options continue to grow. *Dermatology Times, 21*(11), 14–16.

LeRoy, L. (2000). Camouflage therapy. *Dermatology Nursing, 12*(6), 415–419.

McQuaid, D., Barton, J., & Campbell, E. A. (2000). Body image issues for children and adolescents with burns. *Journal of Burn Care Rehabilitation, 21*(3), 194–198.

Morgan, M., McCreedy, R., Simpson, J., & Hay, R. J. (1997). Dermatology quality of life scales: A measure of the impact of skin diseases. *British Journal of Dermatology, 136*, 202–206.

Nelson, L. A., & Thompson, D. D. (1998). Burn injury. *Plastic Surgical Nursing, 18*(3), 159–169.

Pardasani, A. G., Feldman, S. R., & Clark, A. R. (2000). Treatment of psoriasis: An algorithm-based approach for primary care physicians. *American Family Physician, 61*(3), 725.

Van Loey, N. E., & Van Son, M. J. (2003). Psychopathology and psychological problems in patients with burn scars: Epidemiology and management. *American Journal of Clinical Dermatology, 4*(4), 245–272.

Yu, B. H., & Dimsdale, J. E. (1999). Posttraumatic stress disorder in patients with burn injuries. *Journal of Burn Care Rehabilitation, 20*(5), 426–433.

# CHAPTER 16

# Cancers

## NORMAL STRUCTURE AND FUNCTION OF THE CELL

The basic unit of all living things is the cell. The human body contains approximately 75 trillion cells. Although different types of cells perform different functions, all cells have certain basic characteristics in common. All cells require nutrition and oxygen in order to live, and almost all cells have the ability to reproduce. Reproduction of cells is a controlled process so that cells die and form at an approximately equal rate in adults, maintaining a balance in the number of cells present at any time. The precise way in which cell growth and reproduction are regulated within the human body is unknown. Some cells, such as those that make up the layers of the skin or the lining of the intestine, grow and reproduce frequently. Other cells, such as those that make up the musculature of the gastrointestinal tract, may not reproduce for years. Cells that make up neurons, the functional unit of the nervous system, do not reproduce at all. Similarly, little is known about the mechanism that controls the number of each specific cell type that is produced.

Different types of cells make up different parts of body tissue. Cells are named for their different characteristics. For example, *epithelial cells* are cells found in the skin, the lining of body organs (e.g., the lining of the intestine), and glandular tissue (e.g., the breast or prostate). Blood vessels, lymph vessels, and other lymph tissue are composed of *endothelial cells*. Different types of cells are also found in muscle, nerve, bone, and other tissues in the body.

Every cell contains *DNA* (genetic material that is the blueprint for all the body's structures). *Genes*, composed of DNA, carry hereditary information about all characteristics of the organism. Although each cell contains all the genes for a particular organism, it uses only particular genes. This discrimination in the use of genes is the basis for different cell types. Genes determine the growth characteristics of cells, as well as when or whether the cells divide to form new cells. Before cells can reproduce, however, genes must reproduce themselves. After genes reproduce, the cell divides, forming another cell identical to itself. It is through this systematic, organized reproduction of cells that continuity of life is maintained.

## DEVELOPMENT OF CANCER

Cancer is not one disease, but many diseases. There are well over 100 types of *cancers*. Cancers can arise from any type of cell and are classified according to the *cell of origin*. Most frequently, the term *tumor* is assumed to be synonymous with *cancer*; however, not all tumors are cancerous. A tumor, also called a *neoplasm*, is a new and abnormal growth of cells that serves no useful function and may interfere with healthy tissue function. The reason for the proliferation of cells is often unknown. Tumors may be **benign** (noncancerous). Although benign tumors may disturb body function by exerting pressure on surrounding tissues and, thus, preventing surrounding organs from obtaining a sufficient blood supply, they usually grow slowly, do not invade surrounding tissue, remain localized, and do not recur once removed. Generally, cells in benign tumors closely resemble normal cells in the tissue from which they multiplied. **Malignant tumors** are those that are capable of destructive growth and have the ability to invade surrounding tissues and move to other parts of the body. Malignant tumors are *cancerous tumors*.

Cancer develops when there has been an alteration (*mutation*) in the DNA within the normal cell. As a result, the control mechanism that regulates cell reproduction is lost. Because the reproduction of cancer cells is uncontrolled, they reproduce at a rate that exceeds the rate at which the normal cells in the tissue are dying. Some of the more virulent cancer cells are often described as *anaplastic*, meaning that their appearance takes on abnormal characteristics so that they are less differentiated than are the normal cells from which they are derived.

The original site of cancer cell reproduction is called the *primary site*, sometimes referred to as the *primary tumor*. Cancer cells do not remain confined to the original site, but extend and invade surrounding tissues as they reproduce. In addition, cancer cells are less adhesive than are normal cells. Selected cancer cells may break off from the original cluster, enter the bloodstream or the lymph system, and travel to other parts of the body, where they begin another abnormal pattern of reproduction. The movement of cancer cells from the original site to another part of the body is called **metastasis**. Cancer cell reproduction at this additional site is called a *secondary tumor*, meaning that metastasis has occurred and that the secondary tumor is not the original site of cancer growth.

Cancer cells compete with normal cells for nutrients. The reproduction of cancer cells is not well regulated, and some cancer cells reproduce at a more rapid rate than do normal cells. Eventually, available nutrients are taken from the normal cells to nourish the cancer cells.

## CAUSES OF CANCER

The exact cause of cancer is unknown. There are probably many causes, and it may be necessary for a variety of factors to be present for cancer to develop. Although specific causes are unknown, several factors are known to increase the risk of cancer.

- Radiation
- Some chemicals and pollutants
- Smoking and tobacco use
- Some viruses
- Chronic physical irritation to a body part
- Ultraviolet rays (sun)
- Hereditary predisposition

Chemicals or other substances that are thought to cause cancer are called **carcinogens**. Some carcinogens may be present in the environment but not readily evident. Individuals may be exposed to carcinogens within the environment or workplace for a number of years before cancer develops. Some substances may not be carcinogenic in themselves but may serve as co-carcinogens, promoting tumor formation in combination with other carcinogenic agents. Other factors, such as hormonal secretion, diet, and stress, have been implicated as potential factors in the development of or propensity for cancer, but the specific mechanisms that contribute to this relationship are unknown.

## TYPES OF CANCER

Any type of cell in the body may be the source of cancer. Cancers are named for the *type of tissue* from which they originated. Some common types of cancers and the corresponding tissue from which they arise are the following.

- **Carcinoma:** cancer of the epithelial cells
- **Sarcoma:** cancer of the bone, muscle, or other connective tissue
- **Lymphoma:** cancer of the lymphatic system
- **Leukemia:** cancer of blood cells or blood precursor cells
- **Melanoma:** cancer of the pigment-producing cells, usually of the skin

Because the specific behavior of cancer cells depends on the type of cell from which they originated, there can be no generalizations made about cancer. Each type of cancer may progress at a different rate and may respond to different types of treatment in different ways. Consequently, the classification of cancer is important in determining both treatment and prognosis.

## STAGING AND GRADING OF CANCER

When cancer is diagnosed, it is important to determine not only the cancer type but also the extent to which cancer cells have spread. This process is called **staging**. Staging of all cancers not only helps physicians determine the **prognosis** (prediction of the course and outcome of the disease process), but also helps to determine the form of treatment that is most appropriate.

The most common system for staging today is the *TNM system*, which classifies cancer according to tumor size, node involvement, and metastasis. The letter T stands for *tumor;* N, for *node;* and M, for *metastasis*. When there is no evidence of a primary tumor, the stage is defined as *T0*. If cancer cells are present but have not invaded surrounding lymph nodes, the stage is defined as *Tis* (previously called *in situ*). As the tumor increases in size, it may be staged from T1 to T4, depending on the tumor size and involvement. When there is no lymph node involvement, the N staging is *N0*. If cancer cells extend beyond the initial tissue site and involve the lymph nodes in the surrounding area, however, the stage is *N1, N2,* or N3 (previously called *regional involvement*), depending on the degree of involvement and the abnormality of the nodes. If the cancer cells remain at the original site even though the surrounding tissues and lymph nodes are involved, the M staging is *M0*. When cancer cells have metastasized to another area of the body, however, staging is *M1, M2,* or *M3*, depending on the extent of the metastasis.

*Histologic studies* and *grading* are laboratory procedures in which the type and structure of cancer cells are determined microscopically. Histological grading is based on the appearance of cells and the degree of differentiation. Cells are graded as follows:

- Grade I: mild dysplagia (cells are slightly different from normal)
- Grade II: moderate dysplagia (cells are more abnormal)
- Grade III: severe dysplasia (cells are very abnormal and poorly differentiated)
- Grade IV: anaplasia (cells are immature and undifferentiated; cells of origin are difficult to determine)

A **pathologist** (a physician who specializes in the diagnosis of abnormal changes in tissues) examines the cells under a microscope to determine their type and the extent to which they differ from their normal precursors. The histologic type of cell and the grading of the cell are important in the determination of the treatment implemented *and* the prognosis. Individuals with tumor cells that are *well differentiated* (more similar to the cell of origin, with a more organized structure) may have a better prognosis, for example, than does an individual with tumor cells that are considered *anaplastic* (containing more abnormalities in structure).

## GENERAL DIAGNOSTIC PROCEDURES IN CANCER

In general, the earlier the diagnosis of cancer, the better the prognosis. Some cancers grow and invade surrounding tissue without causing physical symptoms. These cancers are called *occult malignancies*. Tests and procedures used to detect abnormalities before symptoms develop are called *cancer-screening procedures*. When symptoms occur or when screening procedures have positive or suspicious results, additional diagnostic testing is necessary.

### Radiographic Procedures (X-ray)

In addition to conventional X-rays, *computed axial tomography*, *magnetic resonance imaging*, *ultrasound*, and, occasionally, *arteriography* may be helpful in identifying an abnormality in normal anatomic structure or the presence of a tumor. *Mammography* is a soft tissue radiographic examination of the breast that is frequently used as a screening and diagnostic procedure because it can reveal cancerous lesions before they can be detected by direct examination of the breast. Although these tests are important in identifying abnormalities, they rarely are used alone in the diagnosis of cancer. A positive diagnosis requires microscopic examination of the tumor cells (*histologic testing*).

### Diagnostic Surgery

In some instances, surgery may be done to confirm or rule out the presence of cancer. Depending on the size and location of the tumor, the surgical procedure may be relatively minor, such as the removal of an external wart or polyp, or a major intervention, such as an *exploratory laparotomy* (the surgical opening of the abdomen for the purpose of investigation).

Regardless of the type of diagnostic surgery performed, an accurate diagnosis of cancer can be made only after a microscopic examination of the tissue. For such an examination, a *biopsy* is performed to remove a small portion of tissue from the body. Biopsies may be done by inserting a needle into the tumor and removing some cells through the needle (*needle biopsy*). Biopsies may also be done by making an incision and removing a portion of the tumor (*incisional biopsy*). The type of biopsy done depends on the size and location of the tumor.

### Cytology

The study of cells that have been scraped from tissue surrounding the area of interest is a *cytologic study*. Perhaps the best-known example of diagnostic cytology is the *Papanicolaou smear* (*Papsmear*). Cells from sputum specimens that have been coughed up from the lungs and other types of fluids may also be examined through diagnostic cytology.

## Endoscopy

An *endoscopic examination* involves the insertion of a tubular device into a hollow organ or cavity to visualize the inside of the structure directly. The procedure may be done through a natural body opening or through a small incision. Examples of endoscopic examinations are *bronchoscopy* (see Chapter 12), *sigmoidoscopy*, *gastroscopy* and *esophagoscopy* (see Chapter 10), and *laryngoscopy* (examination of the larynx or vocal cords). Endoscopy is also a method of obtaining a tissue sample from the internal structure for a histologic examination.

## Nuclear Medicine

In nuclear medicine, small amounts of *radioactive materials* are used for diagnostic procedures, and somewhat larger amounts are used for the treatment of disease. In the diagnosis of cancer, nuclear medicine procedures may be used for the detection and staging of cancers in the *thyroid glands*, *liver*, and *bone*. They may also be used to detect the presence of metastatic disease.

## Laboratory Tests

Although laboratory tests per se may not be diagnostic of cancer, the results of laboratory tests may indicate impaired physiologic function as a result of the cancer, such as the anemia or altered white blood cell count associated with leukemia. In some instances, laboratory tests are used for screening purposes. For example, both alpha-fetoprotein and carcinoembryonic antigens are normally found in embryonic and fetal tissues but disappear after birth. In later life, however, tumors may produce these substances. Consequently, elevated levels of either in adults may be an indication of certain types of cancers, as well as of other diseases.

## GENERAL TREATMENT OF CANCER

Many modalities are available to prevent, control, or cure cancer. Treatment modalities include:

- surgery
- chemotherapy
- radiation (external or internal)
- biological therapy (immunotherapy, hormone therapy, gene therapy)
- bone marrow transplantation

The above treatments may be used alone or in combination. Many therapies involve multiple approaches rather than one. When treatment uses several different types of therapy, treatment is said to be *multimodal*.

A number of factors are considered in determining which procedures are best for the treatment of a particular cancer. A major consideration is the *type* of cancer. Because different cancers grow at different rates, metastasize to different spots, and react differently to various forms of treatment, the *histologic type* of cancer is a major determinant in treatment decisions. The *stage* of cancer is also considered. The extent to which cancer has invaded surrounding tissues and the presence of any metastases determine the aggressiveness, as well as the type, of treatment. The location of the tumor and its relationship to other vital organs determine the accessibility of the tumor for removal or treatment. The goal of intervention also affects the type of treatment.

Goals for treatment of cancer can include:

- cure
- extension of life
- prevention of metastasis
- palliation

In terms of cancer treatment, *cure* is usually defined as *no evidence of cancer for 5 years after treatment*, indicating a normal life expectancy for the individual. Treatment for the prevention of metastasis, also called *adjuvant therapy*, is directed toward eliminating cancer that, although not detectable and not symptomatic, may be present and may cause a recurrence of disease. *Palliative therapy* is directed toward the relief of symptoms or complications of cancer, such as obstruction or severe pain, rather than toward cure.

Factors related to the individual with cancer must also be taken into consideration. *Debilitation* because of disease, *the cancer itself*, or age may compromise individuals' ability to withstand certain treatments. In some cases, individuals may feel that the benefits of some forms of cancer therapy are not worth the risks and side effects; consequently, they may refuse the recommended treatment.

Cancer may be treated *systemically* or *locally*. Often, treatment of cancer consists of a combination of the two. Cancer may be treated *surgically*, *chemically* (chemotherapy), with *radiation*, or with other means—separately or in combination.

### Surgical Procedures

Usually directed toward the local treatment of cancer, surgical procedures may be preventive, curative, palliative, or reconstructive. *Preventive surgery* may be performed when precancerous or suspicious lesions are found. For example, a mole or polyp that, although not malignant, has a high probability of becoming malignant in the future may be removed. *Curative surgery* is generally more extensive. It may involve not only the tumor but also an organ or surrounding tissue. Depending on the size and location of the tumor, curative surgery can affect subsequent function only minimally, can impair function severely, or can cause permanent disfigure-

ment. *Palliative surgery* is directed toward reducing the size or retarding the growth of the tumor, or relieving severe discomfort associated with the presence of the tumor. In all instances, the goal of palliative surgery is to prolong or increase the quality of life rather than to cure the disease. *Reconstructive surgery* is directed toward restoring maximal function or correcting disfigurement.

The surgical procedures used in treatment of cancer may be considered *simple* or *radical*. Simple surgical procedures usually involve removing the tumor while leaving surrounding structures and organs intact. *Radical surgical procedures* are more extensive. In radical surgery not only the tumor is removed, but also some underlying tissue (e.g., muscle or organ). Radical surgery often results in alteration of function or appearance to some degree.

With advances in medical techniques, less radical procedures are now being performed. Surgery now might include *laser surgery* or *cryosurgery* (using low temperatures to devitalize or destroy cells).

### Chemotherapy

Chemotherapy alone is often curative in many cancers, and in others adjuvant chemotherapy used in conjunction with other therapies can augment the survival benefit of the other therapies (Green, 2004). *Antineoplastic medications* (chemical agents that destroy cancer cells) are used in the systemic treatment of cancer. These agents may be used alone or in conjunction with other forms of therapy, such as surgery and radiation. This type of therapy, called *chemotherapy*, can be used for cure, prevention, or palliation. In general, chemotherapeutic agents affect the growth and reproduction of cancer cells.

There are a number of antineoplastic medications used in the treatment of cancer. Although these medications are different and may be administered differently, most affect rapidly dividing cells. Unfortunately, in addition to destroying and damaging cancer cells, these medications can also damage normal cells that grow rapidly, such as the cells of the hair follicles, skin, the lining of the gastrointestinal tract, and bone marrow. As a result, the toxic side effects of chemotherapy may include hair loss (**alopecia**), loss of appetite, nausea, vomiting, diarrhea, fatigue, and suppression of bone marrow function. The altered bone marrow function may interfere with the production of various components of blood. Therefore, individuals undergoing chemotherapy may develop anemia, may bruise easily because of decreased blood clotting ability, and may be highly susceptible to infection because they have fewer white blood cells.

Chemotherapeutic agents may be given intravenously, intramuscularly, subcutaneously, orally, or topically. In other instances, high concentrations of chemotherapeutic agents may be injected directly into a body cavity, such as the bladder or the peritoneal cavity, to treat localized tumors. Treatment may be conducted on either an outpatient or an inpatient basis.

Chemotherapeutic regimens vary with the agent and the disease. Some treatments are given daily; others are given for 1 day every 3 to 8 weeks. Some individuals may use a portable device (*infusion pump*) that pumps small amounts of the chemotherapeutic agent constantly into a vein (*infusion therapy*). In some instances, because the chemotherapeutic agent is administered in small doses over time, toxic side effects may be reduced. This type of treatment delivers maximal dosage of the medication to the tumor site and can also reduce systemic side effects. New agents called chemoprotectants (drugs that protect the body against cancer medications) ameliorate the toxic effects of drugs used in chemotherapy at higher doses.

Not all individuals who receive chemotherapy experience side effects. Those who do not have severe side effects can, for the most part, continue their daily activities. No special precautions are necessary, with the exception of avoiding exposure to individuals with colds or flu because resistance may be lowered during chemotherapy.

## Radiation Therapy

With radiation therapy, high-energy rays are used to damage cancer cells and prevent them from growing and reproducing. This technique may be used to cure cancer, to relieve symptoms, or to keep cancer under control.

Radiation therapy may be delivered externally or internally. During external radiation therapy, a machine beams high-energy rays to the cancer so that the maximum effect of radiation takes place in the tumor itself within the body. Even though the radiation penetrates the skin and underlying tissue, it does minimal damage to these structures. Internal radiation therapy involves inserting small amounts of radioactive material into the body. This is called *brachytherapy*.

There are various types of internal radiation. With intracavity therapy, a radioactive substance is placed in a body cavity for a period of approximately 24 to 72 hours and is then removed; for example, a radioactive implant may be placed into the vagina for the treatment of cervical cancer. With interstitial therapy, a radioactive substance is placed into needles, beads, or seeds and implanted directly into the tumor. The interstitial implant may be removed after a specific period of time, or it may be left in place permanently, depending upon the half-life of the radioactive source.

Like chemotherapy, radiation therapy can affect the growth and reproduction of normal cells, resulting in potentially toxic side effects. The number of normal cells exposed to the radiation, the dosage of radiation, the part of the body receiving radiation therapy, and individual variability determine the side effects experienced. These side effects may appear immediately or weeks or months after the radiation therapy was administered. Some individuals experience generalized symptoms similar to those of radiation sickness: nausea, vomiting, loss of appetite, fatigue, and headache. Other individuals may experience side effects specific to the area irradiated, such as sore throat if the head or neck has been irradiated, or localized skin reactions, such as radiation burn. Like chemotherapy, radiation therapy may also cause bone marrow depression, resulting in anemia, lowered resistance to infection, and possible hemorrhage.

## Biological Therapies

### Immunotherapy

A newer approach to the treatment of cancer is immunotherapy. Since human cancer cells express cancer-associated antigens, the goal of immunotherapy is to strengthen the individual's own immune system so that it recognizes cancer cells as foreign objects and destroys them (Rosenberg, 2004). Thus, the body's own immune system is enhanced to fight cancer cells.

Immunotherapeutic agents can also help to increase the susceptibility of cancer cells to the *cytotoxic agents* (chemicals that are detrimental to or destroy cells). Many immunologic approaches to cancer treatment are already being used. Examples of immunotherapy are the *interferons* and *interleukin-2*. Another example is the use of *bacille Calmette-Guérin (BCG)* in the treatment of superficial bladder cancer.

### Hormone Therapy

*Adjuvant hormone therapy* can be used to increase the benefits of chemotherapy in cancers that are hormone dependent (such as certain breast cancers that are estrogen dependent and prostate cancers that are androgen dependent). Hormones are not used to kill cancer cells, but rather to keep the cancer cells from growing further so that individuals are in remission for extended periods of time. Hormone preparations work by blocking hormone receptors to cells so that estrogen or androgen cannot be used by the cancer cells.

### Gene Therapy

Gene therapy in the treatment of cancer is still in its infancy. Gene therapy works by actually modifying the genetic structure of the cancer cell to suppress or inhibit tumor growth.

### Bone Marrow Transplantation

*Bone marrow transplantation* is performed when the escalation of chemotherapy (chemical substances or drugs used to treat disease) may result in a cure of the cancer, but the dosage would be lethal to the individual's bone marrow. In addition, bone marrow transplants also seem to have an antitumor effect themselves, aside from their use with chemotherapy. Bone marrow transplants are used for a variety of cancers, including *leukemias*, *Hodgkin's* and *non-Hodgkin's lymphomas*, *multiplemyeloma*, and *breast cancer*.

The goal of bone marrow transplantation is to provide healthy cells that can differentiate into blood cells to replace deficient or pathologic cells. The transplanted cells have the ability to completely replace and produce all red blood cells, platelets, T lymphocytes, and B lymphocytes (see Chapter 8) as well as other marrow *stem cells* (cells that can reproduce and differentiate into other types of cells).

In preparation for bone marrow transplantation, individuals receive large doses of radiation and/or chemotherapy that eradicate any viable marrow, as well as kill tumor cells and suppress the immune system to reduce the chance of rejection of the transplant. As a result of immune system suppression, individuals receiving the transplant are susceptible to infection. The individual receives an infusion of cells from the donor, and the bone marrow regenerates using the new cells.

Taking bone marrow from the donor is a surgical procedure in which marrow is removed from the *iliac crests* (hipbone) while the donor is under spinal or general anesthesia. *Allogenic transplants* (taken from another individual) have the advantage of not risking contamination with cancer cells, but the disadvantage of having a higher incidence of transplant rejection, or *graft versus host disease* (GVHD), in which the transplanted cells attack the cells of the individual who received them. To minimize the chance of rejection or GVHD, the more closely matched the donor is to the individual the better, identical twins being the most compatible donors.

Individuals can also receive *autologous transplants* (cells taken from their own body). With autologous transplants, cells are removed from the individual prior to irradiation or chemotherapy and frozen. They are then reinfused. The advantage of autologous infusions is that rejection or GVHD is avoided. The disadvantage is that there is risk of contamination with tumor cells from the individual's body. Also, autologous transplants lack the additional antitumor effect that is seen with allogenic transplants.

In addition to being in the bone marrow, stem cells also circulate in the peripheral blood and may also be used for transplant. Peripheral stem cell transplantation is a procedure by which cells are removed from the peripheral blood, thus avoiding a surgical procedure. For *autologous transplants*, this procedure may be used if the individual is too debilitated to withstand a surgical procedure. The disadvantage in an autologous transplant is, again, the possible contamination with other cancer cells.

For *allogenic transplant*, although the donor is able to avoid a surgical procedure, the recipient may run a greater risk of rejection of the transplant or GVHD because of receiving a greater number of T cells from the donor. The most critical period is 2 to 4 weeks after the bone marrow transplantation. Because of the immunosuppression prior to surgery, individuals may have an increased susceptibility to infections for up to 3 months after the transplant. In addition, because immunosuppressive therapy drastically reduces the components in the blood that control bleeding, complications such as hemorrhage may result.

## COMMON CANCERS AND SPECIFIC TREATMENTS

The diagnostic procedures, treatment, and functional limitations associated with cancer differ depending on the anatomic site involved. In many instances, a combination of treatments, including surgery, chemotherapy, and irradiation, is used. In the treatment of cancer in its very early stages, surgery alone may be sufficient.

### Cancer of the Gastrointestinal Tract

Treatment of cancer of the gastrointestinal tract or accessory organs often consists of the removal or major resection of the organs involved. Because the symptoms of cancers of the esophagus, stomach, liver, and pancreas frequently occur late in the disease, treatment may be directed toward palliation rather than cure.

Surgical treatment for *cancer of the mouth* may include removal of the tumor, as well as removal of the nearby lymph glands to determine whether cancer has spread. If cancer has spread to the neck or other tissues, more radical surgery may be indicated, which can result in facial deformity or disfigurement because of the amount of tissue removed. If the tongue has been partially removed, speech may be affected. Reconstructive surgery may be required later to minimize these effects.

Cancer of the esophagus has been linked to smoking or gastroesophageal reflux disease (Brown, Hoover, Silverman, et al., 2001; Terry, Lagergren, Ye, Nyren, & Wolk, 2000; Wu, Wan, & Bernstein, 2001). Other risks include obesity (Lagergren, Bergstrom, Adami, & Nyren, 2000) and *Barrett's esophagus* (Shaheen & Ransohoff, 2002), which is abnormal tissue extending from the opening of the stomach into the esophagus. Treatment of *cancer of the esophagus* may consist of radiotherapy with or without chemotherapy or surgery. When esophageal cancer is localized, the affected part of the esophagus may be removed and reattached to the remaining part of the esophagus (Enzinger & Mayer, 2003). When the cancer is more severe, **esophagectomy** (removal of the esophagus) may be necessary. If the individual has the esophagus removed, an artificial opening must be made into the stomach and a tube inserted through which liquid feedings can be taken. After the feeding, the opening is then "plugged" to prevent leakage. After removal of the esophagus, individuals lose the ability to eat or drink through the mouth. The ramifications of this type of surgery may seriously influ-

ence individuals' willingness to have surgical versus other forms of treatment for their cancer.

Treatment of **cancer of the large bowel** (colon and rectum) usually involves both surgical removal of the tumor and some resection of the colon itself, through an incision in the abdomen (Pappas & Jacobs, 2004). In many instances, the diseased part of the bowel can be removed and the two remaining ends joined together, enabling the individual to retain normal bowel function. When this is not possible, a colostomy may be performed (see Chapter 10).

## Cancer of the Larynx

Although many other structures in the head and neck can be a site of cancer, one of the most common cancers of the head and neck is cancer of the **larynx** (voicebox). Smoking and alcohol are two leading risk factors for laryngeal cancer and are synergistic in their effects (Wu et al., 2001). Some occupations also appear to have increased risk due to secondary toxic exposures.

### Symptoms of Cancer of the Larynx

The larynx contains the vocal cords. The most common symptom in cancer of the larynx is alteration in voice quality or hoarseness. Other symptoms may include **dysphagia** (difficulty in swallowing) and cough.

### Diagnosis of Cancer of the Larynx

The diagnostic procedures used to identify problems of the larynx often include a procedure called a **laryngoscopy**, in which a hollow tube is inserted into the larynx so that the physician can inspect the structures of the larynx and assess the function of the vocal cords.

### Treatment of Cancer of the Larynx

Although the treatment of cancer of the larynx is dependent on a number of factors, it usually involves irradiation, surgery, or a combination of the two. Although in the past treatment of advanced cancer of the larynx usually involved total removal of the larynx, nonsurgical approaches involving chemotherapy and radiation are now frequently used instead of surgery in many cases (Forastiere et al., 2003). When the tumor is small (stage T1 or T2, N0 and M0), radiation alone may be used rather than surgery to eradicate the tumor (Vokes & Stenson, 2003). Laser treatment, which destroys the tumor by intense light beams, may also be used to treat cancer of the larynx in its early stages. If the tumor is discovered early, before there has been extensive involvement of the surrounding tissues, it may be necessary to remove only part of the larynx. This procedure is called a *subtotal (partial) laryngectomy*. Both subtotal laryngectomy and laser treatment can preserve the capacity for normal speech, although they may affect voice quality to some degree.

When the cancer is more advanced, it may be necessary to remove the larynx completely. This procedure is called a **laryngectomy**. Usually, individuals who have undergone this type of surgery are unable to breathe or speak by normal mechanisms. After the larynx has been removed, the trachea is no longer connected either to the nasopharynx or to the nasal passages (see Chapter 12). The surgeon creates a permanent opening called a **tracheostomy** in the individual's neck and trachea, and the individual breathes through this opening (*laryngostoma*) rather than through the nose and mouth. Although they are able to eat and drink normally, individuals must breathe, cough, and sneeze through the tracheosto-my. The sense of smell, and in turn taste, is diminished because air flows through the opening in the neck instead of through the nose.

### Psychosocial Issues in Cancer of the Larynx

The psychosocial and vocational effects of laryngectomy can be profound. A healthy voice is critical for effectiveness at work as well as in personal and social interactions (Zeitels & Healy, 2003). Individuals immediately lose the ability to make vocal sounds for speech as well as the audible sounds of laughter or crying. Consequently, when at all possible, physicians attempt to preserve as much of the larynx as possible. When this is not possible, individuals must learn new techniques for speaking.

Attempts to improve the ability to speak after treatment of laryngeal cancer have been successful. Surgical techniques have evolved so that much of the larynx can be spared and it doesn't have to be totally removed. In addition, improved methods of voice rehabilitation after total laryngectomy have been devised. There are three basic types of voice rehabilitation techniques after total laryngectomy:

- Tracheo-esophageal speech (shunt speech)
- Esophageal speech
- Electrolaryngeal speech

In tracheo-esophageal techniques a **fistula** (a passageway from one structure to another) is surgically constructed between the trachea and esophagus with a small prosthesis being placed in the fistula. Closing the tracheostomy with the hand or fingers moves air from the trachea to the esophagus, creating a *pseudovoice*. As a result, individuals are able to produce lung-powered speech of better quality than was previously accomplished with other methods such as *esophageal speech*. The prosthesis in the fistula prevents food and liquid from entering the airway when individuals are eating. A limitation of the fistula is the need for periodic removal the prosthesis for cleaning and replacement, and the need to use one hand to occlude the tracheostomy during speech. Special valves that fit into the opening are, however, available to eliminate the need for manual coverage of the opening. During normal breathing the valve remains open; however, when individuals begin to speak, because of increased expiratory pressure, the valve closes.

*Esophageal speech* is a technique of speaking that involves trapping air in the esophagus and gradually releasing it at the top of the esophagus to produce a *pseudovoice*. If sounds produced by esophageal speech are too soft to be heard, a *personal amplifier-speaker* may be used to increase sound volume. Since the air capacity of the upper esophagus is considerably less than that of the lungs, esophageal speech is typically limited in rate, volume, and duration.

*Electrolaryngeal speech* is another speech alternative that may be used by individuals with laryngectomy. It utilizes a battery-powered vibratory device called an *artificial larynx*. There are several types available; however, most are electronic, battery-operated devices that are held against the throat to produce sound. Although the artificial larynx is relatively easy to use, the speech produced has a mechanical, monotone sound that some individuals find objectionable.

Regardless of the type of speech alternative individuals use, *speech-language pathologists* are usually consulted for evaluation and possible treatment based on individuals' specific voice issues. Speech-language pathologists assess factors that have an impact on voice production, identify any problem behaviors, and plan treatment to rectify the problem.

When individuals have a total laryngectomy, they must also adjust to the visible opening in the neck, the laryngeostoma. Any disfigurement, especially when related to the face, may damage individuals' self-concept and self-image. For cosmetic purposes, individuals may wear a scarf or other covering loosely around the neck. This covering can also keep dust and dirt out of the opening. Another type of covering available is a foam filter, which keeps moisture loss to a minimum and also prevents hair, shaving cream, or other particles from falling into the trachea during routine daily hygiene. Since the opening leads directly into the trachea and lungs, individuals must avoid activities such as swimming and water sports in which water could enter the opening. For showering, special laryngectomy shower collars that prevent water from running into the airway are available. With a laryngeostoma, individuals no longer have the benefit of having air humidified as it passes through the upper airway passages. Consequently, they may need to run a humidifier, especially at night, to keep the trachea moist.

Because the quality of speech is also altered, individuals may avoid social situations in which they have to speak, because they perceive their altered speech as distasteful and embarrassing. Although individuals with laryngectomy can carry out most activities of daily living normally, some individuals may notice a decreased ability to lift heavy objects because they cannot close the tracheostomy to build up internal pressure, as those who breathe normally can do, by compressing their lips and holding their breath. Individuals who have had a total laryngectomy should always carry an identification card or wear a medical identification bracelet to inform emergency personnel that they are a total neck breather.

### Vocational Issues in Cancer of the Larynx

Only a few jobs may prove difficult for individuals after a laryngectomy. Those jobs performed in environments with extreme heat or cold, or those that expose individuals to extreme dust or fumes should probably be avoided. Although the physical aspects of laryngectomy may not affect individuals' ability to work, the impact that the use of alternate modes of speech may have on employment can be striking, especially if individuals' use of voice is a necessary component of work. Employers and coworkers may also view individuals as being less socially acceptable because of their speech and therefore avoid interactions. Social support from friends and family or participation in peer support groups like the *Lost Chord Club* can help significantly in the adjustment.

## Cancer of the Lung

Lung cancer is one of the leading causes of cancer death in the United States and tobacco products cause over 80 percent of the lung cancers diagnosed (Miller, 2000). Occupational exposure to carcinogens accounts for approximately 15 percent of lung cancer cases (Cleary, Gorenstein, & Omenn, 1996); however, when exposure is associated with tobacco use, the risk of lung cancer increases dramatically (Miller, 2000).

Lung cancer can be found in a variety of cell types with varied rates of growth, with some types being slow-growing while others are aggressive and fast-growing. Symptoms are often not present until lung cancer has reached an advanced stage. Lung cancer is usually diagnosed through chest X-ray, CT scan, bronchoscopy, or biopsy.

Treatment of lung cancer may be surgical, with removal or resection of the lung, or may consist of radiation therapy, chemotherapy, or a combination. When used in the treatment of lung cancer, radiation therapy is usually for palliation, rarely for cure. For individuals with a type of lung cancer called *small-cell carcinoma*, chemotherapy is generally the treatment of choice. If surgical intervention is used for lung cancer, the primary aim is to remove the total tumor. The extent of the surgery depends on the cancer and its location in the lung. Removal of an entire lung is called a **pneumonectomy**; the removal of only one lobe of the lung is called a **lobectomy**. A *segmental resection* is a surgical procedure in which a segment of the lung is removed. After having a portion of the lung removed, individuals may need to limit their physical activity to some degree, depending on the amount of lung removed and the functional capacity remaining.

Since cigarette smoking is frequently linked to lung cancer, emphysema may also coexist, further limiting respiratory capacity and, consequently, also limiting physical activity.

## Cancer of the Musculoskeletal System

Musculoskeletal cancers frequently result in the amputation of an extremity (see Chapter 14). For some types of bone cancers, however, it may be possible to remove only a section of bone and to avoid amputating the whole extremity. In some instances, bone cancers may be reduced by chemotherapy and then controlled by radiotherapy.

## Cancer of the Urinary System

Cancer can develop in any organ of the urinary system, but the most frequent site is the bladder. There is a high relationship between bladder cancer and cigarette smoking (Droller, 1998).

The most common symptom of bladder cancer is **hematuria** (blood in the urine). When bladder cancer is suspected, the individual generally undergoes a procedure called **cystoscopy** in which a tube called a *cystoscope* is inserted into the bladder, enabling the physician to visualize the inner surface of the bladder and to take a biopsy for laboratory examination.

Bladder cancer is generally classified as *superficial* (in which the cancer cells are confined to the lining of the bladder) or *invasive* (in which the cancer cells have penetrated other tissues). Although cancer of the bladder may be treated in a variety of ways, depending on the stage and type of cancer involved, the most common treatment for invasive cancer is a procedure called *radical cystectomy*, in which the total bladder is surgically removed. Removal of the whole bladder necessitates surgical reconstruction to provide a means for urinary drainage, a procedure called *urinary diversion*. Although removal of the bladder once affected individuals' quality of life, now, because of major advances in urinary diversion, radical cystectomy is a more acceptable option. *Continent urinary diversions* allow individuals to avoid external collection devices and have minimal change in body image with only a small **stoma** (opening) in the abdomen.

When the total bladder is removed, an artificial reservoir for collection of urine must be substituted. Several types of reservoirs may be used. If the entire lower urinary system is removed, including the **urethra** (tube structure through which urine is excreted from the bladder to the outside of the body through the urinary meatus), an internal reservoir is constructed with an opening through which a catheter can be inserted for urinary drainage to the outside of the body. If the bladder alone is removed, leaving the urethra intact, a reservoir may still be constructed, but the individual will be able to continue to excrete urine through the urethra and to have near normal urination function.

At times, only a portion of the bladder may be removed. The removal of a portion of the bladder may greatly diminish the capacity of the bladder, necessitating more frequent urination. Another procedure for urinary diversion is *cutaneous ureterostomy*, in which the *ureters* are brought through the abdomen to the outside of the body, where they drain directly into a bag attached to the outside of the abdomen. A special bag called an *urostomy bag* is worn over the opening to collect urine. Still another urinary diversion procedure is called an *ileal conduit*, which involves removing a segment of small intestine (the *ileum*) and reconnecting the two remaining ends of bowel. Ureters are then connected to one end of the loop of small intestine that has been removed, and the other end of the loop of small intestine is brought to the outside of the abdomen to form an opening through which urine can drain. There is no voluntary control over the drainage of urine through the opening of either the cutaneous ureterostomy or the ileal conduit.

Less common types of urinary diversion include *ureterosigmoidostomy*, in which the **ureters** (tubes that drain urine from the kidneys to the bladder) are connected to the colon so that urine is excreted through the rectum. Because urine mixes with the contents of the colon, bowel movements are liquid, and frequent evacuation of stool is necessary. Because of the potential contamination of the urinary system by organisms of the colon, a major complication of this type of urinary diversion is *chronic pyelonephritis* (see Chapter 13).

When cancer of the bladder is *superficial*, the cancer may be treated with *bacille Calmette-Guérin (BCG)*, a form of *immunotherapy* in which the body's own immune system is stimulated to respond to and fight the cancer cells. BCG therapy consists of instilling the vaccine of BCG into the bladder. When superficial cancer of the bladder is more advanced, chemotherapy may also be used.

Cancer of the kidney may necessitate removal of the kidney (**nephrectomy**). When both kidneys are involved, a portion of one kidney may be left intact to maintain renal function. If both kidneys must be completely removed, individuals must be placed on regular dialysis (see Chapter 13).

## Cancer of the Brain or Spinal Cord

When malignant tumors of the brain are small and accessible and have not invaded surrounding tissue, they may be surgically removed and the individual treated with chemotherapy or radiation. If there are no complications from surgery, individuals may be able to return to active life. Some individuals experience some neurologic deficits after surgery (see Chapter 2). At other times, the tumor may be embedded in the brain or may be located in a part of the brain that is inaccessible, so that surgery is not possible without considerable risk to the individual. In these instances, chemotherapy or radiation therapy alone may be instituted as a means of control or palliation. The degree or type of limitation that results from a malignant brain tumor depends on the type of cancer, its size, and its location within the brain, as well as on any residues that might be experienced from surgery.

Cancers develop less often in the spinal cord than in the brain. Symptoms of a spinal cord tumor may be similar to those experienced with a spinal cord injury, including paralysis (see Chapter 3). Spinal cord tumors are usually treated surgically, with irradiation and chemotherapy as adjunct therapies.

## Lymphomas

The lymphatic system is a connection of lymph nodes and vessels in which a clear fluid called lymph circulates through the body. The lymphatic system acts to fight infection and contributes to the body's immune system (see Chapter 8). Cancers of the lymphatic system are called **lymphomas**.

There are two classifications of lymphomas:

- Hodgkin's disease
- Non-Hodgkin's lymphoma

### Hodgkin's Disease

**Hodgkin's disease** is a chronic, progressive disease in which abnormal cells gradually replace the normal elements within the lymph nodes. The cause of Hodgkin's disease is unknown. Many individuals with Hodgkin's disease are **asymptomatic** (have no symptoms) or have only peripheral **lymphadenopathy** (enlargement of lymph nodes).

Hodgkin's disease is usually diagnosed through an *excisional biopsy* of an affected lymph node. Bone marrow is rarely affected; however, a bone marrow biopsy may also be performed.

Although many individuals' disease is advanced at the time of diagnosis, advances in treatment have made Hodgkin's disease mostly curable (DeVita, 2003). Treatment of Hodgkin's disease varies with the stage at which it is diagnosed. Early stages are usually treated with radiation therapy, and later stages, with chemotherapeutic agents. In the late stage of the condition, a variety of chemotherapeutic agents may be used in combination to treat the disease. Because of the severe toxic effects of this treatment regimen, individuals may have symptoms of nausea and vomiting, bone marrow suppression, and **peripheral neuropathy** (changes of sensation in the extremities). When treated in the early stages, Hodgkin's disease has a high rate of remission, and individuals with this condition have an excellent prognosis.

### Non-Hodgkin's Lymphoma

**Non-Hodgkin's lymphomas** consist of a proliferation of lymph cells that usually disseminate throughout the body. Diagnosis is made through examination of tissue that has been removed. Often bone marrow biopsy is also done because bone marrow involvement is likely.

Unlike with Hodgkin's disease, most individuals with non-Hodgkin's lymphoma are in advanced stages of the disease before diagnosis is made. The most common symptom is generalized **adenopathy** (enlargement of the lymph nodes).The condition may be low grade, meaning that it progresses slowly, or aggressive high grade, meaning that it progresses rapidly and can be fatal in months. Individuals with high-grade non-Hodgkin's lymphoma generally have symptoms of unexplained weight loss or unexplained fever. Non-Hodgkin's lymphomas are usually treated with radiation therapy in the early stages, and chemotherapy in conjunction with radiation therapy in the later stages, with possible bone marrow transplant.

### Multiple Myeloma

Multiple myeloma is a slowly progressive cancer in which there is the uncontrolled reproduction of abnormal plasma cells leading to the destruction of the bone marrow and extending into the bone. Bone marrow produces red blood cells, white blood cells, and platelets, which control blood clotting. As the bone marrow is destroyed, individuals with multiple myeloma may experience anemia and abnormal bleeding. The first symptom of multiple myeloma is often bone pain, which may be concentrated in the back. Bone destruction can also lead to *pathologic fractures* (fractures that occur because of the disease of the bone rather than from injury) and spinal cord compression.

The diagnosis of multiple myeloma may be based on blood tests, radiologic examination of the skeletal system to identify bone destruction, or biopsy of the bone marrow itself. Chemotherapy and, at times, radiation therapy are major forms of treatment.

Because inactivity results in additional breakdown of bone, emphasis is placed on helping individuals remain active. The prognosis is dependent on the stage of the disease when diagnosed; however, multiple myeloma is not currently curable.

### Leukemia

Cancers of tissues in which blood is formed are called leukemias. There are various types of leukemias. Leukemia can be classified as *acute* or *chronic*.

### Acute Leukemia

In most instances there is no known cause of acute leukemia; however, factors such as exposure to radiation, occupational exposure to certain chemicals, and viruses and genetic links have all been cited as possible contributing factors (Appelbaum, 2000). In acute leukemia, there is proliferation of malignantly transformed *stem cells* (cells from which other cells originate) in the bone marrow that suppress the growth and differentiation of normal blood cells. Many abnormal, immature white blood cells are released into the circulatory system. As a result, individuals with acute leukemia frequently experience anemia, **neutropenia** (small numbers of mature white blood cells), and **thrombocytopenia** (abnormal number of platelets). They may also experience fatigue, headache, susceptibility to infection, and bruising or hemorrhage.

Since acute leukemia is a rapidly progressing disease, treatment is usually instituted immediately. The goal of treatment is to induce complete remission. Treatment usually consists of chemotherapy and in some instances bone marrow transplantation.

### Chronic Leukemia

Chronic leukemia consists of a broad spectrum of disorders and involves overproduction of white blood cells, causing **splenomegaly** (enlargement of the spleen). Individuals are often without symptoms initially, so that the condition is first discovered through blood tests during a routine physical, or from medical consultation because of another problem. When symptoms are present, individuals often have fatigue or weight loss.

Chronic leukemia is an unpredictable disease. In some individuals the condition progresses slowly so that they live with it for decades, often dying because of other causes, whereas in others the condition requires frequent and multiple forms of therapy and can result in death within a few years (Rai & Chiorazzi, 2003). Although there are few or no symptoms in the early stages of the disease, if the disease progresses individuals may experience headaches, bone pain, joint pain, or fever. Diagnosis is based on results of blood tests as well as the presence of an enlarged spleen.

Immediate treatment of chronic leukemia is usually not necessary unless there are complications. Initial treatment may consist of oral medication to control the abnormal blood cell proliferation. Later treatment may consist of medications such as interferon (discussed earlier in the chapter) or other types of chemotherapy.

## Cancer of the Breast

As with other types of cancer, early diagnosis of breast cancer is most predictive of prognosis and cure (Fletcher & Elmore, 2003). The use of breast self-examination and mammography can lead to early detection and, thus, permit early treatment. The primary treatment of breast cancer is based on the stage of the disease at the time of diagnosis. The treatment may be local, regional, or systemic. Local/regional control usually involves surgery.

Treatment of breast cancer previously involved removal of the entire breast through either **simple mastectomy** or **radical mastectomy**, in which the entire breast as well as its underlying tissue, including muscle and lymph nodes, was removed. Studies have shown, however, that modified procedures in many cases are just as effective in preventing metastasis or improving survival (Fisher, Bauer, Margolese et al., 1985). These alternative surgical techniques may include:

- **lumpectomy** (removal of the cancerous lesion itself and a small amount of surrounding breast tissue)
- **partial** or **segmental mastectomy** (removal of a quadrant of the breast)

The appropriateness of using more conservative surgical techniques that preserve as much of the breast tissue as possible depends on the size and location of the tumor. In many instances, regardless of the type of surgery, *radiation therapy* and *chemotherapy* are used as adjunct therapies (Burstein, Polyak, Wong, Lester, & Kaelin, 2004).

Depending on the extent of surgery, individuals may experience some limitation in arm motion on the affected side. Individuals may engage in physical therapy or other exercises to gain mobility and range of motion gradually. **Lymphedema** (swelling due to blockage of the lymph system), in which there is a swelling of the arm on the side of the mastectomy, may also occur, usually when the lymph nodes have been removed and the circulation of lymph fluid is slowed. There may also be an increased susceptibility to infection on the operative side.

### Breast Reconstruction

Recent advances in cosmetic surgery have made breast reconstruction a viable option for some individuals. Breast reconstructions that use implants or tissue transfer involve moving or transfering tissue from another part of the body and have become more common in the last few years. Prior to breast reconstruction techniques, women had few choices but to wear an external prosthesis, which could be cumbersome and uncomfortable during physical activity and was not easily incorporated into the women's body image. In breast reconstruction, the entire breast may be reconstructed (a procedure that may require two or more operations over several months' time), or, if there is sufficient chest muscle and the skin remaining after the removal of the tumor is of good quality, a prosthesis may be inserted in a pocket created under the chest muscle. In some instances there may be immediate breast reconstruction at the time of the original surgery, which ame-liorates the experience of breast loss. When the amount of muscle and tissue remaining is insufficient for breast reconstruction, other surgical procedures may be performed in which tissues from other parts of the body are used in the reconstruction of the breast. In some cases tissue expanders may be used. These are adjustable implants filled with a salt solution and inflated to stretch tissue after mastectomy. These implants may be temporary or permanent.

When breast reconstruction is not an option or the individual chooses not to have such a procedure, a permanent breast form called a prosthesis may be used. Breast forms vary in weight and are matched to the size and contour of the remaining breast. Breast prostheses are sold in surgical supply stores, or they may be available in the lingerie departments of large department stores.

### Psychosocial Issues in Breast Cancer

The psychological implications of breast cancer can be devastating for some women. The emotional impact of the loss of breast tissue varies from individual to individual. Not only are there concerns associated with the cancer itself, but there are also concerns regarding changes in appearance. Breast cancer poses a dual threat in the form of risk to life as well as threat to female self-image. Deformity that may be associated with loss of breast tissue is a constant reminder of a life-threatening disease. As a sexually associated structure and societally valued symbol of attractiveness, the breast is also closely linked to a women's self-esteem.

*The Reach to Recovery* program of the American Cancer Society has been in existence since 1969 to help women adjust to breast cancer. The program uses volunteers who have fully recovered from breast cancer to visit the individual and answer questions, provide tips, and offer encouragement. Breast cancer support groups have also been found helpful.

## Gynecological Cancer

### Types of Gynecological Cancer

Gynecological cancers consist of cancer of the *ovary, uterus, cervix,* or *external genitalia.* Regular screenings can be important in early recognition of gynecological cancers and, consequently, early treatment and cure.

*Ovarian cancer,* an insidious disease, generally shows no early detectable symptoms and has therefore often metastasized by the time the cancer is diagnosed. When ovarian cancer is diagnosed, surgery is always required, with probably chemotherapy after surgery.

*Cancer of the cervix* (the neck of the uterus, opening into the vagina) is detected through regular Pap screening in which cancer cells can be identified microscopically. Early-stage cervical cancer usually has no symptoms, so regular screening is important for finding the disease early. If cervical cancer is untreated, it can invade other organs and metastasize. In early disease, and especially if the woman wants to preserve fertility, the cancerous portion of the cervix may be excised, leaving the uterus. If the cancer is more advanced, the cervix and uterus are removed (**total hysterectomy**).

Cancer of the **endometrium** (lining of the uterus) is diagnosed by biopsy of the endometrium. Early symptoms of *endometrial cancer* consist of abnormal uterine bleeding. Treatment usually consists of hysterectomy with accompanying **oophorectomy** (removal of the ovaries). There are generally no physical limitations associated with gynecological cancer and its treatment; however, individuals with advanced disease, or those who undergo chemotherapy or radiation therapy in combination with surgery, may experience fatigue and other side effects related to the therapy itself.

### Psychosocial Issues in Gynecological Cancer

In addition to the stress caused by having a diagnosis of cancer, the psychological issues associated with gynecological surgery may cause some individuals significant distress. Gynecological surgery because of cancer may produce changes in the perception of body image, fertility, or sexuality. Removal of reproductive organs may have emotional and psychological consequences on the perception of sexual function, which affects the relationship with the woman's partner. Although, for the most part, surgery such as hysterectomy should not impair sexual function, considerable misinformation may also surround gynecological surgery and can cause concern for the woman and her significant other. In instances where the cancer involves the external genitalia and necessitates removal, disfigurement and threat to body image may also pose significant emotional distress. Providing the individual and her partner with accurate information about the surgery and its implications can help to alleviate problems.

## Cancer of the Prostate

The prostate is a gland that surrounds the urethra in males and secretes fluid that bathes and nourishes human semen. Prostate cancer may be detected through screening techniques, including physical examination and a blood test for prostate-specific antigen. Other symptoms that individuals may experience are difficulties in urination due to bladder outlet obstruction.

Another condition, *benign prostatic hypertrophy*, although not a malignancy, may cause similar problems. Consequently, *biopsy* of the prostate is generally needed to confirm the diagnosis of cancer.

Treatment, as with other types of cancer, is determined mainly by staging of the cancer. *Radical proctectomy*, in which the prostate gland is removed, may be performed; however, another procedure, *cryotherapy*, in which the prostate is frozen with liquid nitrogen so that tissue **necrosis** (death) occurs, is also used. Individuals may have adjunctive therapy, which includes *hormone therapy* or *radiation therapy*. The complications of surgery in some individuals with prostate cancer include *impotence* and *incontinence*.

### Skin Cancers

Skin cancer is the uncontrolled growth and reproduction of abnormal skin cells. Most skin cancers, if detected and treated early, can be cured. The number one risk factor associated with skin cancer is overexposure to the sun. Individuals with fair skin are more at risk than those with darker skin. Prevention of skin cancer involves protection for ultraviolet exposure, in addition to using sunscreen, covering skin with clothing, and minimizing outdoor activities when the sun is the strongest.

There are several types of skin cancer. *Basal cell cancers* are the most common type of skin cancer and originate in the layer of cells that form the base between the **epidermis** (top layer of skin cells) and the lower level of skin cells called the **dermis** (see Chapter 15). Less common are *squamous cell cancers*, which originate in the uppermost layers of skin. Both types of skin cancer usually do not spread and are easily cured if treated promptly. Treatment usually consists of removal. The most serious type of skin cancer is *malig-nant melanoma*, a cancer that originates from the melanocytes, the cells that produce the skin's pigment or color. Malignant melanoma spreads quickly and is more frequently fatal. Therapy for melanoma is primarily surgical.

## PSYCHOSOCIAL ISSUES IN CANCER

### Psychological Issues

Regardless of the type of cancer or the type of treatment, psychological issues arise in all individuals with cancer. Reactions to the diagnosis of cancer vary according to the individual and often depend not only on the type and extent of the cancer, but also on individuals' particular situation and coping skills.

Despite medical and treatment advances, the word *cancer* still generates fear in many individuals and is stigmatizing for others. Cancer is often perceived as a threat to their mortality and their future, no matter what the actual prognosis. Individuals may fear loss of relationships, independence, job, and integrity of the body and its functions, as well as loss of life. A diagnosis of cancer may also be a symbol of vulnerability, loss of control, or helplessness. Even when the prognosis is good, fear of recurrence lingers with many individuals. When disfigurement due to surgical procedures accompanies the diagnosis of cancer, adjustment to the altered self-image causes further stress and anxiety.

Many individuals with cancer are emotionally overwhelmed when they first learn their diagnosis. Their initial reactions may include depression, irritability, fear, withdrawal, anger and hostility, or denial. Over time, they may come to accept their condition and try to make whatever adaptations are necessary to proceed with life.

Individuals who are younger when diagnosed with cancer may experience greater psychological distress. Body image may be more greatly affected, education and career paths may need to be postponed, and economic and social independence may be thwarted. The cost of treatment may be prohibitive for young adults who have not had the opportunity to establish a financially secure base. Forming or maintaining intimate relationships may also be made more difficult because of the diagnosis, regardless of the prognosis.

Coping with cancer is not static, but rather a dynamic process, evolving over time (Livneh, 2000). Through each clinical stage of cancer, individuals utilize different coping skills to learn how to live with a potentially life-threatening condition. The reactions of individuals during each phase can determine their level of functioning as well as their adherence to the medical protocol.

Holland (1989) described four phases of coping during the clinical course of cancer. Individuals with cancer experience different concerns and different psychological reactions at each phase. The first phase is described as the phase when symptoms are first identified. During this time individuals may experience anxiety, which can either serve as motivation to seek medical attention or, if the anxiety is too great, lead to denial of symptoms and delay in seeking medical diagnosis and subsequent treatment. Phase two is described as the period during which a definitive diagnosis of cancer is made. Depending on their premorbid perceptions of cancer, individuals may experience significant emotional distress or display an attitude of problem solving and determination to do whatever is necessary for cure. The third phase involves the treatment and adjuvant therapy. During this phase individuals may express positive feelings of

empowerment in actively participating in battling the disease, or they may experience feelings of hopelessness and doom. During the fourth phase, when the treatments are completed, individuals may be in remission (free from cancer symptoms). During this time, they may have feelings of uncertainty regarding the possibility of recurrence or the development of another cancer at a future date. In this last clinical phase, individuals may have feelings of vulnerability and uncertainty about future plans or feelings of confidence and optimism about working toward goals for the future.

In some instances, individuals may minimize the seriousness of the illness in an attempt to assimilate its impact and to marshal the resources and coping skills needed to deal with the perceived threat. Clarifying ambiguity and uncertainty while permitting denial is at times a difficult balancing act for all concerned. Some individuals cope by finding a general purpose or meaning to the illness that establishes a framework for the events experienced. Other individuals gain a sense of control by seeking as much information as possible about their disease and treatment. Information can be an important tool in reducing anxiety, but it must be acquired at a rate that is manageable for the individual (Leydon, Boulton, Moynihan, Jones, et al., 2000). As a result of increased cancer survival rates, the quality of the individual's life and the individual's involvement in treatment decisions have become a central issue.

Coping with cancer is an ongoing effort in which the individual reacts to the disease and its implications. Issues for individuals vary across a lifetime, since each life stage has its own opportunities and limitations. Reactions are influenced by outside forces as well as by intrinsic capabilities. Living with the fear of recurrence may promote stress and anxiety

(McGrath, 1999). Individuals may need help in coping with the distress caused by the therapy used to treat their cancer. The uncertainty of not knowing when or if the cancer will recur, or if a new malignancy will develop, can be a constant source of apprehension. Individuals may exhibit a wide spectrum of normal adaptive responses that may change over the course of the disease, or over time.

### Lifestyle Issues

The extent to which cancer affects individuals' everyday activities depends on the type and location of the cancer and its treatment. The side effects of radiation therapy or chemotherapy, such as nausea, loss of appetite, or fatigue, may affect daily activities during treatment or for a short time after treatment. Certain surgical procedures for various types of cancer may also affect individuals' lifestyle to some degree. For example, amputation, colostomy, and laryngectomy all require some adaptation of certain daily tasks.

The effects of cancer on sexuality are diverse. Some individuals experience no difficulty with sexual functioning. Others experience a decrease in sexual desire because of fatigue, pain, depression, or anxiety. Some forms of cancer and its treatment may have direct impact on sexual activity; for example, surgery may directly affect the organs of sexual function. Surgery may also have indirect effects on sexual activity if it alters individuals' physical appearance, thus changing body image and self-esteem. Regardless of whether cancer directly or indirectly affects individuals' ability to engage in sexual intercourse, the need for closeness and demonstration of affection, such as hugging, touching, or kissing, is usually unchanged.

### Social Issues

Despite public education about the new medical advances that render many cancers curable, the general public, and perhaps even the family and friends of individuals with cancer, may still hold the unfounded belief that *cancer* is a synonym for *death*. Such misconceptions may lead to the emotional withdrawal of friends and acquaintances to lessen the impact of loss before it occurs.

Acquaintances may avoid individuals with cancer because the diagnosis reminds them of their own mortality and because it engenders unpleasant feelings. The physical changes that occur because of surgery or treatment may make friends or family uncomfortable and may contribute to aversion and further avoidance. Others may have the mistaken notion that cancer is contagious and avoid close physical contact with individuals or shun them altogether.

Just as alienation may result from the diagnosis of cancer, so may overprotection and enforced dependency, both of which erode individuals' sense of self-esteem and control. Family and friends may feel the need to protect individuals, as well as themselves, from the realities of cancer. Family members may not share their feelings and concerns, creating tension within the family group. As a result, the impact of the condition and the associated emotions may be denied. The individual with cancer, in order to avoid alienation or rejection, may also conceal his or her true emotions.

The challenges that confront family members of individuals with cancer are shaped by the type of cancer, the extent of disease, the type of treatment, and the quality of family relationship prior to diagnosis and the concurrent stressors they may be experiencing (Sherman & Simonton, 2001). Because cancer may change over time, with remissions, relapses, need for additional treatment, or just unpredictability, individuals' place and role in the family may change and require different approaches over time (Moulton, 2000).

The extent to which the cancer affects social activities depends not only on the attitudes and acceptance of the individuals involved, but also on physical factors, such as pain and fatigue. Medical considerations, including the time spent at the hospital and in treatment, may disrupt social and family activities. Special provisions that encourage individuals to participate in social activities can decrease the disruption and the sense of conflict felt by these individuals and their families over time.

## VOCATIONAL ISSUES IN CANCER

There have been a number of reports of employment discrimination and lack of rehabilitation services for persons with cancer (Conti, 1995; Feldman, 1987; Hoffman, 1991). One report sited a survey that found that workers with cancer were fired or laid off five times as often as other workers (Arnold, 1999). Work takes on particular importance, not only from a financial standpoint, but also as a symbol of self-esteem, self-sufficiency, and an affirmation of life.

As with other diseases and disabilities, the most significant barriers to employment after a diagnosis of cancer may be the attitudes of employers and fellow workers, who may have the same misperceptions about cancer that some other social groups have. Attitudes of hopelessness related to cancer diagnosis may be expressed in employers' reluctance to allow individuals with cancer to return to work, their unwillingness to make concessions for any associated limitations, or their rejection of special aspects of treatment. In

some instances employers and coworkers may view cancer as a contagious disease. Employers may also express concern about the ability of these individuals to perform the same work-related tasks for which they had been responsible prior to diagnosis, and may view cancer survivors as a potential economic burden rather than as productive employees.

Although courts have argued about the status of cancer survivors under the American with Disabilities Act (ADA), others have agreed that ADA provides important legal rights for individuals with cancer (Hodges, 1999). As courts continue to discuss the definition of disability, educating and informing employers and individuals with cancer about the protections that ADA provides is an important step in advocacy and in helping individuals obtain or maintain employment for which they are qualified and which they desire (Arnold, 1999).

Vocational planning requires an awareness of the attitudes and prejudice that may exist in the work setting, as well as a specific knowledge about the condition and its treatment requirements, individuals' functional limitations, and the demands of the work setting. Because the limitations and prognosis vary with the type and location of cancer, the type of plan, and whether short-term or long-term planning is most feasible, are dependent to a great extent on these factors. It is also necessary to understand the multidimensional impact of the diagnosis of cancer on the individual and the family. The degree to which individuals' former employment is still suitable is dependent on many variables and must be examined realistically in the context of the demands and implications of returning to the former work setting, as well as in the context of the individual's own particular strengths and limitations.

## CASE STUDIES

### Case I

Mr. R. is a 52-year-old real estate agent. He has worked as a real estate agent for the past 15 years. Previously he was a high school mathematics teacher. He has always been a heavy smoker. Several months ago he sought medical attention because of persistent hoarseness. On evaluation, the physician noted a nodule on Mr. R.'s vocal cord and suggested a biopsy. The nodule was malignant, and as a result, Mr. R. had a total laryngectomy. He is able to talk with an electronic device. He is married to his second wife and has two grown children from his first marriage. The physician is hopeful that the surgery will cure the cancer and has recommended no chemotherapy or radiation.

#### Questions

1. What specific issues related to the laryngectomy would you consider when assessing Mr. R.'s rehabilitation potential?
2. What limitations would Mr. R. experience after his laryngectomy?
3. Is it feasible for Mr. R. to continue in his current line of employment?
4. Are there specific accommodations or assistive devices that may be helpful to Mr. R. in helping him achieve his full vocational potential?

### Case II

Ms. D. has worked as a librarian for the past 20 years. She is currently 45 years old, is married, and has two grown daughters. She recently noted a lump in her left breast. She consulted her physician, and on biopsy the lump was found to be malignant. Ms. D. had a total mastectomy. Twelve lymph nodes were also involved; consequently, the physician recommended a course of chemotherapy. As a result of the chemotherapy Ms. D. has lost all of her hair. She has now completed the course of chemotherapy, however, and her physician says she should be ready to return to work.

#### Questions

1. What issues related to Ms. D.'s medical condition would be important to consider when evaluating Ms. D.'s rehabilitation potential?
2. What psychosocial factors might be important to address in Ms. D.'s rehabilitation plan?
3. What types of services or assistive devices might help Ms. D. reach her full rehabilitation potential?

## REFERENCES

Appelbaum, F. R. (2000). The acute leukemias. In L. Goldman & J. C. Bennett (Eds.), *Cecil textbook of medicine* (21st ed., pp. 953–958). Philadelphia: W. B. Saunders.

Arnold, K. (1999). Americans With Disabilities Act: Do cancer patients qualify as disabled? *Journal of the National Cancer Institute, 91*(10), 822–825.

Brown, L. M., Hoover, R., Silverman, D., et al. (2001). Excess incidence of squamous cell esophageal cancer among US black men: Role of social class and other risk factors. *American Journal of Epidemiology, 153*, 114–122.

Burstein, H. J., Polyak, K., Wong, J. S., Lester, S. C., & Kaelin, C. M. (2004). Ductal carcinoma in situ of the breast. *New England Journal of Medicine, 350*(14), 1430–1441.

Cleary, J., Gorenstein, L. A., & Omenn, G. S. (1996, September 15). Lung cancer: Prevention is the best cure. *Patient Care,* pp. 35, 36, 39, 42, 45–47, 51, 52, 55, 59, 60, 62, 67.

Conti, J. V. (1995). Job discrimination against people with cancer history. *Journal of Applied Rehabilitation Counseling, 26*(2), 12–16.

DeVita, V. (2003). Hodgkin's disease: Clinical trials and travails. *New England Journal of Medicine, 348*(24), 2375–2376.

Droller, M. J. (1998). Bladder cancer: State of the art care. *CA: A Cancer Journal for Clinicians, 48*(5), 269–284.

Enzinger, P. C., & Mayer, R. J. (2003). Esophageal cancer. *New England Journal of Medicine, 349*(23), 2241–2252.

Feldman, F. L. (1987). The return to work: The question of workability. In *Proceedings of the workshop on employment insurance and the patient with cancer, 1987* (pp. 27–35). New York: American Cancer Society.

Fisher, B., Bauer, M., Margolese, R., et al. (1985). Five year results of a randomized clinical trial comparing total mastectomy and segmental mastectomy with or without radiation in the treatment of breast cancer. *New England Journal of Medicine, 312*, 665–673.

Fletcher, S. W., & Elmore, J. G. (2003). Mammographic screening for breast cancer. *New England Journal of Medicine, 348*(17), 1672–1679.

Forastiere, A. A., Goepfert, H., Maor, M., Pajak, T. F., Weber, R., Morrison, W., Glisson, B., Trotti, A., Ridge, J. A., Chao, C., Peters, G., Lee, D. J., Leaf, A., Ensley, J., & Cooper, J. (2003). Concurrent chemotherapy and radiotherapy for organ preservation in advanced laryngeal cancer. *New England Journal of Medicine, 349*(22), 2091–2098.

Green, M. R. (2004). Targeting targeted therapy. *New England Journal of Medicine, 350*(21), 2191–2195.

Hodges, A. C. (1999). The Americans With Disabilities Act: Legal protection for the employment of the cancer patient. Legal Information Network for Cancer. Retrieved June 7, 2004, from http://www.cancerline.org/adact.html.

Hoffman, B. (1991). Employment discrimination: Another hurdle for cancer survivors. *Cancer Investigation, 9*, 589–595.

Holland, J. C. (1989). Clinical course of cancer. In J. C. Holland & J. H. Rowlands (Eds.), *Handbook of psychooncology: Psychological care of the patient with cancer* (pp. 75–100). New York: Oxford University Press.

Lagergren, J., Bergstrom, R., Adami, H. O., & Nyren, O. (2000). Association between medications that relax the lower esophageal spincter and risk for esophageal adenocarcinoma. *Annals of Internal Medicine, 133*, 165–175.

Leydon, G. M., Boulton, M., Moynihan, C., Jones, A., et al. (2000). Cancer patients' information needs and information seeking behaviour: In-depth interview study. *British Medical Journal, 320*(7239), 909–916.

Livneh, H. (2000). Psychosocial adaptation to cancer: The role of coping strategies. *Journal of Rehabilitation, 66*(2), 40–49.

McGrath, P. (1999, July–September). Posttraumatic stress and the experience of cancer: A literature review. *Journal of Rehabilitation, 65*, 17–23.

Miller, Y. E. (2000). Pulmonary neoplasms. In L. Goldman & J. C. Bennett (Eds.), *Cecil textbook of medicine* (21st ed., pp. 449–455). Philadelphia: W. B. Saunders.

Moulton, G. (2000). Cancer survivor issues are all in the family. *Journal of the National Cancer Institute, 92*(2), 101–103.

Pappas, T. N., & Jacobs, D. O. (2004). Laparoscopic resection for colon cancer: The end of the beginning? *New England Journal of Medicine, 350*(20), 2091–2092.

Rai, K., & Chiorazzi, N. (2003). Determining the clinical course and outcome in chronic lymphocytic leukemia. *New England Journal of Medicine, 348*(18), 1797–1799.

Rosenberg, S. A. (2004). Shedding light on immunotherapy for cancer. *New England Journal of Medicine, 350*(14), 1461–1463.

Shaheen, N. & Ransohoff, D. F. (2002). Gastroesophageal reflux, Barrett esophagus, and esophageal cancer: Scientific review. *Journal of the American Medical Association, 287*, 1972–1981.

Sherman, A. C., & Simonton, S. (2001). Coping with cancer in the family. *The Family Journal: Counseling and Therapy for Couples and Families, 9*(2), 193–200.

Terry, P., Lagergren, J., Ye, W., Nyren, O., & Wolk, A. (2000). Antioxidants and cancers of the esophagus and gastric cardia. *International Journal of Cancer, 87*, 750–754.

Vokes, E. E., & Stenson, K. M. (2003). Therapeutic options for laryngeal cancer. *New England Journal of Medicine, 349*(22), 2087–2089.

Wu, A. H., Wan, P., & Bernstein, L. (2001). A multiethnic population-based study of smoking, alcohol and body size and risk of adenocarcinoma of the stomach and esophagus (United States). *Cancer Causes and Control, 12*, 721–732.

Zeitels, S. M., & Healy, G. B. (2003). Laryngology and phonosurgery. *New England Journal of Medicine, 349*(9), 882–892.

# CHAPTER 17

# Assistive Devices

## DEFINING ASSISTIVE TECHNOLOGY

Assistive technology includes any device that is used to promote the functional capabilities of persons with disabilities (Assistive Technology Act of 1998; Blake & Bodine, 2002). An assistive technology device has been defined in the law as "any item, piece of equipment, or product system, whether acquired commercially off the shelf, modified, or customized, that is used to increase, maintain, or improve the functional capabilities of individuals with disabilities" (Assistive Technology Act of 1998, p. 112 STAT. 3631).

Assistive technology enables people to achieve personal goals and to move toward future achievements, as well as to gain employment and be independent in activities of daily living and in society. Technology plays an important role in rehabilitation because it increases the functional capacity of individuals with disabilities. The development of new technologies has made the home, education, and work environments more accessible for persons with a disability and has increased their social, educational, and employment opportunities (Berry & Ignash, 2003). However, the proliferation of technology sometimes makes it difficult to ensure that, as devices are developed, they truly meet the needs of the individuals for whom they are intended (Blair, 2000;

Kroll, Beatty, & Bingham, 2003). It is always important to ascertain whether the assistive device chosen for a specific disability is most appropriate to the individual's needs and is reasonably priced.

Assistive technology and its associated services, if they are to be applied effectively, must be viewed within the context of the life of the individual. Having technology available does not necessarily mean that the resulting assistive device will be useful or that it will be used. Many factors aside from availability are relevant (Hasselbring & Glaser, 2000).

Individuals with disabilities should be actively involved in choosing their assistive devices and in assessing the devices' effectiveness. Devices can range anywhere from do-it-yourself items, such as a paint can opener to help when there is reduced hand strength or low-tech devices such as canes or crutches (Allen, 2001), to sophisticated computer software for individuals with cognitive impairments (Hasselbring & Glaser, 2000). Regardless of the sophistication of adaptive devices, however, the most effective device will still be one that individuals are willing and able to use in their own environment to meet their specific needs. Consequently, before any device is selected, it is important to consider the individual's specific goals and tasks within a given environment, his or her psychosocial incentives

485

and disincentives, his or her personal characteristics, and his or her abilities and preferences (Blair, 2000).

Assistive technology is made to improve functioning in the following areas (Hedman, 1992):

- Accessibility
- Seating
- Mobility
- Augmentative communication
- Environmental control
- Computer access
- Home modification
- Workplace modification

Thus, the assistive devices used for achieving greater functional capacity in these areas can include the following:

- Aids to daily living (Thyberg, Hass, Nordenskiod, & Skogh, 2004)
- Mobility aids (Chen, Chen, Chen, & Lin, 2003)
- Sensory aids (Sokol-McKay, Buskirk, & Whittaker, 2003)
- Communication aids (Neumann et al., 2004).
- Cognitive memory aids (Hammel, 2003)
- Adaptive computer aids (Fichten, Barile, Asuncion, & Fossey, 2000)
- Controls and switches (LoPresti, Brienza, Angelo, & Gilbertson, 2003)
- Environmental accommodations (O'Day, Palsbo, Dhont, & Scheer, 2002)

## INDIVIDUAL ASSESSMENT

Individuals' physical as well as psychosocial environment has an impact on the usefulness of an assistive device. Consequently, the characteristics of the environment must always be considered (Blair, 2000; Hammel, 2003). Both the type and number of assistive devices needed will vary. Few people function in only one set-

ting. Thus, individuals with disabilities may require specific devices for activities of daily living, different devices to be used at work, and still other devices to be used in social and recreational settings.

People with similar disabilities may not require the same type or the same number of assistive devices. The type of assistive device needed depends on where the equipment will be used, the tasks and activities required in each environment, and the extent to which tasks would be enhanced by the use of the device. Architectural accessibility and the amount of environmental support needed for the use of an assistive device also are important considerations. The physical environment in which the assistive device is to be operated must be assessed, and obstacles that could interfere with the device's use must be identified. At times, environmental modification alone may increase the individual's ability to function. As society becomes increasingly aware of the need for universal design so that environments are more accessible for all individuals, many physical barriers that exist today may be nonexistent in the future.

In addition to the physical environment, the psychosocial environment also has an impact on the usefulness of assistive devices. The amount of support and encouragement individuals receive from others in their environment may be a major determinant in the degree to which an assistive device is used.

The cultural environment in which individuals function also plays a major role in the type of device obtained and the extent to which it is used. For example, not all individuals who are deaf or hard of hearing believe that they need to compensate for their decreased ability to hear. Many individuals who are deaf have a strong cultural identity with the Deaf community and may not be receptive to many of the technological advances that are currently available or that may become available in the future.

A thorough assessment of the individual's preferences and needs must be conducted before an assistive device is obtained. If one type of device is inadequate to meet an individual's needs, it should not be assumed that there are no viable alternatives. Likewise, it should not be assumed that all individuals with the same disability require the same type of device. Although it is likely that individuals with severe disability may require high-technology devices, it should not automatically be assumed that individuals want that type of device or that other devices could not be equally useful.

Although access to consumer-responsible assistive devices and services is federally mandated, individuals differ in their needs, values, perspectives, motivations, and expectations, all of which can affect the use of assistive devices. All assistive devices should be matched to individuals' capabilities and temperament. The success of adaptive devices is often determined by the degree to which adaptive devices match individuals' values and perspectives rather than the potential usefulness of the device for day-to-day activities.

## TYPES OF ASSISTIVE DEVICES

Individuals' use of assistive devices and the type of device used may change over time or as they age. If individuals have a progressive disability, different assistive devices may be needed over time to accommodate additional limitations. In other instances, different devices may be required because an individual's lifestyle has changed. Human circumstances are not static. Flexibility must be maintained in evaluating the continuing and changing needs of individuals.

Assistive devices vary in complexity. Whereas some devices are relatively easy to use, others require considerable training and practice before they can be used effectively. The most effective assistive device is one that individuals are comfortable using and one that meets their own particular needs. Technological devices, especially if they are high tech, may be intimidating to some individuals. Anxiety or insecurity about the ability to use a device may cause them to avoid using it or to abandon it. The more sophisticated the device, the more complicated it may be to use.

### Devices for Activities of Daily Living

Devices used in general activities of daily living such as grooming, eating, bathing, toileting, and dressing are generally low-tech aids, and although they usually are less expensive, they are vital to independence and to reaching goals in other areas. They can be as simple as an item purchased from a hardware store, or they can be specially manufactured to meet a specific need.

The type of functional limitations and the environments in which the device is to be used determine the type of device needed for activities of daily living. Individuals' needs may change as they move to different environments. For example, devices used in the home for activities of daily living may not be appropriate on a business trip. The appropriateness of each device should be considered in the context of the setting in which it is to be used.

A variety of devices used by individuals *without disability* also help to increase the functional capacity of individuals *with disability*. Devices such as microwave ovens, electric can openers, and other electronic devices may be convenience items for people without disability, but the same devices also can significantly increase the functional capacity and independence of people with disabilities. The increasing sophistication of computers, robotics, and other electronic devices may also offer more functional independence in activities of daily living for persons with disabilities in the future.

## Mobility Aids

Low-tech aids, such as canes or walkers, or high-tech aids, such as manual or power wheelchairs or scooters, are used to help individuals achieve mobility. Microcomputer-controlled power wheelchairs and powered wheelchairs with puff-sip controls provide increased mobility to individuals with severe disabilities. New technological advances may provide wheelchairs that have instrumentation to alert users that they are too close to objects or that decrease power when there is an object in the path (Galvin & Scherer, 1996). Different wheeled mobility devices may be needed for the same individuals. Some individuals may require one type of wheelchair for indoor use and another type for sports or outdoor use.

Transportation is also an important mobility need, both for getting to work and for increased independence. Hand controls and steering devices to accommodate the needs of individuals with limited use of one or more extremity enable individuals to drive standard motor vehicles. Van conversions such as wheelchair lifts enable individuals to carry wheelchairs or scooters, which can then be used at their point of destination.

The sophistication of mobility and transportation devices will continue to be enhanced in the future. It is possible, however, that without public awareness, environmental constraints will still be a barrier to full adaptation. Wheeled mobility aids as well as transportation aids are only maximally effective when the environment accommodates their use. Both adaptive devices and environmental modifications are necessary for individuals to reach their full independent living and work potential.

## Sensory Devices

A variety of adaptive devices are available for individuals with sensory impairments, ranging in sophistication from simple to complex. For example, an item as simple as a bath thermometer may be important to a person with sensory impairment of the lower extremities in order to prevent burns when bathing, and an optical-to-vibrotactile prosthesis can make it possible for individuals who are blind to distinguish patterns of stimulation so that they can discriminate between certain properties of three-dimensional space.

Assistive devices for individuals with visual impairment may range from glasses to voice recognition computers. A variety of low-vision aids that magnify or enhance visual images may also be used. Assistive devices for individuals with deafness or who are hard of hearing may use amplification, vibrotactile prompts, or visual cues. Assistive devices such as hearing aids and telecommunication display devices can help individuals who are deaf or hard of hearing to function in a hearing world.

## Communication Devices

Communication is a complex activity involving perception and integration of information and includes speaking, writing, reading and hearing, or signing as well as other nonverbal means of communicating. Assistive devices to aid in communication currently range from low-tech devices such as books to high-tech, augmentative communication devices, which are computers. Whether individuals use low-technology or high-technology devices, a certain degree of cognitive and motor ability as well as training is required.

Communication devices can be manual or electronic. Examples of manual devices are communication boards or other systems in which individuals spell out messages or indicate phrases to another person. Electronic systems are often computer based and may filter or manipulate vocalizations or provide synthesized speech.

Because of the complexity of communication and the varying capabilities and needs of individuals in different situations, no one type of device is appropriate for everyone. The device chosen to augment or enhance communication must be one that meets the specifications of the individual who will be using it. Because communication is such an individual and personal function, the individuals using a device are the best qualified to evaluate whether it improves communication outcomes.

### Cognitive Memory Aids

Memory problems, whether related to brain injury or dementia, can impair individuals' quality of life and ability to function independently. Although there are many memory improvement techniques that have been utilized to help individuals increase memory performance, improvement is often short-lived. A number of external devices or systems that serve as memory enhancements have been developed. Some assistive devices permit the user to record and play back messages; others are used as reminders, such as voice-activated reminder calendars; both can be of help to individuals with memory problems.

### Adaptive Computer Aids

Computer technology can help individuals become more independent and can enhance their ability to overcome a wide range of limitations. Some disabilities, however, make computer use difficult. For individuals with these disabilities, a number of assistive devices, such as head controls, can provide an alternative means to computer access. Software has also been developed that automatically adjusts to the needs of the particular individual, especially if the disability limits head or neck movement as well as movement of the upper extremities (LoPresti & Brienza, 2004).

### Controls and Switches

Control mechanisms or switches may be used to operate computers, communication aids, and home environmental controls.

### Environmental Modifications

Accessibility can involve more than architectural structure. Assistive devices for use in the environment can also increase individuals' ability to function within their environment. Simple examples are a Braille labeler to help in identifying items, or a talking smoke alarm as a warning system.

## OTHER TYPES OF ASSISTIVE DEVICES

Although all assistive devices help individuals with disabilities obtain greater functional capacity and independence in some way, not all devices are directly related to an activity or function. Some assistive devices may be used for cosmetic purposes, such as a prosthetic external ear, which may have limited functional use but can be important to the individual's willingness to participate in social inter-actions. In other instances, assistive de-vices help to prevent complications from occurring that may interfere with individ-uals' functional capacity. For example, pressure sores are a major complication for individuals with limited mobility or lack of sensation and can result in extended hos-pital stays, time off from work, and sub-stantial cost. Thus, devices to prevent pres-sure sores from occurring, although not directly related to function, help individ-uals achieve their full functional capacity.

## SERVICE ANIMALS

Although not "devices" per se, service animals can greatly enhance individuals' functional capacity in home, work, or so-cial environments. Although dogs are most often used, simian aids can also be used for a variety of tasks, such as retrieving items that have been dropped, obtaining items that they have been instructed to re-trieve, opening doors, and replacing or storing items in their appropriate place.

Guide dogs can help individuals with visual impairments increase their mobili-ty, and service dogs for individuals with hearing impairments can alert individuals to sounds that require action, such as a baby crying or a doorbell ringing. Larger dogs may assist individuals in wheelchairs to obtain greater mobility by helping to pull a wheelchair when greater propulsion is needed.

## ASSISTIVE DEVICES FOR RECREATION

The assistive devices needed for recre-ational activities, as with all other activi-ties, vary with individual need, interest, and ability. Technology already has creat-ed sports equipment that enables athletes without disability to achieve far greater

records than previously had been expect-ed. Some of the same types of technology applied to recreational devices for individ-uals with disabilities have created a new freedom not previously enjoyed.

The sophistication of the technology used for recreational equipment varies with the activity. The technology needed for assisting individuals in card playing is much different from that needed for help-ing individuals in downhill skiing. Not all individuals want to pursue the same type of recreation they enjoyed prior to their disability, but some embrace the opportu-nity to continue. Frequently, the largest barrier to continuing the recreational ac-tivities of their choice is the bias of those around them, who feel that certain activi-ties are now unrealistic or inappropriate.

## ASSISTIVE DEVICES IN THE WORKPLACE

Additional assistive devices may not be needed in the workplace if appropriate en-vironmental accommodations can be made. For some individuals, modification of the environment through better light-ing, air temperature control, or removal of obstacles may be all that is necessary to enable them to return to their full func-tional capacity. In other instances, finding alternate ways to perform a job function or modifying existing devices may pro-duce the same result.

When assistive devices are needed in the workplace, as in other settings, the type of device is determined by the specific need and the individual's preference. As in oth-er areas of the individual's life, high-tech devices are not always the most appropri-ate or effective way to meet an individual's need or to increase his or her ability to per-form a specific function effectively. Focus-ing on individuals' ability rather than disability and including them in the process of determining what is needed is the most useful approach to determining what, if any, adaptive devices will be beneficial.

## APPRAISAL OF ASSISTIVE DEVICES AND ALTERNATIVES

As new technologies become available, there are more choices of assistive devices to meet specific needs. Ironically, the number of choices available may make it more difficult to choose the device best suited to the individual. Assistive devices must be assessed realistically. It is important that performance claims made by the manufacturer be substantiated by research. New devices on the market should have been appropriately evaluated, and performance results, as well as safety and durability information, should be obtained.

One should also assess the degree to which an assistive device can be upgraded or expanded as new technology becomes available to accommodate new features. In some instances, compatibility with other assistive devices may also be important to determine. The initial cost of the assistive device, its maintenance costs, the availability of resources for repair and associated costs, and the costs of replacement should all be assessed.

It is also important to assess the degree to which a device accurately reflects an individual's preferences, lifestyle, and values. The availability of less elaborate assistive devices should be weighed against more elaborate devices in the context of the specific needs of the individual. Whether or not a device is portable may determine if an individual can use the device in more than one setting. The degree to which assistance is needed to learn to use a device and the extent to which the device can be used independently are also factors that affect utilization.

Although emphasis is placed on the degree to which a device increases functional capacity or quality of life, the aesthetics of the device also cannot be ignored. The appearance of a device, its ease of use, and how disruptive its use may be in certain settings can determine individuals' willingness to use it. If individuals feel conspicuous using a device or believe the device is stigmatizing or interferes with social interaction, it may be abandoned.

The physical and cognitive abilities needed to use an assistive device also are important considerations. Ergonomic aspects, as well as individuals' ability to learn to use a device and maintain it, should be explored. The best assistive device is not always the most expensive. Locating the best assistive device requires closely examining the costs and benefits of the device as opposed to available alternatives and then matching the device to the individual's specific needs and resources.

To maximize the effectiveness of assistive devices, professionals working with individuals need to have comprehensive knowledge of the disability and its limitations (Kroll & Neri, 2003; Wehman, Wilson, Parent, Sherron-Targett, & McKinley, 2000), a good understanding of the multiple consequences of access barriers and barriers to service delivery (Bingham & Beatty, 2003; Neri & Kroll, 2003), and a knowledge of bureaucratic structure that could interfere with appropriate service delivery (Darrah, Magil-Evans, & Adkins, 2002; O'Day et al., 2002). Most of all, however, professionals need to involve individuals with disabilities in the decisions about assistive devices and ask those individuals how they can best help them meet their goals and achieve maximum function and independence.

## REFERENCES

Allen, S. M. (2001). Canes, crutches and home care services: The interplay of human and technological assistance. *Center of Home Care Policy Research and Policy Briefs*, Fall(4), 1–6.

Assistive Technology Act of 1998. PL 105-394 http://www.section508.gov/docs/AT1998.html (retrieved May 16, 2004).

Berry, B. E., & Ignash, S. (2003). Assistive technology: Providing independence for individuals with disabilities. *Rehabilitation Nursing, 28*(1), 6–14.

Bingham, S. S., & Beatty, P. W. (2003). Rates of access to assistive equipment and medical rehabilitation services among people with disabilities. *Disability Rehabilitation, 25*(9), 487–490.

Blair, M. E. (2000). Assistive technology: What and how for persons with spinal cord injury. *SCI Nursing, 17*(3), 110–118.

Blake, D. J., & Bodine, C. (2002). An overview of assistive technology for persons with multiple sclerosis. *Journal of Rehabilitation Research and Development, 39*(2), 299–312.

Chen, Y. L., Chen, S. C., Chen, W. L., & Lin, J. F. (2003). A head oriented wheelchair for people with disabilities. *Disability Rehabilitation, 25*(6), 249–253.

Darrah, J., Magil-Evans, J., & Adkins, R. (2002). How well are we doing? Families of adolescents or young adults with cerebral palsy share their perceptions of service delivery. *Disability Rehabilitation, 24*(10), 542–549.

Fichten, C. S., Barile, M., Asuncion, J. V., & Fossey, M. E. (2000). What government, agencies, and organizations can do to improve access to computers for postsecondary students with disabilities: Recommendations based on Canadian empirical data. *International Journal of Rehabilitation Research, 23*(3), 191–199.

Galvin, J. C., & Scherer, M. J. (1996). *Evaluating, selecting, and using appropriate assistive technology*. Gaithersburg, MD: Aspen Publishers.

Hammel, J. (2003). Technology and the environment: Supportive resource or barrier for people with developmental disabilities? *Nursing Clinics of North America, 38*(2), 331–349.

Hasselbring, T. S., & Glaser, C. H. (2000). Use of computer technology to help students with special needs. *Future Child, 10*(2), 102–122.

Hedman, G. (1992). Assistive technology: A boon to reasonable accommodation. *Private Rehabilitation, 9*, 1–5.

Kroll, T., Beatty, P. W., & Bingham, S. (2003). Primary care satisfaction among adults with physical disabilities: The role of patient-provider communication. *Managed Care Quarterly, 11*(1), 11–19.

Kroll, T., & Neri, M. T. (2003). Experiences with care coordination among people with cerebral palsy, multiple sclerosis, or spinal cord injury. *Disability Rehabilitation, 25*(19), 1106–1114.

LoPresti, E. F., & Brienza, D. M. (2004). Adaptive software for head-operated computer controls. *IEEE Transactions on Neural System Rehabilitation Engineering, 12*(1), 102–111.

LoPresti, E. F., Brienza, D. M., Angelo, J., & Gilbertson, L. (2003). Neck range of motion and use of computer head controls. *Journal of Rehabilitation Research and Development, 40*(3), 199–211.

Neri, M. T., & Kroll, T. (2003). Understanding the consequences of access barriers to health care: Experiences of adults with disabilities. *Disability Rehabilitation, 25*(2), 85–96.

Neumann, N., Hinterberger, T., Kaiser, J., Leins, U., Birbaumer, N., & Kubler, A. (2004). Automatic processing of self-regulation of slow cortical potentials: Evidence from brain-computer communication in paralyzed patients. *Clinical Neurophysiology, 115*(3), 628–635.

O'Day, B., Palsbo, S. E., Dhont, K., & Scheer, J. (2002). Health plan selection criteria by people with impaired mobility. *Medical Care, 40*(9), 725–728.

Sokol-McKay, D., Buskirk, K. & Whittaker, P. (2003). Adaptive low-vision and blindness techniques for blood glucose monitoring. *Diabetes Education, 29*(4), 614–618.

Thyberg, I., Hass, U. A., Nordenskiod, U., & Skogh, T. (2004). Survey of the use and effect of assistive devices in patients with early rheumatoid arthritis: A two-year follow-up of women and men. *Arthritis and Rheumatism, 51*(3), 413–421.

Wehman, P., Wilson, K., Parent, W., Sherron-Targett, P., & McKinley, W. (2000). Employment satisfaction of individuals with spinal cord injury. *American Journal of Physical Medicine and Rehabilitation, 79*(2), 161–169.

# CHAPTER 18

# Managed Care and Chronic Illness and Disability

## THE CONCEPT OF MANAGED CARE

The U.S. General Accounting Office has recently estimated that of the 70.5 percent of Americans younger than the age of 65 with private health insurance, four out of five are covered by a managed care organization (MCO) (Office of Public Policy and Information, 1997). General proliferation of managed care coverage exists in the public health care sector as well. Changes in both Medicare and Medicaid under the Balanced Budget Act of 1997 have dramatically increased the enrollment of beneficiaries in managed care organizations (MCOs) (Office of Public Policy and Information, 1997).

Managed care is not a new concept. Evidence of managed care plans can be found as early as the 1800s, when prepaid medical care through the voluntary participation of employers, workers, and physicians was established for immigrants who were recruited to work on special projects throughout the country (Friedman, 1996). Although managed care has helped contain spiraling medical costs, there is increasing concern that it has also reduced the degree of control health care providers have over treatment and has in some instances limited individual choice and access to certain providers and services.

The impact of managed care on individuals with chronic illness and disability, as well as on those who provide their care, can be significant. Although managed care can increase opportunities for greater access and better care, it also has the potential to shut out some providers of services and to reduce access to care. Professionals providing services to individuals with chronic illness and disability must be familiar with managed care and actively involved in initiatives at the state, federal, and private level to ensure that both consumers and providers are protected.

## DEFINING MANAGED CARE

Managed care is a model of health care in which the financing and delivery of medical care are conducted through a coordinated and integrated system of selected physicians and hospitals that provide comprehensive services to individuals enrolled in a specific health care plan. The purpose of managed care is to control unnecessary cost and use of health care while still providing good access to high-quality health care.

The terms *managed care organization* (*MCO*) and *health maintenance organization* (*HMO*) are used to describe health care plans that deliver specific services to a group of individuals on a prepaid basis. HMOs are managed care organizations (MCOs) whose premise is that future medical problems can be avoided through prevention measures. Consequently, routine medical checks and health promotion activities are encouraged. HMOs operate in designated service areas. If the individual travels outside the service area, coverage is only guaranteed for life-threatening emergencies.

*Point of Service Plans* (*PSOs*) are other kinds of health care plans under managed care. In PSOs, certain characteristics of HMOs are combined with traditional indemnity plans in which physicians are reimbursed for services provided or in which individuals covered in the plan are reimbursed for money spent for services. This type of plan provides individuals with the option at each "point of service" to choose a provider covered under the plan or to choose another individual outside the plan.

Precise definitions of managed care are difficult because the concept is shaped by market forces and thus is continually being modified. Although initially implemented as a cost-containment strategy, managed care has also assumed a greater responsibility for improving the quality of health care to enrolled members. Identifying appropriate treatment, including the type, duration, and location through case management, has become a crucial aspect of service.

## ORGANIZATIONAL MODELS OF MANAGED CARE

A variety of models of managed care organizations exist. The *staff-model HMO* is a system in which the organization owns the facilities in which enrolled individuals receive services, and health care pro-

viders are employees of the organization. This model provides the HMO with more control over services rendered.

The *group-model HMO* is a system in which physicians in one or more group of practices form partnerships or corporations. This group in turn negotiates a flat rate to be paid to the group by an HMO. Health care providers in the group are then responsible for paying employees, paying for hospital care, and paying for care from specialists outside the group. The *network model* is similar to the group model except that a network of group practices contracts with an MCO.

The *IPA* (*individual practice association model*) enables individual physicians to be associated with an HMO without being under a direct contract or being a direct employee of the organization. Physicians in the IPA model can deliver services to individuals who are in the specific HMO plan and those who are not in the plan. In the *direct contract model*, physicians contract directly with the HMO. *Preferred provider organizations* are a predetermined group of health care providers who have agreed to follow specific practice guidelines and accept a specified amount for services. *Provider-sponsored organizations* consist of a group of health care providers who have established their own providers, clinics, hospitals, or other facilities to provide care.

## ADDITIONAL CONCEPTS IN MANAGED CARE

*Capitation* is one type of compensation in managed care through which the health care provider receives a *fixed-rate prepayment* for a designated number of individuals in a group, regardless of the amount of care actually delivered. The *capitation rate* is the negotiated rate per individual enrolled for a specified period. Not all managed care plans are the same. The plan's *Certificate of Coverage* describes the services, benefits, and limitations of the plan, as well as those things excluded from the plan's coverage. The exclusion clause is particularly important because it describes specific services not covered under the plan.

HMOs require that individuals who are enrolled choose a *primary care physician* who will manage their health care and determine when seeing a specialist is necessary. The primary care physician coordinates all routine medical care, hospitalizations, and referrals. If individuals choose to seek care from a provider outside the plan, they are responsible for payment for those services rendered.

Most managed care plans provide benefits that include coverage of prescription drugs. However, to be eligible individuals must use a pharmacy approved by the specific managed care plan in which they are enrolled. Some managed care plans have developed a formulary, that is, a list of drugs that have been evaluated by a committee and approved for coverage. Some managed care plans provide coverage only for drugs that are listed on their formulary.

## CLINICAL PRACTICE GUIDELINES

An increasingly important concept in managed care is accountability through *clinical practice guidelines*. Such guidelines are developed to standardize care in a variety of conditions as a way to control costs and to prevent excessive testing and performance of other procedures. From clinical practice guidelines, clinical protocols are developed that outline the procedures for specific disease conditions that produce the best outcomes. The intent of these standards is to assist health care providers and individuals receiving care to make ap-

propriate health care decisions for specific circumstances and medical conditions.

Clinical practice guidelines are also designed to provide specific outcome expectations and benchmarks for minimal levels of acceptable performance. Theoretically, such guidelines can produce a standard by which quality of care can be accurately measured. Questions can be asked about how and what specific outcomes are developed. A health provider's perception of a successful outcome may be much different from the perception of the individual with a chronic illness or disability. Likewise, a successful outcome may be defined differently from an HMO perspective.

## ETHICAL ISSUES IN MANAGED CARE

Although no concrete ethical issues are related to managed care, the potential for ethical problems rises from the business "for-profit" model of health care and the possible implication of rationing of care. Under the managed care system, health care has the potential to become a corporate structure that is driven by a profit motive, which could be harmful to consumers. Under the capitation model of medical care, health care providers benefit from not providing services. In other words, the fewer services provided to individuals, the greater the profit for the health care provider.

The potential for abuse is present, however, even outside the managed care system in which there is fee for service. The *fee-for-service* model rewards the health care provider for providing services. Consequently, the more services provided, the more financial gain for the health care provider, a system that could encourage overtreatment.

*Rationing of care* is also a potential issue of concern. In some systems, services are provided on the basis of the likelihood of benefit and the availability of resources. In other instances, individuals' access to services is restricted because some procedures are considered experimental or have not been approved because of the cost for the individual versus the overall benefit to society.

Length of hospital stay has also been questionable. Individuals who once would have been discharged from the hospital when they felt able to care for themselves at home are now being discharged on the basis of predetermined guidelines. Specific issues related to hospital stay that have received considerable publicity are postpartum hospital stays for routine deliveries and hospital stays for women who have had mastectomies.

## IMPACT OF MANAGED CARE ON INDIVIDUALS WITH CHRONIC ILLNESS OR DISABILITY

An underlying concept of MCOs is disease management and cost containment. Although disease management is defined as comprehensive treatment of medical conditions, including prevention of disease or disability, and diagnosis, treatment, and management of disease and disability when they occur, the primary aim of managed care is to reduce cost and the amount of services used.

Individuals with chronic illness and disability have complex medical needs requiring extensive health care services (Cutler, 2003) and often require the services of a multidisciplinary team with multiple strategies. Consequently, the managed care model may not always be adequate to meet these complex needs.

*Medicaid* and *Medicare* are federal programs that are primary resources for funding the health care for many people with disabilities. Increasingly, however, these programs are being administered through managed care plans. Many services necessary for individuals with chronic illness or disability are, however, expensive. To control costs, managed care plans may attempt to minimize the utilization of medical services, thus restricting benefits to individuals with chronic illness or disability.

Although there are positive benefits of managed care for individuals with chronic illness and disability, such as care coordination, prevention practices, and low cost of the medications that are on the managed care formulary, there are also limitations. Those that have been reported include (Grabois & Young, 2001):

- delay in getting appointments or test results
- denial of referral to specialists
- inaccessibility of equipment in managed care facilities
- inadequate skill of physicians in managed care facilities to treat specific chronic
- illnesses or disabling conditions
- need for specific approval by an MCO before the most effective medication for treatment of a condition can be obtained if the medication is not listed in the plan's formulary
- limited services for assistive devices

Managed care was first implemented in the health care industry; however, its principles are now being applied to other services. The impact on individuals with chronic illness and disability could be profound.

Because individuals with chronic illness or disability may also experience medical complications and need a variety of allied services, such as homecare, personal assistants, or consultation with a variety of medical specialists, costs can be further increased. For specific disabilities some restriction of service is also included in many managed care plans. For instance, although all managed care plans offer treatment for substance abuse and dependence, varying limits and restrictions apply. Managed care plans also cover treatment of mental disorders; however, limits and restrictions do exist. Specifically, the number of visits to a mental health provider may be limited.

The number of Medicaid recipients in managed care plans has risen dramatically in the past few years (Health Care Financing Administration, 1994). It is evident that the cost of care for individuals with a severe disability is a challenge for a system such as managed care, which emphasizes cost control. Many of the formulas used to determine appropriate services are based on the average needs of able-bodied individuals rather than those with a severe disability or chronic illness. Managing the care of individuals with a chronic illness and disability requires a commitment of financial resources that many managed care plans cannot or will not make. Consequently, the needs of individuals with a chronic illness or disability may not always be identified, and if identified, not adequately served.

## FUTURE ISSUES FACING MANAGED CARE

Managed care is an evolving concept. As market forces change and more data regarding the effectiveness and efficiency of various systems are gathered, the structure and nature of managed care will also change.

Societal values and the impact those values have on public policy cannot be ignored. Likewise, the interplay between private and public sectors regarding managed care must also be considered. The HMO Act of 1973 was a major impetus for HMO development. HMOs, which are private entities, have increasingly become a mechanism for delivery of health care to Medicare and Medicaid recipients. A major question is whether in the future for-profit managed care plans will be able and willing to enroll individuals with a chronic illness or disability, who account for 70 percent of all Medicaid outlays (Ginzberg, 1999; Max, Rice, & Trupin, 1996). As managed care in the private and public sectors becomes more entwined, it is possible that increasing government regulation rather than marketplace competition may drive the managed care enterprise. Although customer satisfaction has become increasingly important in managed care, satisfaction alone may not equate with technical quality. The degree to which quality will enter into contracting decisions and consumer choice is unclear. Thus, the level and quality of services for individuals with chronic illness or disability in the future are still unknown.

Services and procedures considered experimental are currently not covered under many managed care plans; however, as more data are gathered and certain procedures become more common, procedures once considered experimental may become accepted. The question remains: by what criteria will those determinations be made?

Profit margins for MCOs should be closely monitored and evaluated in terms of compliance with established guidelines for care. Practice guidelines that are now being developed to guide care and standardize treatment may contribute to more accountable care if they are developed with multiple stakeholder input, including the input of individuals with chronic illness and disability. Professionals serving individuals with chronic illness or disability must strike a balance between professional responsibility, corporate or agency accountability, and funding resources.

## REFERENCES

Cutler, D. M. (2003). Disability and the future of Medicare. *New England Journal of Medicine, 349*(11), 1084–1085.

Friedman, M. (1996). Capitation, integration, and managed care. *Journal of the American Medical Association, 275*(12), 957–962.

Ginzberg, E. (1999). The uncertain future of managed care. *New England Journal of Medicine, 340*(2), 144–146.

Grabois, E., & Young, M. E. (2001). Managed care experiences of persons with disabilities. *Journal of Rehabilitation, 67*(3), 13–19.

Health Care Financing Administration. (1994). *The Medicare and Medicaid statistical supplement of the Health Care Financing Review*. HCFA Publication #03374. Washington, DC: Author.

Max, W., Rice, D., & Trupin L. (1996). *Medical expenditures for people with disabilities*. Disability Abstract #12. Washington, DC: U.S. Department of Education.

Office of Public Policy and Information. (1997). *Managed care: A primer on issues and legislation*. Arlington, VA: American Counseling Association.

# Medical Terminology

All professions and sciences have their own terminology that give speed, precision, and economy to communication. Medicine is no exception. Medical terms can often seem like a foreign language. Nevertheless, nonmedical professionals working with individuals with chronic illness or disability need to become familiar with commonly used terms so that they can communicate with medical providers and have a better understanding of information contained within medical reports and records. Although each medical term could be looked up in a medical dictionary, the process would be time consuming. Memorizing some commonly used terms can be helpful, but it is unrealistic to memorize all terms with which you may come in contact. Consequently, becoming familiar with prefixes and suffixes commonly found in medical terminology can help you translate unfamiliar terms and provides a framework from which you may be able to figure out a general meaning of a term. Following are common prefixes and suffixes, along with some general terms that are frequently encountered.

## PREFIXES

| Prefix | Meaning |
| --- | --- |
| adeno | glandular |
| angio | vessel |
| ankyl | crooked, growing, together |
| anti | against |
| arthro | joint |
| bi | double, twice |
| bili | bile |
| brachy | short |
| brady | slow |
| broncho | bronchi |
| cardio | heart |
| cephalo | head |
| cervico | neck |
| chole | gall, bile |
| cholecyst | gallbladder |
| chondro | cartilage |
| circum | around |
| craneo | skull |
| cysto | bladder |
| derma | skin |
| dis | negative |
| dors | back |
| duodeno | duodenum |
| dys | difficult, painful |
| ect | outside |
| endo | inside |
| entero | intestine |
| eryth | red |
| ferro | iron |
| fibro | fibers |

## PREFIXES

| Prefix | Meaning |
| --- | --- |
| fore | before, in front of |
| galacto | milk |
| gastro | stomach |
| gingive | gums |
| glyco | sugar |
| gyneco | female |
| hemato | blood |
| hemi | half |
| hemo | blood |
| hepato | liver |
| histo | tissue |
| homo | same |
| hydro | water |
| hyper | increased |
| hypo | decreased |
| hystero | uterus |
| iatr | physician |
| idio | peculiar |
| inter | between |
| intra | within |
| jejuno | jejunum |
| laryngo | larynx |
| latero | side |
| leuko | white |
| lipo | fat |
| lithio | stone |
| macro | big, large |
| mal | bad, poor, abnormal |
| masto/mammo | breast |
| mega | great, large |
| melan | black |
| meso | middle |
| micro | small |
| mono | single |
| muco | mucus |
| multi | many |
| myelo | bone marrow, spinal cord |
| myo | muscle |
| narco | numbness |
| neo | new, recent |
| nephro | kidney |
| neuro | nerve |
| non | not |

## PREFIXES

| Prefix | Meaning |
| --- | --- |
| nos | disease |
| ocul | eye |
| odonto | tooth |
| oligo | few, little |
| opth, optic | eye |
| os | mouth |
| oss, osteo | bone |
| oto | ear |
| pan | all |
| path | disease |
| peri | around |
| pharyng | pharynx |
| phlebo | vein |
| photo | light |
| pneumo | lung |
| pod | foot |
| post | after |
| pre | before |
| procto | anus, rectum |
| pseudo | false |
| psych | the mind |
| pto | fall |
| pyelo | kidney |
| pyo | pus |
| pyro | fever |
| quadri | four |
| radio | radiation |
| recto | rectum |
| retro | backward |
| rhino | nose |
| sacro | sacrum |
| salpingo | fallopian tube |
| sclero | hard or hardening |
| skeleto | skeleton |
| sten | narrow |
| stomato | mouth |
| sub | under, beneath |
| super, supra | above, extreme |
| tachy | fast |
| thermo | heat |
| thoraco | chest |
| thromb | clot |
| uretero | ureter |
| vaso | vessel |

## SUFFIXES

| Suffix | Meaning |
| --- | --- |
| algia | pain |
| ase | enzyme |
| cele | tumor, swelling |
| centesis | to puncture |
| cide | causing disease |
| cyte | cell |
| dynia | pain |
| ectasis | dilation |
| ectomy | excision |
| emesis | vomiting |
| emia | blood |
| esthesia | sensation |
| gram | tracing, mark |
| graphy | record, picture |
| iasis | condition, pathological state |
| itis | inflammation |
| kinesis | motion |
| lithiasis | stones |
| lysis | breakdown |
| mania | madness |
| megaly | enlargement |
| norexia | appetite |
| odynia | pain |
| ology | science or study of |
| oma | tumor |
| osis | disease |
| ostomy | new opening |
| otomy | incision, cutting |
| pathy | sickness, disease |
| penia | lack |
| pepsia | digestion |
| pexy | fixation |
| phage | ingesting |
| phylaxis | protection |
| plasty | repair |
| plegia | paralysis |
| ptosis | prolapse |
| rhagia | hemorrhage |
| rhea | flow, discharge |
| sclerosis | hardness |
| scopy | visually examine |
| sect | cut |
| statis | halt |
| stenosis | narrowing |
| uria | urine |

## TERMINOLOGY RELATED TO POSITION AND DIRECTION

| Term | Meaning |
| --- | --- |
| anterior | before, or in front |
| distal | far away from |
| dorsal | pertaining to the back |
| inferior | below |
| lateral | to the side |
| medial | to the center |
| palmar | pertaining to the palm of the hand |
| plantar | pertaining to the sole of the foot |
| posterior | behind or in back |
| prone | lying face down |
| proximal | nearest to |
| superior | above |
| supine | lying face upward |
| volar | pertaining to the front or abdominal surface |

## TERMINOLOGY RELATING TO BODY AREAS

| Term | Meaning |
| --- | --- |
| carpal | pertaining to the wrist |
| cervical | pertaining to the seven vertebrae in the neck |
| costal | pertaining to the ribs |
| cranial | pertaining to the skull |
| femoral | pertaining to the thigh |
| frontal | pertaining to the front |
| pelvic | pertaining to the pelvis |
| sternal | pertaining to the sternum or breastbone |
| thoracic | pertaining to the 12 vertebrae in the upper portion of the back; chest cavity |

## PREFIXES OF QUANTITY

| Prefix | Meaning |
|--------|---------|
| ambi | both |
| bi | two |
| di | two |
| hemi | half |
| mono | one |
| multi | many |
| olig | few |
| poly | many |
| tri | three |
| uni | one |

## GENERAL TERMS

**complication**: disease concurrent with another disease

**diagnosis**: determination of or naming of a disease

**disease**: structural or functional change within the body judged to be abnormal

**etiology**: study of the cause of disease; also, the cause of a disease

**history**: written description of symptoms in medical record

**idiopathic**: cause unknown

**incidence**: measure of the number of individuals newly diagnosed with a specific condition

**manifestation**: signs, symptoms, laboratory abnormalities

**morbidity**: rate of disease or proportion of diseased persons living in a given locality; frequency of occurrence of a condition within a population

**mortality**: proportion of deaths to the population of a region; the death rate from a particular condition; measure of the number of people dying from a condition in a given period of time

**pathogenesis**: development of disease; sequence of events that lead from cause to structural abnormalities and finally to manifestations of disease

**pathology**: study of disease

**prevelance**: number of people with a disease at any given point in time

**prognosis**: probable outcome of a disease

**signs**: physical observations made by the person examining an individual

**symptoms**: evidence of disease as perceived by the individual experiencing it

**syndrome**: cluster of findings associated with a disease

# Glossary of Medical Terms

**abduction** movement of a body part away from the midline of the body

**abductor** muscle that moves a limb laterally, away from the body

**abrasion** scraping or rubbing off of the skin

**accommodation** change in the shape of the lens to help the eye focus for near or far vision

**achalasia** type of dysphagia in which motility of the lower portion of the esophagus is decreased and food is unable to pass into the stomach efficiently

**acoustic nerve** auditory nerve; eighth cranial nerve

**acoustic reflex** movement of the muscles attached to the malleus and stapes as a response to intense sound

**acquired hearing loss** hearing loss occurring after birth or later in life

**active exercise** individual independent performance of a specified exercise regimen under the direction or supervision of a physical therapist

**adaptation** chemical process in which the eye adjusts to see in the dark

**Addison's disease** condition involving underproduction of hormones by the adrenal cortex

**adduction** movement of a body part toward the midline of the body

**adductor** muscle that moves a limb closer to the body

**adenopathy** enlargement of lymph nodes

**afferent nerves** peripheral nerves that carry messages to the central nervous system

**agnosia** inability to interpret sounds or visual images, or to distinguish objects by touch

**agoraphobia** fear of being in a situation or place from which it might be difficult or embarrassing to escape or in which no help may be available if a panic attack occurs

**agranulocytosis** marked reduction in the level of a specific type of leukocyte

**akathisia** extreme restlessness; inability to sit still for any length of time

**akinesia** complete or partial absence of movement

**allergen** substance that causes an allergic response

**allergy** hypersensitivity to a specific substance or substances from previous exposure

**allograft** graft taken from the same species but not the same person; homograft

**alopecia** hair loss

**alveoli** air sacs in lungs in which exchange of oxygen and carbon dioxide takes place

**Alzheimer's disease** progressive, degenerative type of dementia

**amblyopia** loss of sight or dimness of vision

**amino acids** building blocks of protein

**amnesia** loss of memory

**amputation** removal of a body part

**amyotrophic lateral sclerosis** progressive condition in which degeneration occurs of the nerve cells that convey impulses to initiate muscular contraction

**anaphylaxis** severe systemic reaction resulting from sensitivity to a foreign protein

**anaplastic** term to describe cancer cells that take on abnormal characteristics and become less differentiated than the normal cells from which they are derived

**anasarca** generalized edema

**anastomosis** connection of two tubular structures, through surgery or through a pathological process

**anemia** condition in which a reduction in the amount of hemoglobin or the number of red blood cells occurs

**aneurysm** blood-filled sac formed by a dilation of the walls of an artery or vein

**angina pectoris** chest pain

**anhidrosis** lack of sweating

**ankylosing spondylitis** systemic rheumatic disorder affecting the joints and ligaments of the spine

**ankylosis** immobility or fixation of a joint

**anomia** inability to name objects or remember names

**anophthalmia** congenital absence of the eye

**anorexia** appetite loss

**anosmia** loss of sense of smell

**anosognosia** one-sided neglect (e.g., condition in which individuals are unable to see objects on either the right or the left of the central field of vision)

**anoxia** lack of oxygen

**antibody** an immune substance produced within the body in response to a specific antigen

**antigen** a substance that causes the body to manufacture antibodies against a particular allergen

**anuria** condition in which the kidney is unable to excrete urine

**aorta** largest artery in the body

**aortic semilunar valve** valve through which blood is pumped from the heart into the general circulation

**aphagia** inability to swallow

**aphasia** inability to communicate through speech, writing, or signs due to brain dysfunction

**apnea** cessation of breathing

**apraxia** loss of ability to organize and sequence specific muscle movements to perform a task

**apraxia of speech** articulation disorder characterized by the inability to position and sequence the muscle movements involved in speech

**arachnoid membrane** middle, cobweb-appearing membrane that covers the brain and spinal cord

**arrhythmia** abnormality of the heart rhythm

**arteriosclerosis** thickening and loss of elasticity of arteries

**arthritis** joint inflammation

**arthrocentesis** aspiration of synovial fluid from a joint cavity

**arthrodesis** surgical fusing of two joint surfaces, making them permanently immobile

**arthrogram** radiographic study of a joint

**arthroplasty** surgical replacement, formation, or reformation of a joint

**arthroscopy** visualization of a joint through an arthroscope inserted into the joint

**articulation** coming together of two bones at a joint

**ascites** retention of fluid in the abdominal cavity

**asphyxia** suffocation due to decrease of oxygen and increase of carbon dioxide in the body

**aspiration** withdrawal of fluid or gas from a cavity by means of suction

**aspiration pneumonia** inflammation of the lung resulting from inhalation of foreign substances or chemical irritants

**asthma** chronic inflammatory disease of the airways

**astigmatism** distortion of the visual image resulting from an irregularity in the shape of the cornea or lens

**asymptomatic** without symptoms

**ataxia** impairment of muscle coordination

**atelectasis** collapse of the lung

**atherosclerosis** buildup of plaque on inner walls of blood vessels

**athetosis** slow, writhing, purposeless movement

**atonic** lacking normal tone or strength

**atresia** narrowing or closing of a normal opening; often congenital

**atria** two upper chambers of the heart

**atrophy** shrinkage

**attention deficit/hyperactivity disorder** condition that appears before age 7 that is characterized by inattention, hyperactivity, and impulsivity

**aura** warning (flash of light or other unusual sensation) before a seizure

**auricle** visible portion of the outer ear

**autistic disorder** disorder of brain function with behavioral consequences, including impairment in reciprocal social interactions and impairment in verbal and nonverbal communication

**autograft** graft from individual's own skin

**autoimmune disease** disease in which the immune system directs a response that attacks the body's own cells as if they were foreign substances

**autonomic dysreflexia** condition occurring in individuals with spinal cord injury resulting from excessive neural discharge from the autonomic nervous system and characterized by sudden rise in blood pressure, profuse sweating, and headache

**autonomic nervous system** part of the peripheral nervous system that controls involuntary functions

**axon** process emerging from the neuron that conducts electrical impulses away from the cell body

**bacteremia** presence of bacteria in the bloodstream

**basal ganglia** gray matter imbedded within the white matter of the brain

**benign** noncancerous

**bicuspid valve** mitral valve of the heart

**biliary** term applying to the gallbladder, liver, and their ducts

**binocular vision** coordinated use of both eyes to produce a single image

**biopsy** removal of a small portion of tissue from the body so that it may be examined microscopically (e.g., needle biopsy)

**biosynthetic graft** graft that has been chemically manufactured

**blindness** total loss of light perception

**blood dyscrasias** large group of disorders that affect the blood

**body image** individual's perception of his or her own physical appearance and physical function

**bradycardia** slow heartbeat

**bradykinesia** extreme slowness of movement

**brain stem** portion of central nervous system located at base of the brain between cerebrum and spinal cord

**Broca's aphasia** type of nonfluent aphasia characterized by misarticulation, laborious speech, hesitancy, and reduced vocabulary

**Broca's area** portion of the brain anterior to Wernicke's area and the major area of expressive function

**bronchi** branches leading from the trachea into the lungs

**bronchiectasis** dilation of the bronchi or bronchioles

**bronchospasm** tightening of small muscles around air passages

**burr holes** openings placed in the skull to relieve increased intracranial pressure

**bursa** sac that contains synovial fluid in the synovial joints

**bursitis** inflammation of the bursa

**CABG** coronary artery bypass graft

**calculi** stones

**cancer** cellular tumor; not one disease, but a broad term used to describe many diseases

**candidiasis** yeast infection

**capillaries** minute blood vessels connecting smallest arteries (arterioles) and veins (venules)

**carbuncle** a boil with infiltration into adjacent tissues

**carcinogens** chemicals or other substances that are thought to cause cancer

**carcinoma** cancer of the epithelial cells

**cardiac tamponade** severe constriction of the heart because of accumulation of fluid in the pericardial sac

**cardiomegaly** enlargement of the heart

**cardiospasm** achalasia

**carpal tunnel repair** surgical procedure indicated for carpal tunnel syndrome

**carpal tunnel syndrome** painful condition involving compression of the median nerve in the wrist

**carriers** individuals who harbor germs of a disease and transmit the disease to others, while remaining well themselves

**cartilage** dense type of connective tissue that creates form and maintains structure

**cataract** clouding or opacity of the lens of the eye

**cell body** portion of the neuron

**central deafness** hearing loss resulting from disorder of the auditory center of the brain

**cerebellum** portion of the brain located beneath the occipital lobe of the cerebrum

**cerebral palsy** developmental disability in which injury to the brain occurs during the fetal period, at birth, or in early childhood

**cerebrospinal fluid** fluid bathing the brain and spinal cord

**cerebrovascular accident** stroke

**cerebrum** largest portion of the brain

**cerumen** earwax

**cervix** neck of the uterus, opening into the vagina

**cholecystectomy** removal of the gallbladder

**cholecystitis** inflammation of the gallbladder

**cholelithiasis** gallstones

**chorea** jerky, involuntary movements

**choreoathetosis** abrupt, jerky movements

**chronic bronchitis** defined clinically as a condition in which a chronic productive cough persists on most days for a minimum of 3 months in the year for not less than 2 consecutive years

**chronic obstructive pulmonary disease** collection of diseases including emphysema, chronic bronchitis, and chronic asthma

**cilia** hairlike projections

**circumduction** circular movement

**cirrhosis** progressive disease of the liver in which liver function is altered because of fibrous changes in the structure of the liver

**clonic** pertaining to jerky movement of muscle

**closed head injury** injury in which the skull has not been broken

**coccyx** tailbone

**cochlea** chamber of the inner ear

**colectomy** removal of all or part of the colon

**collateral circulation** alternate blood supply routes

**colon** large intestine

**colostomy** surgical opening in the outer wall of the abdomen through which a portion of the large intestine is brought to the external surface for elimination of fecal material

**coma** state of unconsciousness

**compulsions** persistent actions

**concussion** mild to moderate head injury in which a loss of consciousness occurs, varying from a few minutes to 24 hours after the injury

**conductive hearing loss** damage, obstruction, or malformation in the external or middle ear that prevents sound waves from reaching the inner ear

**confabulation** making up experiences to fill memory gaps

**congenital** present at birth

**congenital hearing loss** hearing loss present at birth

**conjunctiva** membrane that lines the inner eyelid and covers the front part of the eye

**conjunctivitis** inflammation of the conjunctiva

**contracture** deformity in which a permanent contraction of a muscle occurs, resulting in the immobility of a joint

**contusion** soft tissue injury resulting from a blunt, diffuse blow in which the skin is not broken, nor are bones broken, but local hemorrhage occurs with associated bruising and damage to deep soft tissue under the skin

**conversion disorder** disorder in which physical function, often related to neurological function, is lost but no organic cause for the loss can be found

**COPD** chronic obstructive pulmonary disease

**cor pulmonale** right-sided heart failure

**coronary angioplasty** procedure to enlarge a narrowed coronary artery

**coronary arteries** vessels that carry blood directly to the myocardial muscle

**coronary artery bypass** graft procedure to relieve narrowing or constriction of coronary arteries

**coronary artery disease** condition in which arteries that supply blood directly to the myocardial muscle become narrowed or occluded

**cortex** gray matter that makes up the outer portion of the cerebrum

**cranial nerves** peripheral nerves that transmit messages directly to the brain

**craniotomy** surgical procedure in which the skull is opened to remove matter or to control bleeding

**cranium** skull; bony cover surrounding the brain

**creatinine** waste product eliminated by the kidney

**Crohn's disease** inflammation of segments of the small intestine

**cross-tolerance** demonstration of higher tolerances for related substances when tolerance for one substance has been developed

**Curling's ulcer** stress ulcer associated with burns

**Cushing's disease** condition involving overproduction of hormones by the adrenal cortex

**Cushing's ulcer** peptic ulcer associated with head injury

**cyanosis** bluish or gray appearance of skin resulting from lack of oxygen supply

**cyclothymia** mood disorder characterized by symptoms similar to those of bipolar disorders, with both hypomanic and depressive symptoms

**cystic fibrosis** hereditary condition in which mucus-secreting organs in the body become obstructed by abnormal, thick mucus, resulting in degeneration and scarring of the organs involved

**cystitis** inflammation of the bladder

**cytology** study of cells

**deafness** inability to discriminate conversational speech through the ear

**debride** remove dead tissue

**decibels (dB)** sound intensity or loudness

**decubitus ulcers** pressure sores

**delusions** false beliefs

**dementia** deterioration of cognitive abilities

**dendrite** process emerging from cell body of neuron that is involved in transmission of electrical impulses to the cell body

**dental caries** cavities

**dermabrasion** procedure in which scars, wrinkles, or other skin blemishes are worn away to diminish scarring

**dermatitis** superficial inflammation of the skin

**dermis** inner layer of skin lying beneath the epidermis

**diabetes insipidus** condition involving inadequate secretion of the antidiuretic hormone from the pituitary gland

**diabetes mellitus** chronic disorder of carbohydrate metabolism in which an imbalance of the supply of and demand for the hormone insulin occurs

**dialysis** artificial means to replace kidney function

**diaphoresis** excessive sweating

**diaphragm** muscular wall that separates abdominal cavity from thoracic cavity

**diastole** phase of heart activity when the heart is relaxed and the chambers are filling

**diplopia** double vision

**disability** limitation or restriction of activity that results from an impairment

**discography** radiographic study of the cervical or lumbar disks

**diskectomy** removal of a portion of a disk

**dislocation** displacement or separation of a bone from its normal joint position

**distal** farthest from the center of the body

**diuresis** increased urinary output

**diverticulum** small balloon-like sac or pouch

**diverticulitis** infection or inflammation of diverticula

**diverticulosis** presence of numerous diverticula in the intestinal wall

**DNA** genetic material that is the blueprint for all the body's structures

**dormant** inactive

**dorsiflexion** backward movement

**dorsiflexor** muscle that bends a body part backward

**duodenum** first part of the small intestine

**duodenal ulcer** peptic ulcer in the upper portion of the small intestine

**dura mater** outer membrane of the brain and spinal cord

**dysarthria** impairment in the coordination and accuracy of the movement of the lips, tongue, or other parts of the speech mechanism

**dysgraphia** impaired writing ability

**dyskinesia** abnormal involuntary movements

**dyslexia** inability to understand written words

**dyspepsia** indigestion

**dysphagia** difficulty in swallowing

**dyspnea** difficulty in breathing

**dysrhythmia** irregularity of heartbeat

**dysthymia** chronic condition characterized by symptoms similar to those experienced in major depression but in a lesser degree

**dystonia** abnormal muscle tone

**dysuria** painful urination

**ecchymosis** purplish discoloration at the site of injury resulting from bleeding under the skin

**eczema** acute or chronic inflammatory condition of the skin with any of a combination of symptoms, including vesicles, scales, crusts, and redness

**edema** presence of abnormally large amounts of fluid in tissue spaces

**edematous** swollen

**efferent nerves** peripheral nerves that carry impulses away from the central nervous system

**electrolytes** electrically charged particles that are important to many of the body's internal functions (e.g., sodium and potassium)

**embolus** foreign particle or blood clot that travels in the bloodstream until it lodges in a blood vessel too small to allow its passage

**emotional lability** condition in which emotional reactions are inappropriate for the situation and usually unpredictable

**emphysema** permanent enlargement of the alveoli resulting from overinflation of and destructive change in the alveolar walls

**encephalitis** inflammation of the brain

**endarterectomy** removal of plaque or clot in the carotid artery

**endocarditis** inflammation of the inner lining of the heart

**endocardium** lining of the inner surface of the heart

**endometrium** lining of the uterus

**end-stage renal disease** disease or damage to the kidney to the point that it ceases to function

**epidermis** outer layer of skin

**epidural** pertaining to the space between the dura and the skull

**epiglottis** flap at back of throat that closes over opening to trachea when food is swallowed

**epilepsy** chronic neurological condition in which neurons in the brain create abnormal electrical discharges that cause temporary loss of control over certain body functions

**epistaxis** nosebleed

**erythema** redness

**erythrocytes** red blood cells

**eschar** dead tissue resulting from burns

**esophageal reflux** backflow of stomach contents into the esophagus

**esophageal varices** dilated tortuous veins of the esophagus

**esophagectomy** removal of the esophagus

**esophagitis** inflammation of the esophagus

**eustachian tube** tube connecting the throat and the tympanic cavity of the middle ear

**eversion** outward-turning movement

**exacerbation** time period when symptoms become worse

**exertional dyspnea** shortness of breath with activity

**exophthalmos** abnormal protrusion of the eyeball

**expiration** expulsion of air from the lungs

**extension** straightening movement

**extensor** muscle that straightens a limb

**factitious disorder** condition in which individuals voluntarily produce psychological or physical symptoms because of a compulsive need to assume the sick role

**feces** solid waste from the body

**fetal alcohol syndrome** toxic effects of alcohol on developing fetus during pregnancy resulting in deformity of the infant

**fibromyalgia** cluster of signs and symptoms in which individuals experience diffuse aching, pain, and stiffness in muscles and/or joints

**fibrosis** formation of fibrous tissue

**fistula** opening between two tubular structures

**flaccid** limp

**flat affect** showing little emotional responsiveness

**flexion** bending movement

**flexor** muscle that bends a limb

**fluent aphasia** receptive or sensory aphasia

**frontal lobe** portion of the brain located in the front part of each hemisphere

**functional disorder** disorder that has no readily identifiable organic cause

**fused** joined

**gastric ulcer** ulcer in the stomach

**gastritis** inflammation of the stomach

**gastroenterostomy** surgical procedure in which the bottom of the stomach and small intestine are opened, and the two openings are connected to create a passage between the body of the stomach and the small intestine

**gene** unit of heredity that is composed of DNA and carries hereditary information about all characteristics of the organism

**gingivitis** inflammation of the gums

**glaucoma** increase in intraocular pressure

**global aphasia** limited ability to communicate

**glomerular filtration** process by which kidney removes waste products from the blood

**glomerulonephritis** inflammation of the glomeruli of the kidney

**glomerulus** small capillaries located in the nephron of the kidney

**glycosuria** glucose in the urine

**goiter** swelling of the neck resulting from enlargement of the thyroid gland

**grading** system used to describe the structure of cancer cells

**gray matter** nonmyelinated nerve fibers in central nervous system that receive, sort, and process nerve messages

**Guillain-Barré syndrome** acute and progressive condition characterized by muscular weakness usually beginning in the lower extremities and spreading upward

**hallucinations** sensory experiences without environmental stimuli

**handicap** disadvantage because of an impairment or disability that presents a barrier to fulfilling a role or reaching a goal

**hearing impairment** any degree and type of hearing disorder

**hearing loss** impairment in any part of the hearing system that interferes with hearing sound

**hemarthrosis** bleeding in the joint

**hematemesis** vomiting of blood

**hematoma** sac filled with accumulated blood

**hematuria** blood in the urine

**hemianopsia** loss of vision in half the visual field

**hemiplegia** paralysis on one side of the body

**hemoglobin** red pigmented protein that carries oxygen within the erythrocytes

**hemolysis** destruction of red blood cells

**hemophilia** chronic bleeding disorder characterized by a deficiency in or absence of one of the clotting factors

**hemopoiesis** process by which blood cells are formed

**hemoptysis** blood-streaked sputum

**hemostasis** cessation of bleeding from damaged vessels

**hepatitis** inflammation of the liver

**hepatotoxin** substance that is toxic to the liver

**hernia (rupture)** protrusion of an organ through the tissues in which it is normally contained

**herniorrhaphy** surgical procedure used to repair hernias

**Hertz (Hz)** sound frequency or pitch

**heterograft** graft taken from another species; xenograft

**hiatal hernia** protrusion of the stomach through an opening of the diaphragm and into the thoracic cavity

**histology** study of the structure of tissue

**Hodgkin's disease** chronic, progressive disease in which abnormal cells replace normal elements within the lymph nodes

**homeostasis** maintenance of an internal chemical balance within the body

**homograft** graft taken from the same species but not the same person; allograft

**Huntington's chorea** slowly progressive, hereditary disease of the central nervous system characterized by jerky, involuntary movements and intellectual deterioration

**hydrocephalus** buildup of fluid in the brain

**hydronephrosis** buildup of urine in the kidney resulting from backup of urine and blocked outflow

**hyperalimentation** nourishment through infusion of special nutritional solution into a large blood vessel

**hyperbilirubinemia** excess bilirubin in the blood

**hypercapnia** buildup of carbon dioxide

**hyperglycemia** accumulation of large amounts of glucose in the blood

**hyperkalemia** high levels of potassium in the blood

**hyperopia** farsightedness

**hyperproliferation** overgrowth of cells resulting from a tumor

**hypertension** high blood pressure

**hyperthermia** increased body temperature

**hyperthyroidism** overproduction of thyroid hormone

**hypertonia** exaggerated muscle tone

**hypertrophic scars** ropelike configurations of scar tissue that form on the skin surface

**hypertrophy** enlargement

**hyperuricemia** buildup of uric acid in the body

**hypochondriasis** type of somatoform disorder characterized by preoccupation with physical illness

**hypoglycemia** decreased sugar in the blood

**hypothyroidism** insufficient production of thyroid hormone

**hypoxemia** decreased level of oxygen in the blood

**hypoxia** decrease of oxygen

**hysterectomy** removal of the uterus

**ileostomy** portion of small intestine brought through surgical opening to the outside of the abdomen for drainage of fecal material

**ileum** last part of the small intestine

**immune system** complex organization of specialized cells and organs that distinguishes between self and nonself, defending the body against foreign materials

**immunosuppression** suppression of the immune system

**impairment** loss or abnormality of function at the body system or organ level

**in situ** when referring to cancer, the state in which cancer cells are present but remain localized (i.e., they have not invaded the surrounding lymph nodes)

**incisors** teeth at the front of the mouth that provide a cutting action

**incontinence** loss of control of bladder or bowel

**incus** small bone in the middle ear

**infarction** death of tissue resulting from lack of blood supply

**inflammatory bowel disease** a group of disorders that cause inflammation and/or ulceration in the lining of the bowel

**inspiration** breathing air into the lungs

**intermittent claudication** aching, cramping, or fatigue of muscles in the legs when walking

**internal fixation** placement of screws, pins, wires, rods, or other devices through the bone to hold bone fragments together

**intracranial pressure** increased pressure on the brain

**intraocular pressure** pressure within the eyeball

**intravenous** refers to an infusion directly into a vein

**inversion** inward-turning movement

**iridotomy** removal of a portion of the iris of the eye

**irritable bowel syndrome** chronic or intermittent condition of the gastrointestinal tract in which individuals experience spasms of the colon, diarrhea, and/or constipation, cramping, and abdominal pain

**ischemia** inadequate blood supply

**jaundice** yellowish appearance of the skin and whites of the eyes resulting from an excess level of bilirubin in the blood

**jejunum** middle section of the small intestine

**joint** place where two or more bones are bound together

**keratoplasty** plastic surgery of the cornea

**keratotomy** incision in the cornea

**ketoacidosis** condition caused by an excessive level of ketones in the blood that increases the acidity of the blood to toxic levels

**ketone** metabolic product of fat metabolism

**ketoacidosis** acidosis accompanied by a buildup of ketone bodies in the blood (diabetic coma)

**ketosis** buildup of ketone bodies in the blood

**kidney failure** diminished functioning of the kidney

**kyphosis (hump back)** permanent postural deformity of the back

**labyrinth** inner ear

**labyrinthitis** inflammation of the labyrinth of the inner ear

**laceration** injury involving a tear or cut in the skin and underlying tissues

**laminectomy** surgical removal of the posterior arch of a vertebra

**language** set of symbols combined in a certain way to convey concepts, ideas, and emotions

**laparotomy** surgical incision into the abdomen

**laryngectomy** surgical removal of the whole or a part of the larynx

**laryngitis** inflammation of the larynx

**laryngostoma** surgical opening in the neck through which the individual breathes

**larynx** voice box

**legal blindness** central visual acuity not exceeding 20/200 in the better eye with correcting lenses or central field of vision limited to an angle of no greater than 20 degrees

**lens** small transparent disk enclosed in a transparent capsule and located directly behind the iris of the eye

**lethargy** listlessness

**leukemia** cancer of the tissues in which blood is formed

**leukocyte** white blood cell

**leukocytosis** white blood cell proliferation

**leukopenia** abnormal decrease in the number of white blood cells

**ligaments** tough bands of fiber that connect bones at the joint site

**litholapaxy** crushing of a kidney stone in the bladder

**lithotomy** surgical procedure to remove kidney stones

**lobectomy** removal of a lobe (i.e., of the brain; of the lung)

**loosening of associations** no logical progression of thought and rapid shifting from one unrelated idea to another

**lordosis** swayback

**low back pain** pain in the lumbar or sacral region of the lower back

**lymphadenopathy** swollen lymph nodes

**lymphatic system** circulatory system separate from the general circulation and consisting of lymph vessels, lymph fluid, and lymph nodes

**lymphedema** swelling resulting from blockage in lymphatics

**lymph fluid** clear fluid that bathes the body's tissue

**lymph nodes** small glands of the immune system that are located throughout the body and act as filters

**lymphocyte** white blood cell

**lymphoma** cancer of the lymphatic system

**macrophage** phagocyte that ingests dead tissue

**macula** spot on the retina that is the area of most acute vision

**macular degeneration** degeneration of the macula of the eye

**melanin** skin pigment that is responsible for skin color

**melanocytes** cells containing the skin pigment melanin

**malignancy** cancerous growth

**malignant** cancerous, harmful, virulent

**malignant melanoma** cancer that originates in the cells that contain skin pigment

**malingering** producing symptoms intentionally for secondary gain

**malleus** small bone in the middle ear

**mandible** jaw bone

**mastectomy** amputation of the breast

**mastoidectomy** surgical procedure for the removal of infected mastoid air cells located in the mastoid process

**mastoiditis** infection of the mastoid cells within the mastoid process located in the skull

**mastoid process** bony prominence behind the outer ear

**megaloblastic anemia** presence of large abnormal red blood cells

**melanoma** cancer of the pigment-producing cells

**melena** passage of dark, tarry bowel movements, resulting from action of intestines on blood

**Meniere's disease** disorder of the inner ear that includes symptoms of dizziness, hearing loss, and ringing in the ears

**meninges** membranes covering the brain and spinal cord

**meningitis** inflammation of the meninges

**meningocele** type of spina bifida in which membranes surrounding the spinal cord push out through an opening in the spinal column

**metastasis** movement of cancer cells from their original site to another part of the body

**microcephaly** abnormal smallness of the head

**micrographia** reduction in handwriting size

**microphage** a small phagocyte that ingests bacteria

**micturition** urination

**mitral valve** valve between left atria and left ventricle of the heart

**mixed hearing loss** hearing loss involving both conductive hearing loss and sensorineural hearing loss

**molars** teeth at the back of the mouth that provide a grinding action

**motor nerves** peripheral nerves that carry impulses from the central nervous system to other parts of the body

**multi-infarct dementia** condition in which deficits in cognitive function result from small strokes in various locations of the brain

**multiple myeloma** cancer of plasma cells that is characterized by bone destruction

**multiple sclerosis** progressive disease of the central nervous system in which the myelin around message-carrying nerve fibers is destroyed in localized areas of the brain and spinal cord

**mutation** alteration or change of the DNA within the normal cell

**myelin** fatty sheath that surrounds the neuron

**myelomeningocele** most severe form of spina bifida

**myocardial infarction** death of a portion of the heart muscle

**myocardium** heart muscle

**myopathy** disease of the muscle

**myopia** nearsightedness

**myositis** inflammation of the muscle

**myringoplasty** type of tympanoplasty in which damaged eardrum is repaired

**myringotomy** incision into the eardrum to drain pus or fluid

**necrosis** tissue death

**necrotic** dead

**neoplasm** new and abnormal growth of cells that serve no useful function and may interfere with healthy tissue function

**nephritis** inflammation of the kidney

**nephrolithotomy** surgical entry into the renal calix

**nephrosclerosis** condition in which arteries of the kidney become thickened

**nephrosis** general term used to describe conditions, other than direct infection of the kidney itself, that damage the kidney

**nephrotic syndrome** collection of symptoms experienced in nephrosis

**nerve** bundle of fibers outside the central nervous system

**neuroma** bundle of nerve fibers

**neuron** functional unit of the nervous system

**neuropathy** general term to describe functional disturbances or changes in the nerves

**neurotransmitter** chemicals that help transmit nerve impulses between neurons

**neutropenia** small numbers of mature white blood cells

**nocturnal dyspnea** difficulty in breathing while lying down at night

**nonfluent aphasia** expressive or motor aphasia

**non-Hodgkin's lymphoma** proliferation of lymphoid cells that disseminate throughout the body

**nystagmus** involuntary eye movement

**obsessions** persistent thoughts

**occipital lobe** portion of the brain located in the posterior portion of each hemisphere

**occult** hidden

**occupational lung disease** group of lung disorders directly related to matter inhaled from the occupational environment

**oliguria** decreased production of urine

**oophorectomy** removal of the ovaries

**open head injury** injury in which the skull is broken or penetrated

**open reduction** surgical alignment of fractured bone

**ophthalmologist** physician who specializes in conditions and treatment of the eye

**opportunistic infection** infection that would not occur in individuals with normal immune system function

**orthosis** any mechanical device applied to the body to control motion of the joints and to control force or weight distribution on a body part

**orthotist** individual who constructs the orthosis to meet individual needs

**ossicles** small movable bones in the middle ear

**osteoarthritis** local joint disease associated with degeneration of a joint

**osteomyelitis** infection of the bone

**osteophytes** bone spurs

**osteoporosis** reduction in bone mass, causing bones to become weakened, fragile, and easily broken

**otoacoustic emissions** measured reflections in the outer ear of mechanical activity in the cochlea

**otitis media** infection of the middle ear

**otolaryngologist** physician who specializes in disorders of the ear and related structures

**otosclerosis** conductive hearing loss caused by fixing or hardening of the small bones in the middle ear that transmit sound impulses to the inner ear

**ototoxic** describes drugs or chemicals that destroy the hair cells of the inner ear or damage the eighth cranial nerve

**oval** window opening between the middle and inner ear

**pain disorder** preoccupation with pain that is severe enough to cause functional impairment in daily life

**pain expression** individual response to pain

**pain threshold** point at which sensation is perceived as pain

**pain tolerance** point at which individual finds pain unbearable

**palliative** giving temporary relief of symptoms but no cure

**pallor** pale-appearing skin

**palpitations** awareness of beating of the heart

**pancreatitis** inflammation of the pancreas

**panic attack** episode in which the individual has feelings of intense anxiety or terror, accompanied by a sense of impending doom

**paracentesis** puncture of a body cavity with the removal of fluid

**paraparesis** partial paralysis of the lower extremities

**paraplegia** paralysis of the lower extremities

**parasympathetic nervous system** part of the autonomic nervous system

**paresthesia** sensation of numbness or tingling in some part of the body

**parietal lobe** portion of the brain located in the middle of each hemisphere

**Parkinson's disease** slowly progressive disorder of the central nervous system involving extensive degenerative changes in the basal ganglia of the brain with associated loss of or decrease in levels of dopamine

**parotitis** inflammation of the parotid glands

**passive exercise** exercise of a body part by a therapist or by a mechanical device

**pathologic fractures** fractures that occur because of disease of the bone rather than from injury

**pathologist** physician who specializes in the diagnosis of abnormal changes in tissues

**peptic ulcer disease** chronic inflammatory condition characterized by ulcer formation in the esophagus, stomach, or duodenum

**percussion** manual tapping or vibration of the chest or other body cavity

**percutaneous transluminal coronary angioplasty (PTCA)** procedure to enlarge a narrowed coronary artery

**perfusion** blood supply to an organ

**pericardial effusion** accumulation of excessive fluid within the pericardial sac surrounding the heart

**pericardiocentesis** puncturing of the pericardium to drain accumulated fluid

**pericarditis** inflammation of the pericardium of the heart

**pericardium** outer covering of the heart

**periodontal disease** disease of the tissues that surround and support the teeth

**periodontitis** severe form of gum disease

**periosteum** tough outer covering of bone

**peripheral** near the outside or surface of the body

**peripheral nervous system** all nerves extending from the brain and spinal cord

**peripheral neuropathy** disease of the peripheral nerves

**peripheral vascular insufficiency** inadequate blood flow to or from the lower extremities

**peristalsis** rhythmic, muscular movements that move food through the digestive tract

**peritoneum** lining of the abdominal cavity

**peritonitis** inflammation of the peritoneum

**pernicious anemia** complication of surgical resection of the stomach

**personality disorder** disorder characterized by inflexible or maladaptive behaviors that impair interpersonal or occupational functioning

**pervasive developmental disorders** conditions in which impairment occurs in several areas of development, including social interaction and verbal and nonverbal communication or stereotypical behavior

**phagocyte** cell that destroys and ingests foreign material

**phagocytosis** the process of cells ingesting other cells and foreign objects

**phantom limb pain** chronic, severe pain sensation in the amputated extremity

**phantom sensation** sensation that the amputated extremity is still present

**pharyngitis** sore throat

**pharynx** throat

**phlebitis** inflammation of a vein

**phlebotomy** removal of quantities of blood to reduce plasma volume

**phobia** fear and anxiety related to specific situations, persons, or objects

**photosensitive** sensitive to the sun

**pia mater** inner membrane covering the brain and spinal cord

**pinna** visible portion of the outer ear

**plasma** watery, colorless fluid that makes up the liquid portion of the blood

**pleura** membrane lining the chest cavity

**pneumonectomy** removal of the lung

**pneumothorax** collapse of the lung resulting from air entering the thoracic cavity

**poliomyelitis** infectious disease that affects the nerve cells that control muscles

**polycystic kidney disease** hereditary disease characterized by the presence of many cysts in the kidneys

**polycythemia** increase in the number of red blood cells as well as in the concentration of hemoglobin within the blood

**polycythemia vera** form of polycythemia in which an overproduction of both red and white blood cells occurs

**polydipsia** excessive and constant thirst

**polyuria** excessive urination

**posttraumatic stress disorder (PTSD)** disorder that develops after experiencing or observing a traumatic or life-threatening event

**postvocational hearing loss** hearing loss that occurs after the individual has entered the work force

**poverty of speech** diminished use of the spoken word

**prelingual hearing loss** hearing loss that occurs before the individual acquires language, usually before the age of 3

**presbycusis** hearing loss resulting from aging

**presbyopia** loss of the ability of the lens to accommodate to near and far images

**pressure sores** decubitus ulcers

**prevocational hearing loss** hearing loss that occurs after acquiring language but before entering the work force

**prognosis** prediction of the course and outcome of the disease process

**pronation** downward-turning movement

**prosthesis** fabricated substitute for a missing part for activities, occupation, and cosmetic needs

**prosthetist** individual who specializes in making prosthetic devices

**proteinuria** protein in the urine

**pruritus** itching of the skin

**psoriasis** chronic inflammatory disease of the skin in which epidermal cells in the basal layer of the skin are formed too quickly

**psychogenic pain** pain that persists for months or years but has no readily identifiable organic cause

**psychosis** loss of contact with reality

**PTCA** percutaneous transluminal coronary angioplasty

**pulmonary artery** vessel carrying blood from the heart to the lungs

**pulmonary edema** collection of fluid in the lungs

**purpura** condition in which hemorrhage into the skin or other tissue occurs

**purulent** pertaining to pus-containing material

**pyelolithotomy** surgical entry into the pelvis of the kidney

**pyelonephritis** infection of the kidney

**pyloroplasty** widening the opening between the stomach and the small intestine

**quadriplegia** paralysis of all four extremities

**radial deviation** lateral movement of the hand inward toward the body

**radiologist** physician who specializes in radiographic procedures

**radionuclide** radioactive chemical

**Raynaud's phenomenon** spasms of the vessels in the fingers or toes that impair blood flow to those areas

**recruitment** hearing impairment characterized by an abnormal increase in the perception of loudness

**reflex** automatic response to stimuli

**regurgitation** backflow

**remission** period of weeks to years when symptoms subside

**renal** pertaining to the kidney

**reticular formation** groups of cells within the brain stem

**reticulocyte** newly formed red blood cells

**retina** innermost coat of the eye that receives images formed by the lens

**retinitis pigmentosa** slow, progressive loss of peripheral vision

**retinopathy** disease or disorder of the retina

**rheumatic disease** condition that produces symptoms that affect joints, connective tissues, and muscle

**rheumatic fever** condition caused by the body's immune response against a specific organism

**rheumatic heart disease** condition in which the body undergoes a type of allergic response that can cause heart damage

**rheumatoid arthritis** chronic, progressive, and systemic disorder characterized by inflammation and swelling of the synovial joints, resulting in pain, stiffness, and deformity

**sarcoma** cancer of the bone, muscle, or other connective tissue

**sciatica** syndrome of pain that radiates from the lower back into the hip and down the leg

**sclera** white part of the eye

**scoliosis** lateral S-shaped curvature of the spine

**seizure** temporary loss of control over certain body functions

**self-concept** an individual's perceptions and beliefs about his or her own strengths and weaknesses and beliefs about other people's perceptions of him or her

**semicircular canals** part of the vestibular system in the inner ear

**sensorineural hearing loss** hearing loss resulting from damage to nerve pathways that transmit nerve impulses or damage to areas of the brain in which sound is perceived

**sensory nerves** peripheral nerves that carry messages toward the central nervous system

**sepsis** widespread infection throughout the body

**septicemia** presence of toxins in the blood

**sickle cell anemia** severe anemia as a result of sickle cell disease; most severe form of sickle cell disease

**sickle cell crisis** manifestation of sickle cell disease in which blood flow to a body part becomes obstructed by rigid, sickled red cells

**sickle cell disease** a chronic hereditary disorder characterized by abnormal hemoglobin

**sickle cell trait** abnormal gene causing the hemoglobin abnormality in sickle cell disease

**social phobia** phobic disorder in which the individual fears situations that may result in ridicule or humiliation

**somatic nerves** peripheral nerves that innervate body structures that are under voluntary control

**somatoform disorder** experience of physical symptoms for which no organic cause can be found

**spasticity** increased muscle tone, causing stiffness and awkward movements

**speech** verbal expression of language concepts

**spina bifida** congenital disorder of the spinal column in which one or more vertebrae are left open

**spina bifida occulta** mildest form of spina bifida that does not involve damage to the spinal cord

**spinal fusion** the grafting of bone from another area of the body into the disk interspace after laminectomy

**spinal nerves** peripheral nerves that connect and transmit messages directly to the spinal cord

**spleen** organ composed of tissue that disposes of worn-out blood cells

**splenectomy** removal of the spleen

**splenomegaly** enlargement of the spleen

**spondylolisthesis** forward slipping of a vertebra

**spondylolysis** breakdown of a vertebra

**sprain** injury to a ligament and its attachment site because of overstress

**staging** system to describe the extent to which cancer cells have spread

**stapedectomy** surgical procedure in which the stapes is removed and replaced with a prosthesis

**stapes** small bone in the middle ear

**stasis** stagnation

**status asthmaticus** severe, prolonged attack of asthma

**status epilepticus** continuous, uncontrolled seizures

**stem cells** cells that have the potential to become any type of cell in the body

**stenosis** narrowing of a duct or canal (e.g., a blood vessel)

**stoma** artificial opening

**stomatitis** inflammation of the mouth

**strabismus** disorder in which the eyes cannot be directed to the same object or one eye deviates from the central tract

**strain** injury to the tendons and muscles resulting from overstretching or overuse

**stress ulcer** peptic ulcer that develops after an acute medical crisis

**subarachnoid** between the arachnoid membrane and inner membrane covering the brain

**subcutaneous** beneath the skin; oftens refers to fatty tissue

**subdural** pertaining to the space beneath the dura

**subluxation** partial separation of bone from the joint

**supination** upward-turning movement

**sympathetic nervous system** portion of the autonomic nervous system

**synapse** space between neurons where chemical transmission of electrical impulses takes place

**syncope** fainting

**synovectomy** surgical removal of the synovial membrane surrounding a joint

**systemic lupus erythematosus** autoimmune disease of unknown cause

**systole** contraction phase of the heart's work

**tachycardia** fast heartbeat

**tamponade** pathological compression of a part

**tardive dyskinesia** abnormal muscle movements as a side effect of antipsychotic drugs

**temporal lobe** portion of the brain located under the frontal and parietal lobes

**tendinitis** inflammation of a tendon

**tendon** band of tissue that connects muscle to bone

**tenosynovitis** inflammation of the tendon sheath

**tetany** involuntary contraction of the muscles

**thalassemia** group of inherited hemolytic anemias

**thoracentesis** removal of fluid from the thoracic cavity

**thoracic** refers to the chest

**thorax** chest cavity

**thromboangiitis obliterans** rare condition of small and medium-sized arteries of extremities in which blood flow is diminished to a body part

**thrombocyte** platelet

**thrombocytopenia** decrease in platelet number

**thrombocytosis** increase in platelet number

**thrombophlebitis** inflammation of a vein with clot formation

**thrombus** blood clot

**thymus** lymphoid organ lying in upper portion of chest that produces a hormone important in controlling development of lymphocytes

**TIA** transient ischemic attack

**tinnitus** ringing in the ears

**tolerance** with regard to substance use, body adaptation to the substance so that larger amounts of the substance are needed to produce the same effects

**tonic** rigid

**tonometry** measurement of pressure in the eye

**tophi** deposits of crystals in the joints

**trachea** windpipe

**tracheostomy** surgical opening into the trachea

**trachoma** chronic infectious disease of the conjunctiva and cornea

**traction** therapeutic method in which a mechanical or manual pull is used to restore or maintain the alignment of bones or to relieve pain and muscle spasm

**transient ischemic attack (TIA)** temporary blocking of cerebral arteries, causing slight temporary neurological deficits

**traumatic brain injury** injury to the brain from an external physical force to the head

**tricuspid valve** valve between right atrium and right ventricle of the heart

**tuberculosis** infectious disease caused by an organism called the tubercle bacillus

**tumor** new and abnormal growth of cells that serve no useful function and may interfere with healthy tissue function

**tympanic cavity** middle ear

**tympanic membrane** eardrum

**tympanometry** test of acoustic immittance in which the mobility or flexibility of the tympanic membrane are assessed by measuring how much sound energy is admitted into the ear as pressure is varied in the external auditory canal

**tympanoplasty** surgical procedure that involves the middle ear

**ulcerative colitis** inflammatory condition of the large intestine

**ulnar deviation** lateral movement of the hand away from the body

**urea** waste product eliminated by the kidney

**uremia** buildup of waste products (e.g., urea and creatinine) in the blood

**ureterolithotomy** surgical removal of stones from the ureter

**ureterosigmoidostomy** surgical procedure for urinary diversion in which the ureters are connected to the colon so that urine is excreted through the rectum

**ureters** tubes leading from the kidney draining into the bladder

**urethra** single tube leading from the bladder to the urinary meatus

**urinary meatus** outside opening through which urine is eliminated

**urinary tract** collecting system for urine, including the ureters, bladder, and urethra

**urticaria** hives

**vagotomy** cutting of the vagal nerve

**valvuloplasty** procedure to dilate a narrowed or stenosed valve of the heart

**varicose veins** congestion of veins

**vascular insufficiency** inadequate blood and oxygen to a body part

**vena cava** large vessel carrying unoxygenated blood from general circulation to the right atrium of the heart

**venesection** removal of quantities of blood to reduce plasma volume

**ventilation** process by which gases are transported between the atmosphere and the alveoli

**ventricles** two lower chambers of the heart

**vertebrae** bony covering of the spinal cord

**vertigo** dizziness

**vestibular system** part of the inner ear that conducts impulses regarding body balance and movement

**virus** organism that cannot grow or reproduce outside of living cells

**viscosity** thickness

**visual acuity** ability to process visual detail; sharpness of vision

**visual impairment** any deviation of normal vision

**visual spatial deficit** deficiency in depth perception, judgment of distance, size, position, rate of movement, form, and relation of parts to wholes

**vitrectomy** removal of the vitreous humor in the eye

**Wernicke's aphasia** type of fluent aphasia in which effortless speech, relatively normal grammatical structure, and increased verbal output occur, but with reduced information content

**Wernicke's area** portion of the brain located over the temporal and parietal lobes and major area of receptive function

**white matter** myelinated fibers in central nervous system that conduct electrical impulses

**withdrawal** experience of physical symptoms when the amount of a substance is decreased or absent

**xenograft** graft taken from another species; heterograft

# Medications

Prescription medications are an important aspect of treatment of many chronic conditions and many disabilities. It is therefore important to be familiar with major types of prescription drugs and their biological and behavioral effects.

At no time should a nonmedical person advise an individual to stop taking a prescription or to change the dosage prescribed by the physician. If there are questions or doubts about an individual's condition or an individual's reaction to a specific medication, a physician should be consulted.

## ROUTES OF ADMINISTRATION

Medications can be administered in a variety of ways. Knowing the different routes of administration can be helpful in planning effectively so that any special factors regarding medication that may affect an individual's rehabilitation plan can be considered. Routes by which medications can be administered are the following:

I. Oral
   A. Ingested (swallowed)
   B. Sublingual (under the tongue)
   C. Buccal (on mucous membrane on the cheek or tongue)

II. Rectal
   A. Suppository, inserted into the rectum
   B. Liquid, given as a retention enema

III. Parenteral
   A. Intravenous (into a vein)
   B. Intradermal (into the skin)
   C. Subcutaneous (into the fatty layer under the skin)
   D. Intramuscular (into the muscle)

IV. Other
   A. Inhalation (breathing medication in)
   B. Topical (on top of the skin)

## FACTORS INFLUENCING MEDICATION DOSAGE

In order for a medication to act therapeutically, it must be given in sufficient concentration to produce the desired effect. Dosage is based on individual differences among clients. These differences influence how the medication is metabolized and thus absorbed. Factors that influence dosage and metabolism are the following:

1. **Age:** Children are generally more sensitive to drugs than adults, and thus generally require smaller doses.
2. **Body weight:** The ratio of body weight to the amount of drug taken determines the concentration of the drug within the body and therefore affects its potency.
3. **Time of administration:** Oral medications are absorbed more rapidly if

the stomach and upper portion of the intestinal tract are free from food. However, drugs that irritate the stomach lining should be taken with food.

4. **Route of administration:** Medication injected directly into a vein has an immediate effect, whereas medication administered orally or injected into a muscle or subcutaneous tissue has a slower absorption rate, thus taking longer to reach a concentration in the body that will show an effect.

5. **Rate of excretion:** Some drugs build up in the body when they are not excreted or destroyed as fast as they are ingested. If a drug builds up in the body past a certain level of concentration, toxic symptoms can occur.

6. **Drug combinations:** Some drugs are given in combination with other drugs to enhance their action. However, not all drugs are compatible when taken together, and some can seriously affect the action of other drugs. Consequently, it is important that the physician is aware of all medications an individual is taking, even those prescribed by other physicians.

7. **Pathology:** Certain diseases affect the absorption or excretion of different medications, rendering them ineffective or causing toxic symptoms.

8. **Allergies or other drug reactions:** Individuals are at times allergic to different medications or have an abnormal response to them. Once these medications are identified, individu-

als should be encouraged to inform physicians before medications are prescribed of the names of the drugs along with the reactions experienced.

9. **Compliance:** A medication prescribed to treat a condition is only as effective as the client's ability or willingness to take the medication as prescribed.

## METHODS OF CLASSIFYING MEDICATIONS

Drugs may be referred to in three ways:

1. **Chemical name:** This is the precise description of chemical constituents of the medication. An example of a chemical name is N-Methyl-4-carbethoxypiperidine hydrochloride.

2. **Generic name:** This reflects the chemical name to which the drug belongs, but it is simpler. An example of a generic name is *meperidine*. Drugs prescribed by their generic name may be cheaper than those ordered by trade name, but they may not always have all the components of the trade name counterpart.

3. **Trade name:** This represents the brand name of the drug. The trade name is registered, meaning the use of the name is restricted to the manufacturer, who is the legal owner. There may be many trade names of the same generic drug. An example of a trade name is *Demerol*.

## THEREAPEUTIC CLASSIFICATION OF MEDICATIONS

Drugs can be placed into several categories based on the action or therapeutic effect they are expected to produce. These categories are called therapeutic classifications. Some common therapeutic classifications are as follows:

| Category | Therapeutic Effect |
| --- | --- |
| Analgesic | Reduces pain |
| Antacid | Neutralizes stomach acid |
| Antianxiety | Reduces symptoms of anxiety |
| Antiarrhythmic | Corrects abnormal rhythm of the heart |
| Antibiotic | Kills or inhibits growth of microorganisms |
| Anticoagulant | Lengthens the pro-thrombin time and helps to prevent clot formation |
| Anticholinergic | Inhibits action of the involuntary nervous system |
| Anticonvulsant | Prevents convulsions or muscle spasm |
| Antidepressant | Psychic energizers used to treat depression |
| Antidiarrhetic | Prevents diarrhea |
| Antiemetic | Prevents nausea or vomiting |
| Antifungal | Checks the growth of fungi |
| Antihypertensive | Lowers blood pressure |
| Antihistamine | Relieves symptoms of allergic reactions by preventing histamine action |

| Category | Therapeutic Effect |
| --- | --- |
| Anti-inflammatory | Reduces inflammatory reaction such as redness, swelling, etc. |
| Antimicrobial (sulfonamide) | Inhibits growth of microorganisms |
| Antineoplastic | Prevents growth and spread of cancerous cells |
| Antipruritic | Relieves itching |
| Antipsychotic | Reduces psychotic symptoms and halluci-nations |
| Antipyretics | Reduces fever |
| Antiseptic | Inhibits growth of microorganisms |
| Antispasmodic | Relieves muscle spasms |
| Antithyroid | Blocks thyroid hor-mone production |
| Antitussive | Sedative to prevent cough |
| Antiviral | Kills or inhibits growth of virus |
| Astringent | Causes contraction of tissue and halts dis-charge |
| Bronchodilator | Opens airways to permit air to pass more freely in and out of the lungs |
| Cardiotonic | Changes heart rhythm and rate and generally strengthens heart |
| Cathartic | Relieves constipation |
| Cholinergic | Stimulates effect of parasympathetic nervous system |
| Corticosteroid | Produces dramatic short-term anti-inflammatory effects |
| Digestant | Supplements enzyme deficiency |

| Category | Therapeutic Effect |
|---|---|
| Digitalis preparation | |
| | Increases pumping action of the heart muscle |
| Diuretic | Rids body of excess fluid |
| Expectorant | Thins mucus to help expectoration |
| Histamine H2 (receptor antagonist) | |
| | Blocks cells in the stomach lining from producing acid |
| Hypoglycemic agent | |
| | Oral medication that lowers blood sugar |

| Category | Therapeutic Effect |
|---|---|
| Immunosuppressant | |
| | Blocks body's natural response to foreign substances |
| Laxative | Relieves constipation |
| L-dopa | Decreases symptoms of Parkinson's disease |
| Muscle relaxant | Reduces abnormal movement; reduces excess muscle tightness |
| Nitroglycerine | Dilates coronary arteries, enabling the heart muscle to receive more oxygen |

# Glossary of Diagnostic Procedures

**alanine aminotransferase (ALT; former-ly serum glutamic-pyruvic transaminase [SGPT])** blood test to identify liver disease

**angiography (arteriography)** injection of radiopaque contrast material into the arteries to visualize the vessels (see arteriography)

**antinuclear antibodies (ANA)** blood test that identifies the proteins or antibodies that are present with some autoimmune diseases

**arteriogram** (see arteriography)

**arteriography (angiography)** test performed to study the anatomy of vascular structures through injection of radiopaque material into the arteries; may be performed to evaluate vasculature of vessels of the kidney, adrenal gland, brain, heart, or lower extremities

**arthrocentesis** insertion of a needle into a joint cavity for removal of synovial fluid for examination

**arthrography** X-ray study of a joint in which contrast material is injected into a joint, the joint is moved through its range of motion, and X-ray films are taken

**arthroscopy** direct visualization of a joint through insertion of a small instrument called an arthroscope into the joint

**aspartate aminotransferase (AST; formerly serum glutamic-oxaloacetic transaminase [SGOT])** blood test to measure enzyme levels to identify possible coronary occlusive heart disease or liver disease

**audiometric testing** noninvasive procedure involving measurement of the degree of hearing loss through an electronic device called an audiometer

**barium enema (lower GI series)** X-ray examination of the lower gastrointestinal tract

**barium swallow (upper GI series)** X-ray study of the upper gastrointestinal tract

**biopsy** removal of a specimen of tissue from a specified site for examination

**bleeding time** blood test used to measure the length of time it takes for bleeding to stop after a puncture wound; determines how quickly a platelet clot forms

**blood urea nitrogen (BUN)** blood test that measures the level of a waste product of protein metabolism (urea) in the blood; used to evaluate kidney function

**bone marrow aspiration** insertion of a needle into the marrow space of the bone and aspirating a small sample so it may be examined microscopically for various abnormalities in the number, size, and shape of the precursors of blood cells

**bone scan** intravenous injection of radioisotopes that then concentrate in the bone, enabling the concentration to be measured by a special machine called a scanner, which produces a picture of the bone

**bronchoscopy** visual examination of the bronchial tubes through a long hollow tube inserted through the mouth and into the bronchus

**caloric test** test to measure vestibular nerve function

**cardiac angiogram** (see arteriography)

**cardiac catheterization** invasive procedure in which a catheter is passed into the vessel of an arm or leg and then threaded into the heart to study the chambers, valves, and blood supply of the heart and to measure internal pressures

**cardiac stress test** noninvasive exercise test that provides a graphic record of the heart's activity during forced exertion

**chest roentgenography (X-ray)** noninvasive radiographic procedure by which it is possible to visualize organs of the chest cavity on X-ray film

**cholangiogram** a study in which the bile ducts are visualized on X-ray film

**cholecystography** procedure in which the gallbladder is visualized on X-ray film to detect abnormalities, inflammation, or the presence of stones

**complete blood count** blood test that evaluates a variety of components of the blood

**computed tomography (CT scan, CAT scan)** special X-ray procedure that produces three-dimensional pictures of a cross-section of a body part

**C-reactive protein test** blood test used to identify inflammatory processes or tissue destruction

**creatinine clearance test** test that compares the level of creatinine in the blood and the amount of creatinine excreted in the urine over a specified period of time

**cystoscopy** insertion of a special tube called a cystoscope through the urethra into the bladder to directly visualize the bladder wall

**differential** blood test to measure the proportion of each type of white blood cell

**digital venous subtraction** angiography invasive procedure in which a catheter is inserted into a vein, a contrast medium is injected, and a series of X-rays of the blood vessels in the head and neck are taken and visualized on X-ray film

**discography** X-ray study of the cervical or lumbar disks

**echocardiography** noninvasive ultrasound procedure in which the size, motion, and composition of the heart and large vessels are recorded

**electrocardiography (ECG)** graphic representation of electrical activity of the heart muscle

**electroencephalography (EEG)** noninvasive procedure producing a graphic representation of the electrical activity of the brain

**electromyography (EMG)** procedure in which electrical activity of certain muscles is evaluated to diagnose certain muscle diseases

**electronystagmography** procedure to monitor eye movement

**ELISA** initial blood test to screen for HIV antibodies

**endoscopy** (see gastroscopy)

**erythrocyte sedimentation rate (ESR; sed rate)** blood test that measures the rate at which red blood cells settle in a special solution over a certain time period; detects tissue injury or inflammation

**esophageal manoscopy (manometry)** diagnostic procedure in which a catheter is placed through the individual's mouth into the esophagus to evaluate the function of the sphincter between the esophagus and the stomach

**fasting blood sugar (FBS)** blood test to measure the glucose level in the blood when the individual has had nothing to eat

**fluorescein angiography** test used to detect changes in the blood vessels of the retina

**gastroscopy (endoscopy)** diagnostic test in which a lighted, flexible tube called an endoscope or gastroscope is inserted through the mouth, into the esophagus, and into the stomach to enable the physician to visualize the walls of these organs

**glucose tolerance test** blood test in which the individual, after fasting, is given concentrated glucose to drink and then blood samples are drawn at 1-, 2-, and 3-hour intervals

**gonioscopy** examination of the internal structures of the eye

**Halstead-Reitan Battery** neuropsychological test battery

**hematocrit** blood test to measure the percentage or proportion of red blood cells in the plasma

**hemoglobin** blood test to evaluate the amount of hemoglobin content of erythrocytes

**holter monitoring (ambulatory electrocardiography; event recorder)** form of electrocardiography involving continuous recording of the heart's electrical activity; the individual wears the holter monitor externally

**intravenous pyelogram (IVP)** X-ray examination of the kidneys, ureters, and bladder in which a dye is injected into a vein in the arm and then X-rays are taken of the kidneys at intervals over approximately an hour to identify structural abnormalities as well as any problems with passage of the dye through the urinary system

**KUB (kidney, ureters, and bladder roentgenography)** X-ray of the kidney, ureters, and bladder to determine the size, shape, and location of the structures

**laparoscopy** procedure in which a hollow tube called a laparoscope is inserted into a body cavity through a small incision and the contents of the body cavity are examined or surgical procedures are performed

**laryngoscopy** visual examination of the larynx through a tube called a laryngoscope that is inserted into the larynx; enables the physician to inspect the structure of the larynx as well as assess the function of the vocal cords

**LE prep** blood test that examines a specific cell in the blood; useful in diagnosis of systemic lupus erythematosus

**lumbar puncture (cerebrospinal fluid analysis, spinal tap)** insertion of a needle into the subarachnoid space of the spinal column at the lumbar area so that cerebrospinal fluid may be aspirated and studied through laboratory analysis

**Luria-Nebraska Neuropsychological Battery** neuropsychological test battery

**magnetic resonance imaging (MRI; nuclear magnetic resonance imaging [NMRI])** noninvasive procedure in which rapid detailed pictures of body tissue are produced; involves no ionizing radiation, but rather the pictures are formulated when hydrogen atoms in a magnetic field are disturbed by radio-frequency signals

**mean corpuscular hemoglobin concentration** blood test that calculates the amount of hemoglobin in each red blood cell

**mean corpuscular volume (MCV)** blood test to calculate the volume of a single red blood cell

**mental status examination** structured interview used as screening instrument in assessing cognitive impairment

**mini-mental state examination** mental status test to evaluate orientation, memory, attention, and ability to write, name objects, copy a design, and follow verbal and written commands

**Minnesota Multiphasic Personality Inventory (MMPI)** objective personality test

**myelography** X-ray study of the spinal cord

**nerve conduction velocity** (electroneurography) procedure often performed in conjunction with electromyography; measures nerve activity at the nerve-muscle junction to assist in diagnosis of conditions that affect the peripheral nerves

**neuropsychological tests** procedures that are used to assess major functional areas of the brain

**paracentesis** procedure in which a needle is inserted into a body cavity to remove fluid

**partial thromboplastin time (PTT)** blood test to evaluate the special part of the clotting mechanism not evaluated by prothrombin time

**patch test** application to the skin of small amounts of various substances to identify allergic responses

**platelet count** blood test to measure number of platelets in the blood

**positron emission transaxial tomography (PET scan)** radionuclear study in which biochemical or metabolic activities of cells of body tissue are studied

**postprandial blood sugar** blood test in which the glucose level of the blood is measured several hours after eating

**proctoscopy** (see sigmoidoscopy)

**prothrombin time (PT; Pro Time)** blood test to measure the length of time that a blood sample takes to clot when certain chemicals are added to it in the laboratory; tests for specific factors involved in clotting

**pulmonary function tests** procedures to assess the volume of air that can be taken in and expelled from the lungs as well as the ability to move air in and out of the lungs

**radionuclide imaging** intravenous injection of a radioactive substance that localizes in a body tissue so that multiple views of the structure can be taken with a special camera and the images can be evaluated

**red blood cell count (RBC)** measurement of the total number of red blood cells

**reticulocyte count** blood test to assess bone marrow function by measuring production of immature red blood cells

**retrograde pyelogram** procedure in which a small catheter is inserted through a tube that has been inserted into the bladder and then directed into the ureters to the pelvis of the kidney; dye is then injected through the catheter, and X-ray films are taken to visualize the structures and to detect any abnormalities

**rheumatoid factor (latex fixation; agglutination test)** blood test that determines whether an abnormal protein exists in the blood serum; assists in diagnosis of rheumatoid arthritis or other rheumatic diseases

**Rorschach inkblot test** projective personality test

**serum creatinine** measurement of the level of creatinine in the blood to evaluate kidney function

**serum glutamic-oxaloacetic transaminase (SGOT)** (see aspartate aminotransferase [AST])

**serum glutamic-pyruvic transaminase (SGPT)** (see alanine aminotransferase)

**serum thyroxine (T4)** blood test to measure level of thyroid hormone in the blood

**Short Portable Mental Status Questionnaire (SPMSQ)** mental status test to assess orientation, personal history, remote memory, and calculation

**sigmoidoscopy** procedure involving direct visualization of the anus and rectum through a special instrument called a sigmoidoscope

**sonography (ultrasonography)** test in which sound waves passed into the body are converted to a visual image or photograph of a body structure

**speech audiometry** tests to measure the individual's ability to understand speech

**Stanford Binet** intelligence test

**Thematic Apperception Test** projective personality test

**tonometry** measurement of pressure of the eye

**TSH** blood test to measure level of thyroid-stimulating hormone (TSH) in the blood

**tympanometry** technique used to measure the amount of sound energy admitted into the middle ear

**ultrasonography** (see sonography)

**urinalysis** examination of urine under a microscope or through other laboratory procedures to evaluate the concentration, acidity, and presence of components such as protein, sugar, blood, bacteria, or other types of cells in the urine

**urine culture** laboratory examination of sterile urine to determine whether infection is present, and if so, to identify the infectious organism

**venogram** X-ray study in which dye is injected into veins of a body part and X-ray films are obtained at timed intervals to visualize the structure of the venous system

**ventilation/perfusion scan (lung scan)** radiographic procedure that measures transport of gases between the atmosphere and alveoli of the lung and/or the degree to which blood is passed through the vessels into the lungs

**Wechsler Adult Intelligence Scale-Revised (WAIS-R)** intelligence test

**Wechsler Intelligence Scale for Children-Revised (WISC-R)** intelligence test

**Wechsler Preschool and Primary Scale of Intelligence (WPPI)** intelligence test

**Western blot** blood test that is performed as confirmatory test for the HIV antibody

**white blood cell count (WBC)** measurement of the total number of white blood cells

**Wood's light examination** examination of the skin under an ultraviolet light to identify specific types of skin infections

# Functional Limitations

A functional limitation operationally defines the impact of chronic illness or disability on individuals' lives and functional capacity. Functional limitations are those physical, social, or psychological barriers that are associated with a specific condition and that must be considered when developing a rehabilitation plan. Wright (1980) described the categories of limitation associated with loss of function. The following listing of functional limitations uses Wright's schema, with some modifications to provide an orientation that can be used when assessing the functional impact of various chronic illnesses and disabilities.

1. **Sensory limitation:** Refers to any symptom that interferes with an individual's ability to receive information from the outside world. This includes symptoms that limit the individual's ability to feel sensory stimuli, to see, to hear, to smell, or to taste.

2. **Communication limitation:** Refers to any symptom that interferes with an individual's ability to communicate with the outside world. Symptoms would include the inability to speak or to write and the inability to understand spoken or written words.

3. **Atypical appearance:** Refers to manifestations of the condition that tell the casual observer that the individual has a chronic illness or disability. Such manifestations could include change in skin color (cyanosis or jaundice), disfigurements or deformi-

ties, behavioral manifestations, or assistive devices such as canes, wheelchairs, hearing aids, or glasses.

4. **Emotional/behavioral limitation:** Refers to manifestations of the condition that alter individual behavior so that symptoms either interfere with the ability to effectively function within the environment or alert the casual observer to the illness or disability. It should not be confused with normal grief reactions, depression, or other emotional manifestations of adjustment to disability. Emotional or behavioral limitations are symptoms or manifestations that directly result from the chronic illness or disability itself. Examples are impulsivity, aggressiveness, disinhibition, euphoria, inability to control emotions, lack of social skills, or behavior that is offensive to others.

5. **Unapparent limitation:** Refers to conditions in which symptoms or manifestations, although presenting various degrees of limitation, provide no readily observable outward signs of disability, so that the casual observer may be unaware of the chronic illness or disability and its associated limitations.

6. **Cognitive or learning limitation:** Refers to conditions in which symptoms or manifestations interfere with individuals' ability to process or retain information or alter their ability to conceptualize or to attend to information. Included are inability to pay attention or concentrate, difficulty remembering recent or past material or

events, difficulty learning new material, and difficulty grasping concepts.

7. **Substance dependency:** Refers not only to those conditions in which the individual has become psychologically or physically dependent on a substance due to misuse and abuse, but also to all conditions in which individuals are dependent on substances in the treatment of their condition for maintenance of their well-being. Examples of the latter include those conditions that require regular medication use or use of substances such as oxygen.

8. **Pain/sensitivity limitation:** Refers to conditions in which the sensation of pain or perception of pain interferes with the ability to effectively function in the environment. Examples include conditions in which the sensation or perception of pain makes it difficult for individuals to move, interact socially, or concentrate.

9. **Interference with consciousness:** Refers to any condition in which full awareness of the environment is altered at some point in time. Examples would be conditions that produce drowsiness, stupor, or total loss of consciousness.

10. **Deterioration:** Refers to those conditions that are progressive, producing gradual and ongoing deterioration of physical or mental functioning.

11. **Motion limitation:** Refers to any manifestation of a condition that interferes with the ability to move any extremity or the trunk of the body freely. Motion limitations include those conditions in which there is paralysis, but also those conditions in which there is inability to effectively coordinate body movement.

12. **Assistive devices:** Refers to conditions in which individuals need spe-

cial aids to function effectively within their environment, such as hearing aids, crutches, wheelchairs, or assisted breathing devices.

13. **Restricted environment:** Refers to conditions in which individuals are unable to interact fully within the total context of the environment. Examples would be conditions in which exposure to the sun, exposure to crowded environments, exposure to infectious agents, or exposure to certain dusts or molds must be avoided. Included also are conditions in which individuals must be supervised in their activities.

14. **Uncertain prognosis:** Refers to conditions in which there is no way of predicting the outcome or progression of the condition. For example, the same condition in one individual may progress rapidly, producing severe disability, whereas in other individuals the same condition may progress slowly over years, producing little disability. Likewise, in some individuals a condition may be rapidly fatal, whereas others with the same condition may live for years.

15. **Social stigma:** Refers to conditions in which the nature of the condition itself is a source of social stigma, producing barriers to individuals' full functional capacity. This limitation should not be confused with social stigma as a social experience for any person with a disability, but rather should be considered when the diagnosis of the specific condition alone, despite individuals' actual functional capacity, prevents individuals from reaching their goals.

**REFERENCE**

Wright, G. N. (1980). *Total rehabilitation.* Boston: Little, Brown, pp. 83–117.

# INDEX